The SAGES Manual of Robotic Surgery

Sarah Samreen • Omar Yusef Kudsi
Dmitry Oleynikov • Ankit D. Patel
Editors

The SAGES Manual of Robotic Surgery

Second Edition

Springer

SAGES University MASTERS PROGRAM

Editors
Sarah Samreen
Surgery
The University of Texas Medical Branch
Galveston, TX, USA

Omar Yusef Kudsi
Department of Surgery, Brigham and Women's Hospital
Harvard Medical School
Boston, MA, USA

Dmitry Oleynikov
Monmouth Medical Center
Rutgers Robert Wood Johnson Medical School
Long Branch, NJ, USA

Ankit D. Patel
Surgery
Emory University
Atlanta, GA, USA

ISBN 978-3-031-86926-6 ISBN 978-3-031-86927-3 (eBook)
https://doi.org/10.1007/978-3-031-86927-3

This Springer imprint is published by the registered company Springer Nature Switzerland AG
The registered company address is: Gewerbestrasse 11, 6330 Cham, Switzerland

Disclaimer for Society of American Gastrointestinal and Endoscopic Surgeons (SAGES) Manual

The contents of this manual are intended exclusively for educational and informational purposes only, and nothing contained within constitutes medical advice. Neither this manual nor its contents have been subject to formal peer review. The information provided herein does not represent, nor should it be interpreted as, the official position, view, or endorsement of the Society of American Gastrointestinal and Endoscopic Surgeons (SAGES) or its governing body. This manual is not intended for use in diagnosing or treating any health problem, condition, or disease. Individuals seeking personal medical advice should consult an appropriate licensed professional.

Neither SAGES, nor its officers, directors, employees, members, nor any of the contributors to this manual make any representation or warranty, express or implied, regarding the accuracy, completeness, fitness for any intended purpose, or suitability of the information contained herein for any specific use or function. Neither access to, nor use of, this manual creates or implies any physician-patient relationship, and reliance on any information provided, contained, or implied herein is solely at the user's own risk.

Contents

Part I Robotic System Details

1 **The Background of Robotic Surgery** 3
Danyal Fer and Jamil Stetler

Part II Current and Upcoming Robotic Platforms

2 **Current and Upcoming Robotic Platforms: Intuitive da Vinci** 15
Clark Gerhart

3 **Asensus Surgical: Senhance Surgical System** 19
Amit Trivedi and Sarah Wong

4 **The Hugo RAS™** 29
Yoav Mintz and Ronit Brodie

5 **Versius Surgical Robot** 43
Subhash Khanna and Areendam Barua

6 **Virtual Incision: MIRA Surgical System** 63
Dmitry Oleynikov and Shane Farritor

7 **Starting and Developing a Robotic Program** 69
C. Franco-Mesa and Sarah Samreen

8 **Robotic Training and Pathway** 79
Katherine Fay and Ankit D. Patel

9 **Digital Surgery** 87
Jonathan Gootee and Nova Szoka

10 **Navigating Resources for Aspiring and Experienced Robotic Surgeons** 109
Yasamin Taghikhan and Ankit Sarin

Part III Masters Program

11 **Overview of SAGES Masters Program** 119
Daniel B. Jones, Brian P. Jacob, and Linda Schultz

12 **Robotic Paraesophageal Hernia Repair** ... 129
Karan R. Chhabra and Charudutt N. Paranjape

13 **Management of Achalasia: A Disease Hard to Swallow** ... 139
Molly Belisle, Sana Khan, Nicholas Calvo, Alex Lynch, and Abubaker A. Ali

14 **Robotic Esophagectomy** ... 159
Evangelos Tagkalos and Peter P. Grimminger

15 **Robot-Assisted Partial and Total Gastrectomy** ... 175
Raj G. Vaghjiani

16 **Robotic Sleeve Gastrectomy** ... 185
Maria S. Altieri

17 **Robotic Roux-en-Y Gastric Bypass** ... 191
Hany Takla

18 **DS/SADI** ... 215
Paul Anthony Karam, Sarah Samreen, Andrew Lin, and Maher El Chaar

19 **Revisional Foregut and Bariatric Surgery** ... 227
Michelle Nessen and Carlos A. Galvani

20 **Robotic Transabdominal Preperitoneal (TAPP) Inguinal Hernia Repair** ... 257
Samuel Guba and Richard Lu

21 **Robotic Transabdominal Preperitoneal (r-TAPP) and Intraperitoneal Onlay Mesh (r-IPOM) Hernia Repairs for Ventral Hernias** ... 271
Rachel Reed, Savannah Smith, Eli Mlaver, and S. Scott Davis Jr.

22 **Complex Robotic Abdominal Wall Reconstruction** ... 279
Cigdem Benlice, Bilgi Baca, and Omar Yusef Kudsi

23 **Robotic Cholecystectomy** ... 299
Samuel Cass, Jennifer Moffett, and Sarah Samreen

24 **Liver Resection and Biliary Reconstruction** ... 307
Yee Lee Cheah and Caroline J. Simon

25 **Robotic-Assisted Pancreaticoduodenectomy (Whipple)** ... 327
Ahmad Abou Abbass and Mohamad Othman El Helou

26 **Right Hemicolectomy** ... 351
Ibrahim H. Ozata and Emre Balık

27 Left Hemicolectomy and Total Colectomy 365
Kamil Erozkan and Emre Gorgun

28 Low Anterior Resection 387
Cigdem Benlice and Bilgi Baca

Part IV Miscellaneous

29 Robotic Lateral Transabdominal Adrenalectomy 407
Felipe B. Maegawa, Justin Malek, and Snehal G. Patel

30 Thyroid and Parathyroid Surgery 415
Micaela Piccoli, Alice Francescato, and Barbara Mullineris

31 Robotic Pulmonary Lobectomy 427
Andrei I. Gritsiuta, Abbas E. Abbas, and Roman V. Petrov

32 Robotic-Assisted Cardiac Surgery 461
Amalia A. Jonsson and Michael E. Halkos

33 Mediastinal Procedures 471
Brittney Williams and Manu Sancheti

34 Liver Transplantation 493
Yee Lee Cheah, Gi Hong Choi, YoungRok Choi,
and Kwang Woong Lee

Index 523

Contributors

Abbas E. Abbas Department of Thoracic Oncology, Warren Alpert School of Medicine at Brown University, Providence, RI, USA

Ahmad Abou Abbass Directory of Hepatobiliary Surgery, Mission Hospital, Mission Viejo, CA, USA

Abubaker A. Ali Wayne State University, Detroit, MI, USA

Maria S. Altieri Department of Surgery, Hospital of the University of Pennsylvania, Philadelphia, PA, USA

Bilgi Baca Department of General Surgery, Acibadem Mehmet Ali Aydinlar University School of Medicine, Istanbul, Turkey

Emre Balık Maltepe Mahallesi, Zeytinburnu, Istanbul, Turkey

Areendam Barua Minimal Access and Robotic Surgical Oncology, Swagat Super Speciality Surgical Institute and NH, Guwahati, Assam, India

Molly Belisle Wayne State University, Detroit, MI, USA

Cigdem Benlice Department of General Surgery, Acibadem Mehmet Ali Aydinlar University School of Medicine, Istanbul, Turkey

Ronit Brodie Department of General Surgery, Hadassah Hebrew University Medical Center, Jerusalem, Israel

Nicholas Calvo Wayne State University, Detroit, MI, USA

Samuel Cass, MD Department of Surgery, University of Texas Medical Branch, Galveston, TX, USA

Yee Lee Cheah JC Walter Jr Transplant Center, Sherrie and Alan Conover Center for Liver Disease and Transplantation, Houston Methodist Hospital, Houston, TX, USA
Department of Surgery, Houston Methodist Hospital, Houston, TX, USA

Karan R. Chhabra Departments of Surgery and Population Health, NYU Grossman School of Medicine, New York, NY, USA
Division of Bariatric and General Surgery, Bellevue Hospital Center, New York, NY, USA

Gi Hong Choi Division of Hepato-biliary and Pancreatic Surgery, Yonsei University College of Medicine, Seoul, South Korea

YoungRok Choi Division of HBP Surgery, Department of Surgery, Seoul National University College of Medicine, Seoul, South Korea

Maher El Chaar Bariatric Surgery Department, St Luke's University Health Network, Bethlehem, PA, USA

Mohamad Othman El Helou Department of Surgery, Yale New Haven Hospital, Yale School of Medicine, New Haven, CT, USA
Department of Surgery, Henry Ford Providence Hospital, Southfield, MI, USA

Kamil Erozkan Department of Colorectal Surgery, Digestive Disease and Surgery Institute, Cleveland Clinic, Cleveland, OH, USA

Shane Farritor David B. and Nancy K. Lederer Professor of Engineering, Lincoln, NH, USA

Katherine Fay Department of General Surgery, Grady Memorial Hospital, Atlanta, GA, USA
Department of General & Gastrointestinal Surgery, Emory University School of Medicine, Atlanta, GA, USA

Danyal Fer Department of General & Gastrointestinal Surgery, Emory University School of Medicine, Atlanta, GA, USA
Department of General Surgery, David Grant Medical Center, United States Air Force, Fairfield, CA, USA

Alice Francescato Department of General, Emergency Surgery and New technologies, Baggiovara General Hospital, AOU Modena, Modena, Italy

C. Franco-Mesa, MD Division of General Surgery, University of Texas Medical Branch, Galveston, TX, USA

Carlos A. Galvani Department of Minimally Invasive and Bariatric Surgery, Louisiana State University, Baton Rouge, LA, USA

Clark Gerhart General and Bariatric Surgeon, Associate Medical Officer, Intuitive., Sunnyvale, CA, USA

Jonathan Gootee Department of Surgery, West Virginia University, Morgantown, WV, USA

Emre Gorgun Department of Colorectal Surgery, Digestive Disease and Surgery Institute, Cleveland Clinic, Cleveland, OH, USA

Peter P. Grimminger Departmen of General-, Visceral- and Transplant Surgery, University Medical Centre of the Johannes Gutenberg-University Mainz, Mainz, Germany

Andrei I. Gritsiuta Department of Surgery, University of Pittsburgh Medical Center, Pittsburgh, PA, USA

Samuel Guba Department of Surgery, University of Texas Medical Branch, Galveston, TX, USA

Michael E. Halkos Division of Cardiothoracic Surgery, Emory University School of Medicine, Atlanta, GA, USA

Brian P. Jacob Department of Surgery, Icahn School of Medicine at Mount, Sinai, NY, USA

Daniel B. Jones Department of Surgery, Rutgers New Jersey Medical School, Newark, NJ, USA

Amalia A. Jonsson Division of Cardiothoracic Surgery, Emory University School of Medicine, Atlanta, GA, USA

Paul Anthony Karam Bariatric Surgery Department, St Luke's University Health Network, Bethlehem, PA, USA

Subhash Khanna Minimal Access, GI` and Robotic surgery, Swagat Super Speciality Surgical Institute and NH, Guwahati, Assam, India

Sana Khan Wayne State University, Detroit, MI, USA

Omar Yusef Kudsi Department of Surgery, Brigham and Women's Hospital, Harvard Medical School, Boston, MA, USA

Kwang Woong Lee Division of HBP Surgery, Department of Surgery, Seoul National University College of Medicine, Seoul, South Korea

Andrew Lin Bariatric Surgery Department, St Luke's University Health Network, Bethlehem, PA, USA

Richard Lu Department of Surgery, University of Texas Medical Branch, Galveston, TX, USA

Alex Lynch Wayne State University, Detroit, MI, USA

Felipe B. Maegawa Department of Surgery, Emory University School of Medicine, Atlanta, GA, USA

Justin Malek Department of Surgery, Emory University School of Medicine, Atlanta, GA, USA

Yoav Mintz Department of General Surgery, Hadassah Hebrew University Medical Center, Jerusalem, Israel
Faculty of Medicine, Hebrew University of Jerusalem, Jerusalem, Israel

Eli Mlaver Department of Surgery, General and GI Surgery, Emory University School of Medicine, Atlanta, GA, USA

Jennifer Moffett, MD, FACS Department of Surgery, University of Texas Medical Branch, Galveston, TX, USA

Barbara Mullineris, FACS Department of General, Emergency Surgery and New technologies, Baggiovara General Hospital, AOU Modena, Modena, Italy

Michelle Nessen Clinical Instructor of Surgery, Department of Minimally Invasive and Bariatric Surgery, Tulane University, New Orleans, LA, USA

Dmitry Oleynikov Department of Surgery, Monmouth Medical Center, Long Branch, NJ, USA

Department of Surgery, Rutgers Robert Wood Johnson Medical School, Long Branch, NJ, USA

Ibrahim H. Ozata Department of General Surgery, Koç University School of Medicine, Istanbul, Turkey

Charudutt N. Paranjape Department of Surgery, NYU Grossman School of Medicine, New York, NY, USA
Division of Bariatric and General Surgery, Bellevue Hospital Center, New York, NY, USA
Newton-Wellesley Hospital, Newton, MA, USA

Ankit D. Patel Department of General & Gastrointestinal Surgery, Emory University School of Medicine, Atlanta, GA, USA

Snehal G. Patel Department of Surgery, Emory University School of Medicine, Atlanta, GA, USA

Roman V. Petrov Department of Cardiothoracic Surgery, John Sealy School of Medicine at University of Texas Medical Branch, Galveston, TX, USA

Micaela Piccoli, FACS Department of General, Emergency Surgery and New technologies, Baggiovara General Hospital, AOU Modena, Modena, Italy

Rachel Reed Department of Surgery, General and GI Surgery, Emory University School of Medicine, Atlanta, GA, USA

Sarah Samreen, MD, FACS, FASMBS Surgery, The University of Texas Medical Branch, Galveston, TX, USA

Manu Sancheti Emory University School of Medicine, Atlanta, GA, USA

Ankit Sarin Department of Surgery, University of California Davis, Sacramento, CA, USA

Linda Schultz Society of American Gastrointestinal and Endoscopic Surgeons, Los Angeles, CA, USA

S. Scott Davis Jr. Department of Surgery, General and GI Surgery, Emory University School of Medicine, Atlanta, GA, USA

Caroline J. Simon JC Walter Jr Transplant Center, Sherrie and Alan Conover Center for Liver Disease and Transplantation, Houston Methodist Hospital, Houston, TX, USA
Department of Surgery, Houston Methodist Hospital, Houston, TX, USA

Savannah Smith Department of Surgery, General and GI Surgery, Emory University School of Medicine, Atlanta, GA, USA

Jamil Stetler Department of General & Gastrointestinal Surgery, Emory University School of Medicine, Atlanta, GA, USA

Nova Szoka Department of Surgery, West Virginia University, Morgantown, WV, USA

Yasamin Taghikhan Department of Surgery, University of California Davis, Sacramento, CA, USA

Evangelos Tagkalos Department of General, Visceral and Transplant Surgery, University Medical Center Mainz, Mainz, Germany
UGIRA-Fellow 2022–2023 in Chang Gung Memorial Hospital, Taoyuan, Taiwan

Hany Takla, MD, FACS, FASMBS Bariatric and abdominal wall Surgery, Orlando Health Weight loss and Bariatric Surgery Institute, Orlando, Florida, USA

Amit Trivedi Department of Surgery and Bariatric Surgery, Hackensack Meridian Health, Pascack Valley Medical Center, Westwood, NJ, USA

Raj G. Vaghjiani University of Texas Medical Branch, Galveston, TX, USA

Brittney Williams Emory University School of Medicine, Atlanta, GA, USA

Sarah Wong Department of Laparoscopic and Bariatric Surgery, Hackensack Meridian Health, Westwood, NJ, USA

Part I

Robotic System Details

1 The Background of Robotic Surgery

A Journey Through Time: The Evolution and Future of Surgical Robotics

Danyal Fer and Jamil Stetler

Origins of Robotic Telesurgery

At its core, surgical robotics augments surgical care through a fusion of human and machine capabilities to deliver care where and when the patient requires it. Like many endeavors of this type, National Aeronautics and Space Administration (NASA) and US Military provided the brunt of the initial investment. In the 1980s, NASA Ames Research Center explored the concept of transporting one's "awareness" to another environment through what is now known as "virtual reality" or "telepresence," with the intention of reviewing imaging data from the *Voyager* space probe missions while in the NASA labs [1]. Dr. Joseph Rosen, a hand surgeon at Stanford, saw the head-mounted displays and early hand controller as a way to perform complex open microsurgery remotely. This prompted the enlistment of Stanford Research Institute's (SRI) Phil Green, PhD, to bring their robotics expertise to the venture and establish the Green Telepresence System in 1987. Dr. Rosen took a job with Dartmouth, passing the clinical responsibility of the project to US Army Colonel Dr. Richard Satva in 1988, who joined the team at SRI to develop the first "Telepresence Surgery System" consisting of a telepresence surgeon's workstation (Fig 1.1) and remote surgical unit (Fig 1.2).

At SAGES in 1989, Dr. Jacques Perissat debuted a video of laparoscopic cholecystectomy to much controversy. Despite this controversy, Dr. Satava recognized

D. Fer (✉)
Department of General & Gastrointestinal Surgery, Emory University School of Medicine, Atlanta, GA, USA

Department of General Surgery, David Grant Medical Center, United States Air Force, Fairfield, CA, USA
e-mail: danyal.m.fer.mil@health.mil

J. Stetler
Department of General & Gastrointestinal Surgery, Emory University School of Medicine, Atlanta, GA, USA

S. Samreen et al. (eds.), *The SAGES Manual of Robotic Surgery*,
https://doi.org/10.1007/978-3-031-86927-3_1

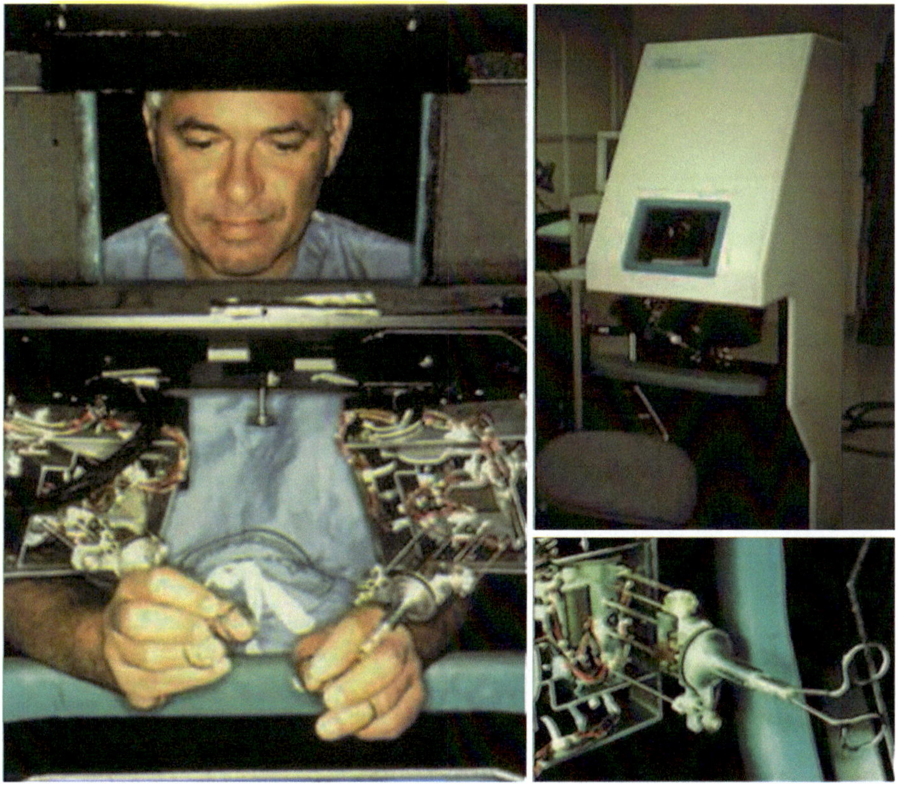

Fig. 1.1 COL Anthony LaPorta operating early telepresence workstation (SRI International)

the potential of laparoscopic surgery and urged the SRI team to develop a laparoscopic platform in addition to open surgery. He saw the advanced visualization and dexterity provided by robotic technology as a critical component to making technically challenging procedures possible [1].

In 1992, a video of the Greene Telepresence system pealing a grape was shown to the Army Surgeon General. Dr. Satava was then assigned to the Advanced Research Projects Agency (ARPA, which subsequently became DARPA), where he would oversee the development of telepresence systems. The military's goal was to develop a mobile surgical unit that could be installed in an armored vehicle and controlled by a surgeon remotely from a mobile army hospital (MASH), allowing then the delivery of immediate surgical care to soldiers in transit from the battlefield. The system was named Medical Forward Advanced Surgical Treatment (MEDFAST), drawing on inspiration from Robert Heinlein's description of medical systems illustrated in his science fiction novel *Starship Troopers* (Fig 1.3). The system successfully repaired swine stomach, intestine, and vascular injuries (Fig 1.4), [2, 3]. While the robotically assisted procedures took longer than traditional open procedures, it was noted the procedures could be completed more quickly

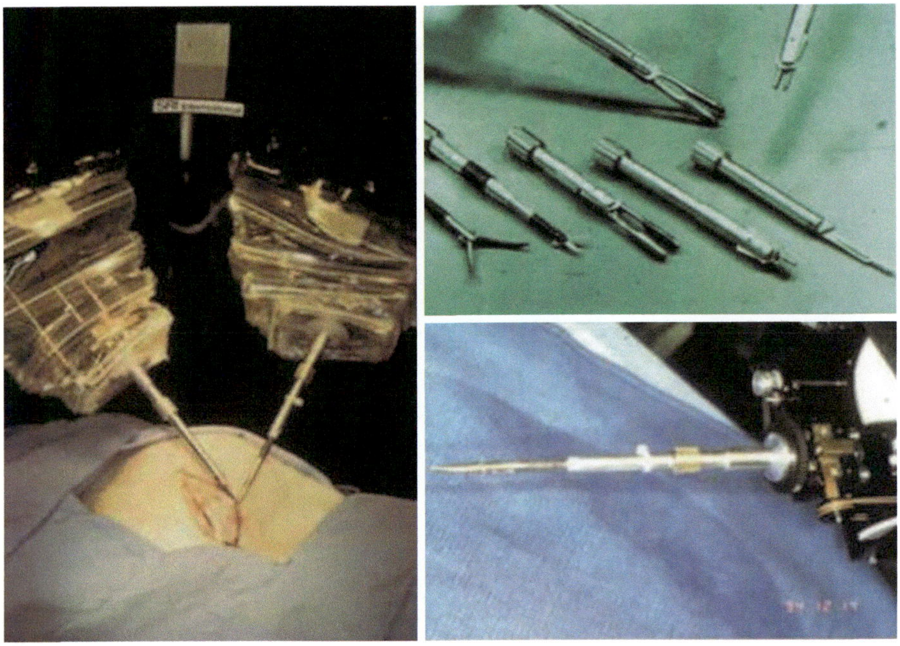

Fig. 1.2 Early remote surgical unit making an incision. Note exchangeable end effectors (SRI International)

Fig. 1.3 Original DARPA concept for remote telesurgery network using microwave communication to transmit surgeon intent

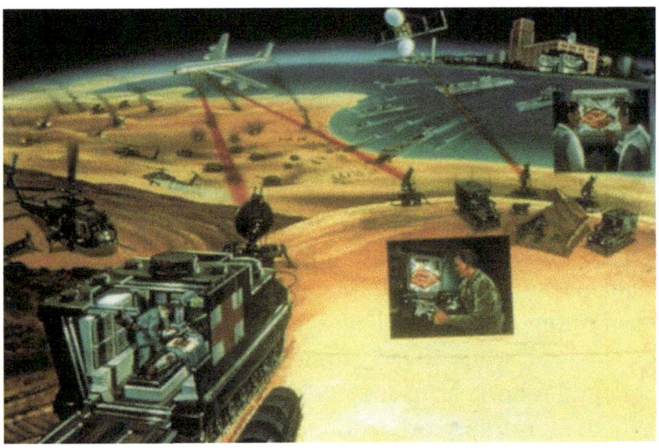

when compared to laparoscopic techniques [4]. The MEDFAST system began incorporating imaging, anesthesia, a robotic scrub tech, and pharmacologic infusion capabilities to form a self-sustaining unit [5]. This concept inspired the TraumaPod program that automated all facets of the operating room, demonstrating these capabilities in full [6](Fig 1.5). As with many DARPA projects, the goal of the project was not to produce a final product but rather to foster the technologies that would make telesurgery a reality, a groundwork that we all benefit from today.

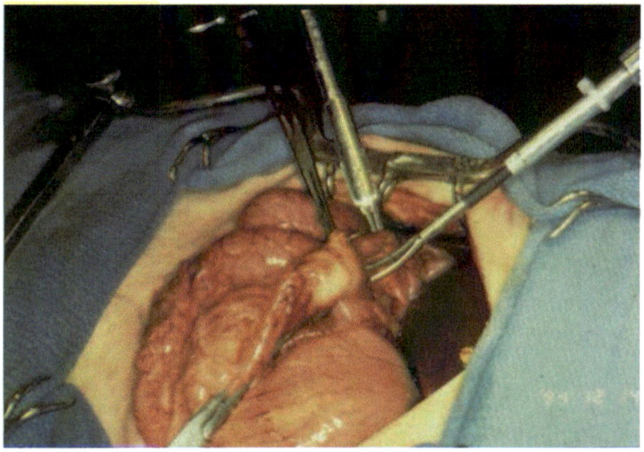

Fig. 1.4 Early bowel open surgery telesurgery using Green Telepresence System (SRI International)

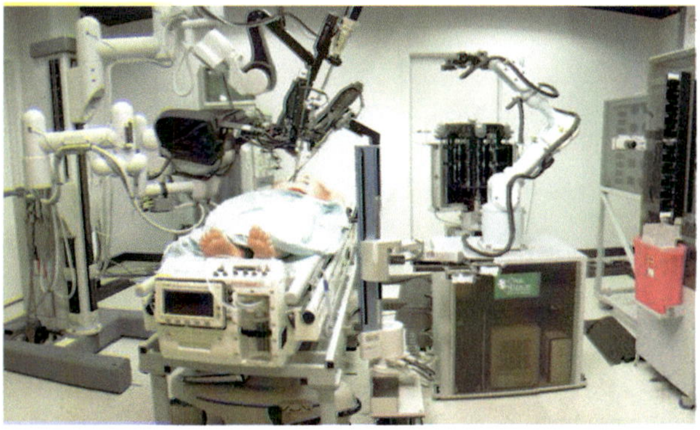

Fig. 1.5 TraumaPod autonomous operating room. This system allowed for complete control of the operating room from the surgeon console. Note autonomous "scrub tech" (right). (Image courtesy of SRI International)

Commercialization

Dr. Yulun Wang founded Computer Motion in 1990 to develop a robotic endoscope holder, initially with funding from NASA. This also attracted funding from ARPA that led to the development of Automated Endoscopic System for Optimal Positioning (AESOP). This system was a voice-controlled endoscope that became the first FDA-approved surgical robot [7]. This system then incorporated bed-mounted robotic arms to become the Zeus surgical system with the intended use in remote telesurgery procedures. The system was used by Dr. Jacques Marescaux to complete a transatlantic surgery ("The Lindbergh" surgery) between New York City and Strausburg France in 2001, removing a woman's gallbladder. This may have been the most expensive surgical procedure to date, with telecommunications costs alone costing over US$1 million [8]. Additionally, the Zeus was the platform that helped facilitate the first national telesurgery program in Ontario, Canada. This group, led by Dr. Mehan Anvari at McMaster University, completed collaborative fundoplications, hemicolectomies, and other general surgery procedures working with less experienced surgeons over 400 km away [9–11].

By 1993, SRI licensed their patents of the Green Telepresence Surgery Program, and they were eventually acquired by Dr. Fred Moll, Dr. John Freund, and Robert Younge, who formed Intuitive Surgical in 1995. The early platform was intended for the minimally invasive market with a bed-mounted system, an open control console, and 3D glasses. The first prototype was named Lenny (short for Leonardo) followed by MONA (short for Mona Lisa), MONA entered initial human trials in 1997, with the first cholecystectomy being performed in Belgium by Dr. Jaques Himpens [12]. While noting the unwieldy setup process, finicky instrument exchanges, and nauseating display, the ergonomic and dexterous benefits of robotic surgery were clear [13]. The lessons learned from this initial period led to the immersive surgeon console and the single cart-mounted robotic arms that would form the Da Vinci Surgical System we know today.

The initial target market for the use of the Da Vinci system was actually in cardiac surgery with plans to incorporate technology to compensate for the heart's motion [14, 15]. While the technology was impressive, there was limited enthusiasm within the cardiac surgery community. A new market was discovered in the urologic community. Dr. Clement-Claude Abbou of Paris had been a pioneer in laparoscopic prostatectomy, working with colleagues in Germany, Dr. Binder and Dr. Kramer. The oncologic equivalence of the minimally invasive approach, compared to open, was demonstrated in clinical trials; however, the procedure had a tremendous learning curve that limited the laparoscopic approach to specialized centers [16]. Dr. Abbou was the first to perform a minimally invasive prostatectomy using a Da Vinci robot on loan from the cardiac surgery department, and his technique was quickly replicated by the Germans [17]. These findings were discussed with Dr. Menon of Detroit, who had been attempting to establish a minimally invasive surgery prostatectomy program but was limited by the technical challenges and poor outcomes [18]. Dr. Menon found the robotic platform flattened his learning to perform minimally invasive surgery. He was able to quickly establish equivalent oncologic and superior functional outcomes as compared to open surgery. He then went on to establish a program at Henry Ford Hospital to popularize the approach [19]. Prior to the introduction of the robotic platform in the United States, few minimally invasive prostatectomies had been performed. As of 2003, 12% of prostatectomies were performed using the robot and as of 2021 around 90% of prostate surgery utilized the robot [20, 21]. There has been rapid uptake in gynecologic, thoracic, and general surgery fields and adoption of robotic platforms rapidly increasing the number and types of procedures performed in a minimally invasive invasive fashion. This trend was possible due to the improved ergonomics, range of motion, and visualization of the robotic platforms.

With innovation, there will always be controversy. In the early days of laparoscopic surgery, opponents pointed to higher costs, high conversion rates, and worse outcomes in certain circumstances [22, 23]. As was argued by proponents of laparoscopic surgery, then, these were all artifacts of both the surgeon and healthcare system learning curve. Minimally invasive approaches to a many surgical procedures have demonstrated equivalent oncologic and functional outcomes with less pain, shorter hospital stays, and fewer postoperative complications [24]. Robotic surgery has expanded access to minimally invasive surgery operations by reducing the technical capacity of the surgeon required to perform these operations. This access did not come without cost. The initial learning curve for operating room teams and surgeons led to significantly longer operating room times in the early days of robotic surgery, though innovations in robot systems and training paradigms have reduced or eliminated these types of delays.

The final barrier to the adoption of these platforms is the enormous cost of these complex systems. Many healthcare systems have been able to bring the cost to parity with laparoscopic surgery. The strategies for making robotic platforms financially feasible the current market paradigm will be discussed in later chapters. As far as the future is concerned, market forces should bring costs down. As of 2021, the global surgical robotics market was valued at US$9.6 billion, which is expected to reach US$18.4 billion by 2027 [25]. This has not gone unnoticed by medical device companies. The previous version of this manual published in 2017 described the host of Intuitive robotic platforms and noted that other companies were considering efforts in the space. This text describes six robotic platforms that are either in the market or near market ready. This excludes homegrown systems such as China's MedBot. Quantifying the potential price distortion caused by Intuitive's dominance in the robotics market presents challenges. Nevertheless, consistent with patterns observed in emerging technologies, initial costs are substantial but are projected to decrease due to factors including rising adoption rates, economies of scale in production, R&D amortization, technological advancements, and, most significantly, increased market competition.

The Future of Surgical Robotics

The initial vision of robotic surgery imagined performing semi-autonomous operations over great distances, reaching areas where surgical expertise was unavailable. Ironically, the gap that surgical robotics filled was the technical expertise lacking in our own operating rooms. Beyond the introduction of new robotics platforms, we will see new tools at our disposal, with the robot console being the hub, as the TraumaPod had initially intended. The next leaps in this technology will be beyond steadying the surgeon's hands and improving our dexterity. Instead, the surgeon console will act as our portal to information and tools to better help patients. Early examples of this are the ability to incorporate fluorescence imaging or endoscopic views into the visual field. Technological progress will continue to take the next steps in helping inform the mind of the surgeon as well as assist in the physical task of surgery.

In the mid-2000s, computer chips called Graphics Processing Units (GPUs), initially meant for producing high-end graphics for video games, began being used for more general-purpose computing. They were found to be very effective at performing tasks known as machine learning or deep learning. Previously, this type of work had to be done with large mainframe computers, but with GPUs the work could be done with a desktop computer. This general innovation and massive reduction in computing costs is what has led to the artificial intelligence (AI) boom we see today. AI systems allow for the rapid ingestion and categorization of information and, if desired, the ability to initiate actions based on that information. AI methods, such as computer vision, allow us to better understand what is happening in the operating room based on using surgical video to autonomously recognize and break down complex procedures, providing guidance and feedback to operating surgeons [26–28]. Robotics add an additional component to this data stream, helping us understand how the movements of surgical robots can contribute to better surgical outcomes [29, 30]. At the forefront, significant work has successfully automated some surgical tasks in the lab. Surgical robots have completed preliminary, high-precision tasks, such as FLS peg transfer, with more speed and accuracy than surgeons [31]. Additionally, there have been impressive demonstrations of autonomous anastomosis and needle handling [32, 33]. Integrating radiographic imaging has enabled virtual barriers to be generated to prevent inadvertent injury to critical structures [34]. The work has continued with the US Military's development of robots to bring autonomous surgical assistance to the battlefield (Fig 1.6). While previous networks could not provide the appropriate cost, bandwidth, or latency for facile teleoperation, 5G and fiber networks are creating the opportunity to allow for seamless telesurgery. In sum, these technologies will aim to augment the capabilities of the surgeon but how surgeons will choose to interact with them remains to be seen.

As we stand on the precipice of the future, the journey of robotic telesurgery from its nascent beginnings in the realms of virtual reality to its current status as a cornerstone of modern medical practice is nothing short of revolutionary. This odyssey, driven by visionary pioneers and transformative technologies, has not only redefined the boundaries of surgical precision and patient care but also set the stage for the next frontier of medical innovation. The integration of AI and machine learning promises to further enhance the capabilities of surgical robots, making procedures safer, more efficient, and accessible to patients around the globe. As we look forward, it is clear that the evolution of robotic telesurgery will continue to be marked by groundbreaking advancements, challenging us to reimagine the limits of

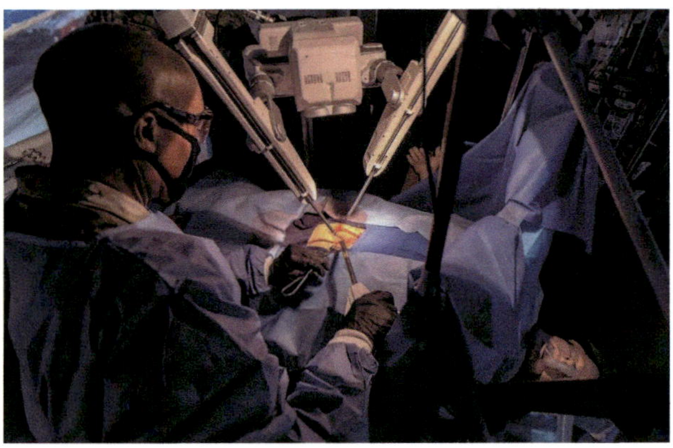

Fig. 1.6 Demonstration of robotic surgical assistance using Taurus-M (designed and manufactured by SRI International) at TATRC. (Used with permission and provided courtesy of the US Army TATRC Public Affairs Office)

what is possible in the operating room and beyond. The legacy of this journey is a testament to the enduring power of human ingenuity and the relentless pursuit of excellence in the service of humanity.

Acknowledgments I acknowledge Dr. Richard Stava for his time and insight into preparing this chapter.

The Green Telepresence surgery project was funded by the Department of Defense under the Bayh-Dole Act (1980), and therefore, all images related to this project are designated as public domain.

References

1. Satava RM. Robotic surgery: from past to future: a personal journey. Surg Clin North Am. 2003;83(6):1491–500. xii
2. Bowersox JC, Shah A, Jensen J, et al. Vascular applications of telepresence surgery: initial feasibility studies in swine. J Vasc Surg. 1996;23:281–7.
3. Bowersox JC, Cordts PR, LaPorta AJ. Use of an intuitive telemanipulator system for remote trauma surgery: an experimental study. J Am Coll Surg. 1998;186:615–21.
4. Bowersox JC, Cornum RL. Remote operative urology using a surgical telemanipulator system: preliminary observations. Urology. 1998;52(1):17–22.
5. Satava R, Jenkins D, Jones S. Advanced biomedical technology program. Arlington: Defense Advanced Research Projects Agency; 2000.
6. Garcia P, Rosen J, Kapoor C, Noakes M, Elbert G, Treat M, Ganous T, Hanson M, Manak J, Hasser C, Rohler D, Satava R. Trauma Pod: a semi-automated telerobotic surgical system. Int J Med Robot Comp Assist Surg. 2009;5(2):136–46. https://doi.org/10.1002/rcs.238.
7. Rosen J, Hannaford B, Satava RM. Surgical robotics: systems applications, and visions. Berlin: Springer; 2011.
8. Marescaux J, Leroy J, Rubino F, et al. Transcontinental robot-assisted remote telesurgery: feasibility and potential applications. Ann Surg. 2002;235:487–92.
9. Anvari M. Reaching the rural world through robotic surgical programs. Eur Surg. 2005;37:284–92.
10. Anvari M. Telesurgery: remote knowledge translation in clinical surgery. World J Surg. 2007;31:1545–50.
11. Anvari M. Robot-assisted remote telepresence surgery. Semin Laparosc Surg. 2004;11:123–8.
12. Himpens J, Leman G, Cadiere G. Telesurgical laparoscopic cholecystectomy. Surg Endosc. 1998;12(8):1091.
13. DiMaio S, Hanuschik M, Kreaden U. The da Vinci surgical system. In: Surgical robotics. New York, NY: Springer; 2011. p. 199–217.
14. Kappert U, Cichon R, Schneider J, et al. Closed-chest coronary artery surgery on the beating heart with the use of a robotic system. J Thorac Cardiovasc Surg. 2000;120:809–11. https://doi.org/10.1067/mtc.2000.109543.
15. Stoyanov D, Mylonas G, Deligianni F, Darzi A, Yang G. Soft-tissue motion tracking and structure estimation for robotic assisted MIS procedures. Medical image computing and computer-assisted intervention. MICCAI … Int Conf Med Image Comput Comput Assist Interv. 2005;8:139–46. https://doi.org/10.1007/11566489_18.
16. Munver R, Volfson IA, Kesler SS, Nazmy M, Sawczuk IS. Transition from open to robotic-assisted radical prostatectomy: 7 years experience at Hackensack University Medical Center. J Robot Surg. 2007;1(2):155–9. https://doi.org/10.1007/s11701-007-0023-0.
17. Abbou CC, Hoznek A, Salomon L, et al. Laparoscopic radical prostatectomy with a remote controlled robot. J Urol. 2001;165:1964.

18. Schuessler WW, Schulam PG, Clayman RV, et al. Laparoscopic radical prostatectomy: initial short-term experience. Urology. 1997;50:854.
19. Menon M, Shrivastava A, Tewari A, et al. Laparoscopic and robot assisted radical prostatectomy: establishment of a structured program and preliminary analysis of outcomes. J Urol. 2002;168:945.
20. Hu JC, et al. Utilization and outcomes of minimally invasive radical prostatectomy. J Clin Oncol. 2008;26:2278–84. https://doi.org/10.1200/JCO.2007.13.4528.
21. Simsir A, Kizilay F, Aliyev B, Kalemci S. Comparison of robotic and open radical prostatectomy: initial experience of a single surgeon. Pak J Med Sci. 2021;37(1):167–74. https://doi.org/10.12669/pjms.37.1.2719.
22. Sinha R, Sharma N. Acute cholecystitis and laparoscopic cholecystectomy. JSLS. 2002;6(1):65–8.
23. Kalata S, Thumma JR, Norton EC, Dimick JB, Sheetz KH. Comparative safety of robotic-assisted vs laparoscopic cholecystectomy. JAMA Surg. 2023;158(12):1303–10. https://doi.org/10.1001/jamasurg.2023.4389.
24. Singh SS, Shinde RK. Minimally invasive gastrointestinal surgery: a review. Cureus. 2023;15(11):e48864. https://doi.org/10.7759/cureus.48864.
25. Fortune Business Insights. Surgical robots market size, share & industry trends analysis | Forecast 2030. 2019.
26. Fer D, Zhang B, Abukhalil R, Goel V, Goel B, Barker J, Kalesan B, Barragan I, Gaddis M, Kilroy P. An artificial intelligence model that automatically labels roux-en-Y gastric bypasses, a comparison to trained surgeon annotators. Surg Endosc. 2023;37:1–8. https://doi.org/10.1007/s00464-023-09870-6.
27. Madani A, Namazi B, Altieri MS, Hashimoto DA, Rivera AM, Pucher PH, Navarrete-Welton A, Sankaranarayanan G, Brunt LM, Okrainec A, Alseidi A. Artificial intelligence for intraoperative guidance: using semantic segmentation to identify surgical anatomy during laparoscopic cholecystectomy. Ann Surg. 2022;276(2):363–9. https://doi.org/10.1097/SLA.0000000000004594.
28. Hashimoto DA, Rosman G, Witkowski ER, Stafford C, Navarette-Welton AJ, Rattner DW, Lillemoe KD, Rus DL, Meireles OR. Computer vision analysis of intraoperative video: automated recognition of operative steps in laparoscopic sleeve gastrectomy. Ann Surg. 2019;270(3):414–21. Note: Co-first author
29. Hung AJ, Ma R, Cen S, Nguyen JH, Lei X, Wagner C. Surgeon Automated performance metrics as predictors of early urinary continence recovery after robotic radical prostatectomy-a prospective bi-institutional study. Eu Urol Open Sci. 2021;27:65–72. https://doi.org/10.1016/j.euros.2021.03.005.
30. Ma R, Ramaswamy A, Xu J, et al. Surgical gestures as a method to quantify surgical performance and predict patient outcomes. npj Digit Med. 2022;5:187. https://doi.org/10.1038/s41746-022-00738-y.
31. Hwang M, Ichnowski J, Thananjeyan B, Seita D, Paradis S, Fer D, Low T, Goldberg K. Automating surgical peg transfer: calibration with deep learning can exceed speed, accuracy, and consistency of humans. IEEE Trans Autom Sci Eng. 2022; https://doi.org/10.1109/TASE.2022.3171795.
32. Saeidi H, Opfermann JD, Kam M, Wei S, Leonard S, Hsieh MH, Kang JU, Krieger A. Autonomous robotic laparoscopic surgery for intestinal anastomosis. Sci Robot. 2022;7(62):eabj 2908. https://doi.org/10.1126/scirobotics.abj2908.
33. Chiu ZY, Richter F, Funk EK, Orosco RK, Yip MC. Bimanual regrasping for suture needles using reinforcement learning for rapid motion planning. In: IEEE conference on robotics and automation. Xi'an; 2021.
34. Zhang H, Gonenc B, Iordachita I. Admittance control for robot assisted retinal vein microcannulation under human-robot collaborative mode. In: 2017 17th international conference on control, automation and systems (ICCAS). Jeju: IEEE; 2017. p. 862–6.

Part II

Current and Upcoming Robotic Platforms

2 Current and Upcoming Robotic Platforms: Intuitive da Vinci

Clark Gerhart

In 1902, Charles Holland Duell, the outgoing Commissioner of the United States Patent Office, commented on the rate at which innovation was progressing saying, "In my opinion, all previous advances in the various lines of invention will appear totally insignificant when compared with those which the present century will witness." [1] I think the same could be said of the dramatic advances that have been made in robotic surgery over the last quarter century.

The story of da Vinci robotic surgery began when SRI International and the Defense Advanced Research Projects Agency (DARPA) set out to develop robotic telepresence surgery systems to address the Department of Defense's need to decrease battlefield casualties [2]. Using a robotic prototype produced by SRI International and DARPA, Intuitive Surgical was later founded in 1995 by Dr. Frederick Moll, M.D., Rob Younge, and John Freund [3]. While microelectronics, virtual reality, and haptic interfaces had been explored since the 1980s, these early robotic technologies had not yet been successfully adapted for use in surgery [4]. "The hard part," Dr. Moll said at the time, "is making a robot that is easy to use by surgeons." [5] But eventually this difficult task was accomplished, and in the year 2000, da Vinci robotic instrumentation received FDA clearance for use in human surgery and the era of robotic-assisted surgery began.

At the outset, Intuitive had hopes of marketing the da Vinci for cardiovascular surgeries [2]. Instead, the wristed instruments were found to enhance urologists' ability to work deep in the pelvis for prostatectomy, and robotic prostatectomy showed improved clinical outcomes compared to both open and laparoscopic approaches [6]. These benefits lead to most prostatectomies being done robotically [7]. Gary Guthart, Intuitive CEO, recalls this episode saying, "We aimed at the heart

C. Gerhart (✉)
General and Bariatric Surgeon, Associate Medical Officer, Intuitive., Sunnyvale, CA, USA
e-mail: Clark.Gerhart@intusurg.com

S. Samreen et al. (eds.), *The SAGES Manual of Robotic Surgery*,
https://doi.org/10.1007/978-3-031-86927-3_2

and hit the prostate."[1] But this was not a missed opportunity. It was an example of the continuous innovation process, which is the foundation of Intuitive's development philosophy. The creation of new robotic technology being guided by surgeons and clinical outcomes is vital for producing technology that is not just novel and exciting but provides improved patient benefits.

As the clinical value story began to unfold, new indications were developed across multiple surgical specialties, and the process of continuous innovation adapted the robotic technology to the new procedures. In 2006, Intuitive's second-generation da Vinci "S" platform simplified the robotic arms on the bedside patient cart, allowing easier setup and instrument exchange. Continued advancements were introduced with the third-generation "Si" da Vinci platform in 2009 with refinements to the surgeon console and advanced instrumentation, including a stapler and vessel sealer, along with instruments for single-site surgery. In 2014, the fourth-generation "Xi" daVinci platform redesigned the robotic arms, freeing them from the column of the beside patient cart, attaching them to a moveable gantry suspended over the patient, which provided greater access to surgical work sites. And longer and more advanced instruments allowed a wider array of surgical procedures to be performed. The latest, fifth generation, "da Vinci 5", was launched in 2024 with improved surgeon ergonomics, enhanced 3D imaging with heads-up display menus so surgeons can manage functions like light intensity, electrocautery and suction, and others with greater efficiency. It introduced first-of-its-kind force sensing technology which enables the system to measure, and surgeons to feel, subtle forces exerted on tissue during surgery. The system also has over 10,000 times the computing power of Xi giving it advanced data capabilities to provide objective performance insights, leverage machine learning, and power AI opportunities into the future.

Throughout the 25-year history since the first FDA clearance of da Vinci robotic systems, surgeons have published over 34,000 peer-reviewed articles. da Vinci robotic systems have been used by more than 66,000 surgeons in 70 countries, and 6 continents to perform more than 17 million procedures.[2]

Continuous innovation has progressed beyond the multiarmed dV5 robotic platforms. In 2018, Intuitive introduced the da Vinci Single-Port "SP" platform, which has three operating arms and a camera that are introduced through one incision that can be as small as 2.7 cm. The 6-mm-diameter instruments have wrists like their multi-armed predecessors, but they also have elbows that provide separation and triangulation of the instruments to reduce clashing. The camera is flexible, articulating much like an endoscope, to rise above or below the instruments to give an unobstructed view of the operative field. While previous laparoscopic single-incision surgical techniques have attempted to do the same operations while reducing the number of laparoscopic port sites from four or five down to one, the SP platform is exploring new ways to access operative sites to preserve healthy tissue and improve outcomes by accessing narrow spaces as in trans-anal, trans-oral, or trans-vaginal

[1] Personal communications.

[2] Intuitive Surgical 2022 earnings report.

procedures, and providing alternate access to the operative site by alternate access within the retroperitoneum, intramuscular, preperitoneal, or subcutaneous planes, as well as using stoma and specimen retrieval sites as points of access.

Intuitive announced another platform innovation, the Ion Endoluminal System, in 2019. This shape-sensing robotic-assisted bronchoscopic biopsy device is directed through the bronchial tree to small and peripherally based lesions. According to the investigators in the PRECIsE study, the early results for this system suggest a high sensitivity for malignancy for nodules with a mean size of 17 mm, and a favorable safety profile, and suggest that it may play an important role in the diagnosis of early-stage lung cancer and metastatic cancers [8].

Robotic-assisted surgery introduces significant computing power into the operating room. Intuitive's Digital platform capitalizes on this by gathering objective data and utilizing it to help support preoperative planning, intraoperative guidance, and postoperative analytics. My Intuitive App allows surgeons to track their robotic practices from their smart device. SimNow provides simulation training for new trainees or surgeons learning new techniques. Integrated Telepresence makes it possible for surgeons to obtain guidance from outside experts while in the operating room or provide educational experiences for surgeons remotely. Instrument movements can be analyzed as Objective Performance Indicators, to understand efficiency, learning curves and improve surgeon performance. The Customer Portal supplies important information about instrument and platform utilization to guide health system time and cost efficiencies.

It appears certain that robotic innovation will continue to flourish as more surgeons and companies explore ways to improve patient care using robotic technology. A review of surgical companies with exciting new surgical robots included a nonexhaustive list of 24 companies offering new robotic solutions for a wide array of surgical specialties ranging from classic intra-abdominal or intrathoracic procedures to orthopedic surgery and dental procedures, tumor ablation, and spine and brain surgery [9]. New imaging devices may overlap the endoscopic visualization with 3D reconstruction of CT and MRI scans to let surgeons see through solid organs to find hidden disease [10]. Injectable molecules may identify cancer or nerves or other critical anatomic structures, allowing them to be seen within the surgical workspace [3]. And throughout it all, the computer-driven robotic devices will provide a wealth of data to be analyzed with machine learning and artificial intelligence to evaluate surgical procedures, allowing surgeons and health systems to improve surgical performance and provide surgical efficiency.

Autonomous surgery, once a thing of science fiction, now appears to be a potential opportunity for robotic surgery. Mahdi Azizian, senior director of the Holoscan Artificial Intelligence sensor processing platform at NVIDIA, suggests that humans will likely remain in the loop for the foreseeable future; however, supervised automation of certain surgical tasks or subtasks is an active area of research, with potential for clinical adoption in future [11]. This may include gradual introduction of guidance and warning features that will require the system to have some knowledge of the surgical task, similar to early aspects of autonomy in automobiles, where the first steps were recognition of road markings, obstacles, cars, and pedestrians [3].

While it may feel like science fiction, considering the computer data that robotic systems provide and recent advancements in AI, we may 1 day see some aspects of robotic surgery become automated.

As Charles Holland Duell concluded his thoughts on the rate of innovation in 1902, he admitted, "I almost wish that I might live my life over again to see the new wonders which are at the threshold." [1] With the amount of advancement that has occurred through the continuous innovation of robotic technology over the last 25 years, I am likewise confident that we stand at a similar threshold, waiting to see what new wonders will be produced in surgical robotics in the next quarter century and beyond.

References

1. Duell CH. Chances for the inventor. The Friend Religious and Literary Journal. 1902;76:28. Accessed via Google Books 13 Dec 23. https://itunes.apple.com/WebObjects/MZStore.woa/wa/viewBook?id=0
2. George EI, Brand TC, LaPorta A, Marescaux J, Satava RM. Origins of robotic surgery: from skepticism to standard of care. JSLS. 2018;22:1–5.
3. Azizian M, Liu M, Khalaji I, DiMaio S. The Da Vinci surgical system. In: The Encyclopedia of medical robotics. 2018;3–28.
4. DiMaio S, Hanuschik M, Kreaden U. Surgical robotics, Chapter 9 The da Vinci surgical system. New York, NY: Springer; 2019. p. 199–217.
5. Moukheiber Z Dr. Robot. Forbes. 2000. https://www.forbes.com/global/2000/0306/0305070a.html?sh=545248225fe1 Accessed 29 Nov 2023.
6. Tewari A, Srivasatava A, Menon M. A prospective comparison of radical retropubic and robot-assisted prostatectomy: experience in one institution. BJU Int. 2003;92:205–10.
7. Oberlin DT, Flum AS, Lai JD, Meeks JJ. The effect of minimally invasive prostatectomy on 90 practice patterns of American Urologists. J Urologic Onc. 2016;34:255e1–5.
8. Ost D, Pritchett M, Reisenauer J, Simoff M, Diaz-Mendoza J, Fernandez-Bussy S, Majid A, Casal R, Keyes C, Parikh M, Folch E. Prospective, multicenter analysis of shape-sensing robotic-assisted bronchoscopy: updates from the PRECISE study. CHEST. 2021;160:A2531–3.
9. Sharp N. Twenty four of the most exciting surgical robotics companies in 2022, September 22, 2022. Escatech. https://www.escatec.com/blog/24-exciting-surgical-robotics-companies. Accessed 13 Dec 23.
10. Boedecker C, Huettl F, Saalfeld P, et al. Using virtual 3D-models in surgical planning: workflow of an immersive virtual reality application in liver surgery. Langenbecks Arch Surg. 2021;406:911–5. https://doi.org/10.1007/s00423-021-02127-7.
11. Azizian M, Khoshnam M, Najmaei N, Patel RV. Visual servoing in medical robotics: a survey. Part I: endoscopic direct vision imaging — techniques and applications. Int. J. Med. Robot. Comput. Assist. Surg. 2014;10:263–74.

3 Asensus Surgical: Senhance Surgical System

Amit Trivedi and Sarah Wong

Asensus Surgical: Senhance Surgical System

Asensus Surgical was formed in 2021 after the rebranding of Transenterix, Inc. Transenterix was founded in 2006 and developed the Senhance Surgical System (Fig. 3.1) that was FDA approved in the United States in 2017. At the time, the Senhance System became only the second FDA-approved robotic surgical system in the United States for abdominal surgery. The System obtained CE mark in 2016 and is now offered for sale in Europe, the Middle East, Africa, Japan, and Taiwan.

The Senhance Surgical System introduced several new concepts to robotic surgery. The system was the first to offer an open-surgeon console that aimed to improve surgeon and operating room ergonomics. Since the system was built on the foundation of laparoscopic surgery, robotic instrument movement is controlled by handles on the console that use traditional familiar laparoscopic motion. These instrument handles were the first to incorporate haptic feedback, allowing for a sense of tactile perception when handling tissue. Another first for the Senhance System is the use of real-time eye tracking to control camera movement. A sensor on the console tracks the surgeon's eyes, and the system is able to move the camera to the point on the screen where the surgeon is focusing. The surgical instrument portfolio for the Senhance System consists of another first in robotic surgery, 3 mm and 5 mm straight stick reusable instruments. Other unique features of the Senhance System include the ability to use any available trocar as the system's instruments and arms are not fixed to the trocar, and the system's use of existing scope and camera systems available in most operating rooms.

A. Trivedi (✉)
Department of Surgery and Bariatric Surgery, Hackensack Meridian Health, Pascack Valley Medical Center, Westwood, NJ, USA

S. Wong
Department of Laparoscopic and Bariatric Surgery, Hackensack Meridian Health, Westwood, NJ, USA

S. Samreen et al. (eds.), *The SAGES Manual of Robotic Surgery*,
https://doi.org/10.1007/978-3-031-86927-3_3

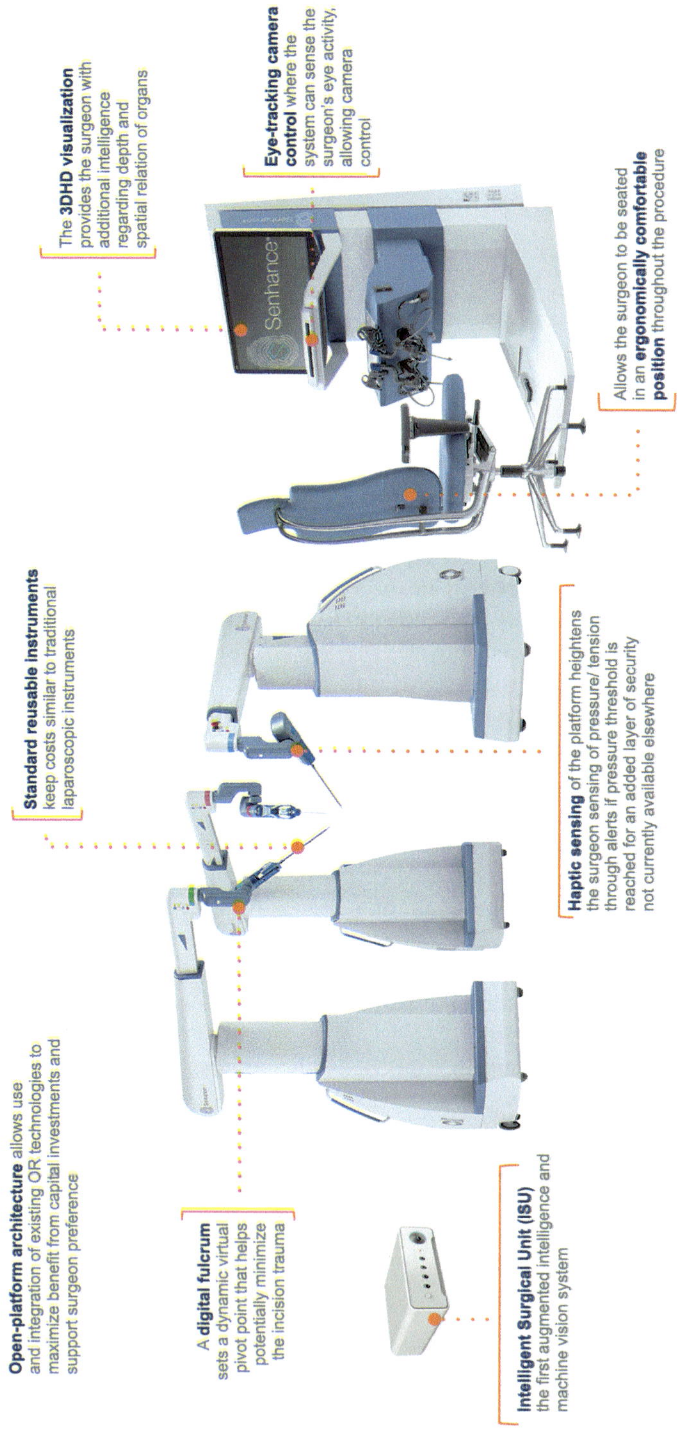

Fig. 3.1 Senhance surgical system

Finally, the Senhance System is built around the concept of digital surgery that aims to digitize the interface between surgeon and patient. With the introduction of the Intelligent Surgical Unit (ISU), the Senhance System has received a major upgrade to include real-time augmented intelligence, enabling the platform to offer a variety of advanced digital capabilities.

Robotic Arms

The Senhance System is approved for three arms in the United States and four arms in Europe. Each arm is the same and is mounted on a movable base. The base can be positioned on either side of the operating table at various angles as long as the excursion of the arm encompasses the expected range of motion of the operative instrument attached to that arm. The arm makes larger motions by raising up or down and cantilevering in and out. Finer motions are made by the distal end of the arm, which has the ability to magnetically attach various instruments and can articulate in several axes at once. When readied for use, the arm is maneuvered into position adjacent to the corresponding trocar. The selected instrument is magnetically attached to the arm, and under visual guidance, it is guided into the operative field. Notably, neither the robotic arm nor the instrument is tethered to the trocar at any stage of the process. Subsequently, the arm undergoes a brief 3-second fulcrum sequence initiated by pressing the fulcrum button located on its side. Once this sequence is completed, the arm is primed for use, and a similar procedure is repeated for the remaining arms.

Senhance System Console

The Senhance Surgical System surgeon console (Fig. 3.2) is based on an open-design concept to facilitate operating room communication and improve surgeon ergonomics (Fig. 3.3). The console consists of an ergonomically designed chair that is attached to the base of the console, a 32 inch 4K 3D monitor, eye tracker for controlling camera movement, and surgeon handles that mimic laparoscopic instrument handles. Similar to the accelerator pedal in a car, robotic motion of the arms and instruments only occurs when a foot pedal located on the base of the console is depressed. Clutching is accomplished by releasing the foot pedal and repositioning the hands to a more comfortable position, followed by depressing the foot pedal to resume operating.

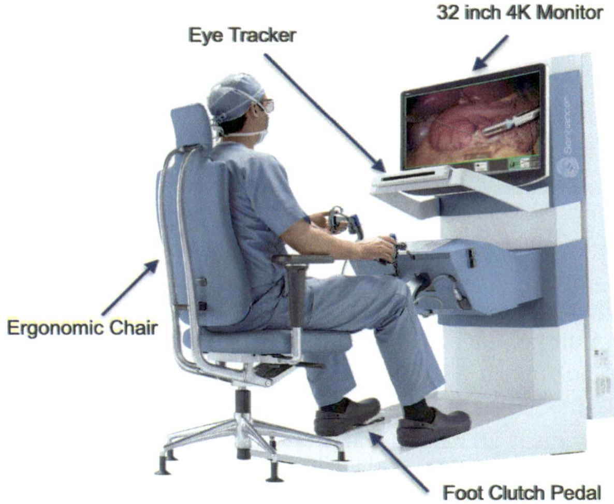

Fig. 3.2 Senhance system surgeon console

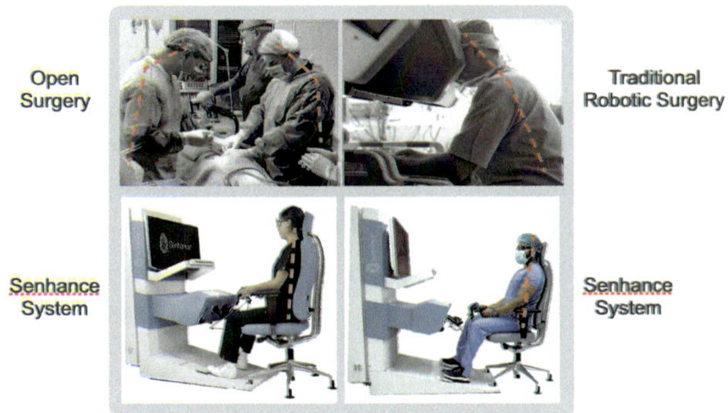

Fig. 3.3 Surgeon ergonomics vs. open surgery and traditional robotic surgery

Straight Stick Instruments

The Senhance System offers a full line of 3 and 5 mm straight stick instruments (Fig. 3.4). These reusable instruments do not have a specific number of lives and like laparoscopic instruments, they can be resterilized, and used again and again. They can also be repaired similar to laparoscopic instruments. At the start of a case, on the back table, the instruments to be used are attached to a corresponding adapter. This adapter magnetically attaches to the robotic arm during use of the instrument. Instrument exchange involves guiding the instrument out of the patient under vision, removing the current instrument from the arm, and attaching the new instrument magnetically to the arm. Once the new instrument is attached, the instrument is guided into the trocar and body under vision. A unique feature of the Senhance System is the rotation dial located on the surgeon handles (Fig. 3.5). The handles have a dial that can be easily rotated by the surgeon to allow for infinite 360-degree rotation of the instrument. This practical feature makes tasks like suturing more ergonomic as the wrists of the

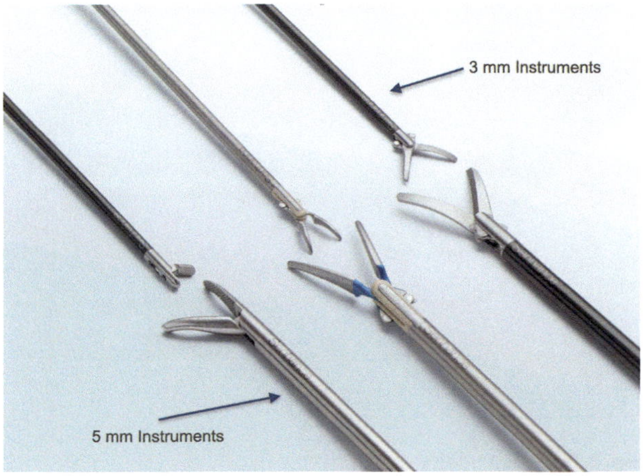

Fig. 3.4 Senhance 3 and 5 mm straight stick instruments

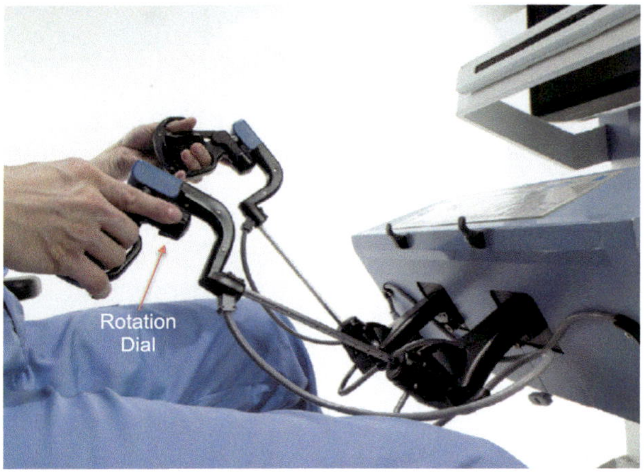

Fig. 3.5 Surgeon handle instrument rotation dial

surgeon do not move and the dial turns the needle holder along the axis of the instrument to drive the needle through the tissue. Needle retrieval and reloading are also made easier by the ability to fully rotate the instrument with the dial.

Articulating Instruments

The Senhance System has introduced a line of 5 mm instruments that partially articulate (Fig. 3.6). The articulating portfolio consists of graspers and needle drivers. The instruments have 7° of freedom, 63° of articulation, and 360-degree independent rotation of the shaft and instrument tip. For tasks like suturing, the independent 360-degree rotation of the tip can be used to drive the needle through tissue following the curve of the needle.

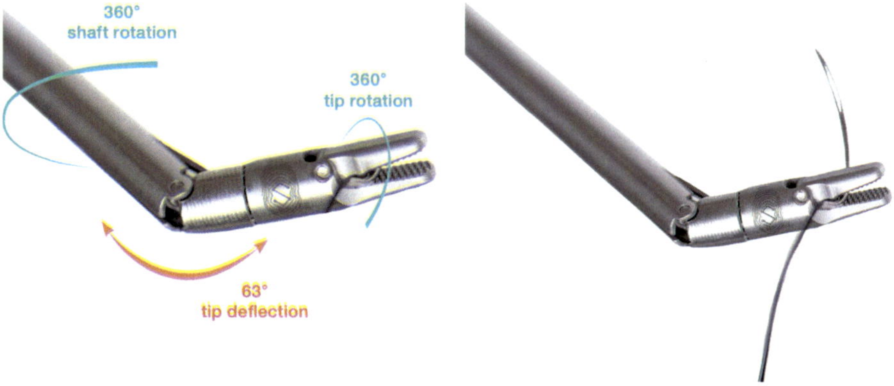

Fig. 3.6 Articulating needle driver

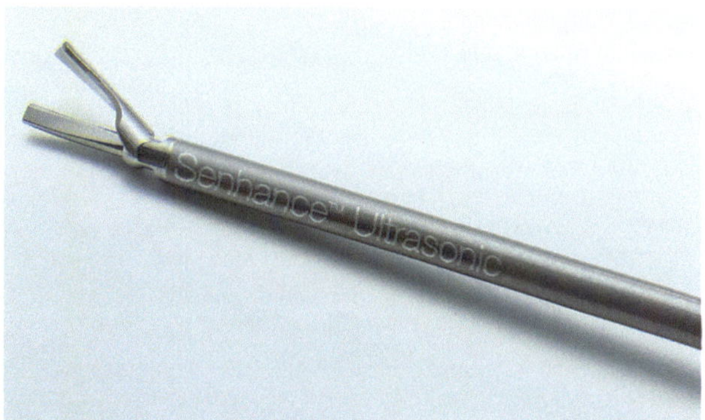

Fig. 3.7 Senhance ultrasonic dissector

Energy

The Senhance System includes monopolar, bipolar, and ultrasonic energy sources. Monopolar instruments include curved scissors, a Maryland dissector, and an L-hook. Bipolar instruments consist of a Maryland dissector and grasping forceps. These instruments are available in both 3 and 5 mm sizes. Advanced energy includes a 5 mm ultrasonic dissector that uses torsional ultrasonic energy to coagulate the tissue (Fig. 3.7).

Scope and Camera

The Senhance System has the unique ability to work with a number of scope and camera systems in both 2D or 3D modes. Existing scope and camera systems used in laparoscopy can be attached to a corresponding adapter that allows the camera to be magnetically mounted on the robotic arm. Adapters are available for both 5 and 10 mm 0, 30, and 45-degree scopes. Currently, the Senhance System has adapters for scopes and cameras from Stryker, Storz, Olympus, and ConMed. The compatibility with a wide variety of differing scopes and cameras allows for the use of

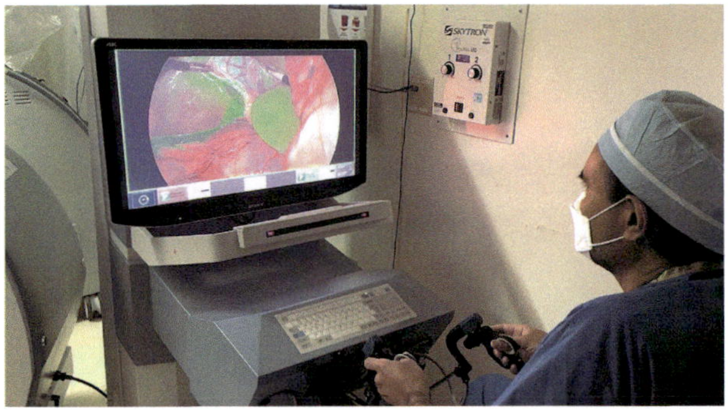

Fig. 3.8 ICG use on Senhance system with Stryker camera and scope

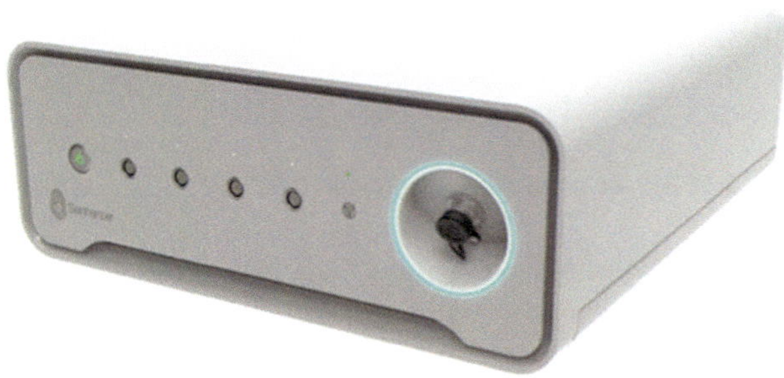

Fig. 3.9 Intelligent surgical unit

features that are specific to that video system such as fluorescence imaging and familiar navigation menus (Fig. 3.8).

Intelligent Surgical Unit

The Senhance Robotic System Intelligent Surgical Unit or ISU was cleared by the FDA, CE Marked, and approved by the PMDA as the first-of-its-kind augmented intelligence machine vision system for use in robotic surgery (Fig. 3.9). The ISU enables the real-time use of an array of digital tools that can be used during live surgery to offer the surgeon clinical insights to improve efficiency, precision, and safety. The ISU processes information in real time from the laparoscope and the surgeon console to enable precise camera control and to add a variety of digital overlays to the live video stream.

Advanced Intelligent Surgical Unit Features

Eye Tracking The addition of the ISU allows for further advancement in the eye-tracking abilities of the Senhance System that are used to move the camera. The ISU allows for the target location in the operative field to remain perfectly centered when zooming in or out while using an angled scope. This feature eliminates the parallax error often encountered in laparoscopy when an angled camera is moved in or out.

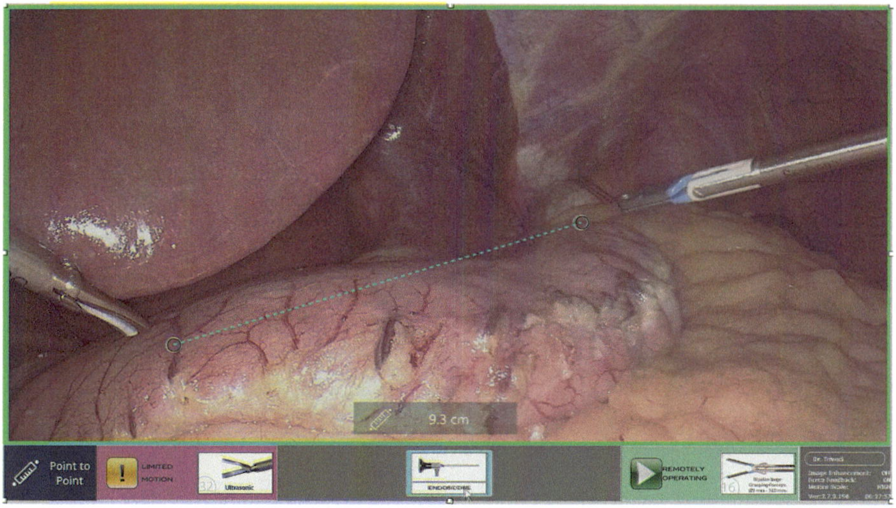

Fig. 3.10 Point-to-point measurement

Point-to-Point Measurement The ISU allows for real-time distance measurements to be performed during surgery. A feature called "point-to-point measurement" can be selected from a menu on the operating screen during surgery (Fig. 3.10). This feature projects a small circle at the tip of two of the working instruments and a real-time measurement of the distance between the circles is displayed at the bottom center of the screen. As each instrument is moved around the operative field, the measured distance between the two circles is updated in real time. This allows for accurate and reproducible distance measurement for any surgery. Examples of use cases include accurately measuring the distance from the pylorus during a sleeve gastrectomy and measuring the exact margin from a tumor during colon surgery.

Go To "Go To" is another feature of the ISU that allows the surgeon to easily reposition the visual field. When the feature is activated, the camera moves automatically to center the visual field around the tip of a selected instrument. This is accomplished by the ISU using digital instrument tracking.

Follow Us "Follow Us" is an ISU feature that digitally identifies the tips of two working instruments and wherever those instruments are moved, the camera will follow keeping the visual field centered between the two instruments. Additionally, if the two instruments are moved apart, the camera zooms back and if the two instruments are brought together, the camera zooms in. This feature allows for efficient movement of the camera to survey the operative field.

Digital Tags The ISU allows for the placement of up to nine digital tags in the operative field to mark tissue and structures (Fig. 3.11). The unique feature of the digital tags is that they remain fixed to the location to which they were originally

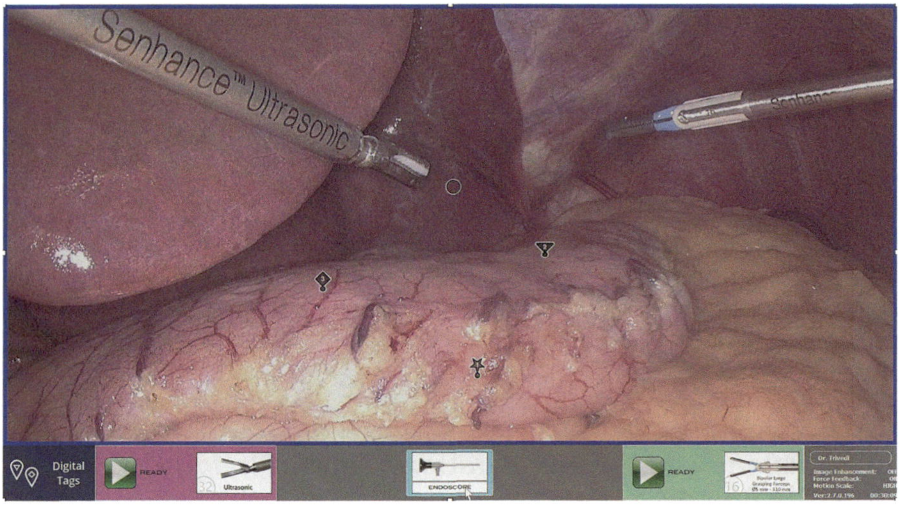

Fig. 3.11 Digital tags

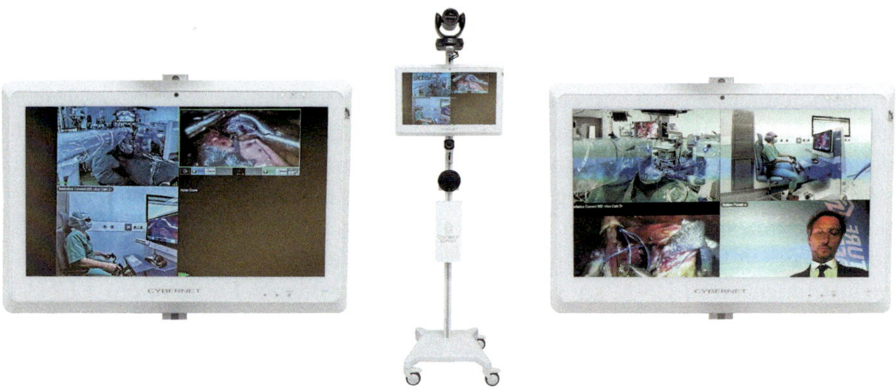

Fig. 3.12 Senhance connect

attached. If the tissue is moved, the tags move with the tissue. This unique feature allows for the marking of important structures and allows the operative team to easily reference the marked areas. The tags can be easily deleted or repositioned as needed.

Senhance Connect

Senhance Connect is a hardware- and software-based product that integrates with the Senhance Surgical System to allow for the live-streaming of surgery and real-time virtual collaboration, tele-mentoring, teaching, and support (Fig. 3.12). The

Senhance Connect system has multistream video capabilities consisting of the surgical video feed as well as two independent cameras that can be placed anywhere in the operating room.

Usage and Indication Guidelines

As the Senhance System gains wider acceptance, its range of applications continues to grow. At present, it is approved for bariatric, colorectal, general surgery, as well as benign gynecological procedures and pediatric applications. Outside the United States, it is also approved for urological procedures, with approval pending within the United States.

Introduction of the Next-Generation Surgical Platform: The LUNA Robotic System

In the early 2023, Asensus Surgical unveiled its second-generation surgical robotic platform, named LUNA (Fig. 3.13). Currently in the developmental stages, LUNA is engineered to enhance and extend the capabilities established by the existing Senhance Robotic System. The LUNA system introduces a suite of advanced features, including an open-surgeon console equipped with innovative unconstrained handles that provide tactile feedback, a 4K Ultra-HD 3D viewing monitor, a standalone interactive touchscreen, and camera control through eye-tracking. The system is designed with up to four independent robotic arms that feature a distinctive instrument drive mechanism that can accommodate a variety of advanced surgical tools. Additionally, Asensus is developing a comprehensive range of 5 mm fully articulating instruments for LUNA, known as TrueWrist Instruments. Furthermore, LUNA's synergy with the Intelligent Surgical Unit (ISU) will allow for real-time machine vision, augmented intelligence, and deep learning capabilities in the operating suite. In 2024, Asensus Surgical was acquired by Karl Storz. The development and commercialization of LUNA will continue under the new partnership.

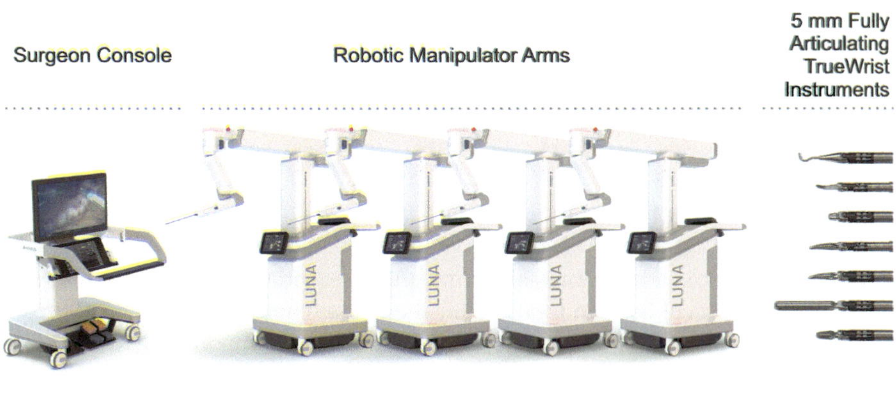

Fig. 3.13 LUNA robotic surgical system

4 The Hugo RAS™

Yoav Mintz and Ronit Brodie

Introduction to Modular Robots

Over the past decade, robotic-assisted surgery procedures have increased dramatically [1]. This trend is associated with the influx of new robotic systems and more robotic designs. The different designs differentiate in the surgeon's console, the configuration of the arm carts, and the concept of single-port or multiport instrument insertion.

Surgeons Console Design

There are two main surgeon console designs: either an immersive view or open-console design. The immersive view design, as in the da Vinci robotic system (Intuitive Surgical, Sunnyvale, CA, USA), emerged in order to enable a reliable 3D view of the operating field, which was crucial not only to have a true three-dimensional view of the organs but also to allow the surgeon to manipulate effectively the articulating instruments that break the boundaries of two-dimensional operation in standard laparoscopy. While the 3D technology of cameras and monitors was not good enough, due to problems with clear vision, areas out of focus, and the necessity to stay straight in front of the monitor, Intuitive Surgical Inc. solved the problem by introducing the immersive view technology. In this concept, the 3D

Y. Mintz (✉)
Department of General Surgery, Hadassah Hebrew University Medical Center, Jerusalem, Israel

Faculty of Medicine, Hebrew University of Jerusalem, Jerusalem, Israel
e-mail: ymintz@hadassah.org.il

R. Brodie
Department of General Surgery, Hadassah Hebrew University Medical Center, Jerusalem, Israel

S. Samreen et al. (eds.), *The SAGES Manual of Robotic Surgery*,
https://doi.org/10.1007/978-3-031-86927-3_4

view is achieved from a 3D laparoscope by transmitting each camera view to its corresponding eye, avoiding any other vision source, and allowing the human brain to achieve the 3D view as if you are looking through a binocular. Once the 3D technology matured to its current form, the open-console option appeared again. In this technology, the 3D monitor displays both cameras' input, while the passive 3D glasses worn by the surgeon filter the view and allow each eye to view the corresponding camera only. The high-definition 3D laparoscopes and monitors with advanced 3D technology deliver an immersive view of the operating field without the need to be totally immersed and disconnected from the operating room.

Arm Cart Design

There are two different concepts for the arm cart design. Either the traditional design where all arms fan out from a single-central column arm cart or the modular design, which include multiple independent arms that each can be positioned and controlled separately. While the traditional arm cart enables a simpler and quicker docking, the axis point of the arm motion is based on the column itself that is outside the surgical table. This results in limited docking options, demanding a large distance between the arms to avoid external collisions, and limits the operation field toward a single abdominal quadrant. The latest design of the da Vinci Xi addressed these limitations with its boom-mounted architecture and the motion axis of the arms. In this design, the arm's pivot point is above the surgical bed and the docking is possible from all sides to target all quadrants without the need for redocking [2].

The modular design of robotic systems such as in the Hugo RAS™ (Medtronic, Minneapolis, MN, USA), the Versius® (CMR Surgical, Cambridge, UK), and the Senhance® (Asenesus Surgical, Durham, NC, USA) allows the positioning of each arm separately. Detaching the arms from a common column enables to choose the best location for each arm and the best direction of instrument insertion without the limitation of being attached to other arms. This design, therefore, improves the docking angles, thereby allowing better maneuverability of the instruments and avoiding external collisions.

The Hugo RAS™ System

The Hugo RAS™ (Medtronic, Minneapolis, MN, USA) is a modular robotic system with an open-surgeon's console. It was designed specifically to address three major issues. The first was to improve the docking angles and instrument maneuverability, the second was to increase the usage versatility and ease of mobilization, and the third was cost reduction.

The development process of the Hugo RAS™ began in 2013 with a collaboration of Medtronic and the German Aerospace Center (DLR). The modular design enables multiple docking options, with 1–4 arms as necessary. Having smaller components

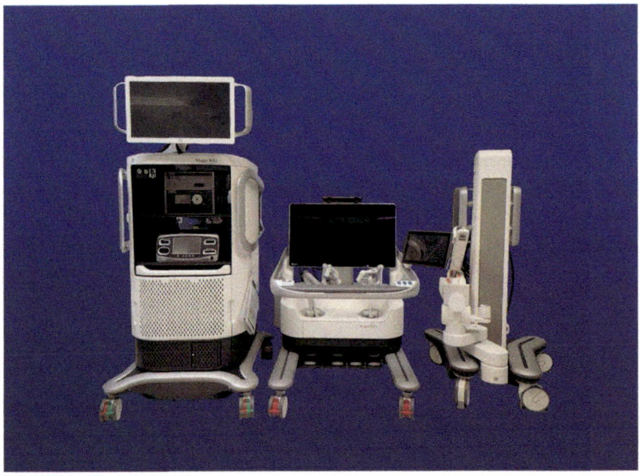

Fig. 4.1 The Hugo RAS™ system is composed of a system tower (left), surgeon console (middle), and up to four arm carts (right)

contributes to the ease of transferring the system from one operating room to the other. The concept of the development of a robotic system that could incorporate laparoscopic devices that are developed and marketed by the same company facilitates cost reduction.

The system is composed of an open console, a system tower, and four independent arm carts (Fig. 4.1). Additional components available are an embedded simulator on the surgeon's console and the Touch Surgery platform for recording and analyzing the surgical videos.

The Surgeon's Console

The surgeon console has an open design, meaning that the vision is based on a standard 3D monitor placed in front of the surgeon and there is no need to be immersed in the vision of the operating field (Fig. 4.2). Once the technology of the 3D monitors has matured to its current form, the ability to achieve a high-definition 3D view of the operative field, without losing focus, or losing the 3D vision, eliminated the need for a separate vision display for each eye. To enable a similar experience, a large 32-inch 3D monitor is positioned in close proximity to the surgeon simulating a theater view. The surgeon wears 3D passive (polarized) glasses, which can be worn on top of standard eyeglasses, transferring the view of each camera to the corresponding eye only to achieve a 3D view. These glasses do not compromise the standard view outside of the monitor and can be worn seamlessly throughout the operation. The large 3D monitor can also be viewed by anyone who wears similar 3D glasses; therefore, the 3D vision is not limited to the console surgeon only.

As a safety feature, there are several trackers (Fig. 4.3) on the surgeon's 3-D glasses that are recognized by an eye-tracking system, and if the surgeon diverts its gaze from the screen, the system automatically disables the control over the robotic arms.

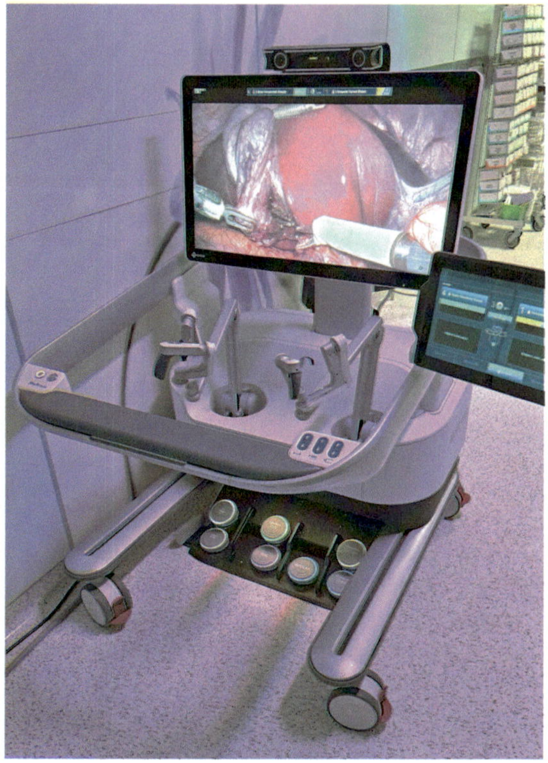

Fig. 4.2 The Hugo RAS^{TM} surgeon console has an open-console design with a 32-inch 3D monitor. The robotic arms are controlled using hand controllers and foot pedals

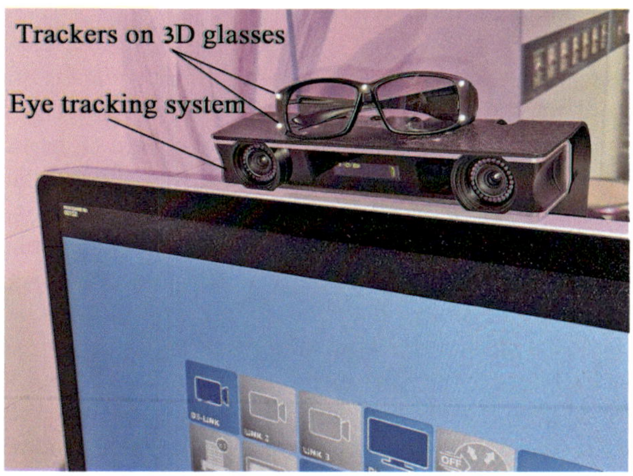

Fig. 4.3 The 3-D glasses have incorporated trackers that are sensed by the eye-tracking system. If the trackers are not facing the eye-tracking system, the controllers are disabled

The controllers are of a pistol grip design, with a double-function trigger (Fig. 4.4). A quick tap on the trigger enables or disables the arms function, while a continuous press on the trigger activates the "clutch" function that enables repositioning of the controllers without moving the robotic arms. Built-in foot pedals

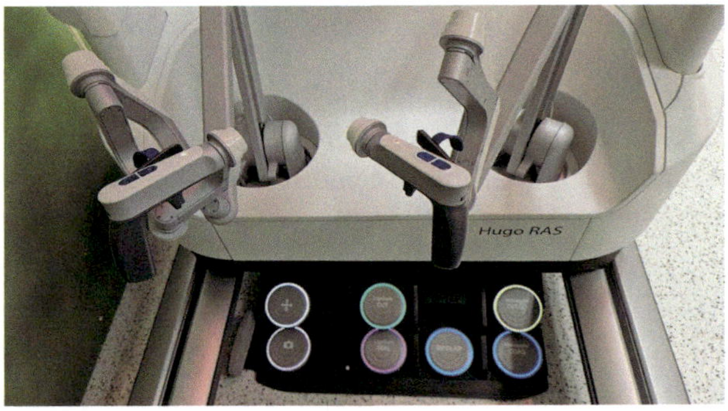

Fig. 4.4 The Hugo RAS™ arms and instruments are controlled by the two hand controllers and the foot pedals. The hand controllers are of a pistol grip design, with a double-function trigger. A quick tap on the trigger enables/disables control over the corresponding arm. A continuous press on the trigger enables a "clutch" mechanism of the corresponding arm. The foot pedals control the activation of the energy instruments, camera movement, simultaneous arms "clutch," and swapping between the third and fourth arm

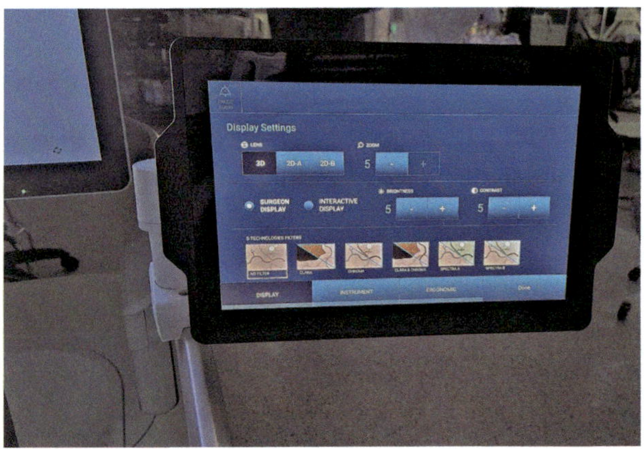

Fig. 4.5 The control pad enables control of the surgeon console ergonomics, the instruments, and the display. It is attached to the arm rest and is used prior to the operation for setup and during the operation if necessary

(Fig. 4.4) activate the monopolar, bipolar, and future advanced bipolar energy instruments and staplers. Moving the camera arm is achieved by a combined action of pressing the camera foot pedal together with moving the controllers. Pressing on the "clutch" pedal frees both of the controllers to move without affecting the robotic arms. A side pedal switches between the third and fourth arms. Switching the control of the arms can also be done from the control pad. The control pad is attached to the arm rest and enables control of the console ergonomics, instruments, and camera display (Fig. 4.5). The control pad enables adjustments of the ergonomics through the height of the arm rest, the monitor, and the reach to the foot pedals. Instrument settings can be adjusted separately to motion scaling and rotation speed as well as enabling camera rotation. The display can be set to either a 3D view or 2D view from each camera, the contrast and brightness can be adjusted, as well as zoom up to X5. Different filters of view are available from the Storz camera.

There are two main advantages in an open-console design:

Improved surgeon ergonomics: the surgeon is sitting down comfortably, with an arm rest to avoid arm fatigue, and without a fixed body position.

Direct visual communication: enables seamless communication with the surgical team and view of the patient as well as the arm's configuration and movement.

System Tower

The system tower is the central processing unit of the Hugo RAS™. The surgeon's console is connected via a data cable to the system, while it is connected to electricity power on its own. Up to four robotic arms can be connected and controlled simultaneously, or less according to the procedure. The arms are connected via a single cable for data and power. The tower is composed of four major components: the interactive display, the vision system, the electrosurgery generator, and the video recording and analytics engine (Fig. 4.6).

The interactive display is a touch screen that serves the OR team for the setup of the system, as well as the operational screen for the assistant surgeon. During the system setup, the screen displays the necessary steps needed to perform and confirm

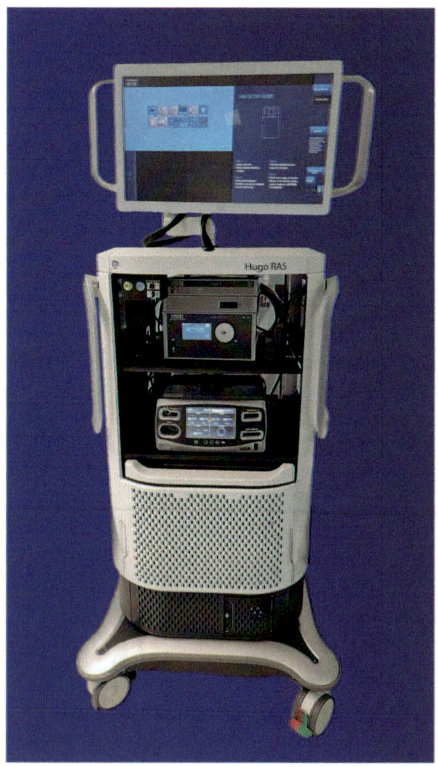

Fig. 4.6 The system tower has an interactive display screen that functions either as the surgeon's view monitor or for setup of the system. The vision system is based on Storz camera and light source, and the electrosurgery generator is based on the Valleylab™ FT10

while monitoring the advancement of the setup, calibration of the arms, and readiness of the system. Once the system is ready and all arms docked, it can be switched to the "surgeons view," which displays a full-screen camera view.

The vision system is based on the Karl Storz 3D HD TipCAM1 S™ (Karl Storz SE & Co KG, Tuttlingen, Germany) with a Storz light source. Either a 0- or 30-degree 3D laparoscope is available, which is connected to the robotic arm using an endoscope adapter. This adapter holds the endoscope in place and enables movements of the endoscope according to the arm movements, as well as rotating the endoscope 180° from 30° up to 30° down by a single switch. Once the rotation is completed, the upside-down image is flipped digitally to maintain the correct surgical view. Flipping the camera, choosing the zoom and filters applied can be controlled from the control pad on the surgeon's console.

The electrosurgical generator is the Medtronic Valleylab™ FT10 enabling connection to the robotic monopolar device and one other monopolar device, as well as to a bipolar device and the LigaSure™. The generator with its tissue sensing technology is specifically adapted to the Hugo RAS™ in order to enable activation from the surgeon's console and deliver energy to the robotic devices.

Arm Cart

The core technology of the Hugo RAS™ is based on the arm carts. The modular system design enables docking from different locations and angles, and the maneuverability of the arm outside and inside the body is determined by the arm's configuration. The arm cart is quite robust; however, it has seven motion hinges and joints to configure it into the desired position when docked, and six more moving joints to maneuver the instruments. A unique feature is the tilting joint that locks the arm within a range of angles from −45 to +30° (Fig. 4.7). This fixed angle serves as the starting point for instrument motion and extends their maneuverability. The tilting angle not only compensates for the patient positioning, for example, tilt and roll of the OR table, but also serves to separate better between the arms to avoid external collisions. Another unique feature of the arm is the alignment of the arm according to the OR table. Once the arm is locked in place, a green/red laser line is projected

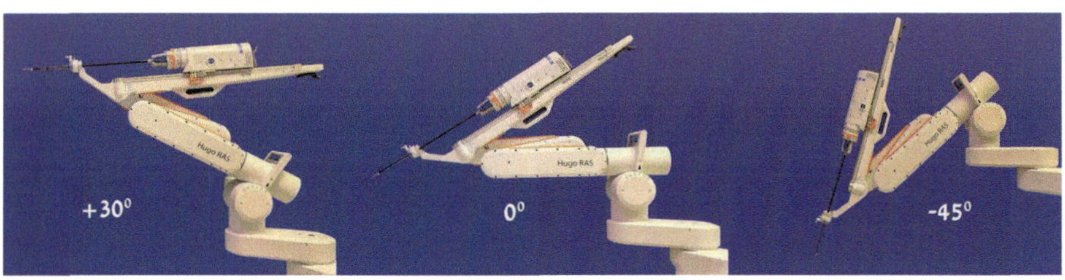

Fig. 4.7 The unique tilting joint of the Hugo RAS™ enables docking from +30° to −45° related to the true horizon. This tilt compensates for the patient's positioning and enables insertion of the instrument without compromising on arm maneuverability

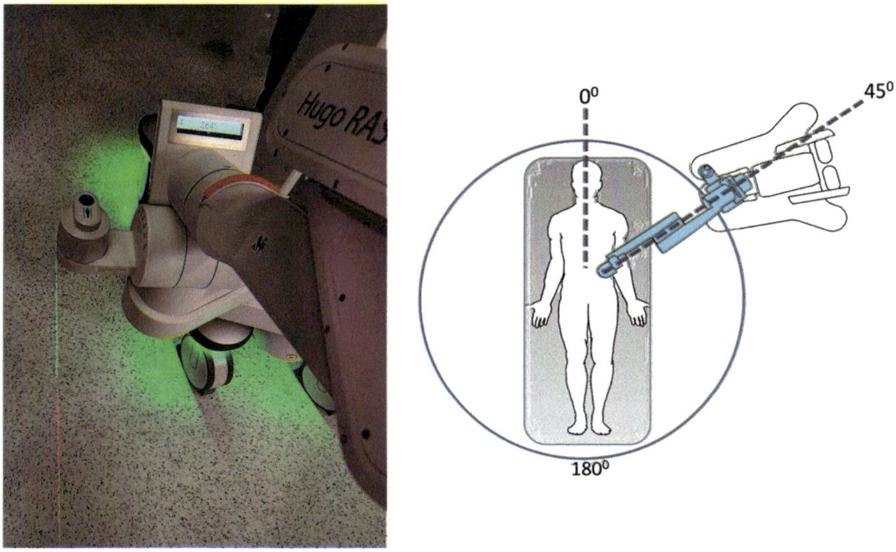

Fig. 4.8 A laser line is projected on the floor once the arm cart is locked in place. Using the laser alignment dial, the laser line is aligned in parallel to the OR table, and then the arm receives it angle in relation to the OR table. The angles of the arms could be from 0 to 360° while the head of the patient represents the 0° and the patients legs represent 180°

on the floor that can be aligned parallel to the OR table using the laser alignment dial (Fig. 4.8). Once aligned and confirmed, each arm receives its angle according to its position, and the angle is displayed on a small screen on the arm itself. This screen serves also to display any alarms regarding that arm. For safety reasons, the arm components are covered with touch sensors that halt the system and send an alarm when activated. This prevents injury to potential fingers or cables entrapped within the arm's components.

Hugo Instruments

All instruments of the Hugo RAS™ can be mounted on any of the arms. Other than the laparoscope, which is 10 mm in diameter, the current instruments are 8 mm. All instruments are wristed with 7° of freedom (Fig. 4.9). The monopolar scissors are currently the main instrument serving for dissection, coagulation, and cutting. A bipolar grasper and a bipolar dissector complement the working energy instruments. Four different graspers are available for tissue handling and two needle drivers for suturing.

Further instruments are anticipated to be released: the robotic Ligasure™, the robotic Signia™, and a wristed hook. These will be available for clinical use once they receive the necessary CE mark.

There are two types of trocars available. Disposable transparent 8 and 11 mm trocars, which are similar to the standard Medtronic trocars, and reusable 8, 11, and

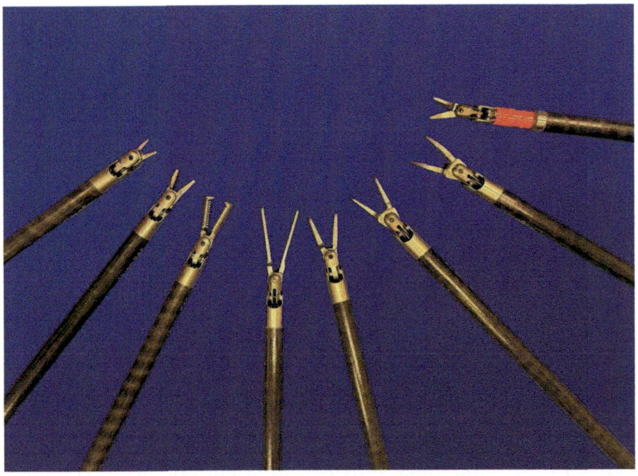

Fig. 4.9 The currently available instruments for the Hugo RAS™ are from left to right: extra large needle driver, large needle driver, toothed grasper, double fenestrated grasper, Cardier forceps, bipolar fenestrated grasper, bipolar Maryland forceps, and monopolar scissors

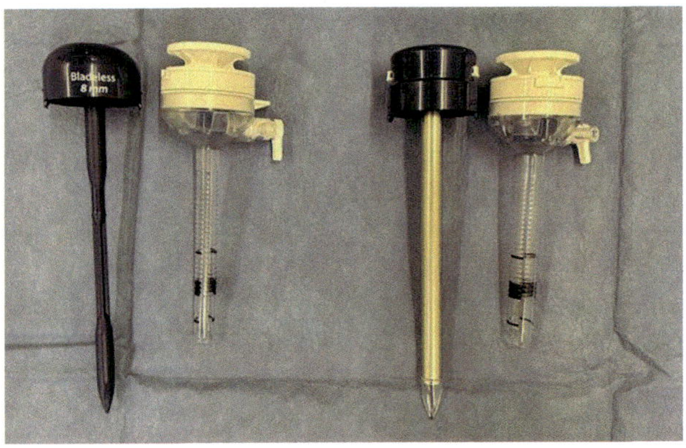

Fig. 4.10 The disposable trocars of the Hugo RAS™. On the left, an 8 mm trocar with its dilating obturator. On the right, an 11 mm trocar with an optical dilating obturator used for the camera port

12 mm metal trocars with a disposable valve mechanism. All trocars have a unique circular head for the attachment to the robotic arm. The 11 mm disposable trocar that is intended for the laparoscope has a bladeless optical canula that enables insertion of the first trocar under visual guidance (Fig. 4.10).

Docking the Arms

Since there are four separate arms, the entire docking of the system is different than the nonmodular robot design. Each arm is docked separately but altogether construct a docking architecture that is suited best and designed specifically to the procedure and patient positioning. In order to facilitate the docking process, the company provides setup guides for each procedure, specifying the location, tilt, and angles of each arm, and the OR table positioning (Fig. 4.11). Since the docking process involves four arms that need to be wheeled in proximity to the patient, this process may take some time; therefore, it should be done in parallel by all the OR team by following the specific instructions in the setup guide.

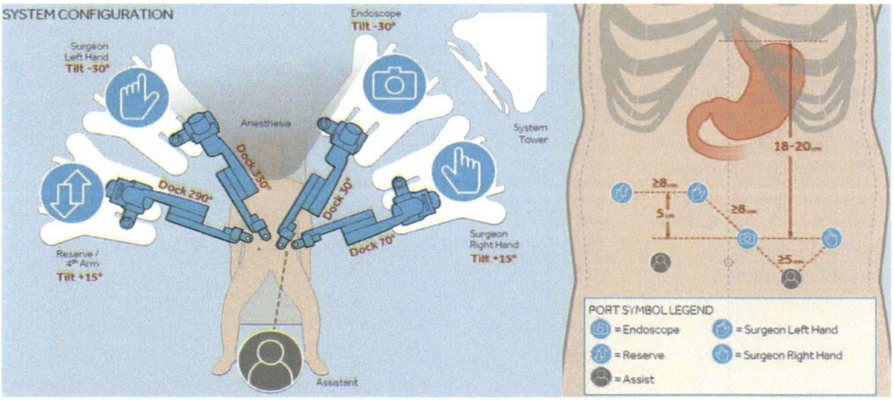

Fig. 4.11 A setup guide provided by Medtronic as a recommendation for docking during left-upper quadrant procedures such as Nissen fundoplication. In the setup guide, the arm's location around the OR table, the tilt and angle of each arm, the trocar positioning, and the OR table tilt and roll are specified

The setup guide creates a standardized and reproducible docking that, once learned, should take up to 5 minutes. The location of the arms, their tilt, and angles are predetermined according to the specific surgery in order to achieve optimal, quick, and reproducible docking. The ability to position the arms anywhere around the OR table, coupled with the tilting joint and the increased maneuverability gained by the six moving joints, yields a superior range of motion of the instruments as well as avoiding external arm collisions (Fig. 4.12).

The stepwise docking procedure begins by positioning the arm carts in place. Once the arm cart is locked in place, it is aligned parallel to the OR table using the laser guiding system. Once aligned, the arm receives its angle. The head of the patient represents the 0-degree angle while the feet represent 180°, thereby creating a complete circle of 360°. The tilt angle is set and the arm is then swiveled until the angle displayed on the arm reaches the docking angle depicted in the setup guide. The port latch is then opened and connected to the trocar to complete the docking. Once all four arms are docked, the angles are reviewed on the interactive display of the system tower and confirmed. This confirmation enables control from the surgeon's console. Trocar positioning is similar to laparoscopic trocar positioning that are determined according to the surgery and body habitus of the patient. Some adjustments are sometimes needed to maintain 8 cm distance from the trocars.

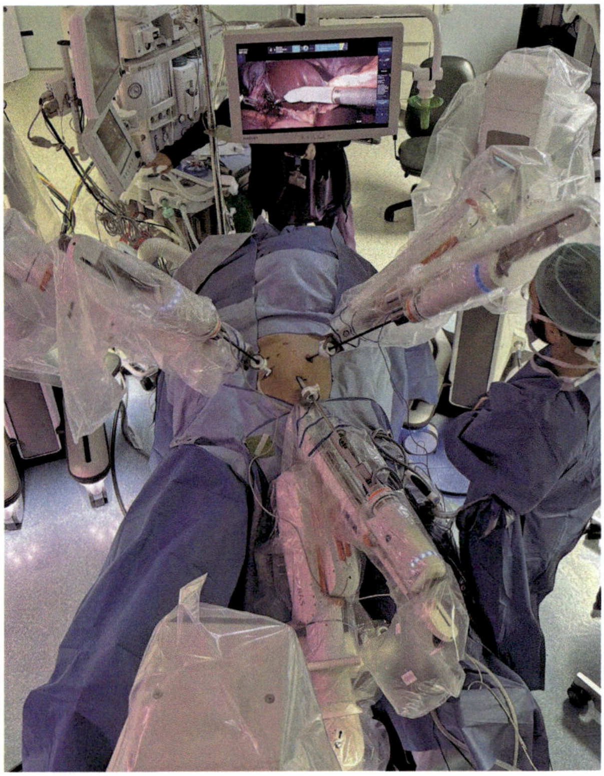

Fig. 4.12 A view of the docking setup of a robotic cholecystectomy using three arms only. The right-hand arm is docked on the left side of the patient, the camera arm is located in between the split legs, and the left-hand arm is docked on the right side of the patient. The gallbladder is retracted using an EndoGrab retractor (Virtual Ports LTD., Hod Hasharon, Israel) prior to docking the robot. In this setup, there is no assistant trocar and the clips are placed through the left upper trocar following temporary undocking of this arm

Clinical Experience with the Hugo RAS™

The Hugo RAS™ system received Conformité Européenne (CE) mark for urologic and gynecologic procedures in 2019 [3]. The first clinical procedures performed with the Hugo RAS™ were in Chile in June 2021. Approval for general surgery procedures was received 2 years later in October 2022.

According to the company, as of December 2023, more than 5600 procedures were performed by the Hugo RAS™ worldwide. These include more than 3000 urologic cases, more than 1200 gynecologic cases, and more than 1200 general surgery procedures.

Academic publications are beginning to emerge with 54 peer-reviewed publications in the English literature, which include 625 patients by December 2023. The operations performed included urologic procedures such as ureterolithostomy, ureteral reimplant, pyeloplasty, nephrectomy [4], partial nephrectomy [5–7], radical prostatectomy [6, 8–16], and radical cystectomy with conduit and neobladder reconstruction [17].

Gynecologic procedures such as sacrocolpopexy [18–21], total hysterectomy and salpingo-oophorectomy [3], and general surgery procedures such as colorectal surgery [22–24], Nissen fundoplication [25], cholecystectomy [23, 26–28], Hiatal hernia repair [23], Heller myotomy [29], transabdominal adrenalectomy [30], inguinal hernia [31], Roux en Y gastric bypass [32], sleeve gastrectomy [23], and subtotal gastrectomy [23].

Generally, in their publications, the authors describe their experience with this new system and conclude that the Hugo RAS™ has significant advantages based on the maneuverability and improved angulation of the arms due to the ability to dock each arm separately. The open console was noted to improve communication between the surgeon and the operating room staff. Additionally, many studies noted that there was not much of a learning curve necessary for those surgeons who were already familiar with and competent in other robotic platforms such as the da Vinci. The prominent disadvantage of the HUGO RAS™ system across all experiences and specialties is the limited variability of instruments, especially an advanced energy instrument and fluorescence imaging capabilities. Questions remain surrounding the true cost-effectiveness of robotic systems that is not unique to HUGO RAS™.

Future Developments

Currently, the Hugo RAS™ is a modular robotic system enabling complete operations such as radical prostatectomy, Heller myotomy, hernia repairs, cholecystectomy, and more. Operations that need advanced energy devices and staplers are performed in a hybrid procedure, that is, using laparoscopic devices through assistant ports. The development of several robotic devices is in the final stages of developments, and some are awaiting CE mark approval. Energy devices in the pipeline include a robotic hook, robotic Ligasure™, and robotic Signia™ stapler. The addition of these instruments will complete the Hugo RAS™ system and enable advanced procedures performed totally robotic. The huge advantage in incorporating these specific instruments, according to the company, will be the comparable cost to their counterparts' laparoscopic devices. Since the Ligasure™ and Signia™ stapler are developed and marketed by the same company, adjustments of these same devices just to be controlled robotically should not significantly affect their cost.

Since the Hugo RAS™ vision system is based on the Storz TipCAM1 S™, upgrading to the Storz Image1 S™ Rubina™ to enable ICG fluorescence is not an engineering challenge, and, according to the company, CE mark approval for the robotic control of the Rubina™ is pending.

References

1. Sheetz KH, Claflin J, Dimick JB. Trends in the adoption of robotic surgery for common surgical procedures. JAMA Network Open. 2020;3(1):e1918911.
2. Morrell ALG, et al. The history of robotic surgery and its evolution: when illusion becomes reality. Rev Col Bras Cir. 2021;48:e20202798.
3. Monterossi G, et al. The first European gynaecological procedure with the new surgical robot Hugo RAS. A total hysterectomy and salpingo-oophorectomy in a woman affected by BRCA-1 mutation. Facts Views Vis Obgyn. 2022;14(1):91–4.

4. Elorrieta V, et al. ROBOT assisted laparoscopic surgeries for nononcological urologic disease: initial experience with Hugo Ras System. Urology. 2023;174:118–25.
5. Gallioli A, et al. Initial experience of robot-assisted partial nephrectomy with Hugo RAS system: implications for surgical setting. World J Urol. 2023;41(4):1085–91.
6. Carneiro A, Andrade GM. Technology description, initial experience and first impression of HUGO RAS robot platform in urologic procedures in Brazil. Int Braz J Urol. 2023;49(6):763–74.
7. Prata F, et al. Robot-assisted renal surgery with the new Hugo Ras system: trocar placement and docking settings. J Pers Med. 2023;13(9):1372.
8. Paciotti M, et al. Nerve-sparing robot-assisted radical prostatectomy with the HUGO robot-assisted surgery system using the 'Aalst technique'. BJU Int. 2023;132(2):227–30.
9. Rocco B, et al. First case of robot-assisted radical cystectomy and intracorporeal neobladder reconstruction with the Hugo RAS system: step-by-step surgical setup and technique. J Robot Surg. 2023;17(5):2247–51.
10. Marques-Monteiro M, et al. Extraperitoneal robot-assisted radical prostatectomy with the Hugo RAS system: initial experience of a tertiary center with a high background in extraperitoneal laparoscopy surgery. World J Urol. 2023;41(10):2671–7.
11. Bravi CA, et al. Robot-assisted radical prostatectomy performed with different robotic platforms: first comparative evidence between Da Vinci and HUGO robot-assisted surgery robots. Eur Urol Focus; 2023.
12. Bravi CA, et al. Outcomes of robot-assisted radical prostatectomy with the Hugo RAS surgical system: initial experience at a high-volume robotic center. Eur Urol Focus. 2023;9(4):642–4.
13. Alfano CG, et al. Implementation and outcomes of Hugo(TM) RAS System in robotic-assisted radical prostatectomy. Int Braz J Urol. 2023;49(2):211–20.
14. Bravi CA, et al. Robot-assisted Radical Prostatectomy with the Novel Hugo Robotic System: initial experience and optimal surgical set-up at a tertiary referral robotic center. Eur Urol. 2022;82(2):233–7.
15. Mottaran A, et al. Robot-assisted simple prostatectomy with the novel HUGO RAS System: feasibility, setting, and perioperative outcomes. Minerva Urol Nephrol. 2023;75(2):235–9.
16. Ou YC, et al. Robot-assisted radical prostatectomy using hugo RAS system: the pioneer experience in Taiwan and Northeast Asia. Int J Med Robot. 2023:e2577.
17. Gaya JM, et al. Robot-assisted radical cystectomy and ileal conduit with Hugo(TM) RAS system: feasibility, setting and perioperative outcomes. Int Braz J Urol. 2023;49(6):787–8.
18. Panico G, et al. The first 60 cases of robotic sacrocolpopexy with the novel HUGO RAS system: feasibility, setting and perioperative outcomes. Front Surg. 2023;10:1181824.
19. Panico G, et al. HUGO(TM) RAS System in urogynaecology: the first nerve sparing Sacral Colpopexy for Pelvic Organ Prolapse. Facts Views Vis Obgyn. 2023;15(1):83–7.
20. Campagna G, et al. Robotic sacrocolpopexy plus ventral rectopexy as combined treatment for multicompartment pelvic organ prolapse using the new Hugo RAS system. Tech Coloproctol. 2023;27(6):499–500.
21. Balestrazzi E, et al. Comparative analysis of robot-assisted simple prostatectomy: the HUGO RAS system versus the DaVinci(R) Xi system. Prostate Cancer Prostatic Dis. 2023;27(1):122–8.
22. Bianchi PP, et al. First worldwide report on Hugo RAS surgical platform in right and left colectomy. Updates Surg. 2023;75(3):775–80.
23. Gangemi A, et al. Surgery of the alimentary tract for benign and malignant disease with the novel robotic platform HUGO(TM) RAS. A first world report of safety and feasibility. Int J Med Robot. 2023;19(4):e2544.
24. Caruso R, et al. New era of robotic surgery: first case in Spain of right hemicolectomy on Hugo RAS surgical platform. BMJ Case Rep. 2023;16(12):e256035.
25. Quijano Y, et al. Robot-assisted Nissen fundoplication with the new HUGO Robotic assisted system: First worldwide report with system description, docking settings and video. Int J Surg Case Rep. 2023;106:108178.
26. Caputo D, et al. Full robotic cholecystectomy: first worldwide experiences with HUGO RAS surgical platform. ANZ J Surg. 2023;94(3):387–90.

27. Vicente E, et al. Robot-assisted cholecystectomy with the new HUGO robotic-assisted system: first worldwide report with system description, docking settings, and video. Updates Surg. 2023;75(7):2039–42.
28. Belyaev O, et al. Safety and feasibility of cholecystectomy with the Hugo(TM) RAS: proof of setup guides and first-in-human german experience. Visc Med. 2023;39(3-4):76–86.
29. Salem SA, et al. Robotic Heller's myotomy using the new Hugo RAS system: first worldwide report. Surg Endosc. 2023;38(3):1180–90.
30. Raffaelli M, et al. The new robotic platform Hugo RAS for lateral transabdominal adrenalectomy: a first world report of a series of five cases. Updates Surg. 2023;75(1):217–25.
31. Mintz Y, et al. Robotic inguinal hernia repair with the new Hugo RAS(TM) system: first worldwide case series report. Minim Invasive Ther Allied Technol. 2023;32(6):300–6.
32. Raffaelli M, et al. Feasibility of Roux-en-Y Gastric Bypass with the novel robotic platform HUGO RAS. Front Surg. 2023;10:1181790.

5 Versius Surgical Robot

Subhash Khanna and Areendam Barua

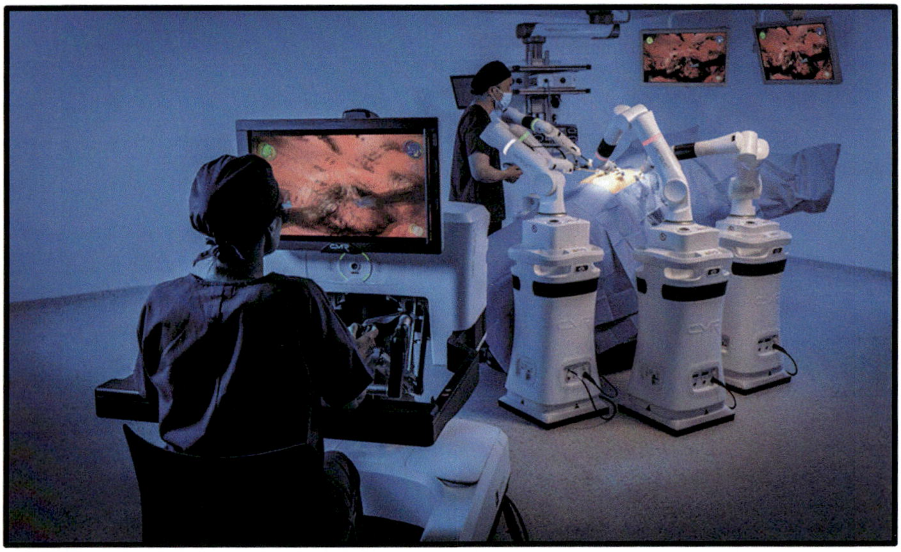

Introduction

The da Vinci surgical system held the fort of robotic surgery for almost two decades since its introduction to the market, with very little competition until the launch of Senhance robotic system in 2016. Unfortunately, Senhance did not fare favorably against da Vinci, and the company TransEnterix hardly could market its system in the global market. It was the first robotic system to introduce independent robotic arms, open platform, haptic feedback, and eye tracking. Even though there were a lot of innovations being put up by TransEnterix, the da Vinci

S. Khanna (✉)
Minimal Access, GI` and Robotic surgery, Swagat Super Speciality Surgical Institute and NH, Guwahati, Assam, India

A. Barua
Minimal Access and Robotic Surgical Oncology, Swagat Super Speciality Surgical Institute and NH, Guwahati, Assam, India

S. Samreen et al. (eds.), *The SAGES Manual of Robotic Surgery*,
https://doi.org/10.1007/978-3-031-86927-3_5

also evolved continually to maintain its market share. This meant that the da Vinci-dominated market was indeed a tough nut to crack and needed much more than innovative technologies only for market appeal. Da Vinci's strong position may be attributed to its early entry advantage, technological advancements, extensive installed base, and market recognition. Versius entered the world of robotic surgery in 2019. It brought some refreshing changes in that the independent arms were sleeker and much less space-consuming, ergonomic seating with an open platform, ease of transport to various operating rooms with smaller overall built, and having both lower initial and lower per-use costs. The number of installed systems in India is around 50, adding to the 160+ installations and over 18,000 procedures performed globally.

System Design

The design of this robotic system is a major game changer in that it has the potential to significantly increase its reach into robotic minimal invasive surgery. Versius claims that it is designed to "give surgeons and hospitals the versatility to operate in the way that's best for patients and to maximise utilisation." Let us dissect into the bold statement of Versius. The Versius is an open-console robotic system, meaning that the surgeon does not need to dip his head into the immersive surgeon console. This open console with its 3DHD head-up display allows surgeons to sit or stand. The surgeons can operate in 3D with the help of polarizing passive goggles. Here, the surgeon does not feel being cut off from the rest of the surgical staff, allows better visual and verbal communication, as well as improved situational awareness between the surgeon and the larger operative teams. It supports three compact robotic-independent mobile instrument arms, apart from the visualization unit that can be shifted between operating theatres (OTs). A big advantage is that it fits in virtually any operating room, given its smaller footprint, which is approximately 4.5 m^2. Also, an assistant surgeon can fit comfortably between the robotic arms in case the need be the robot's wristed tool tip allows for seven degrees of movement inside the patient, enabling more surgical access than traditional laparoscopic surgery. It has a high degree of precision with motion scaling (Fig. 5.1).

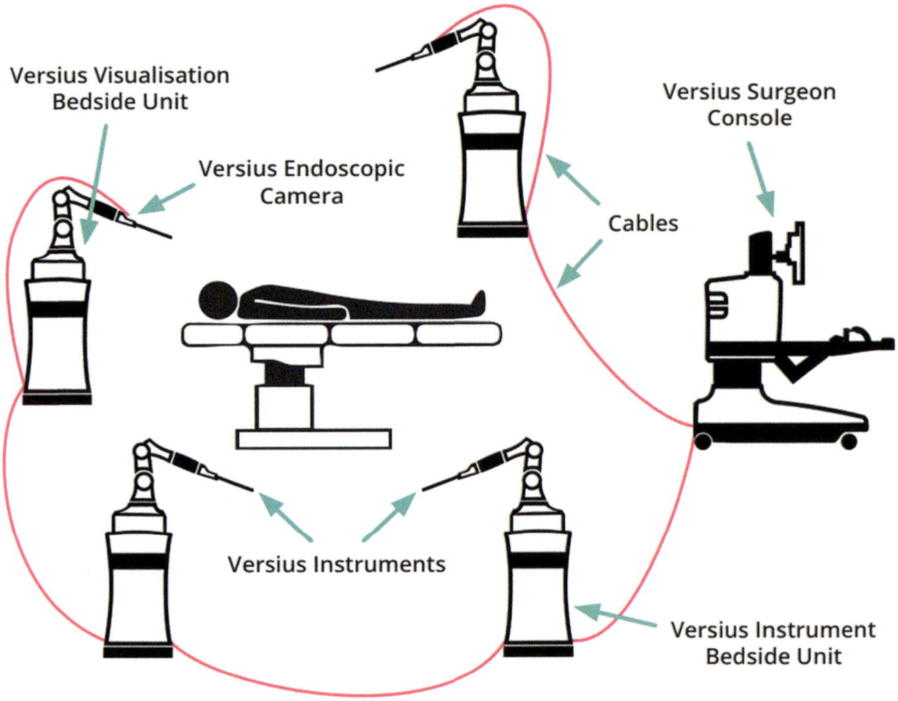

Fig. 5.1 The Versius surgical system components

Components of the Versius Robotic System

1. One surgeon console
2. One visualization bedside (VBSU) unit and an endoscopic camera
3. Three instrument bedside units (IBSUs)
4. A set of six different surgical instruments
5. Accessories such as a virtual training simulator, drapes, and cables

Now let us learn about each of the components in detail.

Surgeon Console

It is the interface via which the robotic system interacts with the surgeon. It doubles up as the power hub of the connected bedside units. The console is outside the sterile field, usually placed at one corner of the operation theatre (OT), at the leg end of the patient, so as to provide a proper view of the surgical setup. The open-console design promotes communication between the surgeon and the rest of the surgical team. The surgeon does not need to scrub for the surgery unless they want to use staplers or energy devices that Versius does not provide. The surgeon console has a

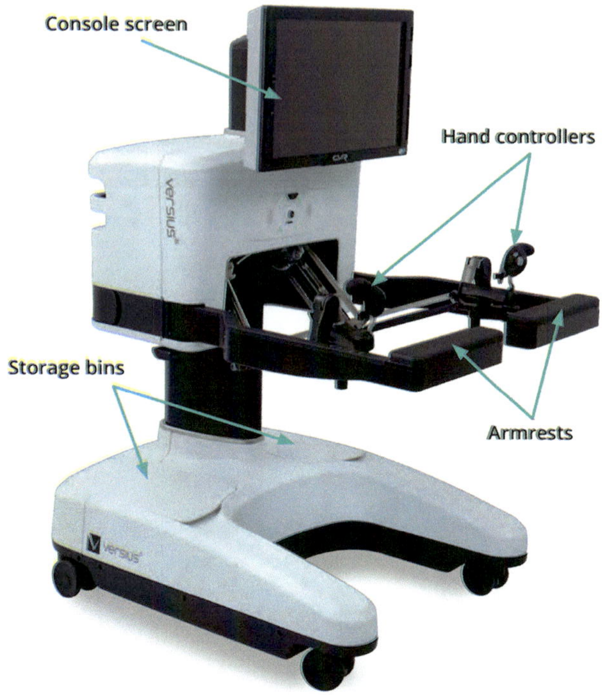

Fig. 5.2 The surgeon console

stop button that stops the surgeon console and any connected bedside unit, which is used to take breaks during long surgeries or to establish communication with the team. The resume button resumes the system operation (Fig. 5.2)

Console Screen The console screen has a 3DHD display, which can be viewed with polarizing 3D passive glasses. There is also the option of changing the video feed to 2D. The surgeon has the independence of sitting in a comfortable chair, for the comfort of the spine, or to stand and operate, given the height-adjustable head-up display, making it ergonomically comfortable for the surgeon. An auxiliary screen (not supplied with the Versius Surgical System) can be connected to the surgeon console to show a 2D replica of the console screen for the bedside team to view. The endoscopic camera video feed can be recorded and saved on an SD card, the slot for which is below the screen.

Updated Console in 2024

Very recently, Versius officially announced the launch of vLimeLite, the imaging technology to visualize ICG, which is integrated to the updated version of Versius surgical robot, Versius Plus. The overlay can be in full color or grayscale. Currently, the advanced version is available only in the European Union. vLimeLite allows surgeons to perform visual assessment of the vessels, blood flow, and related tissue perfusion, as well as biliary anatomy.

Disclaimers

- *Product available in the European Economic Area (EEA) only. Please check the availability of the product with your local sales representative or your local customer service.*
- *Content provided courtesy of CMR Surgical (© CMR Surgical 2024—Do not copy or distribute).*
- *vLimeLite is CE marked. Please check the availability of the product in your country with your local sales representative or your local customer service. The Versius System vLimeLite Instructions for Use, including the approved indications, contraindications, and warnings, can be found in the product labeling supplied with each Versius System. Not available for sale in the United States.*

The Head-Up Display (HUD)

The display, in addition to the 3D video output, gives us important information regarding the system and instrument status. The system icon has a gray background, and the color of the BSU icons corresponds to the colored LED bands in the instrument arms. The visualization unit has a white background. Icons relating to the electrosurgery instruments have an extra feature to set them apart from the non-electrosurgery instruments and allow the surgeon to change between the coagulation (blue) and cut (yellow) modes. The icon color signifies the arm we are referring to, with the same color as the illuminated color bands at the bedside units (Fig. 5.3).

In the above image, the HUD shows that the left-hand controller has a fenestrated grasper mounted on the cyan Versius arm, the orange Versius arm has a needle holder, and pink Versius arm has curved scissors, both of which have not been

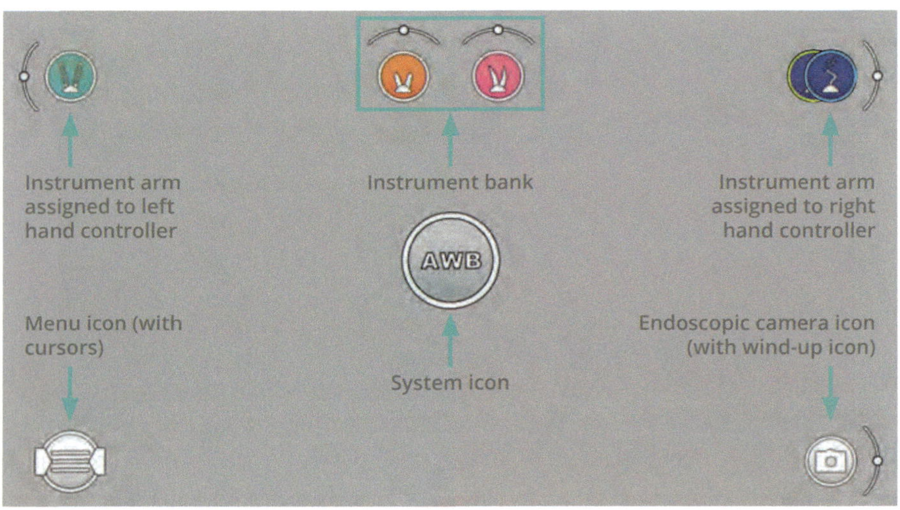

Fig. 5.3 HUD with marked icon locations

assigned to controller and is in the instrument bank, which can be used if need be. The right-hand controller has the monopolar hook, which is assigned in the coagulation mode, as denoted by blue circle around the hook. Other icons are described in the figure.

This information is displayed in the auxiliary screen too so that the important information is displayed for the bedside team too.

Some Important Icons

No Hand-Detected Icon Hand detection is one of the system's safety features. An instrument can be engaged with a hand controller only if the hand controller detects a hand holding it. No hand-detected icons show if one or both the hands are not detected. When a hand is holding a hand controller, the icon disappears from the HUD. The instruments will automatically disengage if the hand controllers are left during the surgery; this is a safety feature (Fig. 5.4).

Wind-Up Icon This icon is next to the instrument icon in the form of an arc and a ball. It gives an indication of the amount of rotation the distal end of the arm has undergone. The ball moves up and down the arc as the distal end of the arm rotates away from the neutral position. Once the ball reaches the end of the arc, the end of the arm cannot rotate any further. This rotation is 360° on either side (Fig. 5.5).

Fig. 5.4 No hand-detected icons

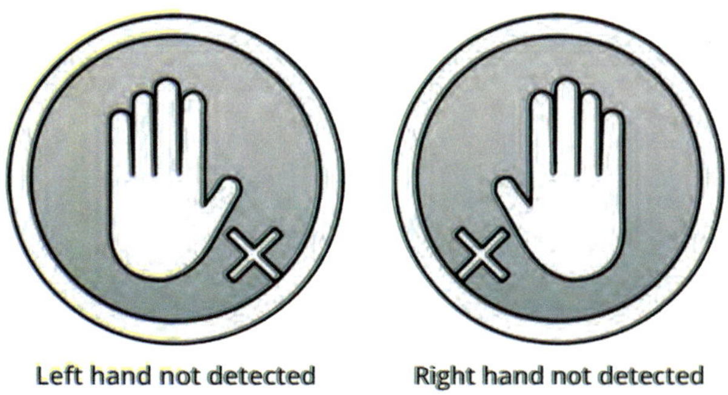

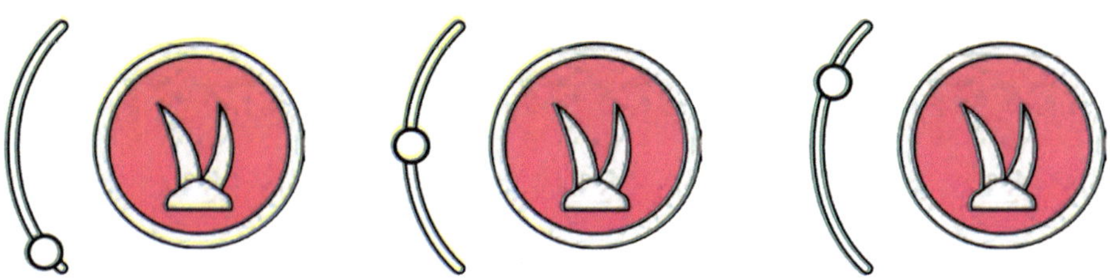

Fig. 5.5 Curved scissors icons for a pink arm, and the corresponding wind-up icons, indicating three different degrees of rotation

Alarm Icons

There are two icons: high- and medium-priority icons (Fig. 5.6).

There are medium-priority alarms for the arms and for the console. If a medium-priority alarm occurs, there is no immediate danger to the patient. We can resume the surgery after taking care of the issue. But we cannot proceed with the surgery if we encounter a high-priority alarm (Fig. 5.7).

Hand Controllers The handgrip is basically like a joystick, with all the controls in the hands as in a game controller. It was based on extensive ergonomic research and further developed with surgeon input, which makes maneuvering the surgical instruments as easy as playing a video game. Also, the console has an arm rest for the elbow to rest while moving the hand controllers in three dimensions. Once the power is on and the system detects that the hand controllers are being held, the hand controllers become as light as a feather, precluding any surgeon fatigue for long-duration surgeries (Fig. 5.8).

Fig. 5.6 Medium-priority alarm icons

Fig. 5.7 High-priority alarm icon. High-priority alarms only occur on arms. This tells us that there has been a major dysfunction and surgery can only proceed post replacing the unit

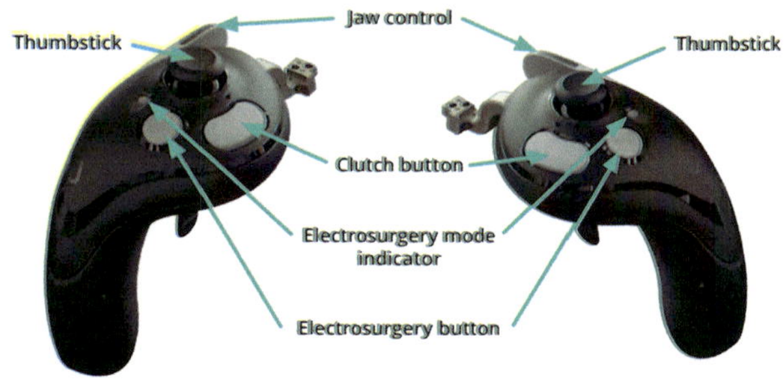

Fig. 5.8 The hand controllers

Versius Instrument and Visualization Bedside Units

The bedside units consist of a Versius cart and a Versius arm. In the visualization bedside unit, the instrument is replaced by the endoscopic camera. The Versius arm is under the control of the surgeon, whereas the cart has to be pushed to the specific position around the patient prior to surgery (Figs. 5.9 and 5.10).

The Versius arm has several parts that are labeled as above. Three key joints allow the Versius arm to mimic a human arm: base, elbow, and V-Wrist. The elbow joint can be moved from its position without disturbing the position of the instrument inside the body to facilitate standing of an assistant surgeon between two bedside units. The black grip band is used to manually position the instrument inside the patient's abdomen/thorax before starting the surgery. The joints are positioned at specific points in space to get specific configurations, each of which has its importance in specific surgeries or to dissect a particular organ from a specific position. There are two illuminated colored LED bands on every arm, which may be any one of the six colors. This helps the surgeon communicate to the surgical staff regarding any issue with the arm. The color of the arm color identifier matches the background color of the HUD icons related to the arm, its bedside unit, and instrument. There are three V-Wrist buttons on the arm and one elbow button that are needed to set up the arm for surgery and change instruments.

The Versius cart is the mobile unit on which the arm is mounted. It has a control panel at its superior aspect and a cart connection panel at its lower part. The control panel has height adjustment buttons, low battery indicator (each bedside unit has its own battery power supply that will support the arm for 20 mins if power from the surgeon console is lost), and orientation buttons (they are used to orient the units to a definite direction, so that the movement of the arms is as desired by the surgeon). The bedside unit status halo is green when the robot is functioning normally, which may turn to yellow or red depending on if the alarm is medium priority or high priority. There are also stop and resume buttons that stop and resume the unit function, respectively. There is a bedside unit sleep button, which puts the arm in such a compact configuration so that it occupies the least space during storage and has the least chance of damage during transportation (Fig. 5.11).

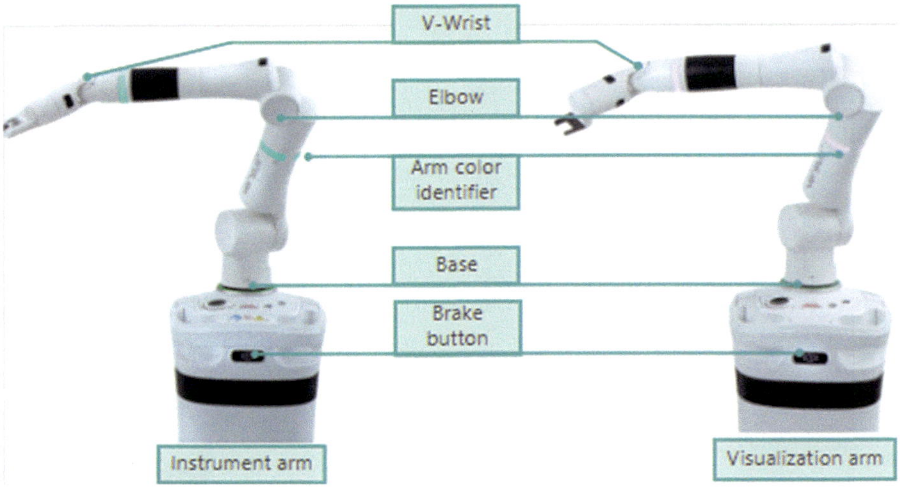

Fig. 5.9 Instrument and visualization bedside units

Fig. 5.10 The Versius instrument bedside unit

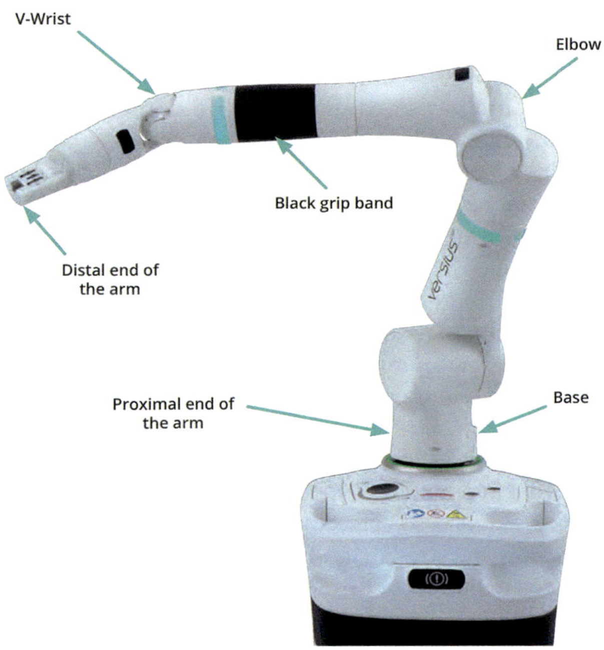

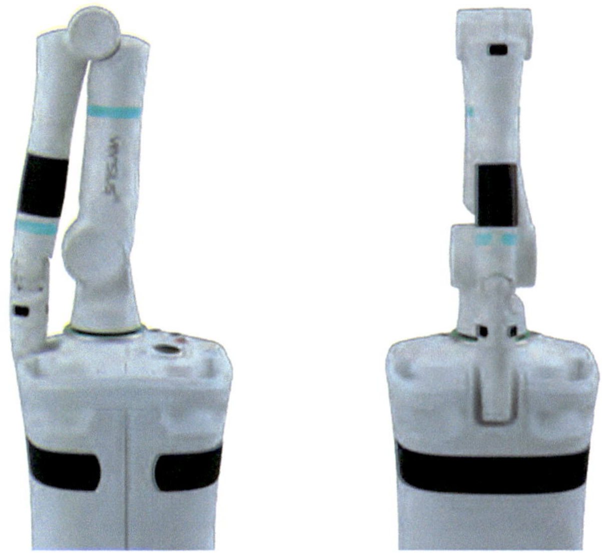

Fig. 5.11 Bedside unit in sleep mode

Arm Modes

Versius arm has seven modes (Fig. 5.12). These modes can be shifted from one mode to another with the help of elbow and V-Wrist buttons placed at the instrument bedside units. These are described in the figure below.

To put the surgical arm from locked to surgical mode, the V-Wrist button is used. The sequence of modes that the arm goes though is depicted in the arm mode map below (Fig. 5.13).

1. **Sleep mode:** In this mode, the arm is in compact storage position, and one needs to awaken the arm by pressing the sleep button to make further use of the same.
2. **Locked mode:** In this mode, only the distal end of the bedside unit can be moved. The rest of the arm stays in position to facilitate attaching the instrument to the arm before port training.
3. **Unlocked mode:** Unlocked mode is used when the bedside team needs to freely move and position the arm, for example, during positioning for draping and positioning the arm into an arc before port training.
4. **Port training mode:** This mode trains the surgical robot so that it knows the location of the pivot around the fulcrum, on which the instruments and endoscope move. This pivot point is located on air, at that specified three-dimensional axis, so that the abdominal wall does not need to be the pivot point as in laparoscopy. This decreases the pain significantly since the trauma to the abdominal wall at the port sites is much lesser.
5. **Instrument adjust mode**: The instrument can be advanced in this mode inside the patient cavity once the port training is complete. The arm can be manually moved with complete freedom of movement while respecting the fulcrum position.

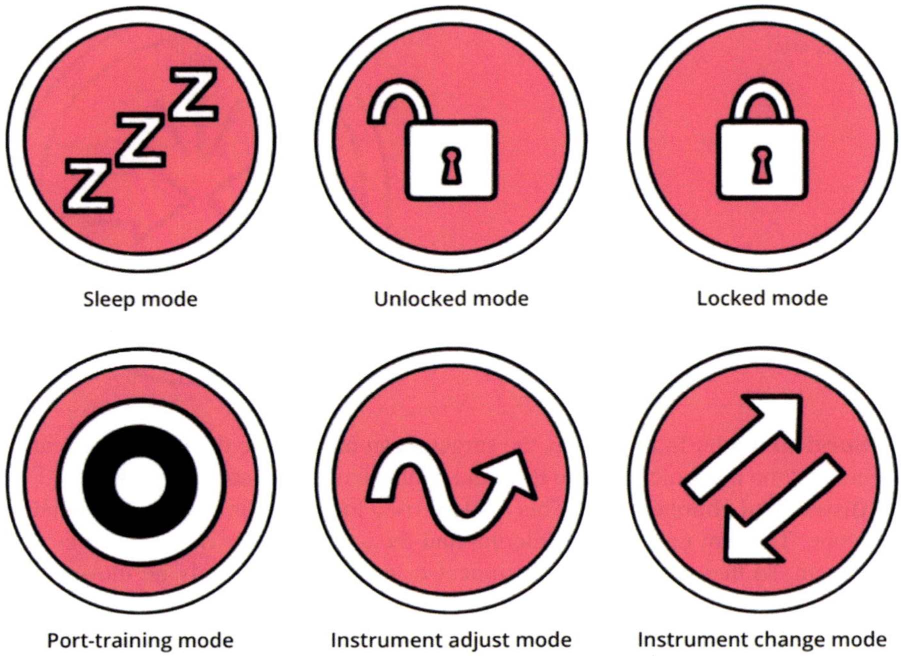

Fig. 5.12 Arm mode icons for a pink arm

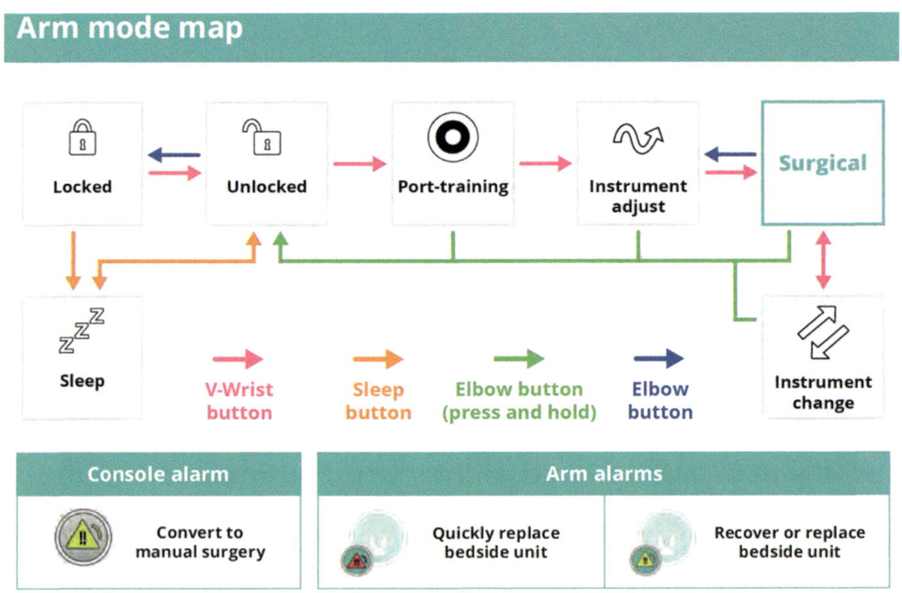

Fig. 5.13 Versius arm mode map showing the use of V-Wrist and elbow buttons to put the arm in various modes

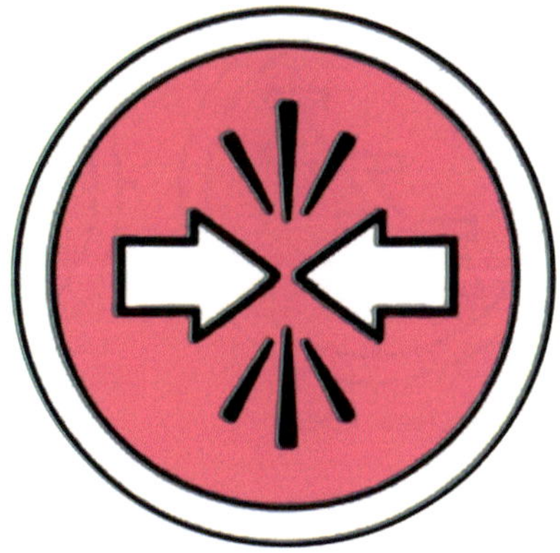

Fig. 5.14 Arm clash icon for a pink arm

6. **Surgical mode:** In this mode, the surgeon can manipulate the endoscopic camera and the instruments using the hand controllers on the surgeon console.
7. **Instrument change mode:** This mode is used to change an instrument or endoscope. The arm respects the fulcrum and the arm's motion is restrained by the system, so that the arm and instrument or endoscope can only be moved in a straight line along the axis of the instrument. In this mode, the system remembers the instrument position upon entering instrument change mode and prevents movement deeper into the patient cavity.

Arm Clash

This robot, having multiple independent arms, has a possibility of frequent clashes if not placed optimally. A Versius arm detects an arm clash if it is pushed too hard by a user pushing or by the arm colliding with an object. If an arm clash occurs, an arm clash icon appears in the icon group of the affected bedside unit (Fig. 5.14).

To resolve the arm clash

- If the clash was from manual pushing, let go of the arm.
- If the clash was from a collision, manually move the arm away from the object in instrument adjust mode.

Instrument Compatibility, User Interface, and Ergonomics

It has all the standard instruments like monopolar hook, monopolar curved scissor, bipolar Maryland grasper, cold scissor, fenestrated graspers, and needle holder, all with a wristed tip. The instruments are attached to the distal end of an instrument arm after the arm drape has been fitted. Each instrument type has the same attachment head and a shaft of 6.8 mm diameter. The attachment head has latches for attaching the instrument to the arm, and fins, which mechanically drive the instrument during surgery. The distal joint can rotate 720° on its own axis for greater maneuverability. The endoscopes have a 10 mm diameter shaft and a 300 mm working length. It comes with 0-degree and 30-degree scopes, which can be attached 30° up or 30° down. It can be moved up–down and left–right. It provides an 81.1° of view. The magnification is 15x with 3D high-definition vision (3DHD). The surgeon needs to put on polarizing 3D glasses for 3D visualization. The head-up display has the option of visualizing in 2D vision also if the surgeon desires so. The visualization unit needs an 11 mm port, while all the instrument ports are 5 mm. Applied Medical balloon ports are one among the validated ports for use with the 10 mm robotic endoscope and 5 mm wristed instruments. Inappropriate port size could lead to an incorrect fulcrum being detected during port training. One of the biggest advantages of this system is that the laparoscopic port placement can be replicated for any surgery and a distance of min 5–6 cm from each port is enough to avoid arm clash. Post training of the arm, the instrument tip has to be a min of 2 cm intracorporeally to start functioning. Apart from the robotic ports, standard laparoscopic ports can be used by the assistant surgeon for additional retraction, suction, mopping with gauze, use of staplers, use of choledochoscope, etc. The assistant surgeon can shift the elbow of the robotic arm without disturbing the intracorporeal position of the instrument and fit in at any position for putting up a port and assistance, with minimal risk of injury to the assistant surgeon due to extracorporeal movement of the instrument arms. In contrast to laparoscopic surgeries, where the standard laparoscopic endoscope needs to be repeatedly cleaned and dipped in hot water to avoid fogging, the problem of fogging of the robotic camera lens is virtually nonexistent due to constant smoke evacuation and achieving the desired electrocautery effect at very low-level settings. Although the Versius Surgical System was validated using a Wolf Endo light system, the light sources of various other companies are compatible. The instruments can be used multiple times, and the life of each instrument varies. All instruments are supplied nonsterile and must be cleaned and steam sterilized before each use. The Versius robotic system requires an Internet connection with an average upload bandwidth of up to 2 Mbps for use in analyzing and improving Versius, and analyzing and improving minimal access surgical techniques. This data is uploaded using a wired Ethernet connection to the Internet. Versius will function normally if there is no connection to the Internet, but data will not be uploaded. This system is indicated for adult use only. The Versius Surgical System requires no routine adjustments to maintain operation and must be serviced only by CMR Surgical or by an appointed agent (Figs. 5.15, 5.16, and 5.17).

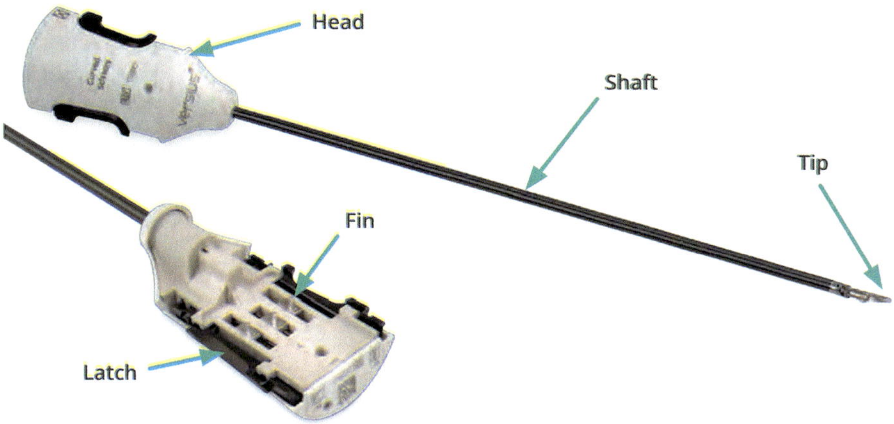

Fig. 5.15 Versius instruments

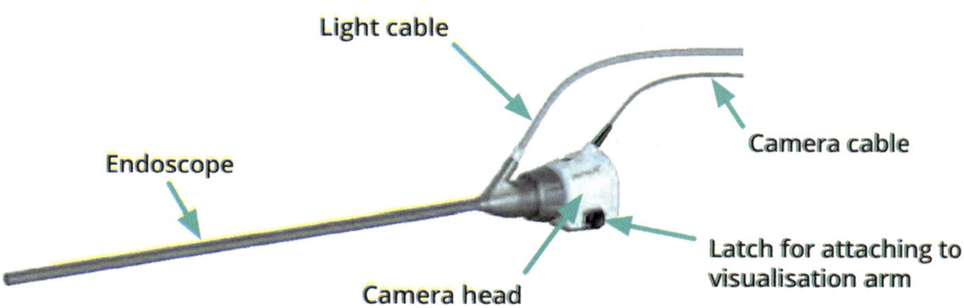

Fig. 5.16 Endoscopic camera

Fig. 5.17 Endoscope angled (30°) and straight (0°)

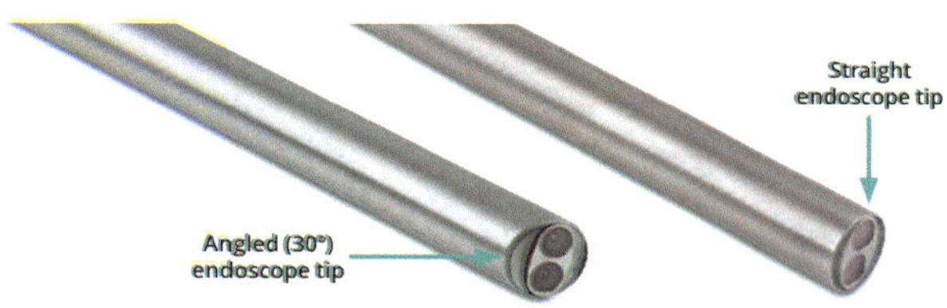

Bedside Unit Positioning Around the Operating Table

The position of the bedside units (BSUs) varies according to the surgical procedure being planned, which again depends on what anatomical region the arms need to reach. They should always be placed parallel to the operating table, with the brake

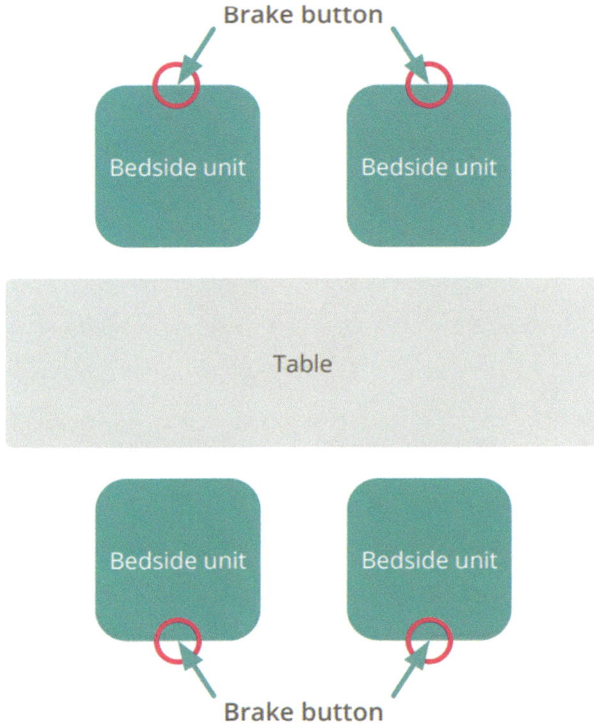

Fig. 5.18 Position of the BSU parallel to the operating table

button away from the table. A maximum of three instrument bedside units can be used along with a visualization bedside unit with the Versius system. The BSUs can be placed close to each other, taking care that the V-Wrists are adequately separated, so that they do not clash on movement during the surgery (Figs. 5.18 and 5.19). The BSUs should be placed so that

- The V-Wrist is not too close to other arms.
- The V-Wrist will not clash with the base.
- The arm does not need to extend any joints fully.

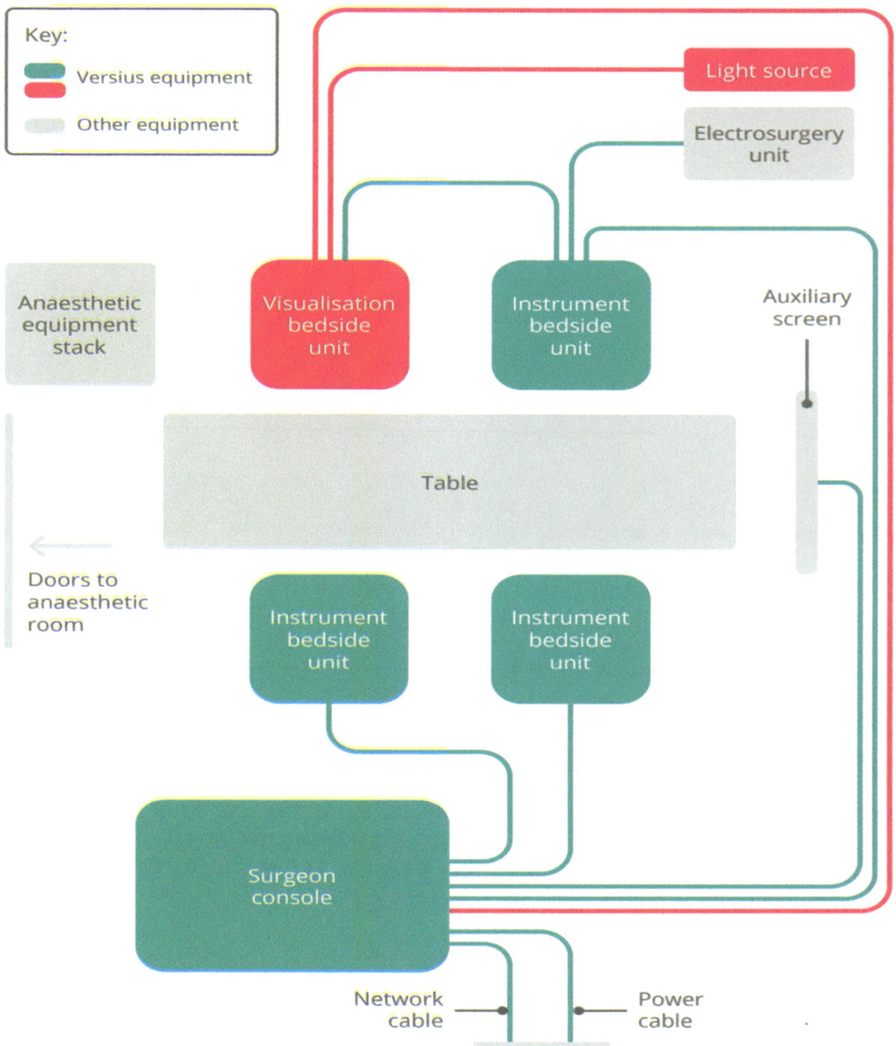

Fig. 5.19 Example of Versius system with four bedside units layout

System Connections

Surgeon console connection panel Located on the base of the surgeon console at the rear, the connection panel is where all the cables are connected to the surgeon console (Fig. 5.20).

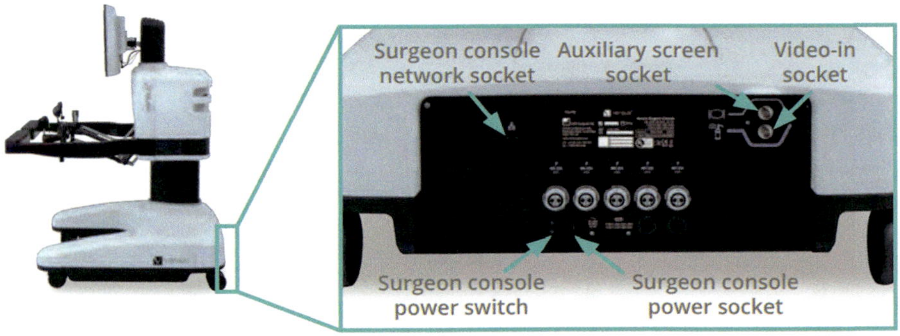

Fig. 5.20 Surgeon console connection panel

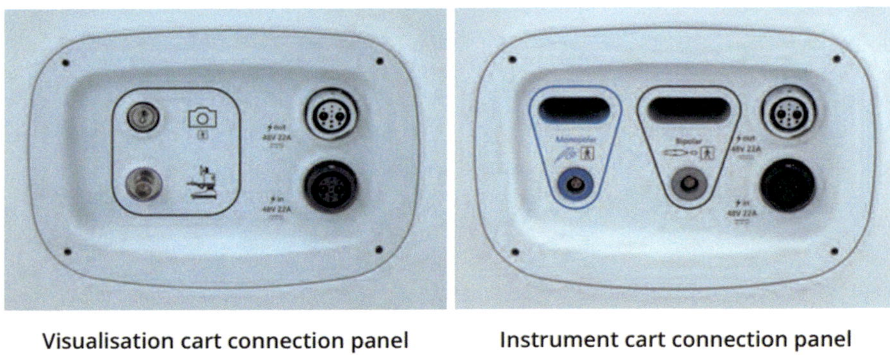

Fig. 5.21 Cart connection panels

The cables connected to the surgeon console are

- Surgeon console power cable (nonsterile)
- Network cable (nonsterile)
- Auxiliary screen cable (nonsterile)
- Video feed cable (nonsterile)
- Bedside unit cable(s) (nonsterile)

Connecting a Bedside Unit to the System

The power-in and power-out sockets available on a cart connection panel are used to connect a bedside unit to either the surgeon console or another bedside unit, based on the system configuration (cabling scheme) chosen: "spider," "daisy chain," or "hybrid" (Figs. 5.21 and 5.22).

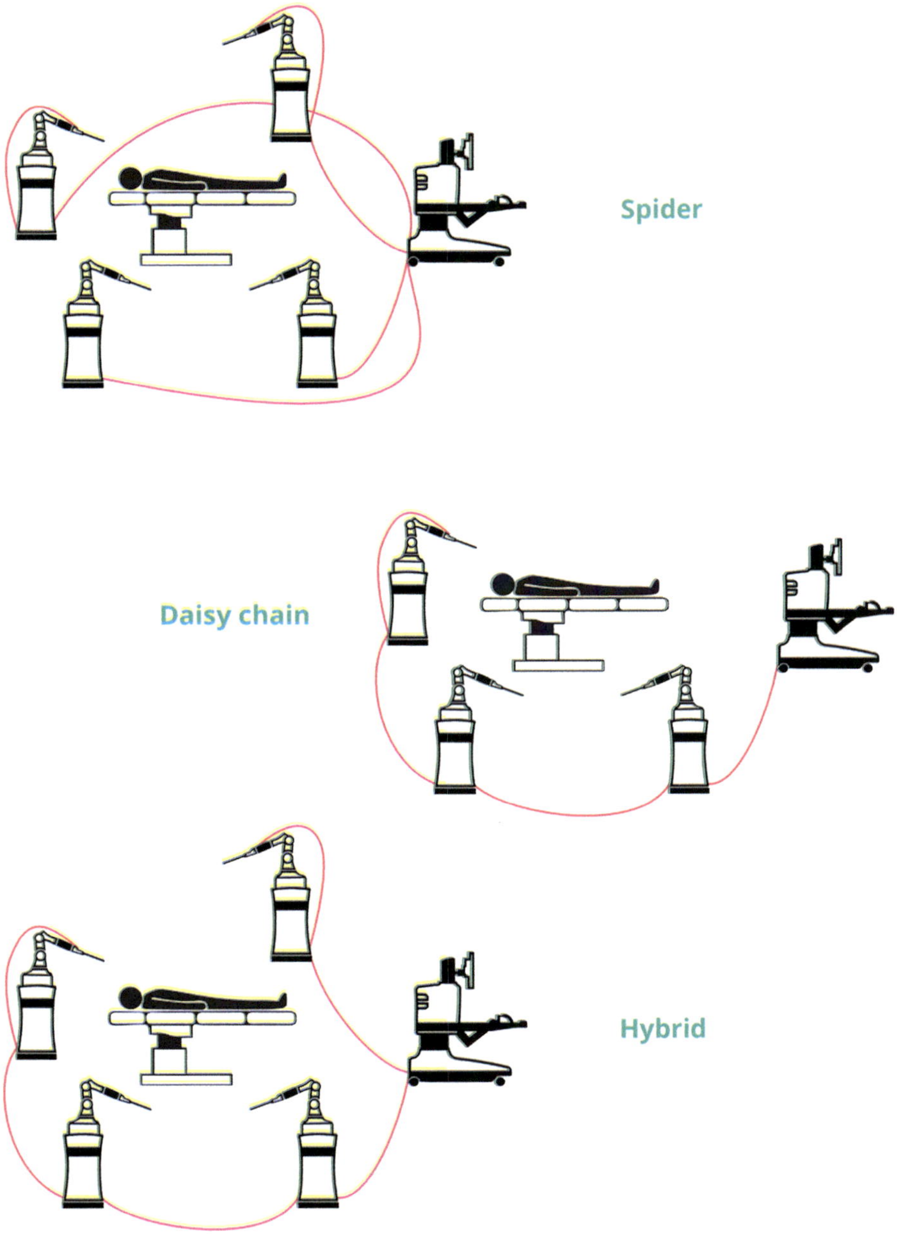

Fig. 5.22 The system cabling configurations

Surgical and Technical Considerations

Before taking up any surgery on this platform, the entire surgical team, including the scrub nurses, has to complete the introductory training course. Before using the system, users should complete basic system training, which includes online and practical training. There are 10 online modules, and the time to complete the entire online training is estimated as 8–10 h. The minimum time for practical training for the surgeon and surgical team is as follows:

Introduction to versius training course		
	Time	
Session	Surgeon	Bedside team
System use: system setup & post-operative task training	12 h 20 min	12 h 50 min
Surgical time – wet lab and dry lab	9 h	8 h 45 min
Team building	1 h 20 min	1 hr 20 min

Where a Versius Surgical System is already in use at a hospital and at least one surgical team in the hospital has been trained in the full training course, additional sterile nurses can be trained in a shorter training course. The online element of this sterile nurse training is estimated as 15 h. The minimum time for practical training in the sterile nurse course is as follows:

Sterile nurse training course	
Session	Time
Team building exercises and troubleshooting	1 h 10 min
System use (set-up and post-operative tasks)	3 h 40 min
Surgical time dry-lab (hands on)	3 h

Approved Procedures

The following are the approved surgical procedures on the Versius robotic platform.

Procedures	
Gynaecology	General
Salpingo-Oophorectomy	Cholecystectomy
Endometriosis resection	Inguinal Hernia
Radical hysterectomy	Hernia repair
Hysterectomy	Gastrectomy
Colorectal	**Urology**
Left & Right hemicolectomy (Low) anterior resection	Nephrectomy
	Pyeloplasty
	Prostatectomy

Although thoracic procedures like esophagectomy can also be done in this system.

Warnings and Precautions

- Prolonged use of the 3D display can lead to side effects such as headache, eye strain, and nausea.
- Versius Surgical System should not be used near an X-ray source.
- The surface of the Versius arm may reach up to 55 °C during use, so direct contact with patient/assistant surgeon's skin should be avoided.
- The robotic arms should be handled only at the areas that are designated safe to hold. There is a risk of hand traps if the arm is touched on a joint when the arm is moving.
- To avoid the risk of permanent damage, the Versius Surgical System must be disconnected and removed before defibrillation.
- The Versius Surgical System should not be used for procedures involving the heart, circulatory system, or central nervous system.

Some Important Safety Features

1. After the arm has been port-trained, the bedside unit brake cannot be deactivated unless the instrument or endoscope is fully retracted out of the port or detached from the arm.
2. If the endoscope camera gets detached accidentally, the control of the surgeon on the movement of the instrument arms is gone and the instruments freeze in that position.
3. If no hands are detected, the instrument gets disengaged, so that the accidental movement of the hand controllers, not made by the surgeon's hands does not injure the patient's organs.
4. In the instrument change mode, the robot memorizes the position of the instrument just prior to getting the arm in that mode. The robot does not let the instrument advance beyond this point to avoid visceral injury.
5. If the brake button is released before the brake is fully activated, the bottom of the bedside unit will rise again. This is a safety feature designed to prevent injuries to the surgical team.

Conclusion

With the Versius taking over the robotic surgery arena rapidly, there has been a significant leap forward in the way minimally invasive surgery is being done globally. However, the true impact of Versius system remains to be seen, how it fares clinically and commercially. Ultimately, the Versius system's success depends on its capacity to bring actual benefits to both healthcare providers and patients. If it can consistently provide better surgical outcomes, lower costs, and a favorable patient experience, it has the potential to transform the area of minimally invasive surgery. However, the question remains unanswered, and only time will tell if the Versius system actually ushers in a new age of surgical care.

6 Virtual Incision: MIRA Surgical System

Dmitry Oleynikov and Shane Farritor

Introduction

Founded in Nebraska in 2006 by Shane Farritor, MS, PhD and Dmitry Oleynikov, MD, FACS, Virtual Incision has become a trailblazer in the realm of minimally invasive surgery. The company was established with a core principle of advancing robotically assisted surgical (RAS) technology allowing surgeries to be more precise, less invasive, and ultimately enhance patient recovery experiences. The company is committed to make every operating room robot ready.

Like other RAS approaches, the MIRA Surgical System offers similar benefits in ergonomics and dexterity. Robotic systems can increase dexterity by eliminating the motion reversal associated with LAP procedures (when the surgeon's hand movements are perceived in the opposite direction when using laparoscopic instruments). MIRA also allows for motion scaling for more consistent and precise manipulation.

Virtual Incision's groundbreaking work revolves around the development of a first-in-class miniaturized robotically assisted surgical platform, designed to navigate a wide range of soft-tissue procedures. The MIRA Surgical System has benefits over other "mainframe" RAS systems that set it apart in a class of its own, namely miniaturized RAS. The MIRA Surgical System was developed to mitigate many of the issues that current "mainframe" robotic systems pose. Mainframe refers to the currently available RAS systems (e.g., Da Vinci Xi) that have a

D. Oleynikov (✉)
Department of Surgery, Monmouth Medical Center, Long Branch, NJ, USA

Department of Surgery, Rutgers Robert Wood Johnson Medical School, Long Branch, NJ, USA
e-mail: Dmitry.Oleynikov@rwjbh.org

S. Farritor
David B. and Nancy K. Lederer Professor of Engineering, Lincoln, NH, USA
e-mail: sfarritor@unl.edu

S. Samreen et al. (eds.), *The SAGES Manual of Robotic Surgery*,
https://doi.org/10.1007/978-3-031-86927-3_6

robust, large, and heavy design to support the external articulation of their robotic arms. These "traditional" RAS systems' large external footprint can lead to cumbersome and long setup times, the need for draping and docking, all while the patient cart and boom are looming over the patient that can interfere with ready access to patient and communication with the operating team. The MIRA Surgical System, on the other hand, can be deployed anywhere, eliminating the need for dedicated robotic rooms and assigned blocks. Its design simplifies setup time and optimizes both access to the patient and communication with the operating team, while allowing seamless operating in multiple quadrants. This lightweight, reusable, "out-of-a-tray" design and potential cost reductions hold the promise to allow wider adoption of robotic surgery programs, allowing for more patients to benefit from better outcomes and faster recovery associated with minimally invasive procedures.

The MIRA Surgical System

Indication

In the United States, marketing authorization was granted by the FDA on February 23, 2024, via the De Novo Classification Pathway (Class II). The MIRA Surgical System is a miniaturized robotic-assisted surgery device indicated for the mobilization of the colon in adults at least 5'0" (1.52 m) tall and having a weight of at least 100 lbs. (45.36 kg) who are undergoing minimally invasive colectomy procedures. It is intended to assist in the visualization of tissues and provide accurate and precise control of surgical instruments to grasp, retract, and dissect while maintaining hemostasis with electrocautery during manipulation of tissues. It is for prescription use only and is to be used by trained physicians in any operating room environment.

Architecture of Platform

The MIRA surgical system consists of an integrated Minibot and Camera, an open-concept surgeon console, and a companion cart (see Fig. 6.1a-c). MIRA is designed to be used with the GelPort® Laparoscopic System made by Applied Medical. The single insertion port is the same device used in hand-assisted laparoscopic surgery (HALS). The Minibot and Camera are inserted into the patient's abdominal cavity through the insertion port and are remotely controlled via the surgeon console located outside the sterile field. The surgeon console includes a main display showing the real-time video feed from the camera, hand input devices, pedal inputs, and an interactive touchscreen. The system is designed to be operated by a minimum of one surgeon and one surgical assistant.

The first-generation system has sterile, single-use bipolar graspers and monopolar scissors instruments. Additional instruments (e.g., needle driver, monopolar hook, vessel sealer) are currently under development.

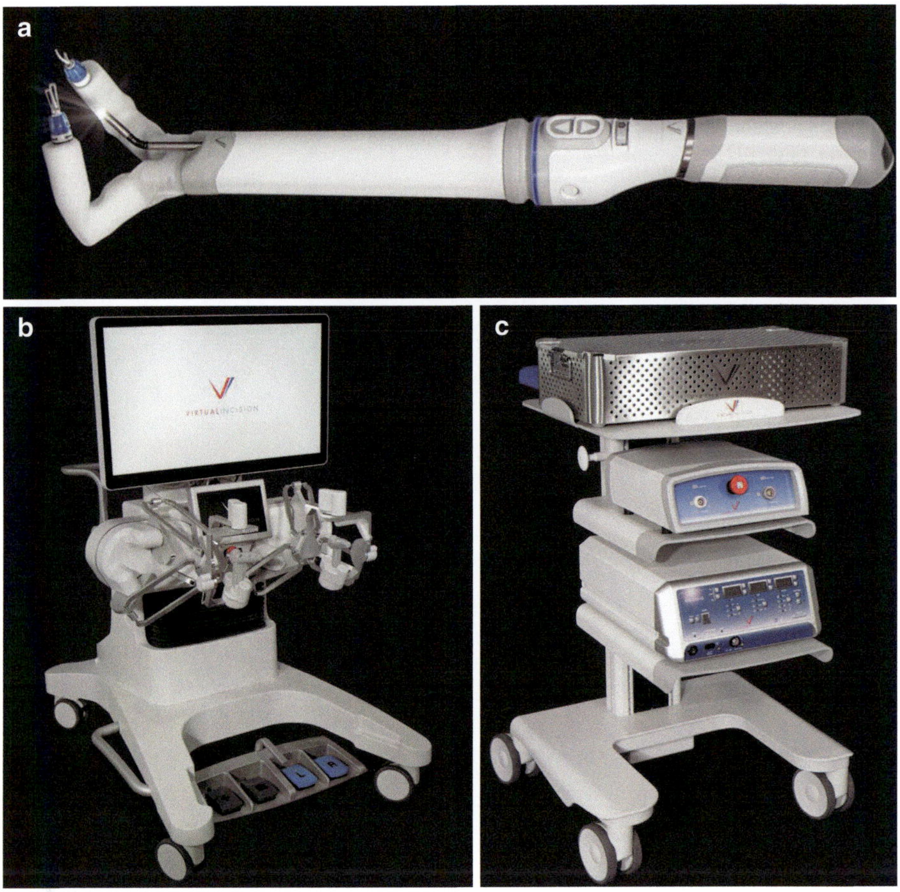

Fig. 6.1 The MIRA surgical system. (**a**) The surgical Minibot and articulating camera, (**b**) The surgeon console, (**c**) The patient cart

Additional Technical Information

The technical differentiator to mainframe robotics is that the motorized robotic arms triangulate inside the patient's abdominal cavity as opposed to externally. Because the instruments triangulate internally, there are no constraints imposed by trocar port placement, which is inherent to the mainframe robotic approach. The MIRA Surgical System has two motorized arms that have six degrees of freedom (Fig. 6.2). Its cross-sectional workspace is 6.7 inches (170 mm) wide and 3.125 inches (80 mm) deep. This cross section is swept approximately 180° about the shoulder pitch joint (Fig. 6.3). The mRASD functions equally over any sweep angle from +90° to −90°, while the articulating camera ensures that the instruments can be in view at all times. Repositioning can be easily performed by adjusting the support arm. This ability to change MIRA's overall position, combined with the reach and dexterity of the arms enable surgery throughout the abdominal cavity.

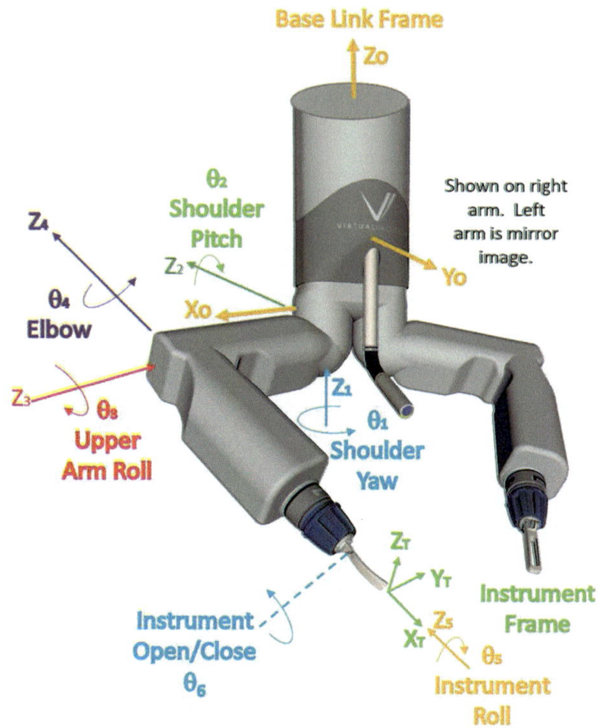

Fig. 6.2 The mRASD arms have six degrees of freedom, including the open/close function of the tool. The shoulder joint can yaw (θ1), pitch (θ2), and roll (θ3) about the upper arm segment. These first three axes of rotation approximately intersect at the shoulder joint. The mRASD elbow allows rotation (θ4) of the forearm with respect to the upper arm. Finally, the instrument can roll (θ5) about the long axis of the instrument with instruments having an open/close actuation capability

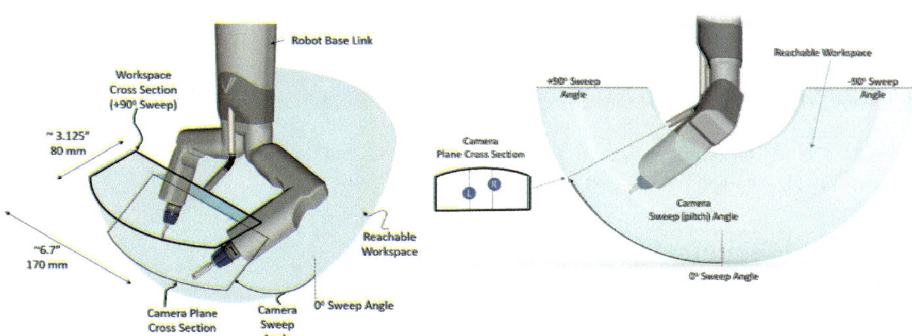

Fig. 6.3 MIRA's reachable workspace: the cross section is swept approximately 180° about the shoulder pitch joint. The workspace cross section is approximately 6.7 inches (170 mm) wide and 3.125 inches (80 mm) deep. The mRASD functions equally over any sweep angle from +90° to −90°. The camera can sweep between +70° to −70°

Clinical Data

The MIRA Surgical System was studied in a prospective, Investigational Device Exemption (IDE) clinical study in three centers in the United States. Based on the patient demographics and clinical characteristics, the study population was found to be representative of the US population for patients undergoing colectomy. The indications for surgery were cancer (40.0%), polyp(s) (40.0%), diverticulitis (16.7%), and cecal mass (3.3%). Seventy percent of patients were overweight or obese, and 53.3% had prior abdominal surgery. Sixty percent had mild systemic disease (ASA II), and 40% had severe systemic disease (ASA III). The cases performed were 15 (50.0%) right colectomy and 15 (50.0%) left colectomy. The overall mean operating time was 163 (SD 56.5) minutes, with an average console time of 77 min. For right colectomy, it was 147 min (range, 80–228), while for left it was 179 min (range, 112–309). One assist port (in addition to the hand-assist gelport) was placed in 63% of patients, and two were used in 37%. The device was manually repositioned a mean six times. Anastomoses were performed extracorporeally in all colectomies. Setup time of the robot was determined to be 5.6 min, median 5 min (range, 1–20 min). All cases had the primary dissection successfully completed and hemostasis achieved with the device. No patients required intraoperative conversion to open surgery. There were no intraoperative adverse events or surgical complications. On pathology, all malignant cases had a complete resection with negative margins and adequate lymph node sampling (median, 26; range, 17–64). Mean intraoperative blood loss was 55.8cc, and one patient received a postoperative transfusion during management of an anastomotic leak.

The median length of stay was 2 days (range, 2–26). There was one unplanned reoperation (3.3%). There were no readmissions. There were no device-related complications and no mortality. According to the Clavien–Dindo classification, 15 surgical complications were observed in nine patients (Gr I: 6; Gr II: 5; Gr IIIa: 2; Gr IIIb: 1; Gr IVb: 1). All major/Clavien–Dindo grade III and greater complications occurred in a single patient. This patient, with severe comorbidities, operated for a stage II sigmoid adenocarcinoma, had an anastomotic leak that required reoperation with a diverting ileostomy. (Figure 6.4 shows an intraoperative view of a colectomy case.)

Telesurgery

Rural and remote populations do not have access to high-quality surgical care, including critical access hospitals, requiring patients to either travel long distances. Remote surgery allows for experts to use the latest robotic technology to assist patients and healthcare providers. Virtual Incision partnered with Savato (CA, USA) telesurgical presence system to perform experimental remote surgery at a distance of 5 miles. The Connectivity System provides highly reliable, low-latency, broad bandwidth connectivity using a

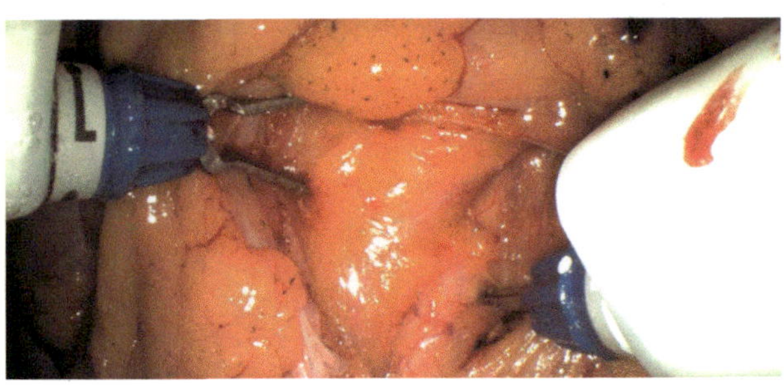

Fig. 6.4 Intraoperative view during left colectomy, dissection of left ureter

dedicated, private network that includes monitoring and immediately available backup networks. The A/V system provides high-quality telepresence that enables clear verbal communication between and among all caregivers and provides multiple video images of the patient and remote operating room for the surgeon who is not in the room. Multiple wet lab procedures across a distance of 5 miles using either public Internet or a dedicated network confirmed reliable connectivity with acceptable latency that enabled completion of hysterectomy, colectomy, and cholecystectomy in a porcine model. The surgeon and remote care team could verbally communicate naturally and effectively. The Sovato App enabled the implementation of the surgical time-out and the preoperative checklists, as well as providing other safety measures. The surgeon and remote care team maintained effective and comfortable verbal and visual communication throughout the setup and completion of the procedures. Remote surgery is safe and feasible, and future use in clinical trials is likely next steps.

MIRA in Space

The MIRA Surgical System is designed to be used in an operating room and to be quickly and easily moved from room to room. The compactness and ease of use of the miniaturized RAS might enable the device to be considered an ideal candidate for remote telesurgery in the future (e.g., for rural areas and military battlefields). Exploring the use of miniaturized RAS in extreme environments helps understand how to remove barriers for patients. An experiment to further validate the proof of concept regarding remote telesurgery was funded by a grant awarded from the National Aeronautics and Space Administration (NASA) to the University of Nebraska through the Established Program to Competitive Research (EPSCoR) program. In January 2024, space-MIRA (a shortened version of MIRA Surgical System) was sent to the International Space Station aboard a Northrop Grumman Cygnus cargo spacecraft carried by a SpaceX Falcon 9 rocket. Testing with space-MIRA on the International Space Station assessed the impact of zero gravity when performing simulated surgical tasks. Six surgeons successfully operated from Virtual Incision's headquarters, utilizing remote-controlled technology to direct the movements of the robot on simulated tissue (Fig. 6.5).

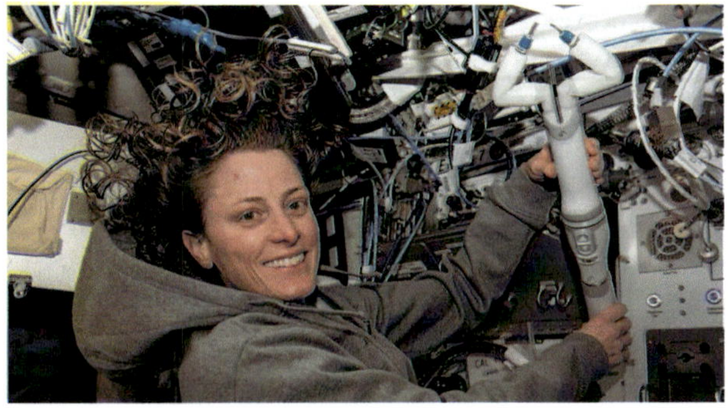

Fig. 6.5 Space-MIRA being shown aboard the International Space Station by astronaut Loral O'Hara (February 2024)

7 Starting and Developing a Robotic Program

C. Franco-Mesa and Sarah Samreen

Purpose

The advantages of minimally invasive surgery (MIS) have been known since the early twentieth century [1]. Nonetheless, the incursion of robotics drastically changed the surgical field. Unlike other MIS tools, these consoles provide countless benefits, including an increase in accuracy, three-dimensional image with depth perception, fully articulated instruments, and improved ergonomics. As a result, surgeons can complete meticulous surgical procedures in unfavorable anatomic locations where open or laparoscopic approaches are unable to be performed or associated with a myriad of complications that outweigh the benefits. While postoperative outcomes with robotic consoles remain comparable to those with other techniques, there is a rising trend in the literature that describes shorter hospital stays, decreased complication rates, and better quality of recovery associated with the use of robotic surgery (RS) [2, 3].

RS is a rapidly growing field in the United States that will continue to expand as training programs incorporate innovative techniques into education curriculums [4]. In the pursuit of providing outstanding patient care, surgeons expand their skill sets to deliver the tools that best fit their patient's needs. Thus, learning additional surgical techniques provides a wider range of options to deliver care. RS has also been known to complement different areas of surgery. For instance, in the setting of acute care surgery (ACS), RS continues to gain favor in cases of cholecystectomy with intraoperative cholangiogram and common biliary duct exploration [5]. In this scenario, patients undergo a one-stage procedure compared to the more common

C. Franco-Mesa · S. Samreen (✉)
Division of General Surgery, University of Texas Medical Branch, Galveston, TX, USA
e-mail: sasamree@utmb.edu

S. Samreen et al. (eds.), *The SAGES Manual of Robotic Surgery*,
https://doi.org/10.1007/978-3-031-86927-3_7

two-stage with endoscopic retrograde cholangiopancreatography. RS is part of the modernization of medicine and will widely spread to complement the general surgeon's armamentarium.

Identifying the Landscape

Before diving into developing a robotic program, it is crucial to understand the current setting and surroundings where such a program will emerge. Factors such as the type of hospital system, number of beds, operating rooms available, and functioning robotic systems will influence the type of program built. The most known FDA-approved system in the United States is the da Vinci Surgical System from Intuitive Surgical [6]. While this may change in the future as different robots are released, it is relevant to identify the strengths and weaknesses that can be encountered in all aspects of project development (logistics, infrastructure, personnel, funding, etc.). Once the starting baseline is recognized, coherent program goals can be established.

Pillars for Starting and Developing a Robotic Surgery Program

Three overlapping phases constitute the tract toward building an RS program (Fig. 7.1). The "adopting" stage encompasses all related to the initial engagement of leadership, basic training, and support. Followed by the "operationalizing" phase, where the learning curve takes place, complexity is escalated, cultural change is promoted, and data collection begins. Finally, during the "standardizing" period, optimization is the priority from both the procedural standpoint and the economic perspective. Other topics such as scheduling priorities, goals, and established teaching curriculums are also approached in the Standardizing phase.

Adopting

The first step of the journey is to identify a leader who is knowledgeable in the field (Fig. 7.2). This "surgeon champion" should have experience with robotic systems and, more importantly, the initiative and desire to participate in the development of the RS program. The leader's goal is to establish a vision of the future of the program and share that vision with other teammates. Furthermore, they are responsible for delivering the knowledge and methods required to manufacture said vision [7].

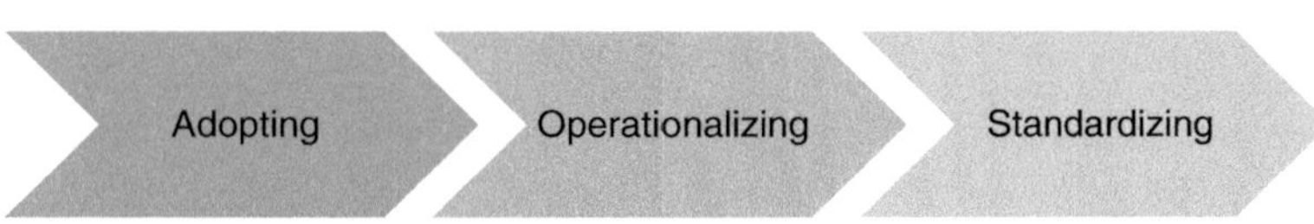

Fig. 7.1 Pillars of building a robotic surgery program

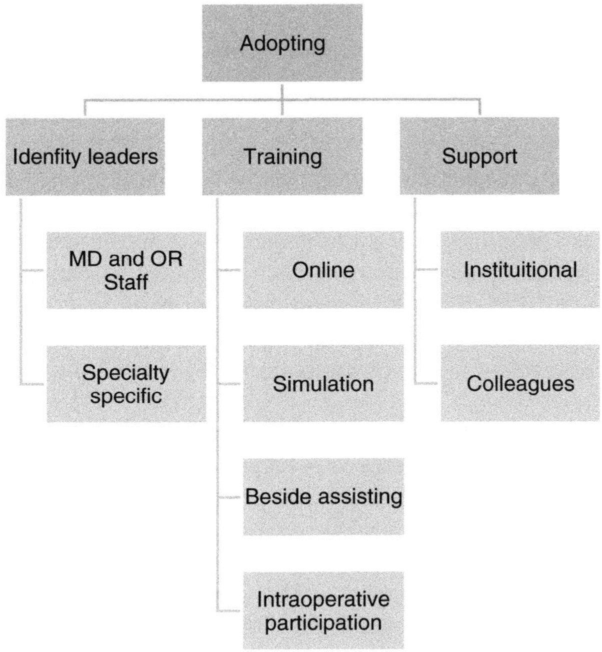

Fig. 7.2 Components of the adopting stage

Finally, the surgeon champion will balance all conflicts and discrepancies along the way. If needed, the leader can appoint trainees to aid with the duties. It is worth noting that in some institutions this role can be targeted by a team rather than just an individual. Once a leading entity has been appointed, a group of learners or apprentices can be selected. This faction is constituted by surgeons who want to be trained in RS and have the availability to do so.

Training in RS is a multimodal endeavor that includes online platform courses, simulator drills, bedside preparation, and intraoperative console experience [8–10]. Each stage targets a different skill set that is valuable to accomplish specific preset milestones. Online modules are completed to become familiar with fundamental concepts of RS such as parts of the console, types of robot equipment, positioning, and energy settings, among others [11]. While some curriculums only use an online platform as an overview of the upcoming education plan, others like the well-known "Fundamentals of Robotic Surgery" employ it for multifaceted and comprehensive training [8, 11]. Virtual RS curriculums range from simple to complex, to tailor to the needs of the rising program.

After a basic understanding of the robotic equipment is acquired, the next step is to participate in console-based simulation. It is well known that simulation-based training has positive outcomes in the surgical education field [12, 13]. This is exemplified by prospective studies demonstrating improvement in performance after these sessions [12]. Regarding RS specifically, simulation exercises upgrade technical fluency, comfort, the notion of the operative field, and pedal coordination

[14–16]. Numerous modules are available in robotic consoles spanning from basic instrument manipulation to the recreation of an entire surgical procedure. For instance, in general surgery RS curriculums, residents start online and simulation drills during the first years of training to be prepared for early intraoperative exposure [9, 10].

After the general concepts and technical skills have been grasped, the next phase is bedside assisting. Although bedside assisting is generally performed by a non-physician first assistant, it is relevant to understand concepts such as patient positioning based on the operation, correct port placement, docking, robotic setup, camera holding, nuances of energy devices, assistant ports, and specimen removal. Additionally setting up robotic components, troubleshooting unexpected situations, and targeting emergency scenarios from the bedside are crucial for safe practice [17].

The last aspect is intraoperative training. In this scenario, an experienced robotic surgeon walks an apprentice through a case. Progressively the apprentice takes on parts of the surgery until they can complete the procedure independently under supervision. While training sessions with a single console are acceptable and many times, the first accessible method in a startup RS program, dual-console systems create an unparalleled opportunity for hands-on learning. Studies in RS comparing single- to dual-console teaching have reported that trainees have longer console time and more frequent interactions with the preceptor when using a dual system [15]. To obtain even more benefits, using HIPAA-compliant video recordings of the procedure for dedicated post-operative debriefing sessions can enhance the overall learning experience [18].

Like any other program on the rise, support from other surgeons must be pursued. Reaching out and recruiting colleagues in the field will guarantee a large enough workforce to accomplish the educational goals established. Additionally, it will be the seed of an environment of teamwork and acceptance of RS within the practice's cultural scenario.

Operationalizing

Operating room (OR) time is one of the largest expenses in healthcare, yet, it is also the principal source of revenue for hospitals [19]. Given the variability of case duration and unpredictable events, developing an efficient yet flexible OR schedule is an essential task. This is no different in the setting of an RS program. To identify the requirements (OR time, personnel, instruments, etc.) for every case, surgeons must establish a pattern of action. In other words, every case should follow a basic configuration or workflow. The more times the case is performed, the more familiar it will become to the team. RS programs start by operationalizing simple cases like nonrecurrent inguinal hernia or elective cholecystectomy for biliary colic and then progress to more complex scenarios such as abdominal wall reconstruction or common biliary duct exploration. While the learning curve varies throughout procedures and surgical centers, studies demonstrate that a reliable curve can be constructed over time [20, 21]. Furthermore, after creating an array of operationalized cases

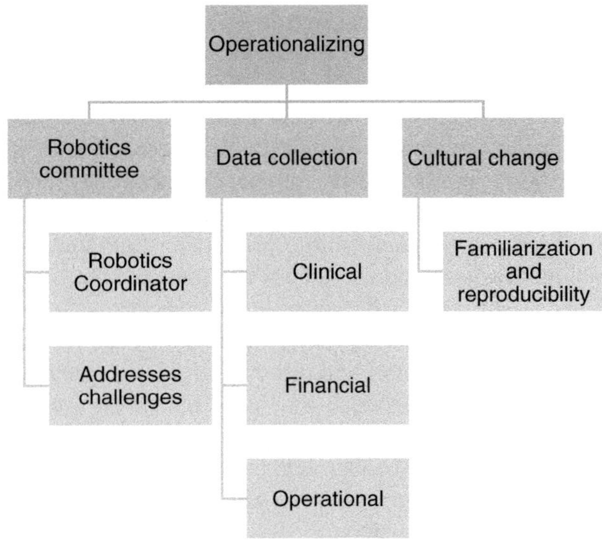

Fig. 7.3 Components of the operationalizing stage

proctoring other physicians becomes an available option to expand the RS program locally or at a larger scale (Fig. 7.3).

Besides creating a pattern for every procedure, a key variable of operationalization is prioritizing safety and teamwork. One cannot take place without the other as everyone has a different role to fulfill. A hospital robotics steering committee that oversees roles, promotes safety, and collects data from procedures is an essential component of the RS program. Through tangible data such as performance indicators, the surgical outcomes of RS can regularly be evaluated. Even more, by developing a framework of key performance indices (KPIs), programs can review liabilities and develop targeted solutions to enhance performance [22]. The permanence and growth of the upcoming RS programs are directly related to the clinical, financial, and operational KPIs. Data this significant can be used to support different types of decisions within the institution in the long run.

Like in any other rising discipline, a cultural environment of collaboration and curiosity is needed for an RS program to flourish. The introduction and acceptance of robotics can be tedious; however, with increasing uptake of robotic technology, it is rapidly becoming a reality. Thus, the goal is to promote a cultural scenario where the use of RS is normalized and regarded as a safe tool for patient care [23].

Standardizing

Standardization is the act of assembling a process throughout time in an organized, efficient, reproducible, and harmonious manner. This practice has been considered fundamental for global development for centuries [24, 25]. Within the medical field, standardization has been essential in areas such as evidence-based medicine, patient safety, and healthcare outcomes [24, 25]. This is the case with the European consensus on robotic mesorectal excision that was published in 2019 and aimed to provide baseline standards for training and technical success in this area of colorectal surgery [26].

The major purpose of standardization in robotic surgery is to reduce variation and optimize efficiency (Fig. 7.4). For instance, employing predetermined instruments and accessory sets for the robot decreases the amount of time preparing the operating room or looking for specific utensils while the procedure is carried out. "Peel packs" (prepackaged sterile robotic instruments) allow for efficiency and establish a predictable sterile processing time and inventory management. Thus, operative time is optimized benefitting the patient, surgeon, staff, and everyone else in the facility involved in operative services.

The standardization journey for an upcoming program is variable. Standardizing on-time first-case start and turnover times are essential parts of the standardization process, along with block time allocation with accurate case scheduling. A study from Stanford attempted to standardize the operative start time for cardiac cases after making a thorough background check of their perioperative data [28]. They noticed that adherence to the start time was associated with increased efficiency, decreased costs, and higher satisfaction [27]. Armstrong et al. described the use of video recordings of numerous microvascular anastomoses to break down key portions of the procedure that could be improved [28]. The videos were analyzed by a multidisciplinary team that provided different perspectives and proposals [28]. While taping and reviewing procedures is not obligatory for standardization, the ability to automatize procedures based on visual documentation is a possibility. No matter what specific strategy for homogenized RS practice is pursued, supporting the robotic scheduling,

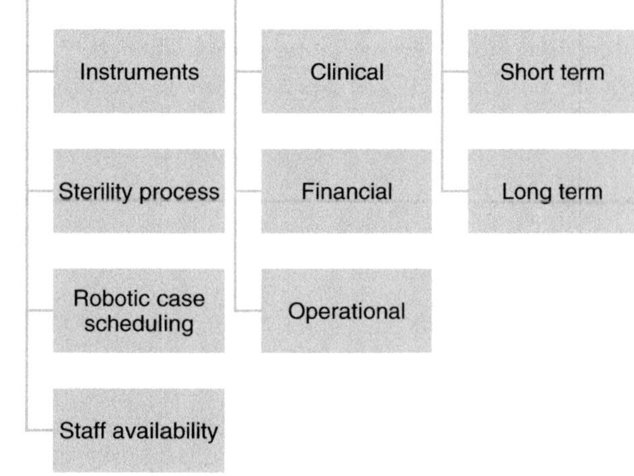

Fig. 7.4 Components of the standardizing stage

allowing block time for certain services, and optimizing turnover time will be beneficial. In the long run, this practice promotes self-sustainability and chronicity with the ability to overcome challenges posed throughout time.

By this point, the RS program is up and running. The success of the course will depend on a well-developed plan for growth. Ideally, this should be designed in a stepwise approach with short-, medium-, and long-term goals. Predicted difficulties should be factored in the proposal as well as alternative solutions. It is crucial to collect data during every stage of the process. These will be useful to construct future projection curves to tailor long-term goals accordingly. Teaching curriculums must be incorporated in forthcoming plans as they will provide structured learning instructions for upcoming surgeons and operative staff.

Lessons

Challenges arise with change and innovation. Building an RS program will come with unparalleled benefits, but also inherent struggles. The path itself is not linear but rather convoluted with peaks and falls. By normalizing and expecting this type of scenery, the unexpected becomes expected. One of the areas that will require time to flourish is cultural change. For this, persistence and patience will be the best allies in the long term. Finally, patient outcomes are the principal tool to determine success; however, financial outcomes matter and will be considered for critical decision-making purposes.

Conclusion

Developing a robotic program is a challenging task. While numerous factors must align to be successful, robotic technology provides numerous benefits associated with patient safety and surgical outcomes in standard and complex procedures. Furthermore, this minimally invasive technique imminently protects the ergonomics of physicians securing a safe practice in the long run. Adopting, operationalizing, and standardizing are the operational pillars of a roadmap to a successful robotic program. The inevitable development of technology challenges physicians to renovate and modernize their surgical practice to guarantee optimal patient care.

Bibliography

1. Radojcić B, Jokić R, Grebeldinger S, Meljnikov I, Radojić N. History of minimally invasive surgery. Med Pregl. 2009;62(11–12):597–602.
2. Yeung TM, Larkins KM, Warrier SK, Heriot AG. The rise of robotic colorectal surgery: better for patients and better for surgeons. J Robotic Surg. 2024;18(1):69. https://doi.org/10.1007/s11701-024-01822-z.
3. Alvarado CE, Worrell SG, Bachman KC, et al. Robotic approach has improved outcomes for minimally invasive resection of mediastinal tumors. Ann Thorac Surg. 2022;113(6):1853–8. https://doi.org/10.1016/j.athoracsur.2021.05.090.

4. Sheetz KH, Claflin J, Dimick JB. Trends in the Adoption of Robotic Surgery for Common Surgical Procedures. JAMA Netw Open. 2020;3(1):e1918911. https://doi.org/10.1001/jamanetworkopen.2019.18911.
5. Alkhamesi NA, Davies WT, Pinto RF, Schlachta CM. Robot-assisted common bile duct exploration as an option for complex choledocholithiasis. Surg Endosc. 2013;27(1):263–6. https://doi.org/10.1007/s00464-012-2431-0.
6. Peters BS, Armijo PR, Krause C, Choudhury SA, Oleynikov D. Review of emerging surgical robotic technology. Surg Endosc. 2018;32(4):1636–55. https://doi.org/10.1007/s00464-018-6079-2.
7. Maykel J. Leadership in surgery. Clinics Colon Rectal Surg. 2013;26(04):254–8. https://doi.org/10.1055/s-0033-1356727.
8. Greenberg AL, Syed SM, Alseidi A, O'Sullivan PS, Chern H. Robotic training for medical students: feasibility of a pilot simulation curriculum. J Robotic Surg. 2022;17(3):1029–38. https://doi.org/10.1007/s11701-022-01508-4.
9. Azadi S, Green IC, Arnold A, Truong M, Potts J, Martino MA. Robotic surgery: the impact of simulation and other innovative platforms on performance and training. J Minim Invasive Gynecol. 2021;28(3):490–5. https://doi.org/10.1016/j.jmig.2020.12.001.
10. Howard KK, Makki H, Novotny NM, Mi M, Nguyen N. Value of robotic surgery simulation for training surgical residents and attendings: a systematic review protocol. BMJ Open. 2022;12(6):e059439. https://doi.org/10.1136/bmjopen-2021-059439.
11. Robotic Task Force SAGES, Chen R, Rodrigues Armijo P, Krause C, Siu KC, Oleynikov D. A comprehensive review of robotic surgery curriculum and training for residents, fellows, and postgraduate surgical education. Surg Endosc. 2020;34(1):361–7. https://doi.org/10.1007/s00464-019-06775-1.
12. De Montbrun S, MacRae H. Simulation in surgical education. Clinics Colon Rectal Surg. 2012;25(03):156–65. https://doi.org/10.1055/s-0032-1322553.
13. Sandeva MG, Tufkova S, Ketev K, Paskaleva D. Evaluating the effectiveness of simulation training in obstetrics and gynecology, pediatrics and emergency medicine. *FM*. 2019;61(4):605–11. https://doi.org/10.3897/folmed.61.e47961.
14. Larkins KM, Mohan HM, Gray M, et al. Transferability of robotic console skills by early robotic surgeons: a multi-platform crossover trial of simulation training. J Robotic Surg. 2022;17(3):859–67. https://doi.org/10.1007/s11701-022-01475-w.
15. Leon MG, Carrubba AR, DeStephano CC, Heckman MG, Craver EC, Dinh TA. Impact of robotic single and dual console systems in the training of minimally invasive gynecology surgery (MIGS) fellows. J Robotic Surg. 2022;16(6):1273–80. https://doi.org/10.1007/s11701-022-01369-x.
16. Wang VL, Pieper H, Gupta A, Chen X, Husain S, Meara M. Expectations versus reality: trainee participation on the robotic console in academic surgery. Surg Endosc. 2021;35(8):4805–10. https://doi.org/10.1007/s00464-020-07874-0.
17. Britton CR, Francis I, Tay LJ, Krishnamoothy B. The role of the bedside assistant in robot-assisted surgery: a critical synthesis. J Perioper Pract. 2022;32(9):208–25. https://doi.org/10.1177/17504589221094136.
18. Cristofari H, Jung MK, Niclauss N, Toso C, Kloetzer L. Teaching and learning robotic surgery at the dual console: a video-based qualitative analysis. J Robotic Surg. 2022;16(1):169–78. https://doi.org/10.1007/s11701-021-01224-5.
19. Denton B, Viapiano J, Vogl A. Optimization of surgery sequencing and scheduling decisions under uncertainty. Health Care Manag Sci. 2007;10(1):13–24. https://doi.org/10.1007/s10729-006-9005-4.
20. Nasseri Y, Stettler I, Shen W, et al. Learning curve in robotic colorectal surgery. J Robotic Surg. 2021;15(3):489–95. https://doi.org/10.1007/s11701-020-01131-1.
21. Soomro NA, Hashimoto DA, Porteous AJ, et al. Systematic review of learning curves in robot-assisted surgery. BJS Open. 2020;4(1):27–44. https://doi.org/10.1002/bjs5.50235.
22. Abdel-Razik MSM, Rizk HI, Zein MM, Abdel-Megeid SMES, Abd El Fatah SAM. Promoting the culture of key performance indicators (KPIs) among primary health care staff at health

district level: an intervention study. Eval Program Plann. 2023;96:102188. https://doi.org/10.1016/j.evalprogplan.2022.102188.
23. Jogerst KM, Coe TM, Petrusa E, et al. Multidisciplinary perceptions on robotic surgical training: the robot is a stimulus for surgical education change. Surg Endosc. 2023;37(4):2688–97. https://doi.org/10.1007/s00464-022-09708-7.
24. Paradis E, De Freitas C, Heisey R, et al. Getting standardization right. Can Fam Physician. 2021;67(5):323–5. https://doi.org/10.46747/cfp.6705323.
25. Lehmann CU, Miller MR. Standardization and the practice of medicine. J Perinatol. 2004;24(3):135–6. https://doi.org/10.1038/sj.jp.7211060.
26. Miskovic D, Ahmed J, Bissett-Amess R, et al. European consensus on the standardization of robotic total mesorectal excision for rectal cancer. Colorectal Dis. 2019;21(3):270–6. https://doi.org/10.1111/codi.14502.
27. Burton É, Medina M, Antonio H. Standardization of operative start times for non-emergent cardiac surgical procedures. J Card Surg. 2022;37(10):3092–8. https://doi.org/10.1111/jocs.16756.
28. Armstrong T, Yu D, Frischknecht A, Minter R, Andreatta P, Kasten S. Standardization of surgical procedures for identifying best practices and training. Work. 2012;41:4673–9. https://doi.org/10.3233/WOR-2012-0108-4673.

Robotic Training and Pathway

8

Katherine Fay and Ankit D. Patel

Introduction

The introduction of minimally invasive surgical (MIS) techniques has been shown to greatly improve surgical outcomes, including lower rates of complications, decreased postoperative pain, and shorter hospital length of stay [1]. However, there are certain limitations inherent to laparoscopy, including reliance on two-dimensional vision, decreased range of motion given the rigidity of instruments, and ergonomic challenges experienced by the operating surgeon. Through the robotic surgery platform, the advantages of MIS are maintained with the added enhancement of three-dimensional vision, further instrument articulation, abolition of tremor, and improved surgeon ergonomics allowing for improved hand–eye coordination and overall surgical precision [2]. Although there are demonstrated surgical benefits and rapidly increasing utilization of the platform, there is no universally adapted training paradigm for robotic surgery. Available programs have significant variation in didactic content and access to technical skill sessions provided. Here, we discuss the key elements of a robotic surgery program to train future and currently practicing surgeons, support continued skill development, and ensure patient safety and optimal outcomes through credentialing and maintenance policies.

K. Fay (✉)
Department of General Surgery, Grady Memorial Hospital, Atlanta, GA, USA

Department of General & Gastrointestinal Surgery, Emory University School of Medicine, Atlanta, GA, USA
e-mail: kat.fay@emory.edu

A. D. Patel
Department of General & Gastrointestinal Surgery, Emory University School of Medicine, Atlanta, GA, USA

S. Samreen et al. (eds.), *The SAGES Manual of Robotic Surgery*,
https://doi.org/10.1007/978-3-031-86927-3_8

Implementation of a Curriculum

Since its integration into modern medicine beginning in the 1980s, the utilization of the robotic surgery platform has steadily increased in the United States across a multitude of surgical disciplines [3–5]. One study showed that as of 2017 use of robotic-assisted surgical techniques had grown exponentially compared to laparoscopic surgical techniques at a relative rate of 10–40-fold [6]. Increasing use has driven the need for the creation of training pathways for currently practicing surgeons as well as the integration of robotic curricula into surgical residency training programs. A survey of general surgery residents in 2015 in the United States indicated that 96% of respondents were training at an institution where a surgical robotic platform was available [7].

Unlike other areas of technical advancement in surgical practice, robotic surgery is one of the few without a surgical society-backed designated curriculum. The adoption of surgical laparoscopy drove the creation of the Fundamentals of Laparoscopic Surgery (FLS) developed by the Society of American Gastrointestinal and Endoscopic Surgeons (SAGES) to ensure that all graduating surgical residents possess the minimum skills to perform laparoscopic procedures safely. Certification in this program has been endorsed by the American Board of Surgery (ABS), the Canadian Association of General Surgeons (CAGS), and American Board of Obstetrics and Gynecology (ACOG) and is a graduation requirement for surgical trainees and necessary for board eligibility. Similarly, the Fundamentals of Endoscopic Surgery (FES), an educational pathway that evaluates basic endoscopic knowledge and skills, is also a requirement within surgical training and board eligibility.

SAGES published a consensus document in 2007 outlining guidelines for the initiation and maintenance of an effective robotic surgery program. Created by an international multidisciplinary consensus group, the document focuses on training and credentialing, clinical applications of robotic surgery, risks of surgery, cost–benefit analysis, and future research [8]. Additionally, the document comments on the key elements of robotic training, credentialing, and program maintenance. While these guidelines are broad and somewhat outdated, they do provide a backbone for future training programs. Recently, several leaders in resident education published recommendations from a robotic surgery working group that we will highlight in the sections below [9].

Curricula Components

The SAGES robotic surgery consensus document highlights combining web-based didactics, virtual reality simulation, in-person course, and cadaveric/animal training models when training new surgeons. When offered in concert, each component allows for the enhancement of certain skill levels that aim to build competency, develop proficient technical skills, and allow for the maintenance of performance in robotic surgery. Each training program then ultimately culminates in training on the robotic platform, including the development of bedside assistant and on-console surgeon skills.

Web-Based Training

Web-based training modules provide significant flexibility to users new to the robotic surgical platform. As the majority of new users are likely in surgical training, self-scheduled learning results in less logistical challenges during the acquisition of foundational knowledge. These courses focus on learning ideal patient selection, instrumentation, patient and system positioning, port placement, and basic troubleshooting. They also review some basics or pre-, intra-, and postoperative care. Expansion of these curricula to include support staff can also allow for greater programmatic efficiency and growth. Eventually, some of this training could be converted to on-demand content or could be accessed in a virtual reality format.

Virtual Simulation

Virtual simulation training has also been shown to play an integral role in the development and maintenance of robotic surgical skills. A variety of simulators are available, including the Fundamentals of Robotic Surgery (FRS) Dome, the da Vinci Skills Simulator (DVSS), and the dV-trainer. As the robotic surgery platform is utilized for more advanced cases, wider application is limited by the fact that many institutions do not see the number of cases needed for proficiency, even for experienced surgeons. The utilization of virtual reality simulation training aims to bridge that gap more effectively and allow for wider application of the robotic platform. Multiple studies support that trainees who participate in virtuality reality simulation perform better on robotic task testing than those who do not [10, 11]. A more recent review compared the more prominent available simulators and demonstrated the ability of a VR training curriculum to improve skills and a proficiency-based training platform being the most effective [12]. For most training programs, these skill simulators will likely be the foundation of any curricula.

Bedside Skills

Once a trainee (either resident/fellow or new user) has indicated proficiency in an online program (defined by most as achievement of a minimum competency score of >90% on written knowledge assessments as well as indicate proficiency of skill on simulators), as well as undergone a bedside teaching session emphasizing basic techniques, they are graduated to in operating room training. While variable by institution, prior to initiation of on-console training, most robotic programs mandate a certain number of bedside assist cases to ensure adequate docking, instrument exchange, and troubleshooting knowledge of the platform. This component of training focuses on the development of clear communication and coordination with the console surgeon. This immediate feedback relationship allows for safe and efficient utilization of the system. Per the current industry standards, the minimum number of cases that need to be completed prior to transitioning to on-console is 10 cases as bedside assist.

Console Training

After the completion of 10 bedside assist cases, the surgeon in training then proceeds with on-console cases. Again, the number of cases that must be completed prior to awarding certification of completion of the robotic surgery program is variable; however, most programs specify the need to perform >50% of at least 20 basic robotic cases. Completion of these cases is achieved in a graduated autonomy approach wherein certain cases or portions of cases are deemed appropriate for certain surgical trainee levels. This is highlighted in the Robotic Surgery Education Workgroup where trainees would progress based on technical proficiency and follow a certain pathway.

Training Programs

While multiple training pathways exist, here we discuss the predominant commercially available training programs.

Fundamentals of Robotic Surgery (FRS)

The FRS is an online, competency-based robotic surgery educational program that trains surgeons on key technical skills that were proposed to be integral to becoming a safe robotic platform user. The curriculum was developed by subject matter experts and funded by a grant through the Department of Defense as well as unrestricted funding from Intuitive Surgical. The curriculum comprises four modules: (1) Introduction to Surgical Robotic Systems, (2) Didactic Instruction for Robotic Surgery Systems, (3) Psychomotor Skills Curriculum, and (4) Team Training & Communication Skills that aim to foster skills that allow a team to safely run a robotic surgical program [13]. The program is applicable across a variety of surgical disciplines and platform agnostic.

A multi-institutional, blinded validation study was conducted at 12 American College of Surgeons (ACS) Accredited Educational Institutes (AEI) between April 2015 and November 2016, where participants were assessed on primary outcome measures of total duration and errors made while performing basic robotic technical skills [14]. Secondary outcomes included cognitive test scores, Global Evaluative Assessment of Robotic Skills (GEARS) rating scale, and robotic familiarity checklist scores. GEARS is a validated rating tool that assesses a performer on six domains, including depth perception, bimanual dexterity, efficiency, autonomy, force sensitivity, and robotic control utilizing a Likert scale [15]. Total scores can be compared during the progression of technical training to track skill acquisition as part of a robotic surgery training program. The study participants followed the FRS curriculum, performed cognitive testing as previously described, and were then tested on proficiency of technical skills utilizing one of three simulators with completion of pre and post testing on avian tissue models. Proficiency skills were tested with one of three simulators: the FRS physical Dome [16], the DVSS, or the dV-Trainer. The control groups were offered the Intuitive da Vinci curriculum, the Robotic Training Network (RTN) curriculum, or participate in existing local training programs with whatever simulator accompanied their program of choice; over 90% of control participants utilized the Intuitive da Vinci curriculum. The study demonstrated noninferiority of the FRS curriculum compared to the control group based on performance metrics. Interestingly, there were differences in performance in the study arm depending on the type of simulator used, suggesting that simulation plays a significant role in technical skill development.

Intuitive Surgical Da Vinci Curriculum

Intuitive Surgical offers an online training pathway specifically for the Da Vinci system, one of the most widely used Food and Drug Administration (FDA)-approved devices on the market. This training course can also be specified to the platform available at the surgeon's given institution. Online modules are available for a variety of roles within the robotic surgery team, including the surgeon, residents/fellows, OR care teams, bedside assists, and robotic program coordinators, which is a unique element to this program. Training of surgical support staff on the fundamentals of communication, operating room set-up, docking/draping, and room turnover can greatly reduce overall operating time and costs [17]. Additionally, surgical staff familiarity with the robotic platform can improve team dynamics, overall job satisfaction, and potentially reduce errors [18]. A prospective study performed evaluating a bedside assistant training course (including surgical technicians, residents, and physician assistants) for robotic-assisted radical prostatectomies demonstrated increased satisfaction with surgical performance [19].

Robotic Training Network (RTN)

The RTN is a standardized robotic surgical education program designed for residents and fellows in training comprised of nine, collaborating academic institutions [20]. It is a multiphased curriculum consisting of robotic platform knowledge, bedside assistant training, on-console training, and development of team dynamics and communication skills. Each phase contains self-guided online modules with built-in assessments, simulator training, and reinforcement of acquired skills through operating room participation. The evaluation of robotic skill competency is achieved through the

Robotic-Objective Structured Assessment of Technical Skills (R-OSATS) that measures performance related to accuracy, tissue handling, dexterity, efficiency, and depth perception [21]. The validity, intra- and inter-reliability of this form of assessment were evaluated at eight different institutions where residents, fellows, and faculty surgeons [the vast majority (84%) from the gynecology department] performed robotic simulation drills [22]. The scores obtained were able to distinguish between novice users and those with robotic surgery experience as well as by PGY level. Additionally, both intra- and inter-reliability were consistently high for all simulation drills, demonstrating it to be a consistent evaluation tool for robotic surgery skill acquisition.

Credentialing: Initialing Privileges and Maintenance

Currently, there are no specific standards for institutional credentialing of robotic surgeons. Additionally, as robotic training is more widely integrated within surgical residency training across a variety of subspecialties, differing levels of experience will need to be accounted for. For most programs, there are three potential pathways as new surgeons undergo the robotic credentialing process—a surgeon new to the robotic platform, a recent surgical residency or fellowship graduate who has completed a robotic training pathway, and a surgeon transferring credentials from one institution to another.

A review of robotic credentialing policies from 42 institutions representing 24 different states across the country indicated that many programs necessitated that all practitioners regardless of prior experience be board-certified or board-eligible (60%) and to have the same privileges for the equivalent open or minimally invasive procedures for which robotic privileges were being requested (83%) [23]. For new users, while 95% of institutions required documentation of completion of a robotic training course through the aforementioned pathways for new robotic surgeons, only 31% required minimum course hours and 21% required a minimum passing score. The significant variation in acceptable pass rates and course components allows for greater variability in the competency of new surgeons to the platform. For more experienced users, the vast majority of programs required a recent case log; however, only a few distinguish a certain number of cases that would indicate proficiency.

Regardless of the level of training, most programs necessitate documentation of proctored cases at the institution for which credentials are sought. Of those with a requirement of proctored cases, the majority mandated a constant number of cases regardless of prior robotic experience and only 14% allowed for a tiered proctored requirement with less proctored cases necessary for more advanced surgeons. Proctor-eligible surgeons must have completed a minimum of 40 of the index cases as recommended by Intuitive.

In addition to initial credentialing, the role of maintenance of privileges is integral to ensuring continued competency in understanding the robotic system and proficiency in technical skill. However, again there is significant variation in the number of cases needed to be completed annually once credentialed as well as a maximum allowable gap between cases.

Conclusion

The robotic surgery platform continues to play an integral role in surgical practice across a myriad of disciplines. Despite its prevalence, no universally accepted training pathway or institutional program exists to support training of and maintenance of surgical users. Here, we have reviewed the key components of such programs as suggested by SAGES as well as the commercially available training pathways. Ultimately to ensure patient safety and program quality through uniformity, a society-endorsed program will need to be developed and adopted widely just as seen with laparoscopy and endoscopy.

References

1. Darzi A, Munz Y. The impact of minimally invasive surgical techniques. Annu Rev Med. 2004;55:223–37.
2. Byrn JC, Schluender S, Divino CM, Conrad J, Gurland B, Shlasko E, Szold A. Three-dimensional imaging improves surgical performance for both novice and experienced operators using the da Vinci Robot System. Am J Surg. 2007 Apr;193(4):519–22.
3. Sheetz KH, Claflin J, Dimick JB. Trends in the adoption of robotic surgery for common surgical procedures. JAMA Netw Open. 2020 Jan 3;3(1):e1918911.
4. Bauerle WB, Mody P, Estep A, Stoltzfus J, El Chaar M. Current trends in the utilization of a robotic approach in the field of bariatric surgery. Obes Surg. 2023 Feb;33(2):482–91.
5. Anderson JE, Chang DC, Parsons JK, Talamini MA. The first national examination of outcomes and trends in robotic surgery in the United States. J Am Coll Surg. 2012 Jul;215(1):107–114; discussion 114-6.
6. Armijo PR, Pagkratis S, Boilesen E, Tanner T, Oleynikov D. Growth in robotic-assisted procedures is from conversion of laparoscopic procedures and not from open surgeons' conversion: a study of trends and costs. Surg Endosc. 2018 Apr;32(4):2106–13.
7. Farivar BS, Flannagan M, Leitman IM. General surgery residents' perception of robot-assisted procedures during surgical training. J Surg Educ. 2015;72(2):235–42.
8. Herron DM, Marohn M; SAGES-MIRA robotic surgery consensus group. A consensus document on robotic surgery. Surg Endosc. 2008 Feb;22(2):313-325; discussion 311-2.
9. Porterfield JR Jr, et al. Structured Resident Training in Robotic Surgery: Recommendations of the Robotic Surgery Education Working Group. J Surg Educ. 2024 Jan;81(1):9–16.
10. Abboudi H, et al. Current status of validation for robotic surgery simulators – a systematic review. BJU Int. 2013 Feb;111(2):194–205.
11. Dulan G, et al. Proficiency-based training for robotic surgery: construct validity, workload, and expert levels for nine inanimate exercises. Surg Endosc. 2012 Jun;26(6):1516–21.
12. Bric JD, Lumbard DC, Frelich MJ, Gould JC. Current state of virtual reality simulation in robotic surgery training: a review. Surg Endosc. 2016;30(6):2169–78.
13. Smith R, Patel V, Satava R. Fundamentals of robotic surgery: a course of basic robotic surgery skills based upon a 14-society consensus template of outcomes measures and curriculum development. Int J Med Robot. 2014 Sep;10(3):379–84.
14. Satava RM, et al. Proving the effectiveness of the Fundamentals of Robotic Surgery (FRS) skills curriculum: a single-blinded, multispecialty, multi-institutional randomized control trial. Ann Surg. 2020 Aug;272(2):384–92.
15. Goh AC, Goldfarb DW, Sander JC, Miles BJ, Dunkin BJ. Global evaluative assessment of robotic skills: validation of a clinical assessment tool to measure robotic surgical skills. J Urol. 2012 Jan;187(1):247–52.
16. FRS Dome. Available at: http://frsdome.wordpress.com.

17. Vetter MH, et al. Incorporating resident/fellow training into a robotic surgery program. J Surg Oncol. 2015 Dec;112(7):684–9.
18. Sgarbura O, Vasilescu C. The decisive role of the patient-side surgeon in robotic surgery. Surg Endosc. 2010 Dec;24(12):3149–55.
19. Thiel DD, et al. Simulation-based training for bedside assistants can benefit experienced robotic prostatectomy teams. J Endourol. 2013 Feb;27(2):230–7.
20. Robotics Training Network. Retrieved from https://www.surgicalexcellence.org/robotic-training-network-rtn. Accessed 4 Mar 2024.
21. Chen R, et al. A comprehensive review of robotic surgery curriculum and training for residents, fellows, and postgraduate surgical education. Surg Endosc. 2020 Jan;34(1):361–7.
22. Siddiqui NY, et al. Validity and reliability of the robotic objective structured assessment of technical skills. Obstet Gynecol. 2014 Jun;123(6):1193–9.
23. Huffman EM, et al. Are current credentialing requirements for robotic surgery adequate to ensure surgeon proficiency? Surg Endosc. 2021 May;35(5):2104–9.

9 Digital Surgery

Jonathan Gootee and Nova Szoka

Introduction

The emerging frontier of surgical innovation, termed digital surgery, follows the eras of open and laparoscopic procedures and builds upon the progress achieved in robotic surgery. Digital surgery introduces a computer interface into the surgeon–patient interaction, encompassing facets such as advanced visualization and augmented reality, enhanced instrumentation, intraoperative data collection, analytics employing artificial intelligence/machine learning, telepresence connectivity, and robotic surgical platforms (Fig. 9.1).

The current growth of digital surgery is propelled by rapid advancements in computational capabilities, Internet connectivity, reduced hardware costs, and increased

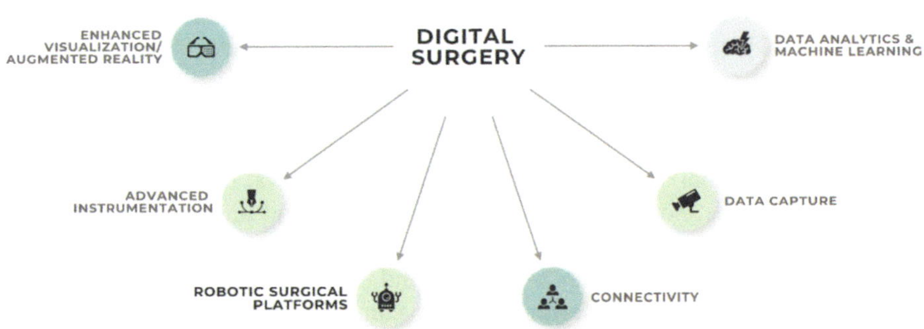

Fig. 9.1 Elements of digital surgery

J. Gootee · N. Szoka (✉)
Department of Surgery, West Virginia University, Morgantown, WV, USA
e-mail: nova.szoka@hsc.wvu.edu

S. Samreen et al. (eds.), *The SAGES Manual of Robotic Surgery*,
https://doi.org/10.1007/978-3-031-86927-3_9

comfort with integrating technology into surgical practice. Its potential spans from enhancing surgical accessibility and transparency in the operating room, to revolutionizing surgical education methodologies and establishing a global framework for surgical advancement. Ultimately, the overarching aim of this technological evolution is to enhance the quality of surgical care [1].

Advanced Visualization

3D Visualization

The utilization of three-dimensional visualization in surgery has shown promising potential in various aspects, including operative planning, procedure execution, acquisition of surgical skills, and patient outcomes. Comparative studies between 2D and 3D vision during the performance of Fundamentals of Laparoscopic Surgery tasks have demonstrated a reduction in time taken for task completion and enhancement in the ease and efficiency of task execution. The majority of robotic surgical platforms now offer 3D visualization capabilities, resulting in improved proficiency, faster task completion, and reduced errors [2, 3].

Fluorescence-Guided Surgery

Fluorescence-guided surgery (FGS) employs a fluorescent dye or a near-infrared-emitting light source in combination with a near-infrared camera to identify specific anatomical structures or assess tissue perfusion during surgical procedures [4, 5].

Visible or "white" light typically cannot penetrate through more than 1 mm of human tissue due to the high degree of diffusion and absorption from hemoglobin and water [6, 7]. NIR light wavelength uses the "optical window" wavelength to maximize light travel through human tissue and can penetrate up to 1–2 cm of tissue [8]. Visible light seen through human tissue appears pink. Pink light against a field of internal organs yields a low signal-to-background noise ratio. NIR light, visualized as green, maximizes the signal-to-background ratio vs. the surrounding red/pink organs. Studies show that a higher signal-to-noise ratio improves surgeon performance in terms of speed and accuracy [9]. Furthermore, multiple surgical camera systems enable views that overlay white light and -infrared light images that allows the surgeon to benefit from seeing the best elements of both types of images (Fig. 9.2).

Recent investigations comparing the use of indocyanine green (ICG) cholangiography to standard cholecystectomy procedures have shown significant benefits. These include reductions in operative time, decreased instances of common bile duct injury, rates of conversion to open surgery, duration of hospital stays, and mortality rates [4, 10]. Furthermore, ICG has been applied to visualize and quantify bowel perfusion in colorectal anastomoses, with certain studies indicating a decrease in anastomotic leak rates when employing this technique [11]. Currently, FGS

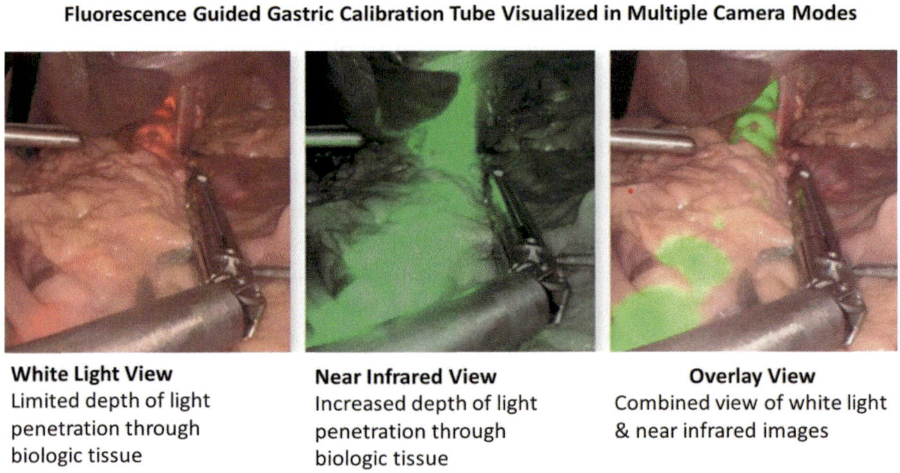

Fig. 9.2 Example of white light versus near-infrared light transmission through biological tissue, and an overlay view that combines white light and near-infrared light images

techniques are being adopted across most surgical specialties with benefits, including providing surgeons with increased visual cues and enabling more precise dissection within the operative field [5].

Augmented Reality

Augmented reality/mediated reality (AR/MR) is a technology that overlays computer-generated objects onto real-world images and video in real time. Positioned on a continuum between the real environment (direct view of the real world) and virtual reality (complete immersion in a digital environment), AR provides an interactive blend of real and virtual elements registered in three dimensions [12, 13]. The application of AR/MR to medical imaging data offers numerous advantages. Utilizing AR/MR-guided surgery, surgeons can maintain focused attention on the procedure without dividing their focus between navigation methods and the patient, leading to improved hand–eye coordination, accuracy, and time efficiency [14]. Moreover, AR/MR platforms facilitate stereoscopic/3D visualization of volumetric data, enhancing physician perception and aiding clinical decision-making.

The current implementation of AR/MR technology in surgery involves several key technologies, including medical imaging segmentation and modeling, tracking, registration, and visualization. These components form the foundation of AR/MR platforms, enabling the seamless integration of virtual elements with real-world surgical environments.

Image segmentation is a crucial process in medical imaging, involving the isolation of regions of interest and the creation of a model for interactive visualization of these areas. The datasets derived from medical imaging are often extensive, presenting challenges in real-time manipulation. Traditionally, the identification of relevant anatomy has relied on marking structures manually or semi-autonomously within each image. Despite the availability of several open-source packages to aid in this process, image segmentation remains a bottleneck for the clinical application of augmented reality (AR) surgical guidance.

Extensive research efforts are underway to develop autonomous image segmentation methods that are generalizable across different cases. However, the establishment of a proven and clinically accepted method is still pending due to multiple challenges, including unclear lesion boundaries, variation in lesion shapes, and difficulty due to similar contrast intensity between neighboring tissues.

Image registration is the process used to establish spatial correspondence between two or more image sets. The precise alignment of virtual images with the real environment is essential for the effective clinical application of augmented reality (AR) platforms. In the context of image-guided surgery, these image sets are typically categorized as static and moving, and algorithms are employed to determine the optimal translation that minimizes differences between the virtual and real environments.

Achieving accurate alignment involves the use of trackers to precisely determine the position and orientation of both the camera and the patient's body. Marker-based registration relies on rigid calibration of markers attached to real objects, enabling precise estimation of their positions as detected by external or internal sensors. Marker-free registration, on the other hand, leverages natural features observed by tracking devices within the real environment, such as the simultaneous localization and mapping (SLAM) technique used in Surgical Endoscopy [15]. Manual registration is also an option. However, registration becomes more challenging when the target organ does not behave as expected, particularly in general surgery where the anatomy is not rigid and undergoes dynamic deformations, such as those caused by respirations or heartbeat [13, 16].

Current Implementation

Augmented reality (AR) systems find optimal application during surgical procedures characterized by minimal movement in the real environment and limited tissue deformation. These scenarios require less complex tracking and processing, unlike surgeries involving mobile organs, where tracking and display present greater challenges. Consequently, AR systems have found successful clinical application in neurosurgery, orthopedics, and otolaryngology, encompassing tasks such as bone dissection, cerebral aneurysm clipping, microvascular decompression, and pedicle screw placement [17–20]. While AR systems demonstrate accurate registration (0.2–3 mm), they have been associated with increased operative time and financial costs [18, 21].

Abdominal surgery has posed challenges for AR implementation due to organ movement. Nevertheless, successful applications have been reported in liver and pancreatic surgery. In these cases, AR facilitates comparison between reconstructed virtual models and intraoperative ultrasound to identify lesions for resection [22]. Studies have also explored the superimposition of 3D representations of hepatobiliary structures onto the surgeon's field of view during open liver surgery [21]. Additionally, intraoperative AR has been utilized to detect sentinel lymph nodes accurately using preoperative SPECT/CT scans, and RSIP Vision has developed RSIP Neph. This is an AR tool used intraoperatively aiding surgeons with partial nephrectomies by precisely locating and resecting intracapsular renal lesions [23, 24].

Enhanced Instrumentation

The advancement and widespread adoption of robotic surgery are closely intertwined with the progression of surgical instrumentation. In traditional open surgery, surgeons directly manipulate conventional surgical tools, engaging with patient tissues firsthand, and receiving direct feedback. However, in minimally invasive surgery, this direct connection between surgeon and tissues is mediated by laparoscopic or robotic instruments, with visuals relayed through a video display [25].

Modern enhanced instrumentation incorporates various elements such as power systems, sensors, automation, and safety features to ensure consistent performance. Key areas of enhancement include intelligent staplers, energy devices, and roboticized instruments.

Recent developments in stapling technology have introduced powered staplers with automated firing mechanisms and tissue compression-sensing capabilities, resulting in well-formed, reliable staple lines [26, 27]. This technology has shown significant benefits, particularly in gastrointestinal surgeries. For instance, studies comparing outcomes between powered and manual staplers in bariatric surgery have demonstrated lower hospital costs and bleeding rates in the powered stapler group [28–30]. Similarly, the use of powered staplers in left-sided colorectal anastomosis has been associated with reduced leak rates, bleeding, ileus, readmission rates, hospital stays, and overall healthcare costs.

Advanced bipolar and ultrasonic energy devices have become standard in the operating room, featuring software algorithms to measure tissue impedance changes and adjust energy output accordingly. These devices offer advantages such as reduced risk of thermal injury, elimination of dispersive electrodes, enhanced sealing capabilities, decreased blood loss, and shorter procedure times [31–33].

Roboticized devices integrate robotic technology with hardware components to enhance surgical capabilities. Examples include the HandXTM, a powered laparoscopic device used for grasping, ligation, and suturing, and the Neoguide endoscope, which employs a computer algorithm to optimize scope movement within the bowel [34].

Data Capture

The operative setting gathers and applies a wealth of data, encompassing various sources. These encompass information from the operating room, such as personnel details, system processes, and quality metrics. Additionally, data from surgical equipment, kinematic data from robotic platforms, and information from the surgical field, such as video streams from image-guided platforms, contribute significantly. Moreover, there is a growing presence of integrated platforms aimed at enhancing data collection and exchange, often referred to as "Integrated Operating Rooms."

Video Data

As digital technology progresses, the opportunities for recording and sharing surgical videos have also advanced. These recordings encompass various aspects of the operative process and serve multiple purposes, including training, coaching, research, assessment, and quality improvement [43–48]. With the introduction of 4K and 8K video resolution, the volume of surgical video data is growing rapidly. Additionally, there are numerous commercially available solutions for secure cloud storage of video data, facilitating the upload of surgical videos without the need for USB drives, DVDs, or encrypted drives.

The efficacy of utilizing video to enhance performance has been extensively documented across various disciplines. Numerous studies highlight the advantages of surgical video recording [38, 47–54]. Medical trainees utilize videos to familiarize themselves with surgical anatomy, procedures, and technical intricacies, thereby preparing for cases more effectively. Curricula based on video content have demonstrated the ability to enhance knowledge base, improve technical performance, and shorten learning curves. Furthermore, a retrospective review of surgeons' videos, supplemented with expert critique, has been shown to positively impact patient outcomes [55, 56].

Surgical videos have also found their way onto social media platforms, where surgeons seek peer feedback or advice on operative approaches. As the benefits of intraoperative surgical video recording become increasingly apparent, surgeons performing open operations have begun adopting technologies to capture such cases. Saun et al. identified 176 clinical applications for open video recording and 125 different types of recording cameras used for capturing open intraoperative cases [48].

Multiple companies, including CMR Surgical, Intuitive, Medtronic, and Stryker, are developing visual medial platforms or "Hubs" that allow for video recording and storage, and enable video sharing or review, as well as virtual collaboration and learning. These systems can facilitate real-time consultation with offsite surgeons during challenging procedures.

Data from Operative Equipment

Kinematics refers to the examination of mechanical motion in points, bodies, and systems. In surgical robotics, kinematics serve the purpose of defining tool positions and joint positions concerning operator control and patient anatomy [40, 41]. Surgical robots have the capability to record precise instrument motion trajectories during procedures, allowing for the analysis of surgical activity beyond what traditional instruments can provide [42]. Understanding surgeon kinematics not only offers insights into operative efficiency but also aids in the development of autonomous robots in the future. Moreover, other operative instruments contributing valuable data include advanced energy devices and powered staplers, as discussed in the preceding section.

Data from the Operating Room and the "Integrated Operating Room"

Several tools are in place to gauge OR efficiency, among them surgical checklists and the Metric for Evaluating Task Execution in the Operating Room (METEOR). These tools undertake data collection, analysis, evaluation, iterative correction, and dissemination to staff and institutions [35–37]. Drawing inspiration from the aviation industry's use of a "black box" recording device to monitor extensive flight data for real-time and future analysis, similar approaches have been adapted for OR settings. Commercially available platforms like the OR Black Box (based in Toronto, ON, Canada) enable the capture of audio, visual, and other data related to various aspects of a procedure, both within the operative field and the operating room itself (e.g., tracking team members). Artificial intelligence and machine learning are employed to assist teams in enhancing quality and efficiency. These systems are designed to detect and redact personal information of patients and providers while retaining clinically relevant data. Additionally, they have the potential to identify intraoperative errors, events, and distractions [38, 39].

Integrated or Digital Operating Rooms are setups designed to seamlessly integrate the OR environment, allowing different equipment sources to interact effectively. These installations often comprise high-resolution video displays, video routing systems, touch-screen controls, digital information archiving capabilities, and a central hub linking multiple ORs internally and externally. Besides streamlining workflows for surgical teams and enhancing safety measures, Integrated ORs facilitate live consultations with medical teams (e.g., pathology), real-time collaboration with virtual surgeons, data exchange with electronic medical record systems, and live feeds for training or educational purposes.

Caresyntax is a vendor-neutral, enterprise-focused surgical data platform that uses proprietary software and AI capabilities, to analyze extensive data streams, including video, audio, images, device data, clinical records, and operational metrics from operating rooms. This real-time information aids surgical teams during procedures and is accessible remotely via a telehealth link. Post-surgery, the platform offers invaluable insights for surgeons to benchmark and refine their practices, enables hospital administrators to optimize resource allocation, supports medical device companies in developing superior products, and assists insurance companies in risk assessment and policy tailoring. Currently, the platform is deployed in over 2800 operating rooms globally, facilitating over 3 million surgical procedures annually [a].

Data Analytics

Artificial Intelligence

The landscape of everyday life has been transformed by data analytics, driven by the convergence of three key trends: advancements in computer processors leading to faster and smaller devices, the application of proven statistical methods, and the availability of vast datasets. This transformation is now extending into healthcare [13].

Artificial intelligence (AI) stands out as a prominent area within analytics, characterized by its aim to develop systems capable of emulating human thought and behavior. In the context of surgery, AI applications often revolve around machine learning (ML), where machines can learn from data and make predictions by identifying patterns. ML techniques, such as supervised and unsupervised learning, enable computers to make predictions based on partial data labeling or the inherent structure within the data [57].

A subset of machine learning called artificial neural networks (ANNs) process signals through layers of simple computational units. ANNs excel in handling multidimensional, covariate data, unlike traditional regression methods. Deep learning, which involves applying one or more ANNs to create systems capable of executing tasks autonomously or semi-autonomously, represents an exciting frontier in AI.

In healthcare, computer vision—a field focused on machines' understanding and interpreting pixelated data, such as images and videos—is gaining traction. While current applications are more prevalent in fields like radiology and pathology, computer-aided diagnosis is a rapidly growing area with significant potential in healthcare [54–59].

In surgery specifically, AI holds promise in various areas, including real-time decision support, surgical education, risk prediction, process optimization, resource management, and even autonomous surgery.

Surgical Decision-Making

Across various surgical subspecialties, AI holds promise in predicting outcomes, preventing complications and missed diagnoses, alleviating the cognitive burden on busy physicians, and facilitating more informed discussions between physicians and patients [60]. AI applications in image recognition have particularly significant implications, aiding both radiologists and surgeons in disease detection and evaluation.

The application of AI in image recognition extends to enhancing endoscopic cancer screening, a technique proven to enhance adenoma detection during colonoscopy [61]. Moreover, computer vision has been employed intraoperatively. Evidence suggests that many surgical adverse events stem from errors in judgment and decision-making during surgery. AI presents a potential solution by augmenting surgeons' mental models during procedures.

Proof-of-concept algorithms have been developed primarily in the context of laparoscopic cholecystectomy. Examples include GoNoGoNet, which identifies safe and dangerous areas of dissection to prevent major bile duct injuries, and CVSNet, which confirms the achievement of a Critical View of Safety [62, 63]. Additionally, ML algorithms are utilized in patient flow and operative resource management tasks, including estimating case length, coordinating between the operating room and post-anesthesia care unit, and predicting case cancellations [64].

Skills Assessment

Peer-rated surgical skill strongly correlates with surgical outcomes, demonstrating predictive power even when surgeries are not rated by other surgeons [65]. Skill assessments can even be performed by trained lay individuals with similar predictive accuracy [66]. The field of automated skill assessment explores whether AI systems can perform similar assessments of surgeon skill automatically. Such systems could play a crucial role in resident training and evaluation, as well as in mentoring or providing remediation for practicing surgeons.

Currently, AI skill assessment systems that have shown promising results in trials typically combine automated kinematic metrics with skill metrics generated by human observers. These metrics are then fed into neural networks (NN) for analysis [67]. However, fully automated skill assessments remain challenging, particularly due to the complexity of evaluating skills such as tissue respect and needle handling.

Despite the challenges, AI-generated assessments of technical skill have demonstrated good agreement with human graders for specific surgical tasks. Nonetheless, issues persist regarding consistency, generalizability, and the ability to provide actionable feedback to surgeons [68, 69].

Patient Care

Utilizing the extensive American College of Surgeons National Surgical Quality Improvement Program (ACS-NSQIP) database, a predictive algorithm based on machine learning was developed to enhance risk prediction [70]. NNs have demonstrated effectiveness in detecting breast, skin and lung cancers, as well as in predicting outcomes for surgical patients [71–73].

In critical care settings, AI-driven tools have the potential to forecast clinical deterioration in patient hours before it occurs. Experimental systems have shown promise in autonomously determining appropriate treatment strategies for patients once they deteriorate [74, 75]. For instance, a machine learning-based hypotension prediction algorithm has been shown to reduce the time spent in a hypotensive state compared to standard care in a randomized single-center trial [76]. AI systems can be utilized to augment and lessen the burden on physician's decision-making [77].

Automated Surgery

Surgery demands proficiency in several fundamental areas: perception (the ability to discern tissues and planes), intelligence (the capacity to decide how to manipulate tissues), and dexterity (the skill to manipulate tissues themselves). Various autonomous or semi-autonomous surgical systems already exhibit some or all of these capabilities, including the CyberKnife system that is utilized for stereotactic body radiotherapy [78].

In the realm of abdominal and soft-tissue surgery, the pliability, distensibility, and complexity of tissues pose challenges to AI autonomy. Present robotic platforms, like the DaVinci Surgical System, primarily function as surgical "assistants," stabilizing instruments and interpreting movements rather than executing movements themselves. Nevertheless, there is optimism regarding the potential for autonomous surgery to expand into gastrointestinal procedures. In laboratory settings, autonomous surgical AIs have demonstrated proficiency in basic tasks such as cutting simulated 2D and 3D tissues and peg transfer [79, 80].

Among these developments, the Smart Tissue Anastomosis Robot (STAR) stands out as one of the most feature-complete AI systems for automated soft-tissue surgery. STAR, an automated suturing robot, has, in porcine models, successfully completed laparoscopic bowel anastomoses [81]. However, it is worth noting that despite these advancements, this AI system still relies on an experienced surgeon to align and suture the bowel for anastomosis.

Connectivity

The digital surgery aspect of connectivity encompasses innovative methods of linking surgeon to surgeon, such as telementoring in educational and clinical settings, as well as connecting surgeon to patient through telesurgery.

Several factors converge to necessitate increased access to surgical care and education beyond the traditional model of in-person surgery. The most apparent factor is the constraints imposed during the COVID-19 pandemic. Virtual access became imperative as in-person attendance became challenging or impossible. This challenge affected everyone from students contemplating a career in medicine to surgical residents and fellows. Practicing surgeons were also impacted. Those motivated to enhance their surgical skills found themselves unable to attend training courses or have proctors visit their facilities. Many sites had to suspend elective operations completely secondary due to equipment limitations or hospital capacity.

Telementoring

Even prior to the onset of the COVID-19 pandemic, there has been a growing disparity between the available learning opportunities and surgical learners. The number of students and trainees surpassing the capacity of hospitals to offer adequate access to operative training experiences. This issue has been exacerbated by the implementation of work-hour restrictions and decreasing autonomy for learners.

Education

Given current surgical training program volumes and population growth rates, projections indicate a potential deficit of nearly 30,000 surgeons by the year 2030 [82]. Addressing this shortfall is estimated to require an additional investment of approximately $10 billion in training efforts. While this presents a significant challenge, it also offers an opportunity to reevaluate training paradigms.

The SAGES Project 6 working group has identified five key areas of basic technical requirements for telementoring: safety, reliability, transmission quality, ease of use, and cost [83]. Additionally, elements of a digital surgery training experience include advanced analysis of surgical video, recording video for later review, and telestration [84].

Telementoring in the context of trainees differs from that for practicing surgeons due to factors such as a more variable skill set, work-hour limitations, the need to meet specific educational requirements, and the presence of a supervising attending.

A telementoring program designed for educational purposes should adhere to evidence-based practices in curriculum development, mentor evaluation, and mentee assessment. Components of a "train the trainer" program and mentee development have been outlined as part of the SAGES Project 6 initiative by Augestad et al [85, 86].

Clinical Practice

Surgical telementoring for clinical practice has been effectively employed for over two decades in various capacities. For instance, in 1998, Rosser et al. utilized teleproctoring to guide doctors in rural Ecuador, a safe laparoscopic cholecystectomy for patients [87]. Fast forward to 2020, amidst the COVID-19 pandemic, telementoring facilitated a valve-in-valve transcatheter mitral valve replacement for an 82-year-old patient through real-time bidirectional audiovisual communication and digital transmission of live videos, enabling direct observation of the operative field by a remote proctor [88]. Numerous other instances of successful surgical telementoring leading to positive clinical outcomes have been documented in the literature [89–92].

Two primary applications of surgical telementoring in clinical practice are virtual intraoperative consultation and skill acquisition. Skill acquisition involves scenarios where a remote mentor surgeon guides the mentee through an entire operation. This application is particularly valuable for performing new or complex procedures, allowing surgeons to undertake such operations with virtual guidance from an experienced proctor. It also enhances the capabilities of local hospitals to offer more complex procedures while mitigating risks associated with performing new or complex procedures without assistance.

Virtual Surgical Assist is another application wherein a surgeon can receive real-time intraoperative consultation during challenging operations, especially when physical consultation is not feasible or would cause delays. This approach can be useful during after-hours, in cases of unexpected findings (such as masses or abnormal anatomy), or in settings where surgeons with the necessary expertise are not physically available. Virtual Surgical Assist brings advanced surgical expertise to local sites, thereby leading to reducing the amount of transfers to tertiary care facilities.

Currently, Skill Acquisition is actively growing, whereas Virtual Surgical Assist is not frequently utilized, primarily due to systemic limitations in implementation [93].

Telesurgery

Telesurgery refers to remote surgeries conducted when the surgeon is not physically present at the patient's location. Manipulation of tissues and equipment and visualization are achieved through teleoperation [94].

The pioneering instance of telesurgery occurred in 2001 with a transatlantic robotic cholecystectomy performed by Dr. Jacques Marescaux. In this groundbreaking procedure, the surgical team was located in New York while the patient was in Strasbourg, France [95, 96]. Subsequently, in 2003, two Canadian hospitals established the first telerobotic surgical service, successfully completing 21 telerobotic surgeries without serious complications or the need for conversions to open operations [97]. Most of the current experience in telesurgery involves the use of inanimate models for simulation and training purposes [98, 99].

Robotic Surgical Platforms

Minimally invasive robotic-assisted surgery (RAS) since the late 1990s has served as a pathway to integrate technological advancements into minimally invasive surgical techniques. Over the past decade, there has been a rapid increase in the number of robotic endoscopic and surgical platforms available [100].

A study conducted in Michigan examining the use of robotic surgery reported a notable rise in the utilization of robotic surgery for general surgical procedures, increasing from 1.8% in 2012 to 15.1% in 2018, accompanied by a decline in laparoscopic surgery [101].

In the surgical field, there are three primary types of robotic systems: active systems, which autonomously perform preprogrammed tasks; semi-active systems, which allow for a combination of surgeon-driven and preprogrammed elements; and fully surgeon-dependent systems.

Robotic surgery platforms typically feature either open or closed consoles. In closed console systems, the surgeon can stabilize their head position for consistent viewing, leading to a standardized field of view. On the other hand, open console systems do not restrict the operator's head position, allowing for free movement during the operation. Although head movement in open console systems may potentially decrease efficiency, it enables improved communication between the surgeon and team members as the surgeon is not confined behind a closed console.

In the United States, currently there are four FDA-approved robotic platforms for general surgery. Table 9.1 shows the aspects of each system that is either FDA or CE approved. The Senhance from Asensus Surgical, MIRA by Virtual Incision (the world's first miniaturized robotic system) and the Da Vinci Xi and Single Port Systems from Intuitive. Additionally, there are two platforms, Versius by CMR Surgical and Hugo by Medtronic, which are currently in use in Europe and awaiting FDA approval. The market for robotic surgical platforms continues to expand, with novel modalities emerging, featuring reduced costs and smaller sizes [102]. Currently, there are over 20 robotic surgical platforms under development, including SPORTTM Surgical System by Titan Medical, Ottava by Johnson & Johnson, Beta 2 by Vicarious Surgical, and MicroSurge by the DLR Institute of Robotics and Mechatronics.

An additional term to become familiar with is robot-assisted "digital laparoscopy," which refers to robotic systems that can utilize familiar laparoscopic instruments and conventional trocars from laparoscopic surgery. This allows for greater control in laparoscopy and increased OR efficiency. Currently, the Senhance and Versius systems enable a digital laparoscopy-type approach.

Significant growth has also been observed in endoluminal robotics, particularly for laparoendoscopic single-port surgery (LESS) and natural orifice transluminal endoscopic surgery (NOTES). These approaches aim to minimize collateral tissue damage. Examples of such systems include the NeoGuide endoscopy system, a computer-aided colonoscope utilizing real-time 3D computerized mapping to navigate the natural curves of the colon; the FlexR robotic system from Medrobotics Corp., a joystick-controlled single-port platform used in surgeries of the oropharynx, hypopharynx, and larynx; and STRAS from iCUBE, a flexible endoscopic system developed for single-port intraluminal surgery.

Table 9.1 Comparison of robotic surgical platforms

Robotic platform	Company	FDA status	Robotic segments	Console	Enhanced visualization	Advanced instrumentation	Data capture/analytics	Connectivity
Da Vinci Xi Multi Port	Intuitive Surgical Inc	Approved	4—Boom mounted	Closed	3D image Firefly—NIR fluorescence imaging	Endowrist instruments including 7 degrees of freedom	Instrument usage Kinematic Analytics	Remote case observation Telemonitoring
Da Vinci Xi Single Port	Intuitive Surgical Inc	Approved	4—Boom mounted	Closed	3D image Firefly—NIR fluorescence imaging	Endowrist instruments including 7 degrees of freedom	Video Instrument usage Kinematic Analytics	Remote case observation Telemonitoring
Senhance	Asensus Surgical	Approved	3—Modular	Open	3D image Eye tracking camera control Intelligent Surgical Unit™ (ISU™) for machine vision available in EU	7 degrees of freedom and haptic sensing	Video	Senhance Connect enables remote case observation & telemonitoring
Mira	Virtual Incision	Approved	2—Table mounted	Open	Robotically controlled camera NIR fluorescence imaging under development	Inserted through a single port	Video Telemetry data	Telementoring & telesurgery under development
Versius	CMR surgical	CE approval, awaiting FDA approval	4—Modular	Open	vLimeLite NIR fluorescence imaging	V-wrist technology gives full wristed instruments	Video Telemetry data Versius Clinical Insights for analytics	
Hugo	Medtronic	CE approval, awaiting FDA approval	4—Modular	Open	3D image	7 degrees of freedom and minimizing hand tremors	Video Touch Surgery for analytics	

NIR near infrared, *EU* European Union

Barriers to Implementation

Multiple barriers are present in all domains of digital surgery, including advanced visualization, enhanced instrumentation, data capture, analytics, increased connectivity, and robotic surgical platforms. One major barrier includes the cost of implementation of newer technological devices and showing that the benefits of these devices offset the increased costs. An additional concern raised with the increased collection of data is concerns for patient confidentiality and sharing patient data.

Conclusion

Digital surgery represents an emerging technology with significant potential to add value across all tiers of the healthcare system. It includes multiple domains, including advanced visualization, enhanced instrumentation, data capture, analytics, increased connectivity, and robotic surgical platforms. These technologies herald a transformative revolution that will profoundly impact the surgical landscape. Surgeons occupy a pivotal role in steering these advancements and collaborating with other stakeholders to uphold the utmost safety and quality within this evolving paradigm. Their unique expertise and insights are crucial for navigating the integration of digital surgical innovations effectively. Through active engagement and collaboration, surgeons can ensure that these technologies are harnessed to their fullest potential, ultimately enhancing patient outcomes and advancing the field of surgery.

Author Disclosures Dr. Szoka is the founder of Endolumik Inc. and a consultant for CSATS.

References

1. Atallah S, editor. Digital surgery. 1st ed. Cham: Springer; 2020.
2. Guanà R, Ferrero L, Garofalo S, Cerrina A, Cussa D, Arezzo A, et al. Skills comparison in pediatric residents using a 2-dimensional versus a 3-dimensional high-definition camera in a pediatric laparoscopic simulator. J Surg Educ. 2017;74(4):644–9. https://doi.org/10.1016/j.jsurg.2016.12.002.
3. Tanagho YS, Andriole GL, Paradis AG, Madison KM, Sandhu GS, Varela JE, et al. 2D versus 3D visualization: impact on laparoscopic proficiency using the fundamentals of laparoscopic surgery skill set. J Laparoendosc Adv Surg Tech A. 2012;22(9):865–70. https://doi.org/10.1089/lap.2012.0220.
4. Reinhart MB, Huntington CR, Blair LJ, Heniford BT, Augen-stein VA. Indocyanine green: historical context, current applications, and future considerations. Surg Innov. 2016;23(2):166–75. https://doi.org/10.1177/1553350615604053.
5. Szoka N, Renton D, Horgan S, editors. The SAGES manual of fluorescence-guided surgery. Springer; 2023. https://doi.org/10.1007/978-3-031-40685-0.
6. Belia F, et al. The Use of Indocyanine Green (ICG) and Near-Infrared (NIR) fluorescence-guided imaging in gastric cancer surgery: a narrative review. Front Surg. 2022;9:880773.
7. Wang TD, Van Dam J. Optical biopsy: a new frontier in endoscopic detection and diagnosis. Clin Gastroenterol Hepatol. 2004;2(9):744–53.
8. Gioux S, et al. Image-guided surgery using invisible near-infrared light: fundamentals of clinical translation. Mol Imaging. 2010;9(5):237–55.

9. Azargoshasb S, Boekestijn I, Roestenberg M, et al. Quantifying the impact of signal-to-background ratios on surgical discrimination of fluorescent lesions. Mol Imaging Biol. 2022;25(1):180–9.
10. Broderick RC, Lee AM, Cheverie JN, Zhao B, Blitzer RR, Patel RJ, et al. Fluorescent cholangiography significantly improves patient outcomes for laparoscopic cholecystectomy. Surg Endosc. 2021;35(10):5729–39. https://doi.org/10.1007/s00464-020-08045-x.
11. Blanco-Colino R, Espin-Basany E. Intraoperative use of ICG fluorescence imaging to reduce the risk of anastomotic leakage in colorectal surgery: a systematic review and meta-analysis. Tech Coloproctol. 2018;22(1):15–23. https://doi.org/10.1007/s10151-017-1731-8.
12. Gupta A, Ruijters D, Flexman ML. Augmented reality for interventional procedures. Digital surgery. Springer; 2021.
13. SAGES Digital Surgery Working Group, Ali JT, Yang G, Green CA, Reed BL, Madani A, Ponsky TA, Hazey J, Rothenberg SS, Schlachta CM, Oleynikov D, Szoka N. Defining digital surgery: a SAGES white paper. Surg Endosc. 2024;38(2):475–87. https://doi.org/10.1007/s00464-023-10551-7.
14. Cham Shuhaiber JH. Augmented reality in surgery. Arch Surg. 2004;139(2):170–4. https://doi.org/10.1001/archsurg.139.2.170.
15. Mountney P, Yang G-Z. Motion compensated SLAM for image guided surgery. Med Image Comput Comput Assist Interv. 2010;13(Pt 2):496–504. https://doi.org/10.1007/978-3-642-15745-5_61.
16. Bernhardt S, Nicolau SA, Soler L, Doignon C. The status of augmented reality in laparoscopic surgery as of 2016. Med Image Anal. 2017;37:66–90. https://doi.org/10.1016/j.media.2017.01.007.
17. Gmeiner M, Dirnberger J, Fenz W, Gollwitzer M, Wurm G, Trenkler J, et al. Virtual cerebral aneurysm clipping with real-time haptic force feedback in neurosurgical education. World Neurosurg. 2018;112:e313–23. https://doi.org/10.1016/j.wneu.2018.01.042.
18. Gsaxner C. Augmented reality in oral and maxillofacial surgery. Computer-aided oral and maxillofacial surgery. Cambridge: Academic; 2021.
19. Kang X, Azizian M, Wilson E, Wu K, Martin AD, Kane TD, et al. Stereoscopic augmented reality for laparoscopic surgery. Surg Endosc. 2014;28(7):2227–35. https://doi.org/10.1007/s00464-014-3433-x.
20. Xin B, Huang X, Wan W, Lv K, Hu Y, Wang J, et al. The efficacy of immersive virtual reality surgical simulator training for pedicle screw placement: a randomized double-blind controlled trial. Int Orthop. 2020;44(5):927–34. https://doi.org/10.1007/s00264-020-04488-y.
21. Gavaghan KA, Peterhans M, Oliveira-Santos T, Weber S. A portable image overlay projection device for computer-aided open liver surgery. IEEE Trans Biomed Eng. 2011;58(6):1855–64. https://doi.org/10.1109/TBME.2011.2126572.
22. Reitinger B, Bornik A, Beichel R, Schmalstieg D. Liver surgery planning using virtual reality. IEEE Comput Graph Appl. 2006;26(6):36–47. https://doi.org/10.1109/mcg.2006.131.
23. Wendler T, Herrmann K, Schnelzer A, Lasser T, Traub J, Kutter O, et al. First demonstration of 3-D lymphatic mapping in breast cancer using freehand SPECT. Eur J Nucl Med Mol Imaging. 2010;37(8):1452–61. https://doi.org/10.1007/s00259-010-1430-4.
24. RSIP Vision. 2023. RSIP Neph announces a revolutionary intra-op solution for partial nephrectomy surgeries. PR News-wire. https://www.prnewswire.com/news-releases/rsip-neph-announces-a-revolutionary-intra-op-solution-for-partial-nephrectomy-surgeries-301731484.html. Accessed 10 Mar 2024.
25. Dario P, Hannaford B, Menciassi A. Smart surgical tools and augmenting devices. IEEE Trans Rob Autom. 2003;19(5):782–92. https://doi.org/10.1109/tra.2003.817071.
26. Gaidry AD, Tremblay L, Nakayama D, Ignacio RC Jr. The history of surgical staplers: a combination of Hungarian, Russian, and American innovation. Am Surg. 2019;85(6):563–6. https://doi.org/10.1177/000313481908500617.
27. Kim J-S, Park S-H, Kim N-S, Lee IY, Jung HS, Ahn H-M, et al. Compression automation of circular stapler for preventing compression injury on gastrointestinal anastomosis. Int J Med Robot. 2022;18(3):e2374. https://doi.org/10.1002/rcs.2374.

28. Roy S, Yoo A, Yadalam S, Fegelman EJ, Kalsekar I, Johnston SS. Comparison of economic and clinical outcomes between patients undergoing laparoscopic bariatric surgery with powered versus manual endoscopic surgical staplers. J Med Econ. 2017;20(4):423–33. https://doi.org/10.1080/13696998.2017.1296453.
29. Pla-Martí V, Martín-Arévalo J, Moro-Valdezate D, García- Botello S, Mora-Oliver I, Gadea-Mateo R, et al. Impact of the novel powered circular stapler on risk of anastomotic leakage in colorectal anastomosis: a propensity score-matched study. Tech Coloproctol. 2021;25(3):279–84. https://doi.org/10.1007/s10151-020-02338-y.
30. Eickhoff A, Van Dam J, Jakobs R, Kudis V, Hartmann D, Damian U, Weickert U, Schilling D, Riemann JF. Computer assisted colonoscopy (the neoguide endoscopy system): results of the first human clinical trial. Am J Gastroenterol. 2007;102:261–6.
31. Rothstein DH, Raval MV. Operating room efficiency. Semin Pediatr Surg. 2018;27(2):79–85. https://doi.org/10.1053/j.sempedsurg.2018.02.004.
32. Mayer EK, Sevdalis N, Rout S, Caris J, Russ S, Mansell J, et al. Surgical checklist implementation project: the impact of variable WHO checklist compliance on risk-adjusted clinical outcomes after national implementation. A longitudinal study. Ann Surg. 2016;263(1):58–63. https://doi.org/10.1097/sla.0000000000001185.
33. Russ S, Arora S, Wharton R, Wheelock A, Hull L, Sharma E, et al. Measuring safety and efficiency in the operating room: development and validation of a metric for evaluating task execution in the operating room. J Am Coll Surg. 2013;216(3):472–81. https://doi.org/10.1016/j.jamcollsurg.2012.12.013.
34. Ayas S, Gordon L, Donmez B, Grantcharov T. The effect of intraoperative distractions on severe technical events in laparoscopic bariatric surgery. Surg Endosc. 2021;35(8):4569–80. https://doi.org/10.1007/s00464-020-07878-w.
35. Jung JJ, Jüni P, Lebovic G, Grantcharov T. First-year analysis of the operating room black box study. Ann Surg. 2020;271(1):122–7. https://doi.org/10.1097/sla.0000000000002863.
36. Okamura AM. ICRA lecture 2: kinematics and control of medical robots. In: ICRA 2016 tutorial on medical robotics. 2016.
37. Kuo C-H, Dai JS, Dasgupta P. Kinematic design considerations for minimally invasive surgical robots: an overview: kinematic design considerations for MIS robots. Int J Med Robot. 2012;8(2):127–45. https://doi.org/10.1002/rcs.453.
38. van Amsterdam B, Clarkson MJ, Stoyanov D. Gesture recognition in robotic surgery: a review. IEEE Trans Biomed Eng. 2021;68(6):2021–35. https://doi.org/10.1109/tbme.2021.3054828.
39. Green CA, Kim EH, O'Sullivan PS, Chern H. Using technological advances to improve surgery curriculum: experience with a mobile application. J Surg Educ. 2018;75(4):1087–95. https://doi.org/10.1016/j.jsurg.2017.12.005.
40. Catchpole K, Perkins C, Bresee C, Solnik MJ, Sherman B, Fritch J, et al. Safety, efficiency and learning curves in robotic surgery: a human factors analysis. Surg Endosc. 2016;30(9):3749–61. https://doi.org/10.1007/s00464-015-4671-2.
41. Weigl M, Weber J, Hallett E, Pfandler M, Schlenker B, Becker A, et al. Associations of intraoperative flow disruptions and operating room teamwork during robotic-assisted radical prostatectomy. Urology. 2018;114:105–13. https://doi.org/10.1016/j.urology.2017.11.060.
42. Law KE, Ray RD, D'Angelo ALD, Cohen ER, DiMarco SM, Linsmeier E, et al. Exploring senior residents' intraoperative error management strategies: a potential measure of performance improvement. J Surg Educ. 2016;73(6):e64–70. https://doi.org/10.1016/j.jsurg.2016.05.016.
43. Ibrahim AM, Varban OA, Dimick JB. Novel uses of video to accelerate the surgical learning curve. J Laparoendosc Adv Surg Tech A. 2016;26(4):240–2. https://doi.org/10.1089/lap.2016.
44. Pollack E, Johnston S, Petraiuolo WJ, Roy S, Galvain T. Economic analysis of leak complications in anastomoses performed with powered versus manual circular staplers in left-sided colorectal resections: a US-based cost analysis. Clinicoecon Outcomes Res. 2021;13:531–40. https://doi.org/10.2147/ceor.s3052960100.

45. Levy B, Emery L. Randomized trial of suture versus electrosurgical bipolar vessel sealing in vaginal hysterectomy. Obstet Gynecol. 2003;102(1):147–51. https://doi.org/10.1016/s0029-7844(03)00405-8.
46. Sutton C, Abbott J. History of power sources in endoscopic surgery. J Minim Invasive Gynecol. 2013;20(3):271–8. https://doi.org/10.1016/j.jmig.2013.03.001.
47. Singleton D, Chekan E, Davison M, Mennone J, Hinoul P. Consistency and sealing of advanced bipolar tissue sealers. Med Devices (Auckl). 2015;8:193–9. https://doi.org/10.2147/mder.s79642.
48. Saun TJ, Zuo KJ, Grantcharov TP. Video technologies for recording open surgery: a systematic review. Surg Innov. 2019;26(5):599–612. https://doi.org/10.1177/1553350619853099.
49. Abdelsattar JM, Pandian TK, Finnesgard EJ, El Khatib MM, Rowse PG, Buckarma ENH, et al. Do you see what I see? How we use video as an adjunct to general surgery resident education. J Surg Educ. 2015;72(6):e145–50. https://doi.org/10.1016/j.jsurg.2015.07.012.
50. Isaacson D, Green C, Topp K, O'Sullivan P, Kim E. Guided laparoscopic video tutorials for medical student instruction in abdominal anatomy. Mededportal. 2017;13(1):10559. https://doi.org/10.15766/mep_2374-8265.10559.
51. Dominguez CO, Flach JM, McKellar DP, Dunn M. Using videotaped cases to elicit perceptual expertise in laparoscopic surgery. In: Proceedings third annual symposium on human interaction with complex systems HICS'96. IEEE Computer Society Press; 2002.
52. Mazer L, Varban O, Montgomery JR, Awad MM, Schulman A. Video is better: why aren't we using it? A mixed-methods study of the barriers to routine procedural video recording and case review. Surg Endosc. 2022;36(2):1090–7. https://doi.org/10.1007/s00464-021-08375-4.
53. Green JL, Suresh V, Bittar P, Ledbetter L, Mithani SK, Allori A. The utilization of video technology in surgical education: a systematic review. J Surg Res. 2019;235:171–80. https://doi.org/10.1016/j.jss.2018.09.015.
54. Hu Y-Y, Mazer LM, Yule SJ, Arriaga AF, Greenberg CC, Lipsitz SR, et al. Complementing operating room teaching with video-based coaching. JAMA Surg. 2017;152(4):318–25. https://doi.org/10.1001/jamasurg.2016.4619.
55. Stulberg JJ, Huang R, Kreutzer L, Ban K, Champagne BJ, Steele SR, et al. Association between surgeon technical skills and patient outcomes. JAMA Surg. 2020;155(10):960–8. https://doi.org/10.1001/jamasurg.2020.3007.
56. Grenda TR, Pradarelli JC, Dimick JB. Using surgical video to improve technique and skill. Ann Surg. 2016;264(1):32–3. https://doi.org/10.1097/sla.0000000000001592.
57. Hashimoto DA, Rosman G, Rus D, Meireles OR. Artificial intelligence in surgery: promises and perils. Ann Surg. 2018;268(1):70–6. https://doi.org/10.1097/sla.0000000000002693.
58. Ward TM, Mascagni P, Ban Y, Rosman G, Padoy N, Meireles O, et al. Computer vision in surgery. Surgery. 2021;169(5):1253–6. https://doi.org/10.1016/j.surg.2020.10.039.
59. Mascagni P, Alapatt D, Sestini L, Altieri MS, Madani A, Wata-nabe Y, et al. Computer vision in surgery: from potential to clinical value. NPJ Digit Med. 2022; https://doi.org/10.1038/s41746-022-00707-5.
60. Loftus TJ, Tighe PJ, Filiberto AC, Efron PA, Brakenridge SC, Mohr AM, et al. Artificial intelligence and surgical decision-making. JAMA Surg. 2020;155(2):148–58. https://doi.org/10.1001/jamasurg.2019.4917.
61. Urban G, Tripathi P, Alkayali T, Mittal M, Jalali F, Karnes W, et al. Deep learning localizes and identifies polyps in real time with 96% accuracy in screening colonoscopy. Gastroenterology. 2018;155(4):1069–1078.e8. https://doi.org/10.1053/j.gastro.2018.06.037.
62. Madani A, Namazi B, Altieri MS, Hashimoto DA, Rivera AM, Pucher PH, et al. Artificial intelligence for intraoperative guidance: using semantic segmentation to identify surgical anatomy during laparoscopic cholecystectomy. Ann Surg. 2022;276(2):363–9. https://doi.org/10.1097/sla.0000000000004594.
63. Zhang X, Chen F, Yu T, An J, Huang Z, Liu J, et al. Real-time gastric polyp detection using convolutional neural networks. PLoS One. 2019;14(3):e0214133. https://doi.org/10.1371/journal.pone.0214133.

64. Bellini V, Guzzon M, Bigliardi B, Mordonini M, Filippelli S, Bignami E. Artificial Intelligence: a new tool in operating room management. Role of machine learning models in operating room optimization. J Med Syst. 2019;44(1):20. https://doi.org/10.1007/s10916-019-1512-1.
65. Wang P, Liu X, Berzin TM, Glissen Brown JR, Liu P, Zhou C, et al. Effect of a deep-learning computer-aided detection system on adenoma detection during colonoscopy (CADe-DB trial): a double-blind randomized study. Lancet Gastroenterol Hepatol. 2020;5(4):343–51. https://doi.org/10.1016/S2468-1253(19)30411-X.
66. Mascagni P, Vardazaryan A, Alapatt D, Urade T, Emre T, Fiorillo C, et al. Artificial intelligence for surgical safety: automatic assessment of the critical view of safety in laparoscopic cholecystectomy using deep learning. Ann Surg. 2022;275(5):955–61. https://doi.org/10.1097/SLA.0000000000004351.
67. Birkmeyer JD, Finks JF, O'reilly A, Oerline M, Carlin AM, Nunn AR, et al. Michigan bariatric surgery collaborative. Surgical skill and complication rates after bariatric surgery. N Engl J Med. 2013;369:1434–42.
68. Katz AJ. The role of crowdsourcing in assessing surgical skills. Surg Laparosc Endosc Percutan Tech. 2016;26:271–7.
69. Hung AJ, Chen J, Gill IS. Automated performance metrics and machine learning algorithms to measure surgeon performance and anticipate clinical outcomes in robotic surgery. JAMA Surg. 2018; https://doi.org/10.1001/jamasurg.2018.1512.
70. Bertsimas D, Dunn J, Velmahos GC, Kaafarani HMA. Surgical risk is not linear: derivation and validation of a novel, user-friendly, and machine-learning-based predictive OpTimal Trees in Emergency Surgery Risk (POTTER) calculator: derivation and validation of a novel, user-friendly, and machine-learning-based predictive OpTimal trees in emergency surgery risk (POTTER) calculator. Ann Surg. 2018;268(4):574–83. https://doi.org/10.1097/SLA.0000000000002956.
71. Loftus TJ, Vlaar APJ, Hung AJ, Bihorac A, Dennis BM, Juillard C, et al. Executive summary of the artificial intelligence in surgery series. Surgery. 2022;171(5):1435–9. https://doi.org/10.1016/j.surg.2021.10.047.
72. Cheng J-Z, Ni D, Chou Y-H, Qin J, Tiu C-M, Chang Y-C, et al. Computer-aided diagnosis with deep learning architecture: applications to breast lesions in US images and pulmonary nodules in CT scans. Sci Rep. 2016;6(1):24454. https://doi.org/10.1038/srep24454.
73. Esteva A, Kuprel B, Novoa RA, Ko J, Swetter SM, Blau HM, et al. Dermatologist-level classification of skin cancer with deep neural networks. Nature. 2017;542(7639):115–8. https://doi.org/10.1038/nature21056.
74. Donald R, Howells T, Piper I, Enblad P, Nilsson P, Chambers I, et al. Forewarning of hypotensive events using a Bayesian artificial neural network in neurocritical care. J Clin Monit Comput. 2019;33(1):39–51. https://doi.org/10.1007/s10877-018-0139-y.
75. CLEW. CLEW Medical receives FDA clearance for AI-based predictive analytics technology to support adult ICU patient assessment. PR Newswire. 2021. https://www.prnewswire.com/il/news-releases/clew-medical-receives-fda-clearance-for-ai-based-predictive-analytics-technology-to-support-adult-icu-patient-assessment-301221173.html. Accessed 10 Mar 2024
76. Wijnberge M, Geerts BF, Hol L, Lemmers N, Mulder MP, Berge P, et al. Effect of a machine learning-derived early warning system for intraoperative hypotension vs standard care on depth and duration of intraoperative hypotension during elective non- cardiac surgery: the HYPE randomized clinical trial: the HYPE randomized clinical trial. JAMA. 2020;323(11):1052–60. https://doi.org/10.1001/jama.2020.0592.
77. Komorowski M, Celi LA, Badawi O, Gordon AC, Faisal AA. The artificial intelligence clinician learns optimal treatment strategies for sepsis in intensive care. Nat Med. 2018;24(11):1716–20. https://doi.org/10.1038/s41591-018-0213-5.
78. Adler JR Jr, Chang SD, Murphy MJ, Doty J, Geis P, Hancock SL. The cyberknife: a frameless robotic system for radiosurgery. Stereotact Funct Neurosurg. 1997;69(1–4 Pt 2):124–8.

79. Gonzalez GT, Kaur U, Rahman M, Venkatesh V, Sanchez N, Hager G, et al. From the dexterous surgical skill to the battlefield – a robotics exploratory study. Robot Explor Study. 2021;186:288–94.
80. Murali A, Sen S, Kehoe B, Garg A, McFarland S, Patil S, et al. Learning by observation for surgical subtasks: multilateral cutting of 3D viscoelastic and 2D orthotropic tissue phantoms. In: 2015 IEEE international conference on robotics and automation (ICRA). IEEE; 2015.
81. Saeidi H, Opfermann JD, Kam M, Wei S, Leonard S, Hsieh MH, et al. Autonomous robotic laparoscopic surgery for intestinal anastomosis. Sci Robot. 2022;7(62):eabj908. https://doi.org/10.1126/scirobotics.abj2908.
82. Williams TE Jr, Satiani B, Thomas A, Ellison EC. The impending shortage and the estimated cost of training the future surgical workforce. Ann Surg. 2009;250(4):590–7. https://doi.org/10.1097/SLA.0b013e3181b6c90b.
83. Bogen EM, Schlachta CM, Ponsky T. White paper: technology for surgical telementoring-SAGES Project 6 Technology Working Group. Surg Endosc. 2019;33(3):684–90. https://doi.org/10.1007/s00464-018-06631-8.
84. Augestad KM, Han H, Paige J, Ponsky T, Schlachta CM, Dunkin B, et al. Educational implications for surgical telementoring: a current review with recommendations for future practice, policy, and research. Surg Endosc. 2017;31(10):3836–46. https://doi.org/10.1007/s00464-017-5690-y.
85. Butt K, Augestad KM. Educational value of surgical telementoring. J Surg Oncol. 2021;124:231–40.
86. Wyles SM, Miskovic D, Ni Z, Darzi AW, Valori RM, Coleman MG, et al. Development and implementation of the Structured Training Trainer Assessment Report (STTAR) in the English National Training Programme for laparoscopic colorectal surgery. Surg Endosc. 2016;30(3):993–1003. https://doi.org/10.1007/s00464-015-4281-z.
87. Rosser JC Jr, Bell RL, Harnett B, Rodas E, Murayama M, Merrell R. Use of mobile low-bandwith telemedical techniques for extreme telemedicine applications. J Am Coll Surg. 1999;189(4):397–404. https://doi.org/10.1016/s1072-7515(99)00185-4.
88. Goel SS, Greenbaum AB, Patel A, Little SH, Parikh R, Wyler von Ballmoos MC, et al. Role of teleproctoring in challenging and innovative structural interventions amid the COVID-19 pandemic and beyond. JACC Cardiovasc Interv. 2020;13(16):1945–8. https://doi.org/10.1016/j.jcin.2020.04.013.
89. Erridge S, Yeung DKT, Patel HRH, Purkayastha S. Telementoring of surgeons: a systematic review. Surg Innov. 2019;26(1):95–111. https://doi.org/10.1177/1553350618813250.
90. Huang EY, Knight S, Guetter CR, Davis CH, Moller M, Slama E, et al. Telemedicine and telementoring in the surgical specialties: a narrative review. Am J Surg. 2019;218(4):760–6. https://doi.org/10.1016/j.amjsurg.2019.07.018.
91. El-Sabawi B, Magee W. The evolution of surgical telementoring: current applications and future directions. Ann Transl Med. 2016;4(20):391. https://doi.org/10.21037/atm.2016.10.04.
92. Hung AJ, Chen J, Shah A, Gill IS. Telementoring and tele- surgery for minimally invasive procedures. J Urol. 2018;199(2):355–69. https://doi.org/10.1016/j.juro.2017.06.082.
93. Shin DH, Dalag L, Azhar RA, Santomauro M, Satkunasivam R, Metcalfe C, et al. A novel interface for the telementoring of robotic surgery. BJU Int. 2015;116(2):302–8. https://doi.org/10.1111/bju.12985.
94. Shahzad N, Chawla T, Gala T. Telesurgery prospects in delivering healthcare in remote areas. J Pak Med Assoc. 2019;69(Supp 1):S69–71.
95. Marescaux J. Code name: "Lindbergh operation". Ann Chir. 2002;127(1):2–4. https://doi.org/10.1016/s0003-3944(01)00658-7.
96. Xu S, Perez M, Yang K, Perrenot C, Felblinger J, Hubert J. Determination of the latency effects on surgical performance and the acceptable latency levels in telesurgery using the dV- Trainer(®) simulator. Surg Endosc. 2014;28(9):2569–76. https://doi.org/10.1007/s00464-014-3504-z.

97. Anvari M, McKinley C, Stein H. Establishment of the world's first telerobotic remote surgical service: for provision of advanced laparoscopic surgery in a rural community. Ann Surg. 2005;241(3):460–4. https://doi.org/10.1097/01.sla.0000154456.69815.ee.
98. Wirz R, Torres LG, Swaney PJ, Gilbert H, Alterovitz R, Webster RJ 3rd, et al. An experimental feasibility study on robotic endonasal telesurgery. Neurosurgery. 2015;76(4):479–84. (discussion 484). https://doi.org/10.1227/NEU.0000000000000623.
99. Acemoglu A, Peretti G, Trimarchi M, Hysenbelli J, Krieglstein J, Geraldes A, et al. Operating from a distance: robotic vocal cord 5G telesurgery on a cadaver. Ann Intern Med. 2020;173(11):940–1. https://doi.org/10.7326/M20-0418.
100. Peters BS, Armijo PR, Krause C, Choudhury SA, Oleynikov D. Review of emerging surgical robotic technology. Surg Endosc. 2018;32(4):1636–55. https://doi.org/10.1007/s00464-018-6079-2.
101. Sheetz KH, Claflin J, Dimick JB. Trends in the adoption of robotic surgery for common surgical procedures. JAMA Netw Open. 2020;3(1):e1918911. https://doi.org/10.1001/jamanetworkopen.2019.18911.
102. Khandalavala K, Shimon T, Flores L, Armijo PR, Oleynikov D. Emerging surgical robotic technology: a progression toward microbots. Ann Laparosc Endosc Surg. 2020;5:3. https://doi.org/10.21037/ales.2019.10.02.

10 Navigating Resources for Aspiring and Experienced Robotic Surgeons

Yasamin Taghikhan and Ankit Sarin

Introduction

As with most emerging technologies, robotic surgery continues to evolve at a rapid pace, making it critical for surgeons to stay updated and skilled in its application. The increasing complexity and diversity of robotic systems have resulted in a growing demand for comprehensive, high-quality training resources. These resources cater to both novices and experienced surgeons, offering opportunities to build foundational knowledge, enhance technical skills, and foster professional growth.

While most training resources currently focus on the Intuitive da Vinci robotic platform, an increasing number of platform-agnostic resources are emerging as the field diversifies. This chapter provides a structured and detailed overview of key resources available for robotic surgeons, covering foundational knowledge, practical skills, professional networking, and continuing education opportunities. It serves as a roadmap for navigating the wealth of information and tools essential for excelling in this innovative field.

Foundational Knowledge

It is imperative for aspiring and current robotic surgeons to continue to build upon their foundational knowledge through reviewing books, latest journals, and via online platforms and communities as they advance through various stages of their careers. In this section, you will find resources that offer theoretical knowledge, practical tips, and visual aids for all levels of surgeons.

Y. Taghikhan · A. Sarin (✉)
Department of Surgery, University of California Davis, Sacramento, CA, USA
e-mail: ytaghikhan@ucdavis.edu; axsarin@ucdavis.edu

S. Samreen et al. (eds.), *The SAGES Manual of Robotic Surgery*,
https://doi.org/10.1007/978-3-031-86927-3_10

1. **Books**
   a) *Robotic Surgery* by Farid Gharagozloo and others. A comprehensive multi-specialty robotic surgery volume that can serve as a reference for all robotic surgeons. [1]
   b) *Atlas of Robotic General Surgery* by Yuri W. Novitsky. An inclusive atlas that covers a wide range of robotic techniques for general surgery by 50+ experts in the field. It includes many high-quality colored illustrations that complement the text. [2]
   c) *Principles and Practice of Robotic Surgery* by Eduardo A. Sagarin. A great reference covering adult and pediatric robotic surgeries with step-by-step instructions for new and experienced surgeons. [3]
   d) *Essentials of Robotic Surgery* by Matthew Kroh and Sricharan Chalikonda. Excellent reference from 2015. [4]
   e) *Robotic General Surgery* by Yuman Fong and others. A newly released reference for surgeons at all levels of training with discipline-based chapters showcasing many robotic procedures in general surgery. [5]
2. **Journals and Publications**
   a) ***Journal of Robotic Surgery***

A peer-reviewed journal that creates a platform for surgeons and researchers to review and exchange knowledge and expertise in the field of robotic surgery. [6]

b) ***International Journal of Medical Robotics and Computer-Assisted Surgery***

A diverse international cross-disciplinary journal focusing on advancements, techniques, and clinical outcomes in robotic surgery. [7]

c) ***Surgical Innovation (SRI)***

Although not exclusively covering robotic surgery topics, this journal covers emerging topics and offers peer-reviewed articles highlighting the advances in minimally invasive surgery. [8]

d) ***Annals of Surgery***

A highly respected journal that frequently publishes significant studies on robotic surgeries, randomized trials, and systematic reviews. [9]

e) ***Surgical Endoscopy***

Focuses on minimally invasive surgery, including robotic-assisted procedures, and is known for publishing cutting-edge research and reviews. [10]

Educational Websites and Platforms

Society of American Gastrointestinal and Endoscopic Surgeons (SAGES)

i. Offers a variety of resources including videos and guidelines, including detailed manuals and atlas. [11]

WebSurg

ii. A comprehensive platform created by surgeons that includes online modules, live demonstrations, and interactive session from international experts. This platform offers the opportunity to learn from experts all over the world. [12]

Surgical Council on Resident Education (SCORE)

iii. A great resource for residents and newly practicing surgeons as it provides didactic materials as well as quizzes to reinforce learning. [13]

Crowdsourced Assessment of Technical Skills (C-SATS)

iv. A unique platform that offers personalized feedback on performance by allowing robotic surgeons to upload procedure videos to be reviewed by experts. [14]

Intuitive Surgical Online Learning Platform (My Intuitive)

v. My intuitive surgical program offers a wide selection of material, including video tutorials, interactive stimulations, as well as access to the da Vinci Surgical System learning. [15]

Podcasts and Beyond

a) **Global Robotic-Assisted Surgery Podcast (GRASP)**

Leading robotic surgeons appear as guests on this podcast and offer their expertise within their field. [16]

b) **Behind the Knife (BTK)**

While not exclusively focused on robotics surgery, this podcast covers a variety of topics related to robotic and minimally invasive surgeries through guest speaker discussions. Additionally, their YouTube channel offers content on robotic procedures. [17]

Practical Skills

1. Surgical Videos Libraries and Live Streams
   a. **Journal of Medical Insight (JOMI)**

A unique library of videos including robotic surgery taken from the perspective of surgeons that allow for on-demand virtual shadowing experiences for all levels of surgeons including trainees. [18]

b. **Csurgeries**

A collection of peer-reviewed surgical videos including robotic surgeries designed for educational purposes. [19]

c. **GIBLIB**

An assortment of curated surgical videos and lectures on demand for current and aspiring surgeons. [20]

d. **Intuitive Telementoring**

A unique way to learn from other surgeons by remotely observing or broadcasting live procedures. [15]

2. **Simulation Training**

a) **Da Vinci SimNow**
   An online simulation training platform that provides a range of exercises to help improve robotic surgery skills, available for surgeons at various levels of experience. **[15]**
b) **Surgical Science**

   A medical simulation company that offers an extensive library of stimulated surgeries as well as the ability to customize surgeries. It is intended for organizations seeking to further advance the training level of their surgeons. [21]

3. **In-Person Proctoring**
   a. **SAGES Robotics Resident and Fellows Courses**
   A nationwide course offered to residents and fellows throughout the year with prerecorded lectures on robotic general surgery topics as well as hands-on skills training on the robotic console. [22]

b. **Institute for Research into Cancers of the Digestive System (irCAD)**

An international organization offering both on-site and online courses across various disciplines, including robotic surgery aiming to enhance skills in robotic and minimally invasive surgery. [23]

c. **Association of Program Directors for Colon and Rectal Surgeons Robotic Training Courses**

An association providing resources for both colorectal surgery residents and program directors, specifically offering surgeon led robotic training course to fellows both virtually and on-site. [24]

d. **American Urological Association (AUA) Robotic Surgery Courses**

These include hands-on workshops and courses specifically designed for urological surgeons interested in robotic-assisted surgery. [25]

e. **Da Vinci Training Passport**

A wide-ranging set of training courses focusing on furthering technical knowledge as well as skills through hands-on lab work. This program also included a proctoring series where surgeons can get one-on-one coaching from experienced robotic surgeons. [26]

Professional Communities and Networking

1. **Professional organizations**

Society of American Gastrointestinal Endoscopic Surgeons (SAGES)

i. The society strives on developing and promoting standards, guidelines, and best practices in robotic surgery through many different methods, including courses, guidelines, and library of robotic surgery content. [27]

Society of Robotic Surgery (SRS)

ii. A global organization dedicated to advancement of robotic surgery with yearly annual meetings to educate and further develop best practices among robotic surgeons. [28]

European Association for Endoscopic Surgery (EAES)

iii. A global community of surgeons in Europe and beyond that focuses on endoscopic and minimally invasive surgery, including robotic surgery with educational programs and conferences. [29]

2. **Social Media and Networking**

a. **LinkedIn Groups**

Groups such as "Robotic Surgery Network," "Surgical Innovation and Robotics," and many other provide a great platform for networking among various surgeons. [30]

b. **Facebook Groups**

Groups such as "Robotic Surgery Discussion Groups," "Robotic Surgery—Clinical Cases and Discussion," and others are typically private groups where surgeons and healthcare professionals share experiences, ask questions, and discuss robotic surgery techniques and technologies. [31]

c. **X (Formerly Known as Twitter)**

Ability to interact with robotic surgeons from all over the globe in order to gain insight into the latest robotic advancement. [32]

@roboticsurgery: an example of a Twitter handle that shares news, research updates, and developments in the field of robotic surgery.

#RoboticSurgery: A popular hashtag where users share articles, research, and discussions related to robotic surgery.

#MinimallyInvasiveSurgery: a broader hashtag that often includes posts about robotic surgery as part of the minimally invasive surgery community.

d. **Reddit- r/Surgery**

An online community where surgeons discuss many topics, including robotics surgery. A platform for sharing, exchanging ideas, and seeking advice from peers in the field. [33]

Continuing Education

Many of the previously mentioned societies such as SAGES offer opportunities through meetings, online content, and courses for physicians to earn CMEs. Below are highlights of some lesser-known CME opportunities for aspiring and current robotic surgeons.

Continuing Medical Education Opportunities

a. **American College of Surgeons (ACS)**

Offer CME-accredited robotic surgery courses as well as grand round series on robotics and surgical education. [34]

b. **Society of Laparoscopic and Robotic Surgeons (SLS)**

A multispecialty society that offers an open forum for surgeons interested in robotics and minimally invasive surgery. They offer education recordings that qualify for CME credits in many specialties. [35]

c. **Master of Science in Robotic Surgery (Advent Health University)**

This program offers a master's degree within 2 years to physicians (attendings, residents, and fellows) in robotic surgery. The program includes both self-study and in-person coursework focusing on a variety of surgical subspecialties such as bariatrics, thoracic, and urology. [36]

d. **Annual SSF Robotics Course**

An annual symposium with target audience of neurological and orthopedic surgeons covering the latest topics on robotic surgery within each respective field. [37]

e. **Mayo Clinic Advanced Surgical Technologies and Robotics**

An annual symposium that focuses on the latest updates on robotic and other technological healthcare advances through expert presentations and panel discussions. [38]

Conclusion

As the field of robotic surgery continues to advance, so does the wealth of resources available to surgeons. It is imperative for surgeons to continue to seek out new resources to further their foundational knowledge and enhance their practical skills. Many of these resources were covered in this chapter from books and journals to social media and networking opportunities. Each resource helps novice and experienced surgeons enhance their expertise to stay at the forefront of robotic surgery field and improve patient outcomes while advancing in their careers.

References

1. Gharagozloo F, Patel VR, Giulianotti PC, Poston R, Gruessner R, Meyer M, editors. Robotic surgery. Cham: Springer; 2021. [Crossref]
2. Novitsky YW. Atlas of robotic general surgery E-book. Elsevier Health Sciences; 2021. [Crossref]
3. Costello T. Principles and practice of robotic surgery – E-book. Elsevier Health Sciences; 2023. [Crossref]
4. Kroh M, Chalikonda S. Springerlink (Online service. Essentials of robotic surgery). Cham: Springer; 2015. [Crossref]
5. Fong Y, Erhunmwunsee L, Pigazzi A, Podolsky D, Portenier DD. Robotic general surgery. Lippincott Williams & Wilkins; 2024. [Crossref]
6. Journal of Robotic Surgery [Internet]. SpringerLink; 2024. [Crossref]
7. Wiley Online Library. Wiley online library | Scientific research articles, journals, books, and reference works [Internet]. Wiley.com. 2019. [Crossref]
8. Sage Journals. SAGE Journals: Your gateway to world-class research journals [Internet]. Sagepub.com. 2023. [Crossref]
9. Annals of Surgery [Internet]. Lww.com. 2024. [Crossref]
10. Surgical Endoscopy [Internet]. SpringerLink. [Crossref]
11. SAGES Manuals – SAGES [Internet]. SAGES. 2023. [Crossref]
12. WebSurg, the online university of IRCAD [Internet]. websurg.com. [Crossref]
13. SCORE | General Surgery Resident Curriculum Portal [Internet]. Surgicalcore.org. 2019. [Crossref]

14. A Post-operative Surgical Insights Platform | C-SATS. C-SATS [Internet]. C-SATS. 2021. [Crossref]
15. Intuitive.com. 2023. [Crossref] [Crossref]
16. The Global Robotic Assisted Surgery Platform (GRASP) [Internet]. Global Robotic Assisted Surgery Platform. 2024. [Crossref]
17. Behind The Knife: The Premier Surgery Podcast | Surgical Education [Internet]. behindtheknife.org. 2024. [Crossref]
18. Journal of Medical Insight | Peer-Reviewed Surgical Videos for Video-Based Surgical Education [Internet]. Journal of Medical Insight. [Crossref]
19. CSurgeries [Internet]. CSurgeries. 2024. [Crossref]
20. GIBLIB [Internet]. Giblib.com. 2024. [Crossref]
21. Medical training simulation in virtual reality | Surgical Science [Internet]. Surg Sci. 2017. [Crossref]
22. SAGES Robotics Residents and Fellows Courses – SAGES [Internet]. SAGES. 2024. [Crossref]
23. Course specialties – IRCAD [Internet]. IRCAD. 2023. [Crossref]
24. Robotics – APDCRS [Internet]. Apdcrs.org. 2023. [Crossref]
25. AUA Annual Meeting [Internet]. Auanet.org. 2024. [Crossref]
26. Da Vinci Training Passport [Internet]. [Crossref]
27. Society of American Gastrointestinal and Endoscopic Surgeons (SAGES) [Internet]. SAGES. 2013. [Crossref]
28. Society of Robotic Surgery | SRS [Internet]. Society of Robotic Surgery | SRS. [Crossref]
29. Robotics subcommittee – EAES [Internet]. EAES. 2024. [Crossref]
30. LinkedIn. LinkedIn [Internet]. LinkedIn. 2024. [Crossref]
31. Facebook [Internet]. Facebook. 2019. [Crossref]
32. x.com [Internet]. X (formerly Twitter). [Crossref]
33. Reddit. reddit [Internet]. reddit. 2019. [Crossref]
34. Robotics and Surgical Education [Internet]. ACS. [Crossref]
35. Education SLS [Internet]. Sls.org. 2024. [Crossref]
36. Online Master of Science in Robotic Surgery [Internet]. AdventHealth University. [Crossref]
37. 9th Annual SSF Robotics Course 2024 – Seattle Science Foundation CME – Continuing Education (CE) [Internet]. Cloud-cme.com. 2024. [Crossref]
38. Mayo Clinic School of Continuous Professional Development [Internet]. Mayo.edu. 2019. [Crossref]

Part III

Masters Program

11 Overview of SAGES Masters Program

Daniel B. Jones, Brian P. Jacob, and Linda Schultz

The SAGES Masters Program organizes educational materials along clinical pathways into discrete blocks of content that could be accessed by a surgeon attending the SAGES annual meeting or by logging into the online SAGES University (Fig. 11.1) [1]. SAGES Masters Program has 12 pathways: Acute Care Surgery, Bariatric, Biliary, Colorectal, Flexible Edoscopy, Foregut, Hernia, Leadership & Professional Development, Liver, Pancreas, Robotics, Solid Organ. Flexible Endoscopy, and Robotic Surgery (Fig. 11.2). Each pathway is divided into three levels of targeted performance: Competency, Proficiency, and Mastery (Fig. 11.3). The levels originate from the Dreyfus model of skill acquisition [2], which has five stages: novice, advanced beginner, competency, proficiency, and expertise. The SAGES Masters Program is based on the three more advanced stages of skill acquisition: competency, proficiency, and expertise. *Competency* is defined as what a graduating general surgery chief resident or MIS fellow should be able to achieve; *Proficiency* is what a surgeon approximately 3 years out from training should be able to accomplish; and *Mastery* is what more experienced surgeons should be able to accomplish after seven or more years in practice. Mastery is applicable to SAGES surgeons seeking in-depth knowledge in a pathway, including the following: areas of controversy, outcomes, best practice, and ability to mentor colleagues. Over time, with the utilization of coaching and participation in SAGES courses, this level should be obtainable by the majority of SAGES members. This edition of the

D. B. Jones (✉)
Department of Surgery, Rutgers New Jersey Medical School, Newark, NJ, USA
e-mail: dj477@njms.rutgers.edu

B. P. Jacob
Department of Surgery, Icahn School of Medicine at Mount, Sinai, NY, USA

L. Schultz
Society of American Gastrointestinal and Endoscopic Surgeons, Los Angeles, CA, USA

S. Samreen et al. (eds.), *The SAGES Manual of Robotic Surgery*,
https://doi.org/10.1007/978-3-031-86927-3_11

Fig. 11.1 Masters Program logo

Fig. 11.2 Masters Program clinical pathways

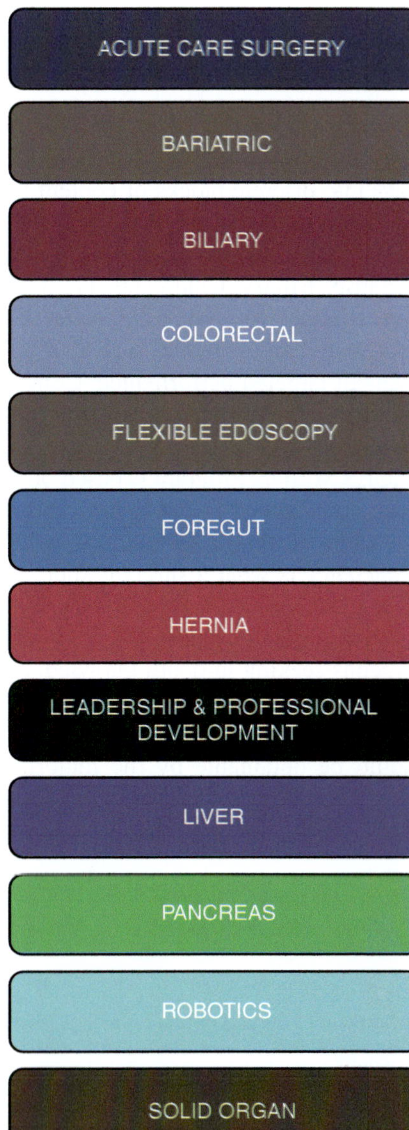

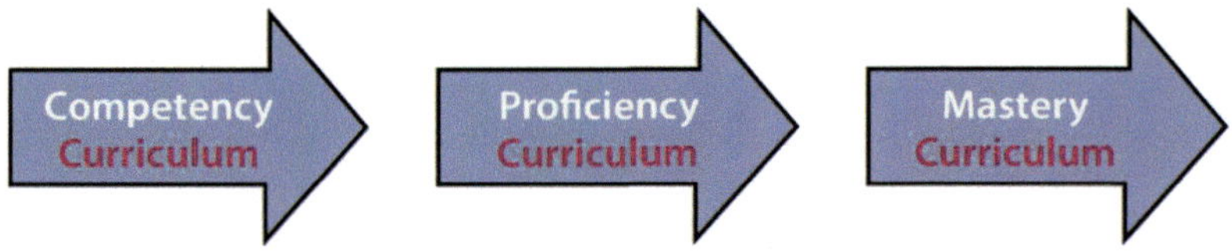

Fig. 11.3 Masters Program progression

Table 11.1 Robotic curriculum

Curriculum elements	**Competency**
Anchoring procedure—Competency	2
CORE LECTURE	1
CORE MCE 70%	1
Annual meeting content	8
Guidelines	1
SA CME hours	6
Sentinel articles	2
Social media	2
Hands-on robotic proficiency verification	12
Credits	*35*
Curriculum elements	**Proficiency**
Anchoring procedure—Proficiency	2
CORE LECTURE	1
CORE MCE 70%	1
Annual meeting content	5
FUSE	12
Outcomes database enrollment	2
SA CME hours (ASMBS electives, SAGES or SAGES-endorsed)	3
Sentinel articles	2
Social media	2
Credits	*30*
Curriculum elements	**Mastery**
Anchoring procedure—Mastery	2
CORE LECTURE	1
CORE MCE 70%	1
Annual meeting content	3
Fundamentals of surgical coaching	4
Outcomes database reporting	2
SA CME credits (ASMBS electives, SAGES or SAGES-endorsed)	5
Sentinel articles	2
Serving as video assessment reviewer and providing feedback (FSC)	4
Social media	6
Credits	*30*

SAGES Manual—Robotic Surgery aligns with the current version of the new SAGES University Masters Program Robotic Surgery pathway (Table 11.1).

Robotic Surgery Curriculum

The Robotic Curriculum is a little different from the other SAGES Masters Program pathways. To complete the robotic pathway, a robotic surgeon should complete requirements in the corresponding pathway. For example, for successful completion of the Robotic Competency Curriculum for Hernia, the learner should be able to demonstrate a robotic ventral hernia for competency, a robotic inguinal hernia for proficiency, and a robotic complex abdominal wall reconstruction or a recurrent hernia repair to accomplish mastery. This recognizes the importance of understanding disease and also unique technical expertise of mastering the robot technology.

The key elements of the Robotic Surgery curriculum include core lectures for the pathway, which provides a 45-min general overview, including basic anatomy, physiology, diagnostic workup, and surgical management. As of 2018, all lecture content of the annual SAGES meetings are labeled as follows: basic (100), intermediate (200), and advanced (300). This allows attendees to choose lectures that best fit their educational needs. Coding the content additionally facilitates online retrieval of specific educational material, with varying degrees of surgical complexity, ranging from introductory to revisional surgery.

SAGES identified the need to develop targeted, complex content for its mastery-level curriculum. The idea was that these 25-min lectures would be focused on specific topics. It assumes that the attendee already has a good understanding of diseases and management from attending/watching competency and proficiency-level lectures. Ideally, in order to supplement a chosen topic, the mastery lectures would also identify key prerequisite articles from *Surgical Endoscopy* and other journals, in addition to SAGES University videos. Many of these lectures will be forthcoming at future SAGES annual meetings.

The Masters Program has a self-assessment, multiple-choice exam for each module to guide learner progression throughout the curriculum. Questions are submitted by core lecture speakers and SAGES annual meeting faculty. The goal of the questions is to use assessment for learning, with the assessment being criterion referenced with the percent correct set at 80%. Learners will be able to review incorrect answers, review educational content, and retake the examination until a passing score is obtained.

The Masters Program Robotic Surgery curriculum taps much of the of SAGES existing educational products including FLS, FES, FUSE, SMART, Top 21 videos, and Pearls (Fig. 11.4). The Curriculum Task Force has placed the aforementioned modules along a continuum of the curriculum pathway. For example, FLS, in general, occurs during the Competency Curriculum, whereas the Fundamental Use of Surgical Energy (FUSE) is usually required during the Proficiency Curriculum. The Fundamentals of Laparoscopic Surgery (FLS) is a multiple-choice exam and a skills assessment conducted on a video box trainer. Tasks include peg transfer, cutting, intracorporeal and extracorporeal suturing, and knot tying. Since 2010, FLS has been required of all US general surgery

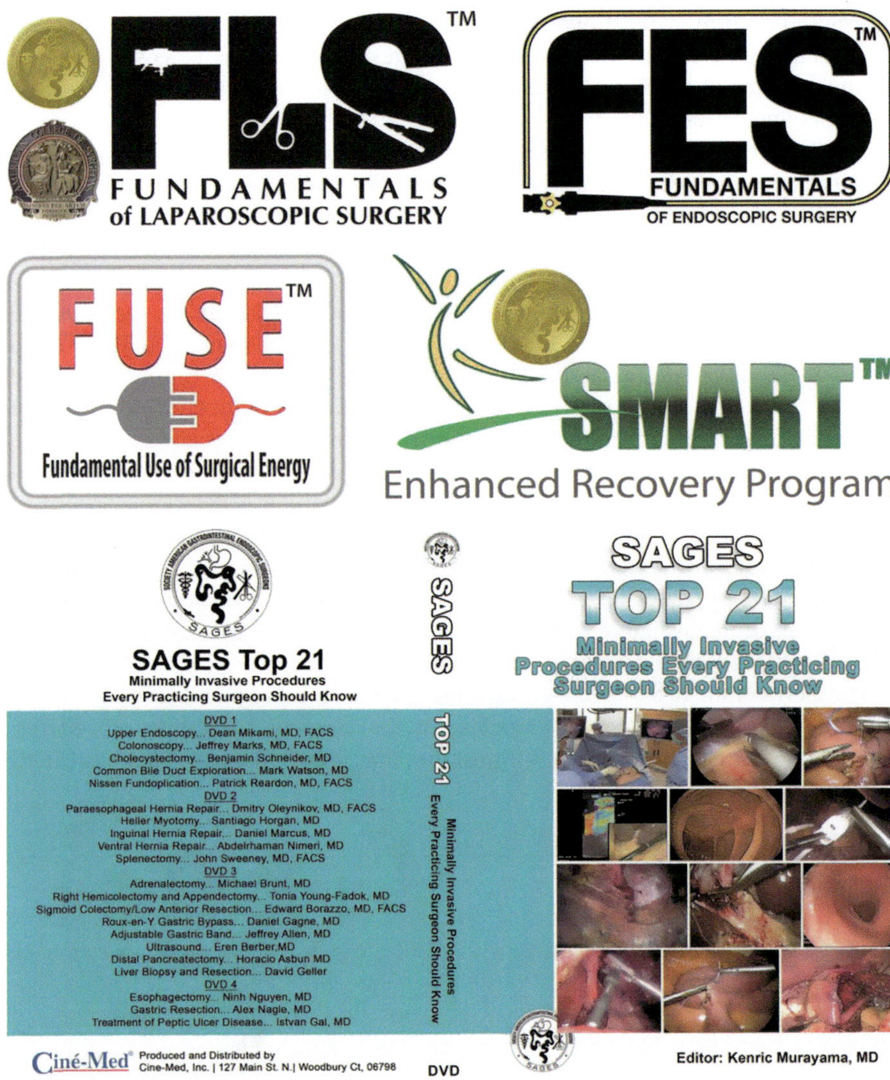

Fig. 11.4 SAGES educational content: FLS, FUSE, FES, SMART, Top 21 videos

residents seeking to sit for the American Board of Surgery qualifying examinations. The Fundamentals of Endoscopic Surgery (FES) assesses endoscopic knowledge and technical skills in a simulator. FUSE teaches about the safe use of energy devices in the operating room and is available at FUSE.didactic.org. After learners complete the self-paced modules, they may take the certifying examination.

The SAGES Surgical Multimodal Accelerated Recovery Trajectory (SMART) Initiative combines minimally invasive surgical techniques with enhanced recovery pathways (ERPs) for perioperative care, with the goal of improving outcomes and patient satisfaction. Educational materials include a website with best practices, sample pathways, patient literature, and other resources such as videos, FAQs, and an implementation timeline. The materials assist surgeons and their surgical team with implementation of an ERP.

Top 21 videos are edited videos of the most commonly performed MIS operations and basic endoscopy. Cases are straightforward with quality video and clear anatomy.

Pearls are step-by-step video clips of 10 operations. The authors show different variations for each step. The learner should have a fundamental understanding of the operation.

SAGES Guidelines provide evidence-based recommendations for surgeons and are developed by the SAGES Guidelines Committee following the Health and Medicine Division of the National Academies of Sciences, Engineering, and Medicine standards (formerly the Institute of Medicine) for guideline development [3]. Each clinical practice guideline has been systematically researched, reviewed, and revised by the SAGES Guidelines Committee and an appropriate multidisciplinary team. The strength of the provided recommendations is determined based on the quality of the available literature using the GRADE methodology [4]. SAGES Guidelines cover a wide range of topics relevant to the practice of SAGES surgeon members and are updated on a regular basis. Since the developed guidelines provide an appraisal of the available literature, their inclusion in the Masters Program was deemed necessary by the group.

The Curriculum Task Force identified the need to select required readings for the Masters Program based on key articles for the various curriculum procedures. Summaries of each of these articles follow the American College of Surgeons (ACS) Selected Readings format.

Facebook™ Groups

While there are many great platforms available to permit online collaboration by user-generated content, Facebook™ offers a unique, highly developed mobile platform that is ideal for global professional collaboration and daily continuing surgical education (Fig. 11.5). The Facebook groups allow for video assessment, feedback, and coaching as a tool to improve practice, and their use to enhance professional surgical education has been validated by Dr. Brian Jacob's International Hernia Collaboration closed Facebook group.

Based on the anchoring procedures determined via group consensus (Table 11.2), participants in the Masters Program will submit video clips on designated SAGES closed Facebook groups, with other participants and/or SAGES members providing qualitative feedback. Using crowdsourcing, other surgeons would comment and provide feedback.

Eight, unique vetted membership-only closed Facebook groups were created for the Masters Program, including a group for bariatrics, hernia, colorectal, biliary, acute care, flexible endoscopy, robotics, and foregut. The SAGES Robotic Surgery group is independent of the other groups already in existence and will be populated

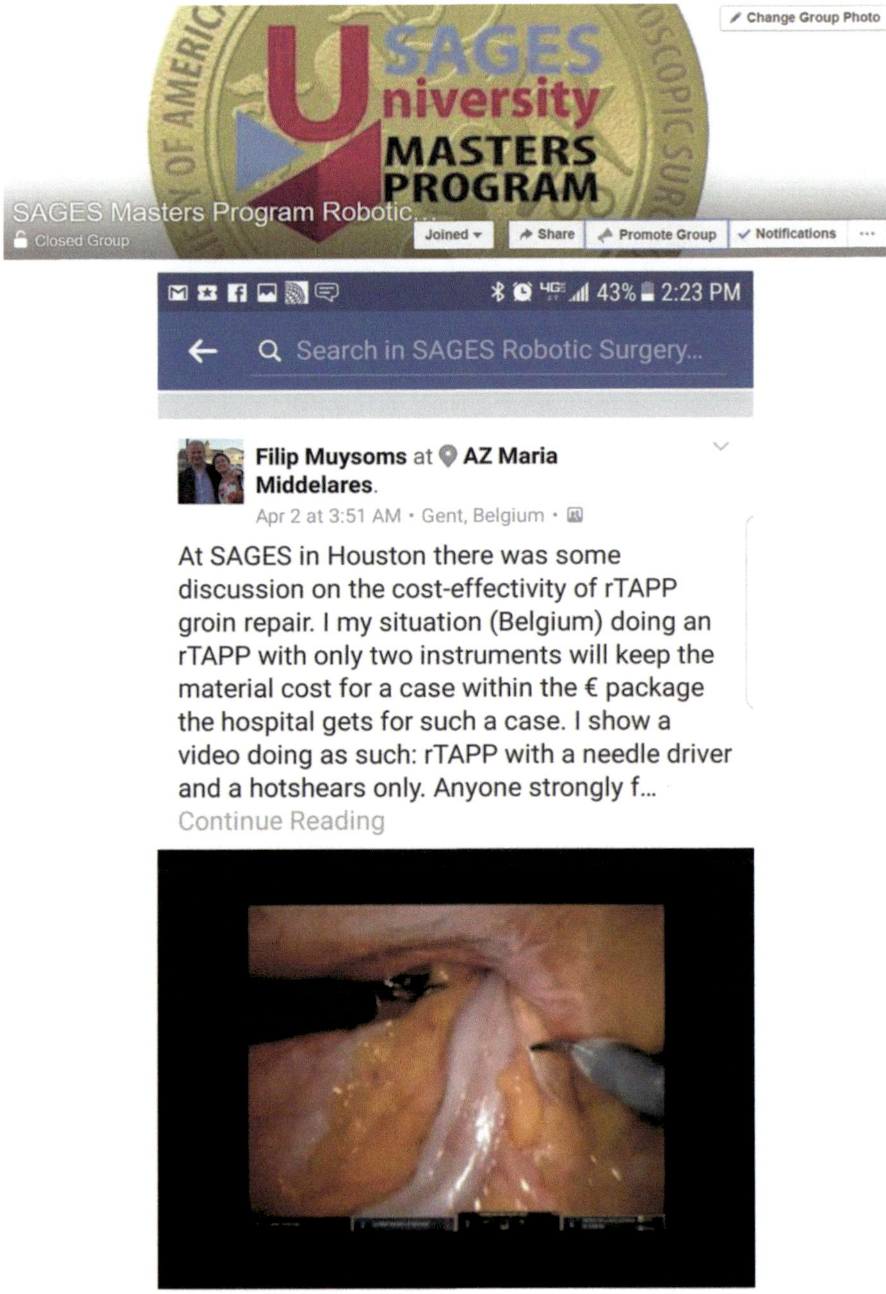
Change Group Photo
SAGES University MASTERS PROGRAM
SAGES Masters Program Robotic...
Closed Group
Joined
Share
Promote Group
Notifications
43% 2:23 PM
Search in SAGES Robotic Surgery...
Filip Muysoms at AZ Maria Middelares.
Apr 2 at 3:51 AM · Gent, Belgium ·
At SAGES in Houston there was some discussion on the cost-effectivity of rTAPP groin repair. I my situation (Belgium) doing an rTAPP with only two instruments will keep the material cost for a case within the € package the hospital gets for such a case. I show a video doing as such: rTAPP with a needle driver and a hotshears only. Anyone strongly f...
Continue Reading

Fig. 11.5 Robotic Surgery Facebook group

Table 11.2 Anchoring procedures for Robotic Surgery pathway

Robotic Surgery anchoring procedure by pathway	Level
Biliary	
Multiport cholecystectomy	Competency
Cholecystectomy with IOC or for uncomplicated acute cholecystitis	Proficiency
Cholecystectomy for difficult/severe acute cholecystitis or common bile duct exploration (CBDE)	Mastery
Foregut	
Nissen fundoplication	Competency
Paraesophageal Hernia Repair or Heller Myotomy	Proficiency
Redo fundoplication	Mastery
Hernia	
Primary ventral hernia repair	Competency
Primary inguinal hernia repair	Proficiency
Redo hernia or complex hernia (transversus abdominis release)	Mastery
Bariatric	
Sleeve gastrectomy or lap band	Competency
Roux-en-Y gastric bypass	Proficiency
Revisional bariatric surgery	Mastery
Colorectal	
Right colectomy	Competency
Left colectomy	Proficiency
Left colectomy with splenic flexure release, colectomy for complex inflammatory disease or advanced cancer	Mastery

only by physicians, mostly surgeons or surgeons in training interested in a wide range of robotic surgery applications.

The group provides an international platform for surgeons and healthcare providers interested in optimizing outcomes in a surgical specialty to collaborate; share; discuss; and post photos, videos, and anything related to a chosen specialty. By embracing social media as a collaborative forum, we can more effectively and transparently obtain immediate global feedback that potentially can improve patient outcomes, as well as the quality of care we provide, all while transforming the way a society's members interact.

For the first two levels of the Masters Program, Competency and Proficiency, participants will be required to post videos of the anchoring procedures and will receive qualitative feedback from other participants. However, for the mastery level, participants will submit a video to be evaluated by an expert panel. A standardized video assessment tool, depending on the specific procedure, will be used. A benchmark will also be utilized to determine when the participant has achieved the mastery level for that procedure.

Once the participant has achieved mastery level, he will participate as a coach by providing feedback to participants in the first two levels. Masters Program participants will therefore need to learn the fundamental principles of surgical coaching. The key activities of coaching include goal setting, active listening, powerful inquiry, and constructive feedback [5, 6]. Importantly, peer coaching is much different than traditional education, where there is an expert and a learner. Peer coaching is a "co-learning" model where the coach is facilitating the development of the coached by using inquiry (i.e., open-ended questions) in a noncompetitive manner.

Surgical coaching skills are a crucial part of the Masters curriculum. At the 2017 SAGES Annual Meeting, a postgraduate course on coaching skills was developed and video recorded. The goal is to develop a "coaching culture" within the SAGES Masters Program, wherein both participants and coaches are committed to lifelong learning and development.

The need for a more structured approach to the education of practicing surgeons as accomplished by the SAGES Masters Program is well recognized [7]. Since performance feedback usually stops after training completion and current approaches to MOC are suboptimal, the need for peer coaching has recently received increased attention in surgery [5, 6]. SAGES has recognized this need and its Masters Program embraces social media for surgical education to help provide a free, mobile, and easy-to-use platform to surgeons globally. Access to the Masters Program groups enables surgeons at all levels to partake in the Masters Program curriculum and obtain feedback from peers, mentors, and experts. By creating surgeon-only private groups dedicated to this project, SAGES can now offer surgeons posting in these groups the ability to discuss preoperative, intraoperative, and postoperative issues with other SAGES colleagues and mentors. In addition, the platform permits transparent and responsive dialogue about technique, continuing the theme of deliberate, lifelong learning.

To accommodate the needs of this program, SAGES University is upgrading its web-based features. A new learning management system (LMS) will track progression and make access to SAGES University simple. Features of the new IT infrastructure will provide the ability to access a video or lecture on-demand in relation to content, level of difficulty, and author. Once enrolled in the Masters Program, the LMS will track lectures, educational products, MCE, and other completed requirements. Participants will be able to see where they stand in relation to module completion and SAGES will alert learners to relevant content they may be interested in pursuing. Until such time that the new LMS is up and running, it is hoped that the SAGES Manual will help guide learners through the Masters Program Curriculum.

Conclusions

The SAGES Masters Program Robotic Surgery Pathway facilitates deliberate, focused postgraduate teaching and learning. The Masters Program certifies completion of the curriculum but is NOT meant to certify competency, proficiency, or mastery of surgeons. The Masters Program embraces the concept of lifelong learning after fellowship and its curriculum is organized from basic principles to more complex content. The Masters Program is an innovative, voluntary curriculum that supports MOC and deliberate, lifelong learning.

References

1. Jones DB, Stefanidis D, Korndorffer JR, Dimick JB, Jacob BP, Schultz L, Scott DJ. SAGES University Masters program: a structured curriculum for deliberate, lifelong learning. Surg Endosc. 2017;31(8):3061–71.
2. Dreyfus SE. The five-stage model of adult skill acquisition. Bull Sci Technol Soc. 2004;24:177–81.
3. Graham R, Mancher M, Miller Woman D, Greenfield S, Steinberg E. Institute of Medicine (US) committee on standards for developing trustworthy clinical practice guidelines. In: Graham R, Mancher M, Wolman DM, Greenfield S, Steinberg E, editors. Clinical practice guidelines we can trust. Washington, DC: National Academies Press (US); 2011.
4. Guyatt GH, Oxman AD, Vist GE, Kunz R, Falck-Ytter Y, Alonso-Coello P, Schünemann HJ, GRADE Working Group. GRADE: an emerging consensus on rating quality of evidence and strength of recommendations. BMJ. 2008;336:924–6.
5. Greenberg CC, Ghousseini HN, Pavuluri Quamme SR, Beasley HL, Wiegmann DA. Surgical coaching for individual performance improvement. Ann Surg. 2015;261:32–4.
6. Greenberg CC, Dombrowski J, Dimick JB. Video-based surgical coaching: an emerging approach to performance improvement. JAMA Surg. 2016;151:282–3.
7. Sachdeva AK. Acquiring skills in new procedures and technology: the challenge and the opportunity. Arch Surg. 2005;140:387–9.

12 Robotic Paraesophageal Hernia Repair

Karan R. Chhabra and Charudutt N. Paranjape

Hiatal hernias have a significant correlation with gastroesophageal reflux disease (GERD), and their management is vital in antireflux surgery. Paraesophageal hernias, a specific category of hiatal hernias, often necessitate surgical intervention due to their distinct symptoms and treatment requirements.

Classification and Pathophysiology of Hiatal Hernias

In a typical anatomical arrangement, the gastroesophageal junction (GEJ) and the stomach are positioned below the diaphragmatic hiatus. Hiatal hernias are categorized as follows, with types II, III, and IV classified as "true" paraesophageal hernias. It is estimated that hiatal hernias may be present in approximately 10–15% of adults, as determined by radiological studies [1].

Type I (Sliding Hiatal Hernia): In this type, the GEJ ascends through the hiatus into the mediastinum. Constituting 70–90% of all hiatal hernias, they may not have clinical significance unless associated with severe GERD or other symptoms.

Type II: Here, the fundus of the stomach moves into the mediastinum, while the GEJ remains within the abdomen. These are less common.

K. R. Chhabra (✉)
Departments of Surgery and Population Health, NYU Grossman School of Medicine, New York, NY, USA

Division of Bariatric and General Surgery, Bellevue Hospital Center, New York, NY, USA

C. N. Paranjape
Department of Surgery, NYU Grossman School of Medicine, New York, NY, USA

Division of Bariatric and General Surgery, Bellevue Hospital Center, New York, NY, USA

Newton-Wellesley Hospital, Newton, MA, USA

S. Samreen et al. (eds.), *The SAGES Manual of Robotic Surgery*,
https://doi.org/10.1007/978-3-031-86927-3_12

Type III: This type involves herniation of both the GEJ and a portion of the stomach and is the most prevalent among the "true" paraesophageal hernias.

Type IV: In this category, the stomach, along with another intra-abdominal organ, such as the colon or spleen, constitutes the hernia contents.

Surgical Decision-Making

Not all sliding hiatal hernias necessitate surgical intervention. Surgery is advised for sliding hiatal hernias only if patients otherwise meet the criteria for foregut surgery following objective physiological tests and persistent symptoms despite comprehensive medical treatment. For true paraesophageal hernias, it was once believed that surgery was mandatory for all cases (even asymptomatic ones) due to the risk of sudden and severe complications like gastric volvulus. However, current understanding indicates that the annual risk of such acute complications is relatively low, around 1% [2]. Consequently, SAGES from 2013 guidelines currently recommend surgery only for paraesophageal hernias with related symptoms or complications [3]. However, more recent guidelines from the European Association for Endoscopic Surgery (EAES, published in 2023) favor repair for asymptomatic patients who are otherwise reasonable surgical candidates based on improvements in surgical outcomes in the last decade [4].

Surgical Technique

Laparoscopic and robotic transabdominal approaches are now the predominant methods for treating paraesophageal hernias. Transthoracic approaches represent less than 2% of these procedures and are outside the scope of this text [5]. Of transabdominal approaches, laparoscopic repairs remain nearly 10 times more common than robotic repairs in the United States, though this difference is likely to narrow with time [6].

There is currently little high-quality evidence comparing the results of laparoscopic and robotic hiatal hernia repair. The existing literature consists largely of single-center studies with low sample size and designs that are subject to unmeasured confounding. Generally, robotic approaches have been associated with longer operative time, shorter length of stay, and mixed results with regard to complications and recurrences [6–9]. The robotic approach does not change our decision-making regarding whether to offer paraesophageal hernia repair, but we have found robotic repair to be preferable to laparoscopic repair in several scenarios: high BMI, large (including type IV) hernias, or reoperative repairs. In these cases, the visualization and dexterity afforded by the robot are preferable to that achieved laparoscopically. In addition, the length of the robotic arms means that one can use similar port placement regardless of the size of the hiatal hernia.

Positioning and Setup

The following instructions are applicable to the Da Vinci Xi Surgical System (Intuitive Surgical, Sunnyvale, CA), the predominant platform used throughout the United States. Compared to its predecessor the Si, the Xi can be docked in a variety of arrangements depending on the setup of the operating room. A typical OR setup is depicted in Fig. 12.1. We typically dock the robot from the patient's left side, with a liver retractor post placed on the patient's right. The patient is positioned supine, with arms extended, and a footboard to enable steep (15 degree) reverse Trendelenburg positioning. An orogastric tube is placed for gastric decompression but a Foley catheter is typically not placed. If visualization is adequate, we limit insufflation pressure to 10 mm Hg in order to minimize the subcutaneous emphysema that can develop during an extended mediastinal dissection.

Our preferred port placement is depicted in Fig. 12.2. We begin with a Hasson technique through or above the umbilicus, but other approaches to peritoneal access are also reasonable. The four robotic working ports are spaced across the abdomen at the level of the umbilicus. The ports are aimed toward the patient's left shoulder to limit torque and postoperative pain. The bedside assistant sits at patient's right with a 12 mm Airseal assistant port (optional) placed slightly below the level of the robotic ports, between arms 1 and 2. A Nathanson liver retractor is placed in the

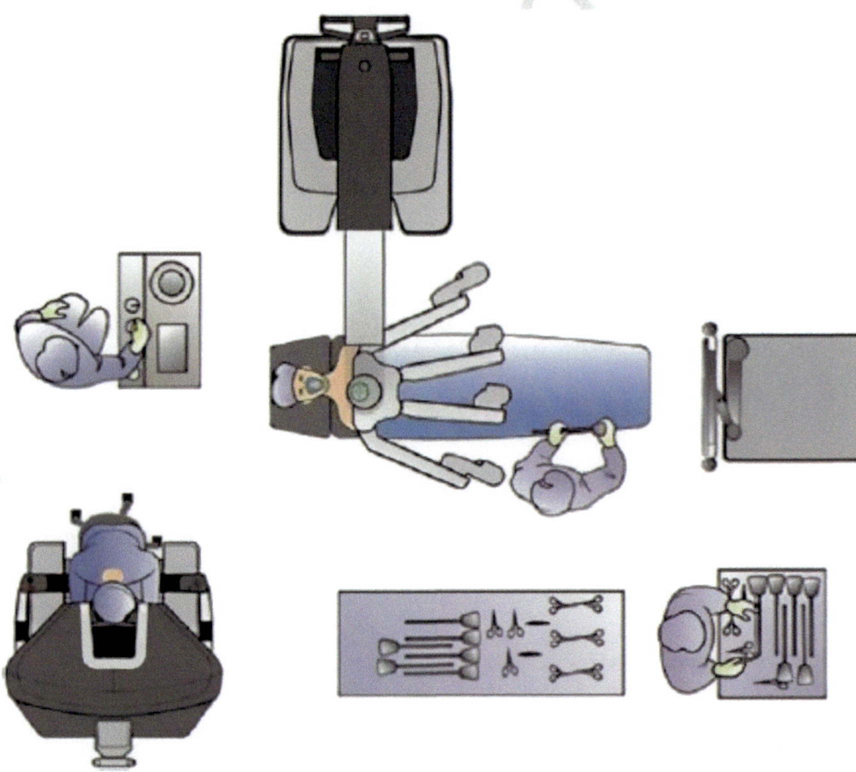

Fig. 12.1 An operating room setup for robot-assisted laparoscopic paraesophageal hernia repair using a side docking technique

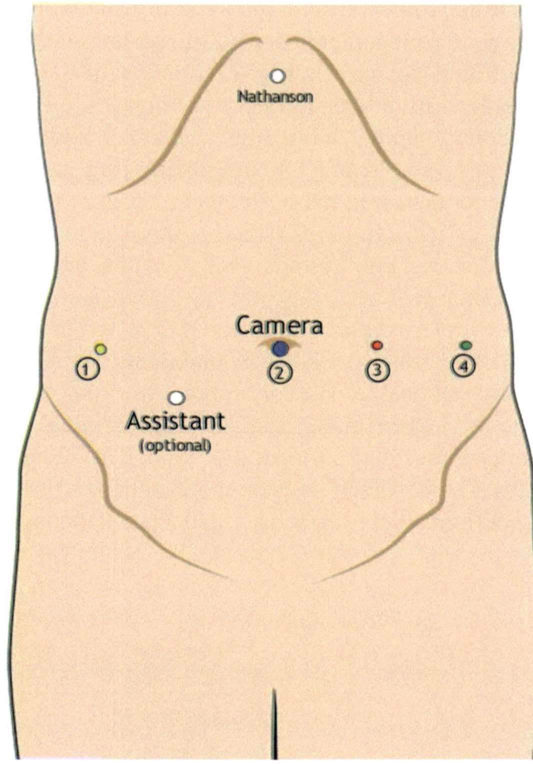

Fig. 12.2 The authors' preferred port placement. Robotic ports are spaced equally across the abdomen, a minimum of 1 hand-breadth apart, at the level of the umbilicus

right upper quadrant. We recommend using a short arm for the Nathanson liver retractor to avoid arm collisions. Our preferred instruments are as follows:

Arm 1. Cadiere or another atraumatic grasper.
Arm 2. 8 mm 30-degree camera.
Arm 3. Energy device—either Synchroseal or Vessel Sealer Extend. We prefer the Synchroseal because it has a faster cycle time and a finer dissecting tip, but it has a longer learning curve than the Vessel Sealer Extend and requires a separate energy generator.
Arm 4. Cadiere or another atraumatic grasper.

Additional instruments are rarely needed. To omit the assistant port, sutures and other supplies can be placed into the peritoneal cavity prior to docking the robotic arms.

Operative Technique

Once the arms have been docked, the liver retractor has been placed, and the patient has been positioned in steep reverse Trendelenburg position, we manually reduce the hernia contents using atraumatic graspers. We then enter the lesser sac using an energy device through the pars flaccida on the right. It is critical to enter the plane between the medial hernia sac and the lateral crura, preserving the fascia over the crura for easier closure and while staying outside the hernia sac (Fig. 12.3). This dissection is extended anteriorly across to the left crus. At this point, we mobilize the short gastric vessels as needed in order to facilitate the later fundoplication.

The dissection proceeds posteriorly around the esophagus, using a Penrose drain or one of the robotic arms for retraction and ensuring total mobilization of the sac from the chest and mediastinum (Fig. 12.4). As the stomach and esophagus are repositioned into the abdomen, the vagus nerves are identified and preserved. The dissection continues, freeing esophageal attachments to the mediastinum to achieve at least 2–3 cm of tension-free intra-abdominal esophagus. The hernia sac is generally resected using an energy device.

After ensuring sufficient esophageal length, we close the hiatus. No single suturing method has been deemed superior; however, a posterior repair with permanent suture is commonly favored. Our preference is to use permanent barbed suture (specifically 9" 0 V loc®, Medtronic, Minneapolis, MN). We suture this in a running horizontal mattress pattern, in order to distribute tension across the crura. Interrupted sutures are also commonly used. Key considerations include avoiding aortic injury when suturing near the left crus, and avoiding the inferior vena cava when suturing the right crus. It is ideal to incorporate some of the fascia overlying the crura to decrease the risk of sutures pulling through. The wristed robotic instruments facilitate careful yet efficient closure while minimizing tissue trauma (Fig. 12.5).

In general, even large defects are usually closable with sutures alone, without undue tension. If not feasible, relaxing incisions on the right or left hemidiaphragm can be performed. The use of mesh is controversial, with the best studies showing mixed results on long-term hiatal hernia recurrence rates with possible harms, including chest pain and dysphagia [10–12]. Current guidelines from the EAES include a "weak" recommendation in favor of mesh to reduce recurrence rates [4].

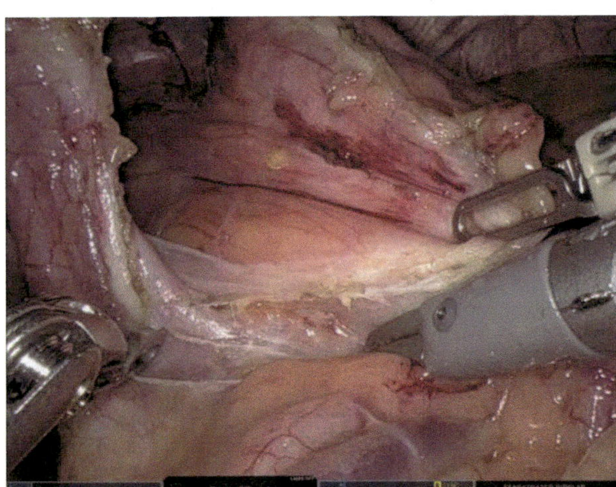

Fig. 12.3 Developing the plane between the crura and hernia sac, while preserving the diaphragmatic fascia, the left gastric vessels, and the integrity of the hernia sac

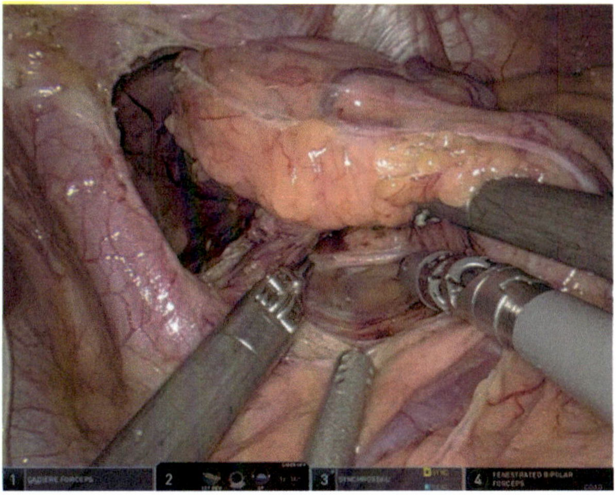

Fig. 12.4 Developing the retroesophageal window using blunt dissection. A Penrose drain can be used for anterior retraction of the esophagus once this window is fully developed

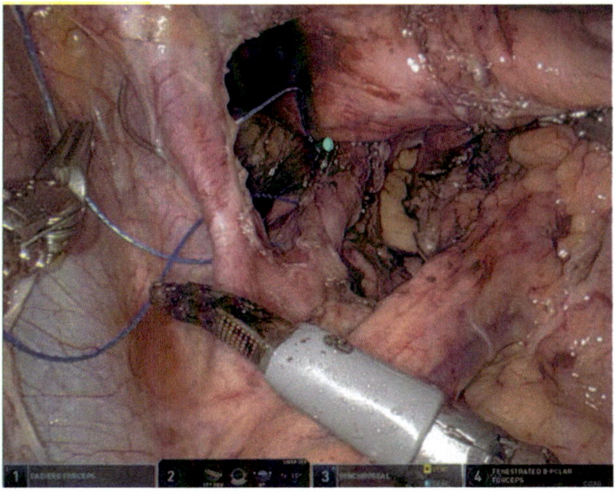

Fig. 12.5 Running horizontal mattress closure of the hiatus

However, there are no large, multicenter randomized trials of mesh versus primary repair, and no robust trials comparing the results of various types of mesh. We use mesh selectively based on the mobility of the crura and for defects >5 cm. When using mesh, biologic material (such as Phasix ST or Bio-A, at our center) is preferred over permanent to reduce the risk of erosion into the esophagus (Fig. 12.6).

Following hiatal closure, a fundoplication is typically performed. We perform fundoplication by placing a marking suture 6 cm lateral and 6 cm caudal to the angle of His (Fig. 12.7). A 54 Fr bougie is then passed through the esophagus into the stomach. The surgeon passes their left hand posterior to the esophagus, then brings the fundus with the marking suture through this space to perform a shoeshine maneuver (Fig. 12.8). If the patient has normal esophageal manometry, we perform

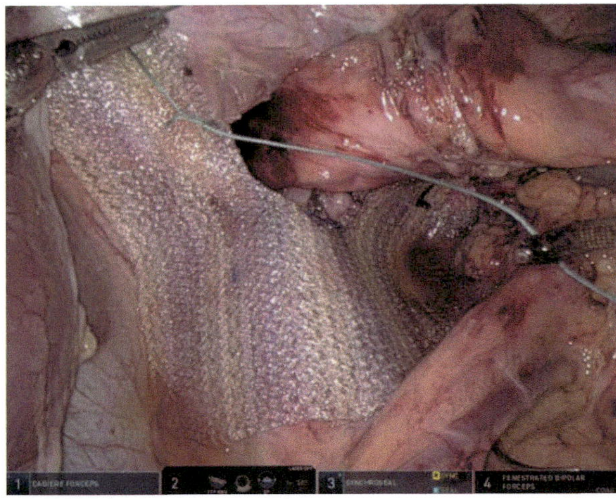

Fig. 12.6 Absorbable mesh is used selectively to reinforce the posterior hiatal closure

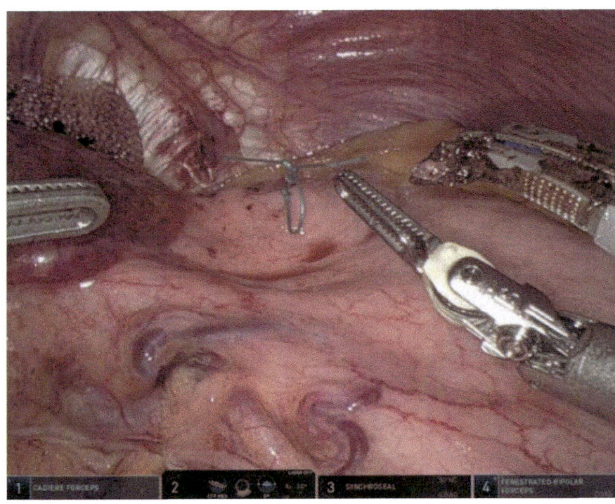

Fig. 12.7 A marking suture placed 6 cm lateral and 6 cm distal to the Angle of His can facilitate creating a fundoplication

a loose and floppy Nissen fundoplication. If the patient's motility is abnormal or unclear, we perform a partial (Toupet) fundoplication. A recent meta-analysis indicated that fundoplication in the setting of paraesophageal hernia repair may be associated with reduced recurrence of GERD (relative risk [RR] 0.64, $p = 0.07$) and paraesophageal hernia (RR 0.53, $p = 0.06$), although these results did not reach statistical significance.[16] We often perform a gastropexy suture to further anchor the stomach in the abdomen.

We perform a completion endoscopy at the conclusion of every case. We pay particular attention to the ease of the scope's passage through the lower esophageal sphincter, as well as the appearance of the fundoplication on retroflexed view. We also perform a transversus abdominus plane (TAP) block under laparoscopic visualization.

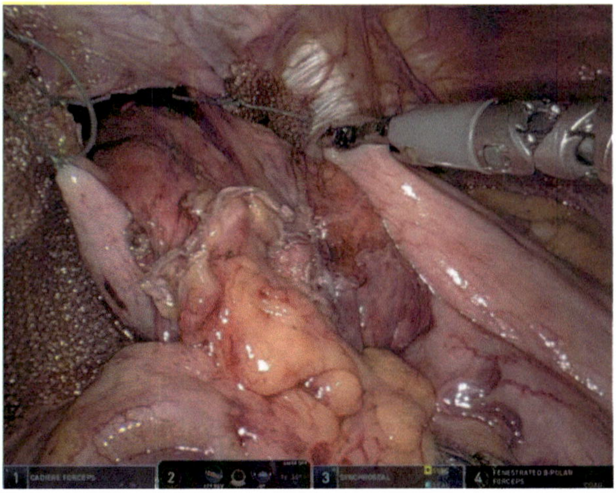

Fig. 12.8 Shoeshine maneuver prior to completing the fundoplication

Postoperative Care

Postoperatively patients are allowed a clear liquid diet on postoperative day zero with the following exceptions: no carbonation, no gelatins, no chewing gum, no straws, and no caffeine. Patients are typically discharged home on the day of surgery or the day afterward on a full liquid diet for 2 weeks. We continue proton pump inhibitors for 2 weeks after surgery then attempt to wean them in the outpatient setting. We routinely measure gastrointestinal quality-of-life scores in the preoperative and postoperative setting, including the GERD-HRQL and Eckardt scores. Patients are also encouraged to work with a registered dietician preoperatively and postoperatively to optimize diet choices.

References

1. Kim J, Hiura GT, Oelsner EC, et al. Hiatal hernia prevalence and natural history on non-contrast CT in the Multi-Ethnic Study of Atherosclerosis (MESA). BMJ Open Gastroenterol. 2021;8(1):e000565. https://doi.org/10.1136/bmjgast-2020-000565.
2. Stylopoulos N, Gazelle GS, Rattner DW. Paraesophageal hernias: operation or observation? Ann Surg. 2002;236(4):492–501.
3. Kohn GP, Price RR, DeMeester SR, et al. Guidelines for the management of hiatal hernia. Surg Endosc. 2013;27(12):4409–28. https://doi.org/10.1007/s00464-013-3173-3.
4. Markar SR, Menon N, Guidozzi N, et al. EAES Multidisciplinary Rapid Guideline: systematic review, meta-analysis, GRADE assessment and evidence-informed recommendations on the surgical management of paraesophageal hernias. Surg Endosc. 2023;37(12):9013–29. https://doi.org/10.1007/s00464-023-10511-1.
5. Mungo B, Molena D, Stem M, Feinberg RL, Lidor AO. Thirty-day outcomes of paraesophageal hernia repair using the NSQIP database: should laparoscopy be the standard of care? J Am Coll Surg. 2014;219(2):229–36. https://doi.org/10.1016/j.jamcollsurg.2014.02.030.
6. Kooiker P, Monnett S, Thompson S, Richmond B. Robotic-assisted versus laparoscopic repair of type II, III and IV hiatal hernias: a retrospective study comparing adverse outcomes. Laparosc Endosc Robot Surg. 2023; https://doi.org/10.1016/j.lers.2023.12.004.

7. O'Connor SC, Mallard M, Desai SS, et al. Robotic versus laparoscopic approach to hiatal hernia repair: results after 7 years of robotic experience. Am Surg. 2020;86(9):1083–7. https://doi.org/10.1177/0003134820943547.
8. Nocera F, Wilhelm A, Schneider R, et al. Robot-assisted vs. laparoscopic repair of complete upside-down stomach hiatal hernia (the RATHER-study): a prospective comparative single center study. Br J Surg. 2021;108(Supplement_4):znab202.001. https://doi.org/10.1093/bjs/znab202.001.
9. Ma L, Luo H, Kou S, et al. Robotic versus laparoscopic surgery for hiatal hernia repair: a systematic literature review and meta-analysis. J Robot Surg. 2023;17(5):1879–90. https://doi.org/10.1007/s11701-023-01636-5.
10. Watson DI, Thompson SK, Devitt PG, et al. Five year follow-up of a randomized controlled trial of laparoscopic repair of very large hiatus hernia with sutures versus absorbable versus nonabsorbable mesh. Ann Surg. 2020;272(2):241. https://doi.org/10.1097/SLA.0000000000003734.
11. Analatos A, Håkanson BS, Ansorge C, Lindblad M, Lundell L, Thorell A. Hiatal hernia repair with tension-free mesh or crural sutures alone in antireflux surgery: a 13-year follow-up of a randomized clinical trial. JAMA Surg. 2023; https://doi.org/10.1001/jamasurg.2023.4976.
12. Oor JE, Roks DJ, Koetje JH, et al. Randomized clinical trial comparing laparoscopic hiatal hernia repair using sutures versus sutures reinforced with non-absorbable mesh. Surg Endosc. 2018;32(11):4579–89. https://doi.org/10.1007/s00464-018-6211-3.

13 Management of Achalasia: A Disease Hard to Swallow

Molly Belisle, Sana Khan, Nicholas Calvo, Alex Lynch, and Abubaker A. Ali

Introduction

Achalasia originates from the Greek *a-* (not) *khalasis* (relaxation), translating to failure of relaxation [1]. It is a rare esophageal motility disorder characterized by impaired relaxation of the lower esophageal sphincter (LES) with absent or spastic contractions of the esophagus [2]. Relaxation of the esophageal smooth muscle is impaired by a loss of inhibitory nerve function of the esophageal myenteric plexus. The prevailing hypothesis is that of an autoimmune reaction targeting an unknown antigen within the esophageal myenteric neurons in genetically predisposed patients. This is challenged by findings that antibodies against myenteric neurons identified in patients with achalasia do not selectively target esophageal myenteric neurons and have also been identified in patients with gastroesophageal reflux disease (GERD) [3]. Infectious and degenerative hypotheses have also been postulated, but no theory has been definitively accepted. The annual incidence of achalasia is estimated at 1–5 cases per 100,000 individuals [4]. There is no predilection for sex or race. Achalasia can occur at any age, but its incidence and prevalence show an age-related increase, predominantly affecting patients over the age of 60 [4]. The most common symptoms of achalasia are dysphagia, regurgitation of undigested food, heartburn, chest pain, and weight loss [2]. The evaluation of a patient suspected to have achalasia involves the barium esophagram and upper endoscopy to rule out structural causes of dysphagia and a definitive diagnosis is made with high-resolution manometry [5]. Endoluminal functional lumen imaging probe (EndoFLIP) measures the dimensions, movement, and pressure inside the esophagus and can be used as an adjunct to high-resolution manometry for diagnosis in equivocal cases [6]. Medical and surgical treatments aim to palliate symptoms of achalasia as there is no curative therapy available. Treatment involves

M. Belisle · S. Khan · N. Calvo · A. Lynch · A. A. Ali (✉)
Wayne State University, Detroit, MI, USA
e-mail: aaali@med.wayne.edu

S. Samreen et al. (eds.), *The SAGES Manual of Robotic Surgery*,
https://doi.org/10.1007/978-3-031-86927-3_13

nonsurgical management such as LES botulinum toxin injection and pneumatic dilation, and surgical management such as per-oral endoscopic myotomy and laparoscopic Heller myotomy [1].

Pathophysiology

The esophagus is a muscular hollow tube that transports food from the mouth into the stomach using gravity and peristalsis. The transfer of food from the esophagus into the stomach is controlled by the lower esophageal sphincter (LES), a 2–4 cm thickened circular muscle layer at the distal end of the esophagus. The LES prevents reflux of gastric contents back into the esophagus by maintaining a resting sphincter tone of 10–30 mmHg. Relaxation of the LES facilitates passage of food into the stomach. This is triggered by swallowing and esophageal wall distention that activates nonadrenergic noncholinergic neurotransmitters, most commonly nitric oxide and vasoactive intestinal peptide (VIP) [3].

Achalasia is characterized by the functional impairment of inhibitory postganglionic neurons in the myenteric plexus ganglion cells of the distal esophagus and the lower esophageal sphincter [7]. The inciting event is unknown, but is hypothesized to be autoimmune in nature, possibly triggered by a viral infection. Individuals with achalasia are more likely to have concurrent autoimmune diseases compared to the general population with an increased prevalence of serum neural autoantibodies [2]. The progressive degeneration of postganglionic neurons in the distal esophagus is caused by an inflammatory response, largely by T-cell lymphocytes [8]. The inflammation of the myenteric plexus impairs the release of nitric oxide and VIP, resulting in unopposed cholinergic stimulation that impairs esophageal and LES relaxation while increasing contractility of the esophagus [2].

Clinical Features

The development of symptoms of achalasia is insidious, with patients typically experiencing symptoms for years prior to seeking formal evaluation [9]. The most common symptoms are progressive dysphagia to both solids and liquids, heartburn from fermentation of carbohydrates in the esophagus, regurgitation of undigested food, which can be mistaken for vomiting, weight loss, and chest pain [10]. Regurgitation of food while lying flat can lead to pulmonary sequelae such as cough and pneumonia [2]. The Eckardt symptom score (ESS) is a widely used tool in clinical and research settings to evaluate symptom severity by measuring weight loss in kilograms, chest pain, regurgitation, and dysphagia [11].

Many patients with achalasia are initially misdiagnosed with GERD. The American College of Gastroenterology recommends a diagnostic workup for achalasia in patients suspected of having GERD who do not respond to acid-suppressive therapy [5].

Diagnosis

Once achalasia is suspected in patients with the symptoms described above, diagnostic modalities, including the barium esophagram, upper endoscopy, manometry, and Endoflip, can be used to confirm the diagnosis.

Barium esophagram is a complementary study that can show a dilated esophagus with a classic "bird-beak" appearance of a narrow gastroesophageal junction in late-stage disease. Timed barium esophagram (TBE) is a simple and cost-effective study that can identify aperistalsis and delayed emptying of barium into the stomach, allowing for the assessment of post-therapy results. A retrospective cohort study by Blonski et al. used TBE with liquid barium to differentiate untreated achalasia from other groups of gastroesophageal junction outflow obstruction and non-achalasia dysphagia with a 79.5% predictive accuracy. This accuracy was improved to 100% using tablet barium. However, they noted that patients with non-achalasia dysphagia also retained liquid and tablet barium 39.3% of the time [12]. Barium esophagram is not specific for achalasia and should not be used alone in diagnosis [5].

Upper endoscopy is used to rule out more common structural disorders of the esophagus, including strictures and neoplastic processes. In patients with achalasia, upper endoscopy can show a dilated esophagus with retained food products. The LES can be traversed by the scope with gentle pressure, unlike in cases of esophageal obstruction by stricture or neoplasm [5]. Patients with achalasia have an increased risk of developing esophageal cancer due to chronic stasis, typically squamous cell type. Those with alarming clinical features such as symptoms of less than 6 months duration, elderly patients with new-onset dysphagia, rapid weight loss, or abnormal endoscopic evaluation raising suspicion for malignancy should undergo further evaluation with endoscopic ultrasound and fine-needle aspiration [13].

Manometry is used to confirm the diagnosis. Manometry findings of achalasia are incomplete relaxation of the lower esophageal sphincter and absence of peristalsis in the distal two-thirds of the esophagus. High-resolution manometry (HRM) has largely replaced conventional manometry due to superior specificity and is the gold standard test for diagnosing achalasia [5]. The Chicago Classification is a system that uses HRM findings to diagnose achalasia and further divides it into three clinically relevant subtypes that vary in treatment types and response. An elevated median integrated relaxation pressure, along with failed peristalsis or spasm on HRM, is consistent with a diagnosis of achalasia. Type I achalasia is characterized by absent peristalsis and pressurization in the distal esophagus, type II by absent peristalsis but with panesophageal pressurization, and type III by abnormal peristalsis with premature contraction [14]. Heller myotomy is indicated for type I and II achalasia, while type III achalasia has shown the best response with peroral endoscopic myotomy. Patients with type II achalasia have the best prognosis with treatment and patients with type III have the worst [1].

The endoluminal functional luminal imaging probe (EndoFLIP) is an adjunctive study that provides a three-dimensional image of the esophageal lumen by measuring diameter, volume, and pressure changes [15]. It can be used to diagnose achalasia in patients where manometry is inconclusive and intraoperatively to assess treatment results. Upper endoscopy may be required to guide the EndoFLIP catheter into the stomach if it is unable to be passed through the gastroesophageal junction [16].

Endoscopic Functional Luminal Imaging Probe (EndoFLIP)

Endoscopic functional luminal imaging probe (EndoFLIP) is a balloon-based catheter that uses impedance planimetry technology to assess the cross-sectional area and distensibility of any sphincter and has been used to determine esophagogastric junction (EGJ) geometry, physiology, and pressure in response to volume distension [17]. A growing body of literature suggests that EndoFLIP can be used in the diagnosis of achalasia and a tool to measure the effectiveness of therapeutic intervention [16]. Manometry remains the current gold standard to diagnose achalasia; however, there are times when obtaining accurate manometric results is not possible or the results do not correlate with patient symptoms. If the EGJ cannot be traversed with the probe, which can occur in a large hiatal hernia (50%) and achalasia (24%), precise conclusions cannot be determined. Likewise, a large hiatal hernia can show elevated integrated relaxation pressure (IRP), yet the LES relaxation may not be impaired, due to the anatomic angulation of the EGJ secondary to the intrathoracic position of the stomach. Multiple studies have shown that the distensibility index (DI) in patients with achalasia falls below 1 $mm^2/mmHg$, which was supported by Law et al., who found that patients with DI <0.8 have a 99% probability of having a diagnosis of achalasia. They also found that values of DI of 0.8–1.3 had a 95% probability of having achalasia and not a hiatal hernia. Thus, for patients with symptoms of dysphagia and upper endoscopy or esophagram consistent with achalasia, the EndoFLIP DI value can provide additional confirmation of improvement with myotomy. Of note, a DI >2.3 $mm^2/mmHg$ with 30cc in the 8 cm balloon was consistent with 99% probability of having a hiatal hernia and DI 1.4–2.2 $mm^2/mmHg$ had a 94% probability of having a hiatal hernia and not achalasia [17].

Treatment

Pharmacotherapy

Calcium channel blockers and nitrates are the mainstay medical therapies for achalasia. However, their use is limited due to adverse effects and poor long-term symptom relief. Beta-agonists, anticholinergics, and phosphodiesterase inhibitors have also shown efficacy in treating achalasia but are not widely used due to poor tolerance. All agents for achalasia are usually taken before meals due to the short duration of relief.

Nitrates release nitric oxide, which leads to smooth muscle relaxation at the lower esophageal sphincter. Isosorbide dinitrate is the most common agent for achalasia. It transiently improves dysphagia, but its efficacy is limited by tachyphylaxis and side effects such as headache, palpitations, and dizziness [18, 19]. Calcium channel blockers inhibit calcium influx into smooth muscle cells, which leads to smooth muscle relaxation. Nifedipine is the agent of choice and reduces sphincter pressures but does not alter esophageal emptying. The main side effects are headaches and peripheral edema [18, 19].

Pharmacotherapies are the least effective treatment option for achalasia and carry a high incidence of adverse effects. Furthermore, there is a lack of high-quality literature evaluating these agents. Thus, several societies recommend reserving pharmacotherapy for poor endoscopic or surgical candidates or for patients who have failed botulinum toxin injection [5, 20, 21].

Endoscopic Treatment

Botulinum Toxin Injection

Botulinum toxin works to decrease LES pressure by inhibiting the presynaptic release of acetylcholine. A total of 80–100 units of botulinum toxin is injected into four quadrants at the lower esophageal sphincter. In a meta-analysis, Leyden et al. showed that 78% of patients treated with a single injection of botulinum toxin injection had initial remission of symptoms. However, 52% were in remission at 6 months and 38% in remission at 12 months [22]. Zaninotto et al. injected botulinum toxin twice 1 month apart, which showed 78% remission at 6 months, 60% at 12 months, and 34% at 24 months [23]. Botulinum toxin injections have poor long-term efficacy compared to alternative therapies [22, 23]. Thus, its use is limited to patients who are not candidates for pneumatic dilation or myotomy. Repeat injections are often required in patients undergoing sole treatment by botulinum toxin injection. Botulinum toxin injection is well tolerated, with mild side effects occurring in only 8% of procedures. These included transient chest pain and heartburn. Severe complications include acute mediastinitis, but this is rare [24]. There are concerns that repetitive botulinum injections can result in a fibrotic reaction that obscures the submucosal plane and increases the complication rates of future myotomy [25]. However, more recent studies call these concerns into question [26]. While there is not yet a consensus, some organizations believe that botulinum toxin injection does not significantly affect myotomy outcomes [5].

Pneumatic Dilation

Pneumatic dilation is a nonsurgical option for achalasia that functions to dilate the LES using air pressure, disrupting the sphincter's circular muscle layer. The procedure can be performed under endoscopic or fluoroscopic guidance. There is variability in technique, but typically a 3 cm transparent polyethylene balloon is inflated to 10–12 psi for 60 s. The most serious complication is perforation, which can occur in 2–4% of patients [27, 28]. These can be managed with observation, covered stents, or operative intervention depending on the nature of the perforation. Some advocate limiting its use only to patients who are surgical candidates due to the risk of perforation and subsequent operation [5]. Symptom remission for a single pneumatic dilation at 1 year has been reported in the range of 55–90% [23, 27, 28]. Pneumatic dilation is preferred to botulinum toxin injection due to improved long-term efficacy [23]. A randomized control trial by Boeckxstaens et al. showed similar long-term remission rates at 2, 5, and 10 years between pneumatic dilation and laparoscopic Heller myotomy [28–30]. However, 25% of pneumatic dilation patients required repeat dilation after 5 years. Further studies and meta-analyses have demonstrated the noninferiority of pneumatic dilation to laparoscopic Heller myotomy [31]. Thus, some advocate that either treatment can be used for the initial treatment of achalasia. However, like botulinum toxin injection, there is concern that scarring and inflammation from pneumatic dilation can complicate future myotomy [32].

Per-oral Endoscopic Myotomy (POEM)

POEM is a hybrid therapy performed under general anesthesia to create a surgical myotomy. First, the gastroesophageal junction is identified, and then diluted methylene blue is injected 10–15 cm proximally. Next, a 1.5 cm longitudinal incision is made on the mucosa to create a submucosal tunnel. A myotomy is then performed along the circular muscle fibers, extending 2–3 cm onto the gastric cardia. The endoscope is then withdrawn and passed through the gastroesophageal junction to assess the adequacy of the myotomy. Finally, the mucosal incision is closed with endoscopic clips, endoscopic sutures, or endoscopic stents.

POEM is indicated for patients who are surgical candidates but wish to avoid surgery or those who failed prior treatments. Patients undergoing POEM achieved 2-year clinical success rates of 80–90% [33, 34]. POEM has been found to be superior to pneumatic dilation for treatment-naive patients [33]. However, Werner et al. showed similar rates of treatment success for naive patients treated with POEM compared to laparoscopic Heller myotomy with Dor fundoplication [34]. POEM can also be used as salvage therapy after the failure of laparoscopic Heller myotomy. Saleh et al. found that patients with recurrent symptoms after laparoscopic Heller myotomy had 1-year treatment success rates of 62% with POEM compared to 27% with pneumatic dilation [35]. It should be noted that there are significantly increased rates of postoperative GERD associated with POEM compared to other therapies. Other less common adverse effects include mucosal perforation, pneumomediastinum, pneumoperitoneum, and *Candida esophagitis*.

Heller Myotomy and Its Evolution

The surgical treatment of achalasia is not a cure; instead, its goal is to enhance the functionality of the EGJ, facilitating the emptying of the esophageal contents in the absence of peristalsis [36]. The first documented treatment of dysphagia was in 1674 with anterograde dilation using a whalebone [37]. It was not until centuries later that the concept of cardioplasty of the EGJ was first proposed by Gottstein in 1901. In 1914, Ernst Heller went on to describe an "extramucosal cardioplasty" involving an anterior and posterior 8 cm vertical esophageal myotomy for the treatment of idiopathic dilation of the esophagus. Zaaijer modified this technique using only an anterior myotomy with promising results in eight patients in 1923 [38]. This myotomy was performed via an open approach, either trans-thoracic or trans-abdominal. The myotomy incision, as described by Ellis et al., extended to only 5 mm on the gastric wall [38]. Through a "short" myotomy on the gastric wall, he was able to achieve an improvement rate of 89% with marked reflux in 5% of patients. Notably, a trans-abdominal approach resulted in a significantly higher incidence of postoperative reflux, which is attributed to a longer myotomy on the gastric wall, division of the phrenoesophageal ligament, and greater mobilization of the esophagus. In 1962, Dor introduced a partial fundoplication to an extended myotomy to decrease postoperative reflux. Bonavina et al. supported this technique finding that in 206 patients who had an anterior myotomy (8 cm on the esophagus and 2 cm on the stomach) with Dor fundoplication 93.8% of patients had complete or near-complete resolution of symptoms [38]. The addition of a Dor fundoplication after a Heller myotomy reduced pathologic reflux demonstrated by Richards et al. finding a 47–9% measurable decrease in 24-h pH studies without impact on dysphagia [39].

The myotomy with fundoplication remained the tenet of surgical treatment for achalasia; however, the approach underwent modernization in the 1990s with the introduction of laparoscopic techniques to esophageal surgery. The first laparoscopic cardiomyotomy was performed by Dr. Cushieri in 1991 [40]. In 1992, Dr. Pelligrini described the results of 17 patients who underwent a thoracoscopic 7 cm myotomy on the left side of the esophagus extending only 5 mm on the gastric wall. The goal was to balance dysphagia relief with reflux prevention. While the short- and long-term outcomes were excellent in 90% of cases, this approach had drawbacks, including intraoperative lung exclusion, a postoperative chest tube, and high incidence of reflux given the absence of fundoplication [38]. The ability to perform a myotomy and a partial fundoplication could be achieved with a laparoscopic approach, making this the standard of care by the late 1990s. Comparisons of these approaches by Patti et al. found that the laparoscopic group had shorter median hospital stay (42 hours laparoscopic vs. 84 hours thoracoscopic group), better resolution of dysphagia (90% laparoscopic vs. 87% thoracoscopic group), and improved 24 h pH testing (10% laparoscopic vs. 60% thoracoscopic group) [38].

Regarding the type of fundoplication, Rawlings et al in 2012 found no significant difference in terms of relief of dysphagia and reflux control when comparing a Dor to a Toupet fundoplication. Albeit, Rebecchi, and colleagues found a significant difference in the dysphagia symptoms when a Nissen wrap was performed [38]. The advent of robotic surgery has rivaled the previous laparoscopic techniques arguing the absence of a tremor and 3D magnified view can reduce the incidence of esophageal perforation. In 2005, Horgan et al. demonstrated a perforation incidence of 0% in the robotic group versus 16% in the laparoscopic group. Huffman et al. supported these findings in 2007 with a perforation rate of 0% in the robotic group versus 8% in the laparoscopic group. The development of cardiomyotomy, as envisioned by Heller over a century ago, performed minimally invasively with a partial fundoplication, remains the surgical treatment of choice for achalasia today [37].

The key component of selecting patients for surgical management of achalasia is to differentiate it from other motility disorders such as pseudoachalasia, malignancy, and mechanical obstruction. This should be performed in the preoperative setting by the surgeon reviewing the history of the patient's symptoms and review of previous studies, including the results of esophageal manometry, endoscopy, and contrast esophagram. The patient needs to understand that this is a palliative surgery meant to relieve the symptoms and is not a cure. A laparoscopic myotomy, when combined with an antireflux procedure, provides better symptom relief (90%) than all endoscopic and other surgical approaches and carries a lower complication rate of 6.3% [40]. This information should be communicated to the patient during the preoperative clinic visit.

Heller Myotomy

Operative Steps

Anesthesia Induction and Robot Docking

Patients are advised to stay on a liquid diet preoperatively for 1 week, especially if they have an end-stage esophagus, that is, sigmoid esophagus. During this time, they are placed on a high-protein shake. Preoperative enoxaparin is given prior to intubation. Care is taken by anesthesia to minimize the risk of aspiration by performing a rapid sequence intubation and the patient not laying completely flat.

After induction of general anesthesia, the patient is placed on the operating table in supine position, with both arms tucked and a foot board in place. The arm is tucked to allow the robot to be docked with no interference with the arm board. Having the arm out is an acceptable practice. The patient is given prophylactic antibiotics, usually a first-generation cephalosporin, within 1 h of the incision. An orogastric tube and an optional Foley catheter is inserted. Sequential compression devices are turned on and functioning throughout the case.

The procedure is commenced by making a stab incision in the left upper quadrant at Palmer's point. A Veress needle is inserted and pneumoperitoneum established to 15 mmHg of CO_2. The authors use the Davinci Xi platform. All trocars are lined in a horizontal line that is no more than 15 cm below the xiphoid process. The abdominal cavity is then entered along the right mid-clavicular line using a 30-degree 5-mm laparoscope housed in a robotic 8-mm trocar, using the Optiview technique. Under direct visualization, an 8-mm trocar is then placed two fingerbreadths to the left of the umbilicus, approximately 15 cm below the xiphoid process. Two additional 8-mm trocars are inserted roughly 8 cm apart along the left midclavicular and left anterior axillary lines. An optional additional 5-mm assistant port is placed in the right lower quadrant. The patient is then placed in reverse Trendelenburg position. The authors utilize two right hands and one left hand. The Davinci Xi robot is then docked with a Maryland bipolar in (right midclavicular trocar), camera in arm two, Vessel sealer/hook/syncroseal in (left midclavicular trocar), and Cardiere grasper in (left anterior axillary trocar). At this point, the orogastric tube is removed once the stomach is confirmed to be deflated and suction is left on while it is being withdrawn slowly to suction all esophageal content.

Liver Retraction

Next, the left lateral segment of the liver is retracted. This has been described with a Nathonson retractor or pretzel retractor. Both of which require an additional incisional with an epigastric incision with the former and 5 mm trocar in the latter. The Nathanson retractor should be positioned so it does not interfere with robot arms. Alternatively, a suture hammock with a #1 V-lock 18-inch suture as described by Dr. Havaleshko's, "Dima stitch," to suspend the left lateral segment of the liver anteriorly in order to expose the hiatus.

Hiatal Dissection

The dissection toward the crus can be initiated with a right-first approach or a left. If the surgeon plans to perform a Toupet fundoplication as the choice of partial wrap or the patient has a hiatal hernia (rare), then a left approach is more logical. This will allow for the placement of a penrose/umbilical tape for esophageal retraction from the patient's left. This can be retrieved from the right side once the retroesophageal window is created. However, if the plan is to perform a Dor fundoplication or not to perform a wrap at all (in the case of sigmoid esophagus, i.e., end esophagus), it is better to start with the right-first approach. A person may wonder why with a Dor wrap to start on the right side. When creating a Dor wrap, the retroesophageal attachment is kept intact. Also, if the fundus is very floppy, the short gastric arteries do not need to be taken down, although preserving the short gastrics with a Dor wrap is not the author's preferred approach as it can create tension at the gastroesophageal junction.

To begin the left-first approach, the gastrocolic ligament is incised, and dissection is continued toward the left crus, taking down the short gastric vessels and mobilizing the gastric fundus. This can be performed using the vessel sealer or Synchroseal. Care is taken to avoid avulsing the splenic capsule or splenic vessels by aiming the tip of the bipolar device toward the left crus and never toward the splenic hilum. To expose the left crus, the stomach should be grasped by the posterior wall and retracted toward the patient's right side, that is, away from the spleen. This provides better exposure than grasping the anterior wall or the greater curve.

Attention is then carried to incising the pars flaccida along the lesser curvature, heading toward the right crus. Care should be taken as sometimes a replaced left hepatic artery can arise from the left gastric artery. The vessel can be clamped and the liver observed for color change. If none are observed, the vessel is transected. The phrenoesophageal membrane and peritoneum overlying the esophagus is incised, with care to not injure the esophagus or anterior vagus nerve. Then, the pillar of the left crus is separated from the esophagus. Dissection is then carried into the mediastinum. This is done mostly in a blunt fashion, anteriorly and laterally to the esophagus, so that at least 9 cm of esophagus is exposed for esophageal myotomy later, or dissected roughly to the level of the inferior pulmonary vein. The lateral esophageal dissection can help straighten the esophagus, whether this provides better emptying or not is unknown.

Next, the fat pad is excised from the anterior surface of the esophagus taking care not to injure the anterior vagus nerve. It is best to start taking the fat pad starting on the greater curve, heading toward the lesser curve with frequent, gentle pulling of the fat pad caudally to locate the vagus nerve.

Myotomy

The myotomy can be performed with or without a bougie in place. If utilized, a 56 French or similar-sized lighted Bougie is carefully inserted into the esophagus, to facilitate the myotomy. The lighted bougie can be seen entering the abdominal cavity both on white mode and near-infrared mode. The anesthesia team can perform or the surgeon can insert the bougie to avoid the complication of an esophageal perforation. The myotomy can be performed in a blunt fashion (Fig. 13.1a), using scissors, a hook (Fig. 13.1b), or bipolar device (vessel sealer or Synchroseal). The magnification, stability of the robot platform, and 3D magnification allow this critical portion of surgery to be performed with precision. Initially, the longitudinal outer muscle of the esophagus is bluntly separated (Fig. 13.2a). This facilitates exposure of the circular muscle of the esophagus, which is then incised with the vessel sealer, which is our preferred approach (Fig. 13.2b). The esophageal myotomy is then extended 7–9 cm proximally along the esophagus, exposing the underlying mucosa (Fig. 13.3). The lighted bougie helps with the mucosal transillumination to ensure myotomy completion (Fig. 13.4). It is important to note there is currently no consensus on the length of the myotomy. Currently, SAGES recommends a 4 cm esophageal myotomy, extended on the stomach for 2 cm. The 2018 International Society of Diseases of the Esophagus guidelines recommend at least 6 cm proximal to the gastroesophageal junction, with 2 cm distal to the junction [41].

The myotomy is then extended distally along the stomach, for a length of 3 cm (Fig. 13.5). Wright et al. compared 52 patients with achalasia undergoing a Heller myotomy, extending for 1–2 cm onto the gastric wall and Dor fundoplication to 63 patients who underwent an extended myotomy (3 cm) with Toupet fundoplication, and found that the extended 3 cm myotomy gave patients better relief of dysphagia [42]. This is done with blunt dissection, exposing the underlying mucosa. The robot, with its articulating instruments, allows this portion of

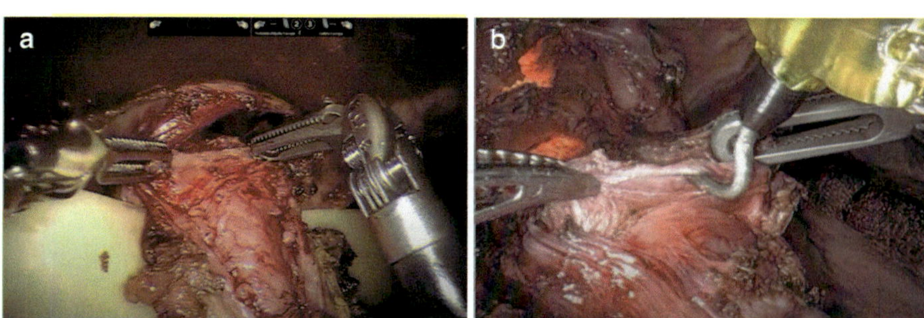

Fig. 13.1 The myotomy can be performed using various techniques, including blunt dissection (**a**), or with the aid of instruments such as scissors, a hook (**b**), or a bipolar device like the Synchroseal or a vessel sealer

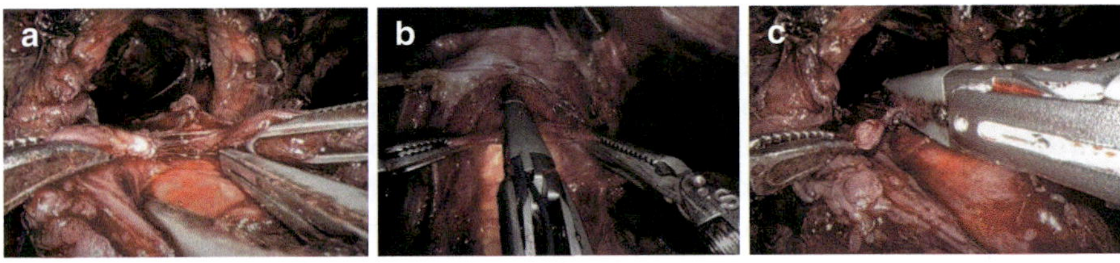

Fig. 13.2 The procedure begins with blunt separation of the longitudinal outer muscle of the esophagus (**a**), allowing clear exposure of the underlying circular muscle. The circular muscle is then incised using the vessel sealer (**b** and **c**)

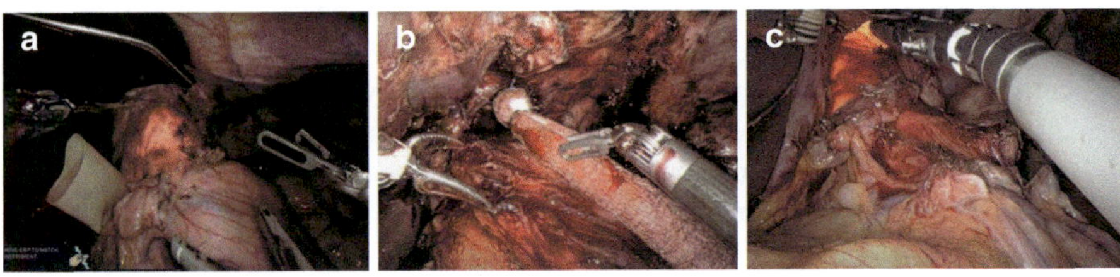

Fig. 13.3 The esophageal myotomy is then extended 7–9 cm proximally along the esophagus, exposing the underlying mucosa. In image "b" an epinephrine-soaked sponge is used to clear the blood and facilitate visualization. In image "c" you can see the anterior Vagus nerve crossing from left to become the anterior Vagus nerve in the abdomen. This should be preserved and retracted during the myotomy

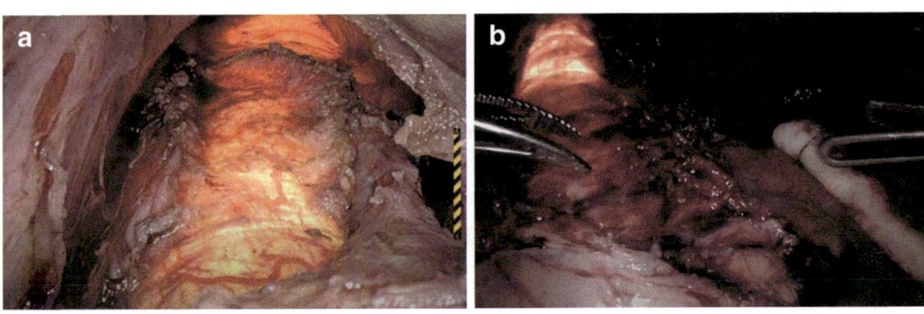

Fig. 13.4 A lighted bougie helps with the mucosal transillumination to ensure myotomy completion

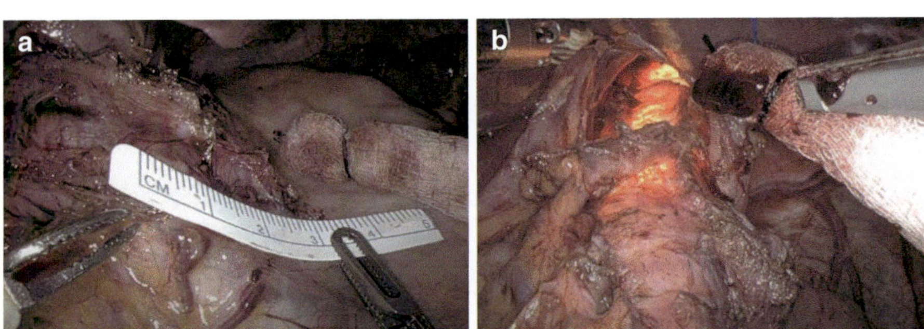

Fig. 13.5 The myotomy is further extended distally along the stomach, for a length of 3 cm

surgery, which is the most difficult due to the high risk of perforation on the gastric side due to the insertion of the oblique fibers. Unlike during laparoscopy, there is no tactile feedback and the surgeon relies heavily on visual cues. Also, unlike laparoscopy, this portion can be performed with a hook in a top-down fashion from the esophagus toward the stomach because the instruments articulate. Completion of gastric myotomy should be confirmed by visualizing the cardinal vein, which can sometimes bleed during this portion of the procedure (Fig. 13.6). Care should be taken not to use energy sources as to avoid gastric mucosal injury that can result in immediate versus delayed perforation. It is best to control any bleeding from the myotomy with soaked epinephrine gauze and gentle pressure (Fig. 13.7). The length of both esophageal myotomy and gastric myotomy is measured with a ruler that is inserted intra-abdominally.

The lighted bougie is then removed and intraoperative upper endoscopy is performed. We like to perform a picture-in-picture endoscopy, that is, Tile Pro, where the surgeon can see both the laparoscopic view of abdomen and the endoscopic image at the console. The purpose of endoscopy is to

1. Examine the ease by which the scope passes the GE junction prior to and after the wrap.
2. Confirm the GE junction and, therefore, confirm the length of gastric myotomy and esophageal myotomy.
3. Examine the completion of myotomy by noticing mucosa bulging.
4. Examine for any bougie injury or mucosal perforation. The latter is performed by emerging the mucosa underwater and performing a leak test.

Partial Fundoplication

Attention is then paid to the partial fundoplication; the type of partial fundoplication performed, Dor versus Toupet, is still under debate. Tomasko et al. retrospectively compared patient outcomes for laparoscopic Heller myotomy with either Dor versus Toupet and found overall patient satisfaction was similar (93.8% vs. 87.5%)

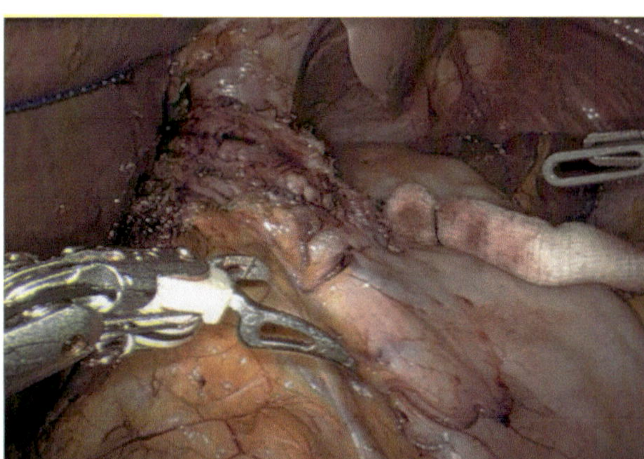

Fig. 13.6 The completion of the gastric myotomy is confirmed by visualizing the cardinal vein

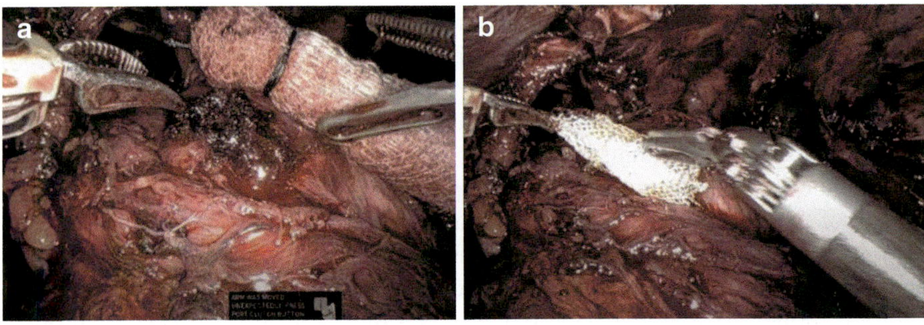

Fig. 13.7 Bleeding from the gastric myotomy is managed using epinephrine-soaked gauze and gentle pressure, which helps prevent delayed thermal injury to the mucosa

[43]. They found no difference in regards to the incidence or severity of postoperative heartburn, dysphagia, or bloating. The mean operative time for the Toupet fundoplication was 137.3 min while the mean time for the Dor fundoplication was only 111.5 min (p = 0.006). Torres et al. had similar findings with their randomized control trial comparing laparoscopic Heller myotomy with Dor versus Toupet fundoplication in regards to patient symptom scores and high-resolution manometry long term [44]. These studies provide support that either option is acceptable.

The goal of surgical intervention of achalasia is to provide an adequate myotomy while reducing the risk of reflux. This lies with an intraoperative assessment of the LES during the myotomy and fundoplication that can be done with EndoFLIP. Law et al. were able to report changes in EndoFLIP prior to and after myotomy and after fundoplication. There was a measurable difference in mean DI from 0.7 mm^2/mmHg prior to myotomy to 3.2 mm^2/mmHg after ($p < 0.001$). Following fundoplication, the DI decreased to 2.2 mm^2/mmHg following Dor fundoplication, which is consistent with previous studies finding a decrease in DI to 3.3 from 4.5 mm^2/mmHg. This distensibility has been correlated to an Eckardt score with a DI <3 associated with an Eckardt score of >3, indicating treatment failure. The median Eckhardt score in this study utilizing intraoperative EndoFLIP after myotomy and fundoplication was 0 from 4.5 prior to surgery, still with no reported symptoms of postoperative reflux. Therefore, EndoFLIP can be a beneficial adjunct during surgery to reduce the risk of reflux symptoms and provide optimal patient outcomes [17]. In cases where the patient has an end-stage esophagus, that is, sigmoid esophagus, no wrap is performed. In these patients, we only reconstitute the angle of His to reduce reflux without compromising the EGJ. Endoflip is a great adjunct that is currently available at some institutions and can help tailor the choice of wrap; however, the authors do not currently use this technology.

Our institution typically performs the Dor procedure. The initial and possibly most important step is to reapproximate the angle of His, by suturing the medial portion of the fundus to the left crus with a #2-0 Ethibond suture (Fig. 13.8a, b). The fundoplication is then performed by suturing the medial portion of the fundus to the left pillar of the crus and the left edge of the myotomy. Then, two additional sutures are placed distally, approximately 1 cm apart, securing the medial portion of the fundus to the left edge of the myotomy (Fig. 13.8c). The most lateral part of the fundus is then secured to the right edge of the myotomy and the right pillar of the crus. Two additional sutures are then placed distally, securing the lateral fundus to the right edge of the myotomy, ensuring no mucosa is incorporated. Finally, one last stitch is placed between the upper two stitches and the crus, completing the Dor fundoplication.

After the wrap is completed, repeat upper endoscopy is performed to ensure patency of the gastroesophageal junction and the scope is retroflexed to assess the wrap (Fig. 13.9). Richards et al. performed a prospective, randomized, double-blind, control trial comparing surgical outcomes in patients who underwent Heller myotomy alone versus Heller myotomy plus Dor fundoplication [39]. They enrolled 43 patients and found pathologic reflux, defined as distal esophageal acid exposure

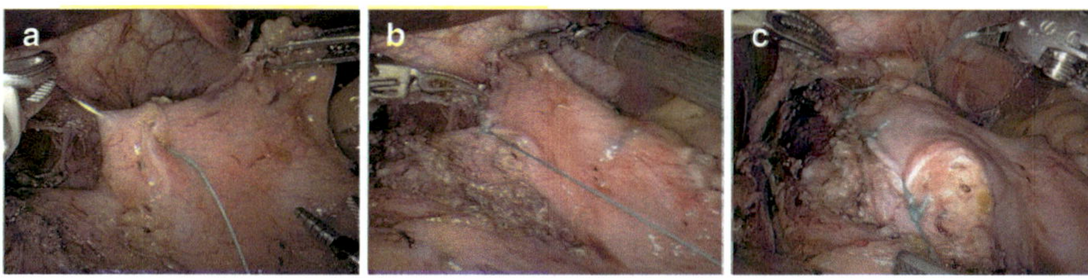

Fig. 13.8 Dor fundoplication is performed to re-establish the angle of His. This involves suturing the medial portion of the fundus to the left crus using a #2-0 Ethibond suture (**a** and **b**). Total of three sutures are placed separated 1 cm apart. The fundoplication is then completed by securing the the anteriolateral fundus to the right pillar of the crus and the right edge of the myotomy with three sutures separated 1 cm apart

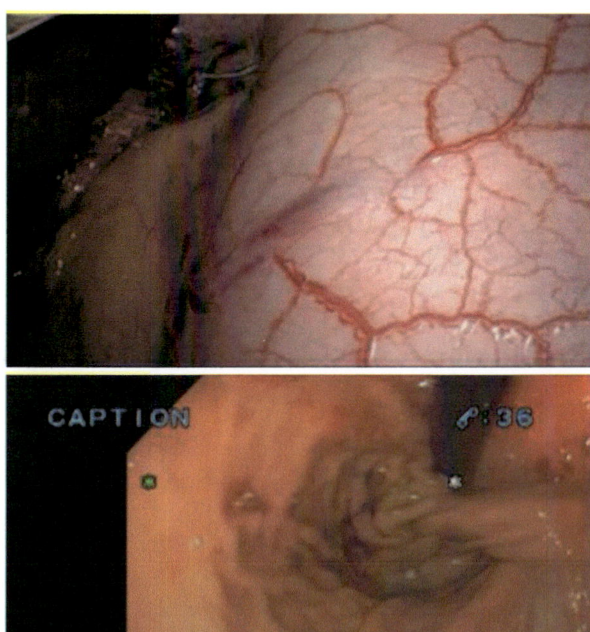

Fig. 13.9 A repeat upper endoscopy with retroflexion is performed to assess the integrity and positioning of the wrap after its completion. It's important to make sure the wrap although partial is not too tight when the scope is traversing the GE junction. The latter can lead to postoperative dysphagia

time of more than 4.2% per 24-hr period 6 months postoperatively, was significantly reduced in the Heller plus Dor group (47.6% vs. 9.1%). There was no difference found in postoperative dysphagia. These findings were investigated for long-term effects by Broman et al., who contacted the previous cohort 10 years later, and found the dysphagia scores were slightly worse for Heller alone than Heller plus Dor, but the findings were not statistically significant [45]. Interestingly, 96% of patients contacted stated they would undergo the operation again.

Intraoperative Complications

Esophageal Perforation

Iatrogenic esophageal perforation can occur while creating the myotomy. This should be noticed intraoperatively with the assistance of the lighted bougie (Fig. 13.10a) or during upper endoscopy with or without a leak test. This can be repaired with a 5-0 PDS suture, in a figure-of-eight fashion (Fig. 13.10b). A leak test should be performed after repair (Fig. 13.10c).

Gastric Perforation

Gastric mucosal perforation is more common than esophageal mucosal perforation due to the oblique muscles. This can occur while extending the myotomy into the cardia of the stomach. This can be repaired with a 5-0 PDS suture, in a figure-of-eight fashion (Fig. 13.11). A leak test should be performed after repair.

Vagal Nerve Injury

Care should be taken to identify anterior vagus nerve intraoperatively. If one vagal nerve is transected, this should be disclosed to the patient after completion of the case (Fig. 13.12). Unilateral vagal nerve injury can lead to delayed gastric emptying;

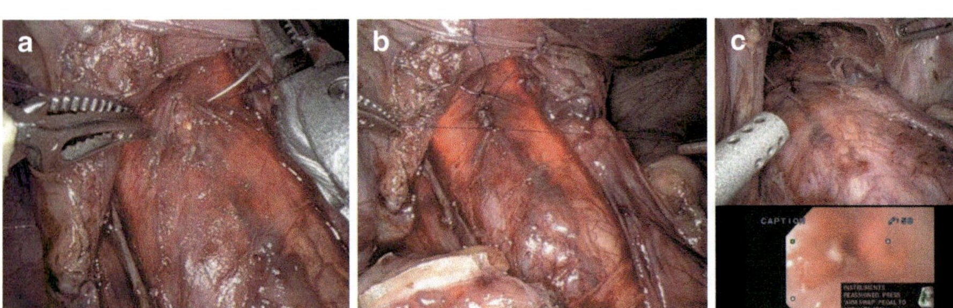

Fig. 13.10 An iatrogenic esophageal injury is identified intraoperatively with the assistance of the lighted bougie (**a**). The injury is repaired using a 5-0 PDS suture (**b**), followed by a leak test to ensure the repair's integrity (**c**)

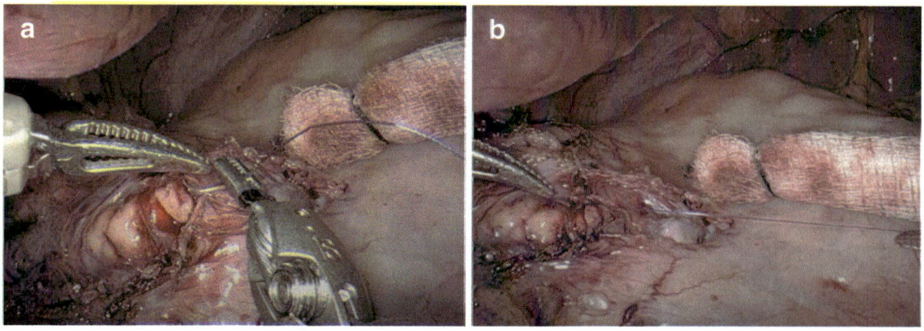

Fig. 13.11 An iatrogenic gastric perforation is repaired using a 5-0 PDS suture in an interrupted fashion

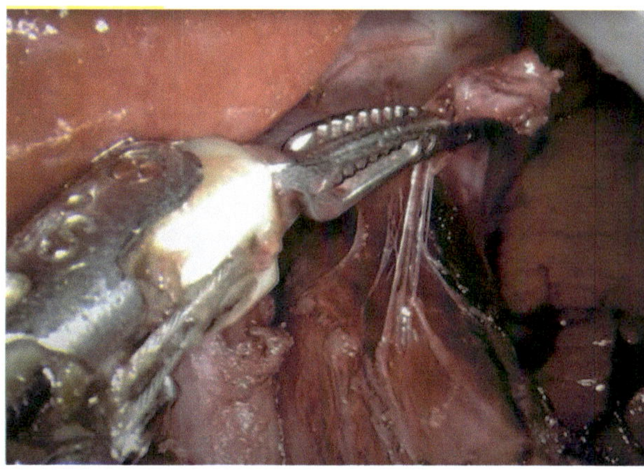

Fig. 13.12 Unilateral anterior vagal nerve injury is noted intraoperatively

however, Lindeboom et al. have shown that fundoplication itself may significantly accelerate gastric emptying [46]. This may be due to alteration in gastric compliance. Postprandial accommodation of the proximal stomach is impaired, which may lead to more rapid transport of the meal to the antrum, thereby accelerating gastric emptying. Oelschlager et al. recently investigated the use of an intentional vagotomy to lengthen the esophagus during complex esophageal surgery [47]. They found no difference in the severity of abdominal pain, bloating, diarrhea, or early satiety between the vagotomy and no vagotomy groups. They propose it as an alternative to a Collis gastroplasty when extensive esophageal mobilization fails to provide adequate esophageal length.

Postoperative Care

Postoperatively, patients are admitted to the surgical team and are started on a clear liquid diet immediately, even if the patient had a mucosal injury that was repaired intraoperatively. Scheduled antiemetics are given for 5 days postoperatively. Patients also receive 10 mg of Decadron every 8 h for 48 h. This helps reduce the swelling from the bougie being inserted and has antiemetic properties. Emesis can generate a high pressure within the esophagus, leading to perforation of the mucosa. Analgesia can be provided with oral narcotics such as Hycet. No intravenous pain medication is needed. A multimodal approach for analgesia is used. In our practice, it is not necessary to obtain a postoperative swallow study unless the patient was noted to have an intraoperative mucosal injury, in which case a contrast esophagram should be obtained with gastrografin followed by barium. Patients can be discharged within 24 h on a clear liquid diet and advance to a soft diet at home. Patients should be provided with education to return for evaluation in the emergency department with symptoms of chest pain, shortness of breath, or persistent nausea. Patients are seen in clinic postoperatively, and a Eckardt score is performed comparing it to preoperative score. Our practice is to place these patients on a proton pump inhibitor. While not a standard recommendation, this approach remains common practice. Acid reflux is a known occurrence after surgical or endoscopic myotomy, resulting from the disruption of the natural antireflux barrier. Although the incidence of postintervention acid reflux is well documented, the lack of a precise definition stems from varied diagnostic criteria. Moreover, both subjective and objective measurements of acid reflux in these patients tend to decrease over time. Considering this information, current guidelines suggest conducting endoscopic surveillance around 12 months after myotomy and POEM procedures [48].

References

1. Pandolfino JE, Gawron AJ. Achalasia: a systematic review. JAMA. 2015;313(18):1841–52.
2. Savarino E, Bhatia S, Roman S, Sifrim D, Tack J, Thompson SK, Gyawali CP. Achalasia. Nat Rev Dis Primers. 2022;8(1):28.
3. Furuzawa-Carballeda J, et al. Achalasia – an autoimmune inflammatory disease: a cross-sectional study. J Immunol Res. 2015;2015:1.
4. Mayberry JF. Epidemiology and demographics of achalasia. Gastrointest Endosc Clin N Am. 2001;11(2):235–47.
5. Vaezi MF, et al. ACG clinical guidelines: diagnosis and management of achalasia. Am J Gastroenterol. 2020;115:1393–411.
6. Triggs JR, et al. Functional luminal imaging probe panometry identifies achalasia-type esophagogastric junction outflow obstruction. Clin Gastroenterol Hepatol. 2020;18(10):2209–17.
7. Gregersen H, Lo KM. Pathophysiology and treatment of achalasia in a muscle mechanical perspective. Ann New York Acad Sci. 2018;1434(1):173–84.
8. Kraichely R, et al. Neural autoantibody profile of primary achalasia. Digest Dis Sci. 2010;55:307–11.
9. Eckardt VF, et al. Risk factors for diagnostic delay in achalasia. Digest Dis Sci. 1997;42:580–5.
10. Tsuboi K, et al. Insights gained from symptom evaluation of esophageal motility disorders: a review of 4,215 patients. Digestion. 2012;85(3):236–42.
11. Taft TH, et al. Evaluating the reliability and construct validity of the Eckardt symptom score as a measure of achalasia severity. Neurogastroenterol Motil. 2018;30(6):e13287.
12. Blonski W, et al. Timed barium swallow: diagnostic role and predictive value in untreated achalasia, esophagogastric junction outflow obstruction, and non-achalasia dysphagia. Off J Am Coll Gastroenterol|ACG. 2018;113(2):196–203.
13. Portale G, et al. Pseudoachalasia: not only esophago-gastric cancer. Dis Esophagus. 2007;20(2):168–72.

14. Rohof WOA, Bredenoord AJ. Chicago classification of esophageal motility disorders: lessons learned. Curr Gastroenterol Rep. 2017;19:1–6.
15. Donnan EN, Pandolfino JE. EndoFLIP in the esophagus: assessing sphincter function, wall stiffness, and motility to guide treatment. Gastroenterol Clin. 2020;49(3):427–35.
16. Law YY, et al. Intraoperative diagnosis and treatment of Achalasia using EndoFLIP during Heller Myotomy and Dor fundoplication. Surg Endosc. 2022;36(4):2365–72.
17. Donnan EN, et al. EndoFLIP in the esophagus: assessing sphincter function, wall stiffness, and motility to guide treatment. Gastroenterol Clin N Am. 2020;49(3):427–35. https://doi.org/10.1016/j.gtc.2020.04.002.
18. Tustumi F. Evaluating the non-conventional achalasia treatment modalities. Front Med (Lausanne). 2022;9:941464. https://doi.org/10.3389/fmed.2022.941464.
19. Nassri A, Ramzan Z. Pharmacotherapy for the management of achalasia: current status, challenges and future directions. World J Gastrointest Pharmacol Ther. 2015;6(4):145–55. https://doi.org/10.4292/wjgpt.v6.i4.145.
20. Nijhuis O, et al. European guidelines on achalasia: United European Gastroenterology and European Society of Neurogastroenterology and Motility recommendations. United Eur Gastroenterol J. 2020;8(1):13–33. https://doi.org/10.1177/2050640620903213.
21. Jung et al. Korean Society of Neurogastroenterology and Motility. 2019 Seoul consensus on esophageal achalasia guidelines. J Neurogastroenterol Motil. 2020;26(2):180–203. https://doi.org/10.5056/jnm20014. Erratum in: J Neurogastroenterol Motil. 2021;27(3):441–442
22. Leyden, et al. Endoscopic pneumatic dilation versus botulinum toxin injection in the management of primary achalasia. Cochrane Database Syst Rev. 2014;2014(12):CD005046. https://doi.org/10.1002/14651858.CD005046.pub3.
23. Zaninotto, et al. Randomized controlled trial of botulinum toxin versus laparoscopic heller myotomy for esophageal achalasia. Ann Surg. 2004;239(3):364–70. https://doi.org/10.1097/01.sla.0000114217.52941.c5.
24. Van Hoeij, et al. Complications of botulinum toxin injections for treatment of esophageal motility disorders. Dis Esophagus. 2017;30(3):1–5. https://doi.org/10.1111/dote.12491.
25. Smith CD, et al. Endoscopic therapy for achalasia before Heller myotomy results in worse outcomes than heller myotomy alone. Ann Surg. 2006;243(5):579–84; discussion 584–6. https://doi.org/10.1097/01.sla.0000217524.75529.2d.
26. Tan S, et al. Efficacy and safety of peroral endoscopic myotomy in achalasia patients with failed previous intervention: a systematic review and meta-analysis. Gut Liver. 2021;15(2):153–67. https://doi.org/10.5009/gnl19234.
27. Javed, et al. Durability of pneumatic dilation monotherapy in treatment-naive achalasia patients. BMC Gastroenterol. 2019;19(1):181. https://doi.org/10.1186/s12876-019-1104-z.
28. Boeckxstaens, et al. European Achalasia Trial Investigators. Pneumatic dilation versus laparoscopic Heller's myotomy for idiopathic achalasia. N Engl J Med. 2011;364(19):1807–16. https://doi.org/10.1056/NEJMoa1010502.
29. Moonen A, et al. Long-term results of the European achalasia trial: a multicentre randomized controlled trial comparing pneumatic dilation versus laparoscopic Heller myotomy. Gut. 2016;65(5):732–9. https://doi.org/10.1136/gutjnl-2015-310602.
30. Boeckxstaens G, et al. 10-year follow-up results of the European Achalasia Trial: a multicentre randomized controlled trial comparing pneumatic dilation with laparoscopic Heller myotomy. Gut. 2023:gutjnl-2023-331374. https://doi.org/10.1136/gutjnl-2023-331374.
31. Cheng, et al. Laparoscopic Heller myotomy is not superior to pneumatic dilation in the management of primary achalasia: conclusions of a systematic review and meta-analysis of randomized controlled trials. Medicine (Baltimore). 2017;96(7):e5525. https://doi.org/10.1097/MD.0000000000005525.
32. El-Magd EA, et al. Pre-operative endoscopic balloon dilatation and its impact on outcome of laparoscopic Heller cardiomyotomy for patients with achalasia: does the frequency and interval matter? Surg Endosc. 2023;37(10):7667–75. https://doi.org/10.1007/s00464-023-10314-4.
33. Ponds, et al. Effect of peroral endoscopic myotomy vs pneumatic dilation on symptom severity and treatment outcomes among treatment-naive patients with achalasia: a randomized clinical trial. JAMA. 2019;322(2):134–44. https://doi.org/10.1001/jama.2019.8859.

34. Werner, et al. Endoscopic or surgical myotomy in patients with idiopathic achalasia. N Engl J Med. 2019;381(23):2219–29. https://doi.org/10.1056/NEJMoa1905380.
35. Saleh, et al. The efficacy of peroral endoscopic myotomy vs pneumatic dilation as treatment for patients with achalasia suffering from persistent or recurrent symptoms after laparoscopic Heller myotomy: a randomized clinical trial. Gastroenterology. 2023;164(7):1108–1118.e3. https://doi.org/10.1053/j.gastro.2023.02.048.
36. Pesce M, et al. Modern achalasia: diagnosis, classification, and treatment. J Neurogastroenterol Motil. 2023;29(4):419–27. https://doi.org/10.5056/jnm23125.
37. Fisichella PM, et al. From Heller to POEM (1914–2014): a 100-year history of surgery for achalasia. J Gastrointest Surg. 2014;18:1870–5. https://doi.org/10.1007/s11605-014-2547-8.
38. Chiruvella A, et al. Masters program foregut pathway: robotic Heller. The SAGES manual of robotic surgery. Cham: Springer; 2018. https://doi.org/10.1007/978-3-319-51362-14.
39. Richards, et al. Heller myotomy versus Heller myotomy with Dor fundoplication for achalasia: a prospective randomized double-blind clinical trial. Ann Surg. 2004;240(3):405–12; discussion 412–5. https://doi.org/10.1097/01.sla.0000136940.32255.51.
40. Campos GM, et al. Endoscopic and surgical treatments for achalasia: a systematic review and meta-analysis. Ann Surg. 2009;249(1):45–57. https://doi.org/10.1097/SLA.0b013e31818e43ab.
41. Zaninotto G, et al. The 2018 ISDE achalasia guidelines. Dis Esophagus. 2018;31(9):doy071. https://doi.org/10.1093/dote/doy071.
42. Wright AS, et al. Long-term outcomes confirm the superior efficacy of extended Heller myotomy with Toupet fundoplication for achalasia. Surg Endosc. 2007;21(5):713–8. https://doi.org/10.1007/s00464-006-9165-9.
43. Tomasko, et al. Quality of life comparing dor and toupet after heller myotomy for achalasia. JSLS. 2014;18(3):e2014.00191. https://doi.org/10.4293/JSLS.2014.00191.
44. Torres-Villalobos, et al. Dor vs Toupet fundoplication after laparoscopic Heller myotomy: long-term randomized controlled trial evaluated by high-resolution manometry. J Gastrointest Surg. 2018;22:13–22. https://doi.org/10.1007/s11605-017-3578-8.
45. Broman K, et al. Heller myotomy versus Heller myotomy with Dor fundoplication for achalasia: long-term symptomatic follow-up of a prospective randomized controlled trial. Surg Endosc. 2018;32(4):1668–74. https://doi.org/10.1007/s00464-017-5845-x.
46. Lindeboom M, et al. Gastric emptying and vagus nerve function after laparoscopic partial fundoplication. Ann Surg. 2004;240(5):785–90. https://doi.org/10.1097/01.sla.0000143124.30911.0f.
47. Oelschlager BK, et al. Vagotomy during hiatal hernia repair: a benign esophageal lengthening procedure. J Gastrointest Surg. 2008;12(7):1155–62. https://doi.org/10.1007/s11605-008-0520-0.
48. Joelson AM. Management of GERD after myotomy for achalasia. Foregut (Thousand Oaks, Calif.) (2634–5161). 2022;2(4):425.

14 Robotic Esophagectomy

Evangelos Tagkalos and Peter P. Grimminger

Introduction

Worldwide, esophageal cancer is one of the most common tumors, with approximately 600,000 new cases each year [1, 2]. The highest incidence rates are found in China, Iran, Kazakhstan, South Africa, and South America, with rates of up to 545 per 100,000 population per year. It is also the sixth leading cause of cancer-related death, with nearly 550,000 deaths worldwide each year, compared to 400,000 deaths in 2012 [1, 2]. Both squamous cell carcinoma (SCC) and adenocarcinoma (AC) are responsible for the increasing prevalence of esophageal cancer, representing the two most common types. While SCC remains the most common type of esophageal cancer worldwide, there has been a decline in this type in Western countries and a significant increase in AC, including AC of the esophagogastric junction [1]. Esophageal carcinoma has a tendency to metastasize to regional lymph nodes in its early stages. The likelihood of regional lymph node metastases occurring is directly correlated with the depth of invasion into the esophageal wall. Distant metastases are more frequent in the liver, but can also occur in other organs such as the lungs, brain, adrenal glands or bones, as well as nonregional lymph nodes, depending on the location of the carcinoma. The surgical approach for the esophagus depends on its anatomical course from the pharynx to the upper abdomen. Reconstruction can be done using the stomach, a segment of the small intestine (only for short-segment

E. Tagkalos
Department of General, Visceral and Transplant Surgery, University Medical Center Mainz, Mainz, Germany

UGIRA-Fellow 2022–2023 in Chang Gung Memorial Hospital, Taoyuan, Taiwan
e-mail: evangelos.tagkalos@unimedizin-mainz.de

P. P. Grimminger (✉)
Departmen of General-, Visceral- and Transplant Surgery, University Medical Centre of the Johannes Gutenberg-University Mainz, Mainz, Germany
e-mail: peter.grimminger@unimedizin-mainz.de

S. Samreen et al. (eds.), *The SAGES Manual of Robotic Surgery*,
https://doi.org/10.1007/978-3-031-86927-3_14

defects), or a section of the colon, in order of their suitability. The stomach is the most suitable replacement organ from a surgical and anatomical point of view for a reconstruction by means of a gastric pull-up. Furthermore, it requires only a single anastomosis (esophagogastrostomy).

The risk of surgery, especially the transthoracic esophageal resection, is relatively high due to several factors [3–5]. Patients often have comorbidities such as chronic obstructive pulmonary disease or previous cardiac disease, which are linked to risk factors such as smoking and alcohol consumption. The required abdomino-thoracic 2-cavity-procedure places a significant burden on the body. The duration of an abdomino-thoracic esophageal resection typically ranges from 4 to 6 h, depending on the level of difficulty. This places it in the upper third of the spectrum of operating times for visceral surgery. The procedure is carried out in close proximity to sensitive structures such as the aorta, coeliac trunk, pulmonary veins, azygos vein, pars membranacea of trachea, right main bronchus, pericardium, left atrium, vagus nerve, recurrent laryngeal nerve, and thoracic duct. Structures can be damaged either directly or indirectly (e.g., through thermal means) during surgery or in the early postoperative period due to leakage of aggressive gastric acid, bile acid, pancreatic enzymes, or due to inflammatory processes. Complications of the transthoracic esophagectomy with gastric pull-up reconstruction include anastomotic insufficiency, pneumonia, hemorrhage, chylothorax, lesion of the recurrent laryngeal nerve causing hoarseness, esophago-tracheal or esophago-bronchial fistula, conduit-necrosis, arrhythmia, and enterothorax [3, 4, 6, 7]. The incidence of anastomotic insufficiency, a common surgical complication, is estimated to be between 7.2% and 35%. Large cohort analyses report 30- and 90-day mortality rates of 2.4–8.9% depending on the expertise and frequency of the clinic in performing esophageal resections, although leading world centers demonstrate 90-day rates below 1% [8–12]. Esophagectomy is a technically demanding operation that produces substantial trauma for the patient. The open procedure has been the only relevant approach for many decades, but it was associated with high morbidity and mortality rates exceeding 20% in small-volume centers during the last decade [1]. However, the shift from open surgery to minimally invasive approaches has resulted in reduced morbidity and mortality rates. Curative therapeutic strategies for esophageal AC and AC of the esophagogastric junction mainly involve transthoracic esophagectomy with abdominal and thoracic lymph node dissection after chemotherapy or chemoradiation in the case of locally advanced disease.

The Shift to Minimally Invasive Esophagectomy

In the last decade, a number of randomized control trials have shown that minimally invasive techniques, such as hybrid (HE), minimally invasive (MIE), and robotic-assisted (RAMIE) esophagectomy, provide significant benefits compared with open procedures. The studies from Haverkamp et al. [13] and the updated version from de Groot et al. [14], which investigated the worldwide trends in surgical techniques for the treatment of esophageal- and gastroesophageal-junction cancer, showed a clear shift to minimally invasive techniques—from only 15% in 2007 to 79% in 2021—which mirrors the results of the following RCTs.

The MIRO trial, which compared open esophagectomy (OTE) and HE, concluded that the HE group had a 50% lower risk of major pulmonary complications compared to the OTE group. After 3 years of follow-up, the HE group showed a trend toward improved overall and disease-free survival (67.0% versus 55%, and 57% versus 48%) [15].

MIE, first described in 1995, was an evolution of HE that aimed to reduce surgical trauma, including the thoracic minimally invasive access. The first RCT comparing MIE with OTE, the TIME trial, was published in 2012. The study showed significantly fewer postoperative complications after MIE [16].

The ROBOT trial, the first RCT to compare OTE with RAMIE, was published in 2019. The authors concluded that RAMIE was associated with fewer postoperative complications than OTE, with 59% of the RAMIE group experiencing postoperative complications compared to 80% of the OTE group ($p = 0.02$). In addition, RAMIE was associated with a lower median blood loss (400 ml vs. 568 ml, $p < 0.001$) and a lower incidence of postoperative pulmonary (RR 0.54; 95% CI, 0.34–0.85; $p = 0.005$) and cardiac (RR 0.47; 95% CI, 0.27–0.83; $p = 0.006$) complications [17].

The RAMIE trial, a multicenter Chinese RCT comparing MIE and RAMIE in patients with SCC, showed that both RAMIE and MIE were safe and feasible for the treatment of SCC and that RAMIE achieved shorter operative times with higher lymph node dissection ($p = 0.016$) in patients who received neoadjuvant therapy [18].

The second completed RCT comparing MIE to RAMIE in SCC patients was also a multicenter Asian study (Taiwan/China). Preliminary results reported at the first Upper-GI Robotic Association (UGIRA) Congress in Taipei in 2023 reported lower RLN palsy rates for RAMIE.

The third RCT comparing MIE to RAMIE and the first to include Western patients with AC of the intrathoracic esophagus or gastroesophageal junction, the ROBOT-2 trial, is still recruiting. Primary endpoint is the number of resected lymph nodes according to the TIGER protocol [19].

In anticipation of the long-term results of the last three RCTs on overall and disease-free survival between MIE and RAMIE, a small number of nonrandomized studies suggest a potential advantage of RAMIE. A very recent two-center study between Taiwan and Germany, which compared 945 consecutive patients who underwent MIE or RAMIE for esophageal cancer— the largest in the literature to date comparing these two techniques—according to Textbook Outcome Procedure (TBO) achievement rates, showed that RAMIE produced statistically significantly higher TBO rates (53.3% vs. 42.2%; $p < 0.001$). In the same study, patients who achieved a TBO had a statistically significantly longer median overall survival (109 months vs. 21 months; $p < 0.001$) as well as disease-free survival (87 months vs. 13 months; $p < 0.001$) than those who did not achieve a TBO [20].

Another neuralgic issue with RAMIE is its learning curve. The first assessments of RAMIE learning curve were published by Hernandez et al. and Sarkaria et al [21, 22]. They concluded that the learning effect was observed after 20 and 30–45 cases, respectively. The latter studies did not provide a clear cut-off point for completion of the learning curves. Van der Sluis et al. evaluated the learning curve of RAMIE using the cumulative sum method (CUSUM) for a proctor and a novice surgeon undergoing proctoring in 312 cases. According to the authors, the proctor required 70 procedures and 55 months to achieve proficiency, while the proctored novice surgeon completed the learning phase after 15 supervised and 9 unsupervised/independent cases (24 cases in 13 months) [23]. The authors conclude that proctoring can significantly reduce the number of cases and the time required to complete the learning curve. It should be noted that RAMIE is a procedure with standardized settings in many centers worldwide.

In light of the above data, we will describe the two most commonly used minimally invasive robotic-assisted techniques for esophageal resection: Ivor-Lewis and McKeown esophagectomy.

Robotic-Assisted Ivor-Lewis Esophagectomy

The fully robotic minimally invasive "one surgeon–one assistant" 4-arm transabdominal and transthoracic esophagectomy with D2 lymph node dissection and gastric pull-up reconstruction is presented [24–26]. The two phases, the abdominal and the thoracic, are described in detail. We recommend this procedure for tumors located in the mid and distal esophagus or at the gastroesophageal junction (Siewert types I and II).

Abdominal Phase

The patient is placed in a normal supine position with a 15° reverse Trendelenburg. The da Vinci® Xi patients' cart is positioned on the right side of the patient and the surgical assistant on the left. As each patient's anatomy is different, it is recommended that trocar placement be tailored to the patient. To determine this, the camera trocar should be placed in the midline in a position that allows the abdominal phase to be performed without maximum extension of the robotic arm in the upright position (like a flip-up action). After placing the camera trocar (T3), the remaining three robotic trocars are placed as shown in Fig. 14.1. The next trocar to be placed is a 12 mm (T2) on the upper right at the same level as T3 and almost 6–8 cm away from it. The next trocar to be placed is T1 in the right lateral subcostal area at least 6–8 cm (and at least 2 cm below the 10th intercostal space) to the right of T2. T4 is placed in a mirrored position to T2 according to the midline, and finally the assistant port is placed in the left lateral position 1–2 cm above T4. After docking the camera to T3, the remaining robot arms 1, 2, and 4 are docked to T1, T2, and T4, respectively (Fig. 14.1).

Instrument Placement

T1: Fenestrated tip-up grasper.

T2: Fenestrated bipolar forceps using the 8 mm reduction cap and robotic stapler (Sureform→; 12 mm).

T3: Camera.

T4: Vessel Sealer or SynchroSeal, monopolar hook or scissors.

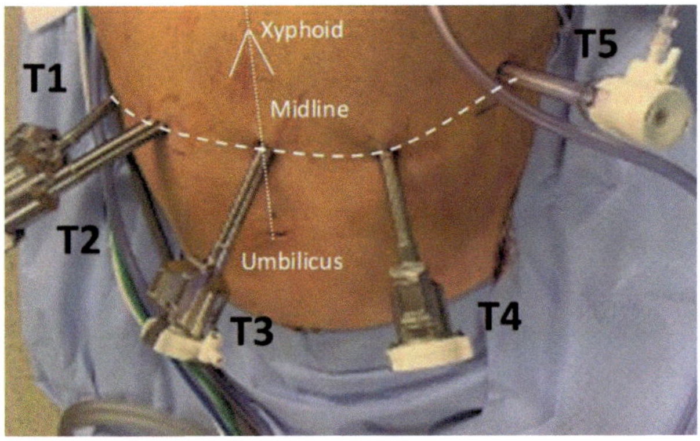

Fig. 14.1 Trocar placement for the abdominal phase. The distances between T2-T3 and T3-T4 should be the same if possible

To start, the fenestrated tip-up grasper is used to retract the liver. After opening the pars flaccida of the hepatogastric ligament, the dissection is extended toward the right diaphragmatic crus. To facilitate a good surgical plane, the assistant should retract the pericardial fatty tissue to the left of the patient. The right side of the distal esophagus and the gastroesophageal junction should be fully mobilized from the diaphragm. Remember to prepare the lymph nodes at station 1 so that they can be retrieved with the specimen. Pay particular attention to the right pleura, as opening it (if not necessary, e.g., in the case of a bulky gastroesophageal junction tumor) may result in the need for thoracic drainage on the right side. If this is the case, place it in a position where it can later be exchanged with a robotic trocar in the thoracic phase. The next step is to identify the gastroepiploic arcade (right gastroepiploic artery) and carefully dissect the greater omentum. The assistant retracts the omentum to the left of the patient and the surgeon provides countertraction to the right (in relation to the gastroepiploic artery, which should always be medial to the surgeon's instruments to avoid traumatic injury to the vessel). The key to this step is that both the surgeon and the assistant should move gradually, always correcting the plane by adjusting the traction and countertraction. To avoid unnecessary movements that could slow you down or even cause injuries, both the assistant and the surgeon's left arm can move once the right arm of the surgeon has grasped and secured the tissue to be sealed and cut, providing a stable plane. After repositioning, the tissue can be divided and so on. The short gastric vessels are dissected after the partial omentectomy. Try to dissect these vessels away from the stomach to avoid damaging the intramural vascular network of the gastroepiploic arteries. To facilitate better visualization of the plane, the stomach should be gently retracted from T1 to the right of the patient using the tip-up grasper. After mobilization of the gastric fundus, the left crus can be freed from the esophagus and the gastroesophageal junction. Try to avoid opening the left pleura at this stage if not necessary. The lymph nodes at station 2 are prepared so that they can be retrieved with the specimen. When mobilizing the diaphragmatic crus, take particular care not to traumatize the parietal peritoneum to avoid bleeding of the diaphragmatic muscle tissue (Fig. 14.2).

The next step is to mobilize the stomach from the transverse colon and pancreas. To do this, the assistant should grasp the posterior wall of the stomach and move it upwards toward the abdominal wall. After dissecting the adhesions to the pancreas

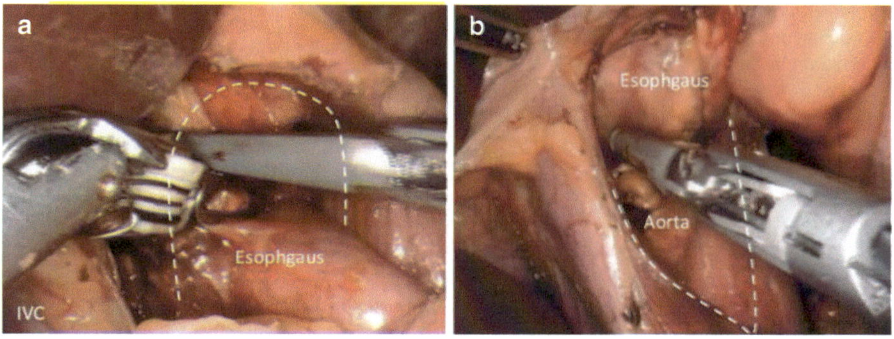

Fig. 14.2 The mobilization of the abdominal esophagus. The ventral (**a**) and dorsal (**b**) situs after complete mobilization. With interrupted lines are demonstrated the diaphragmatic arch (**a**) and the crus (**b**). IVC: inferior vena cava

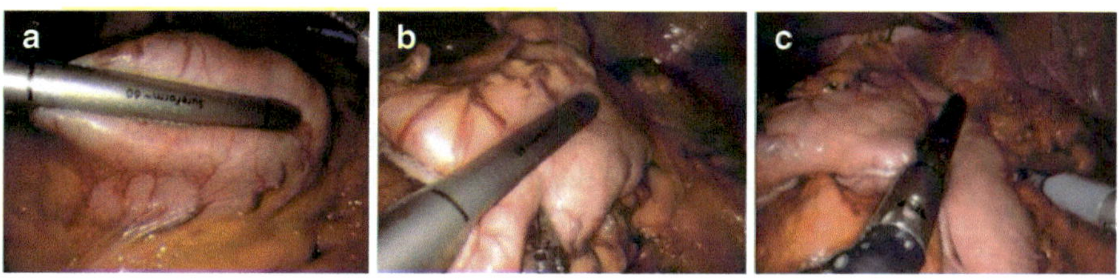

Fig. 14.3 The creation of the gastric conduit. (**a**) The first stapler is inserted sparing the first branches of the right gastric artery. (**b**) The second stapler should be positioned parallel to the greater curvature to ensure that the conduit will be neither too narrow nor too wide. (**c**) The last stapler should leave a 3–4 cm tissue connection to the fundus to enable the anastomotic creation in the thoracic part

and freeing the stomach from the mesocolon, the plane moves to the pylorus. This step requires extreme caution as injury to the right gastroepiploic vessels (vascularization of the gastric conduit) may be irreparable, making the use of the stomach for reconstruction unnecessary. The assistant (T5) lifts the posterior antrum wall, while the fenestrated bipolar forceps (T2) can be utilized to provide the required countertraction of the mesocolon (try to have the right gastroepiploic vessels at a 90° angle to your visual axis).

After completing the mobilization of the posterior stomach wall from the pancreas and separating the adhesions to the mesocolon, the stomach should be mobilized from the gallbladder leading to the visualization of the duodenum (pars I). The gastric conduit can now be prepared. Try not to dissect the first branches of the right gastric artery as they vascularize the intramural network of the lesser curvature. The fatty tissue of the lesser curvature should be dissected down to the stomach so that the stapler can be inserted in a clear gastric front. Through T2, the robotic stapler (SureForm™ Stapler, Intuitive, Sunnyvale, USA) is placed in a position as shown in Fig. 14.3 in the distal third of the lesser curvature. The conduit should be neither too narrow to avoid the risk of ischemia, nor too wide to avoid its dilatation in the thoracic cavity. At this point, a 3–4 cm tissue connection to the fundus should not be dissected, a step that is crucial for the anastomotic technique described later in the thoracic part.

Once the conduit has been constructed, lymph node dissection of the lesser curvature and the hepatoduodenal ligament can be performed. To obtain a clear plane, the partially dissected lesser curvature should be lifted cranially. For a more controlled dissection, a monopolar hook or scissors can be used at this point. Dissection begins medial to the gastric artery, which is held at a 90° angle to our 6-h axis. After identification of the proper hepatic artery, the gastroduodenal artery, and the common hepatic artery, the lymph node harvest from stations 12 and 8 can be completed. Try not to separate the lymph nodes from the specimen. To obtain the lymph nodes from stations 7, 9, and 11p, the celiac trunk and the splenic artery as well as the cranial pancreatic border are used (Fig. 14.4).

The left gastric artery should be prepared and divided at its origin together with the left gastric vein to facilitate dissection. On completion of this step, the stomach, the gastroesophageal junction, and the abdominal esophagus should be fully mobilized, allowing a clear view of the aorta, pericardium, and right and left pleura. Once the instruments have been retrieved, the da Vinci® Xi patient trolley undocked, and all trocars removed, the wounds can be closed and the abdominal phase completed.

Thoracic Phase

The patient is placed in the semi-prone position (45° tilt). Collapse of the right lung is achieved by an endotracheal block or a double lumen endotracheal tube. The da Vinci® Xi patient's cart is positioned to the right side of the operating table and the assistant to the left.

Trocar placement is shown in Fig. 14.5. You can start with either the assistant's 12 mm port (T5), which is placed in the 5th intercostal space along the anterior axillary line, or the camera trocar T3, which is placed in the 6th intercostal space, 3 cm to the left of T5 and a few cm higher. After establishing an intrathoracic pressure of

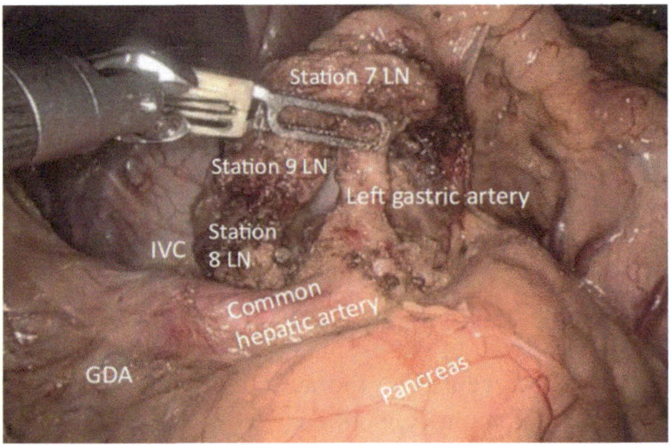

Fig. 14.4 The preparation of the common hepatic artery as well as the left gastric artery. *GDA* gastroduodenal artery, *ICV* inferior vena cava, *LN* lymph nodes

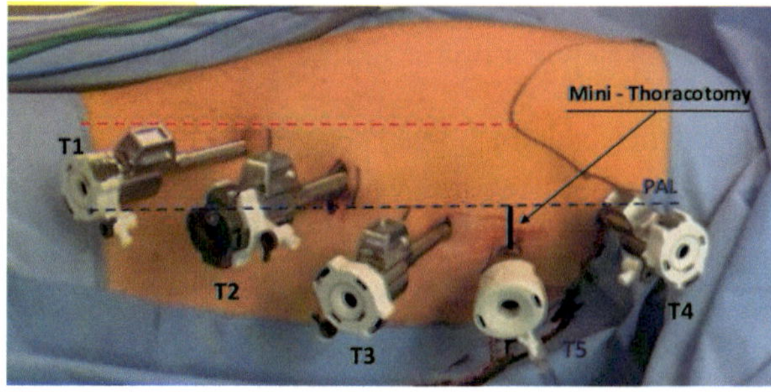

Fig. 14.5 Trocar placement of the thoracic phase. The red interrupted line is the recommended upper border for placement of a trocar. The black vertical line above the T5 shows the recommended mini-thoracotomy site. *PAL* posterior axillary line

8 mmHg and checking the operative site, T2 is placed in the 8th intercostal space (if a robotic stapler is used, it is advisable to use the 12 mm trocar), followed by T4 in the 4th intercostal space, facing the esophageal hiatus and slightly higher than T3 (this axis is very important for the placement of this trocar). Finally, T1 is placed laterally to T2 in the 10th intercostal space above the posterior axillary line. Try to leave enough space between the robotic trocars to avoid collisions.

Instrument Placement

T1: Fenestrated tip-up grasper.

T2: Fenestrated bipolar forceps using the 8 mm reduction cap and the robotic stapler (Sureform→; 12 mm).

T3: Camera.

T4: Vessel Sealer or SynchroSeal, monopolar hook or scissors.

Mobilization of the esophagus begins with an incision of the parietal pleura at the inferior pulmonary ligament along the anterior esophageal border. The operative plane is extended cranially in relation to the subcarinal lymph nodes, which should be harvested with the specimen up to the azygos arch. Fine dissection of the pleura should extend above the azygos arch. At this point, the right vagus nerve is the lateral border. For this step, the surgeon can be assisted by the assistant (try to position the assistant's instrument in the 6th row of your screen to avoid unnecessary movement) or the T1 (tip-up grasper) (Fig. 14.6).

The azygos arch should be carefully prepared and the small bronchial artery (posterolateral to the azygos vein) should be dissected. The monopolar hook or scissors are instruments that allow fine dissection up to this point. The azygos can be resected at this point with Hem-o-lok (Telefex Medical, Weck Drive, NC) clips (using T2) or with hand-held clips using T5 (Fig. 14.7).

Try not to dissect the azygos vein too close to the chest wall as a stump of 2–3 cm may provide better traction in the following steps. Alternatively, a hand-held vascular stapler can be used. Once this step has been completed, the right paratracheal lymph nodes can be dissected separately. The next step is to dissect the pleura down to the esophageal hiatus. The plane should be extended parallel to the azygos vein. The thoracic duct should be visualized and dissected at the lower mediastinum (Fig. 14.8).

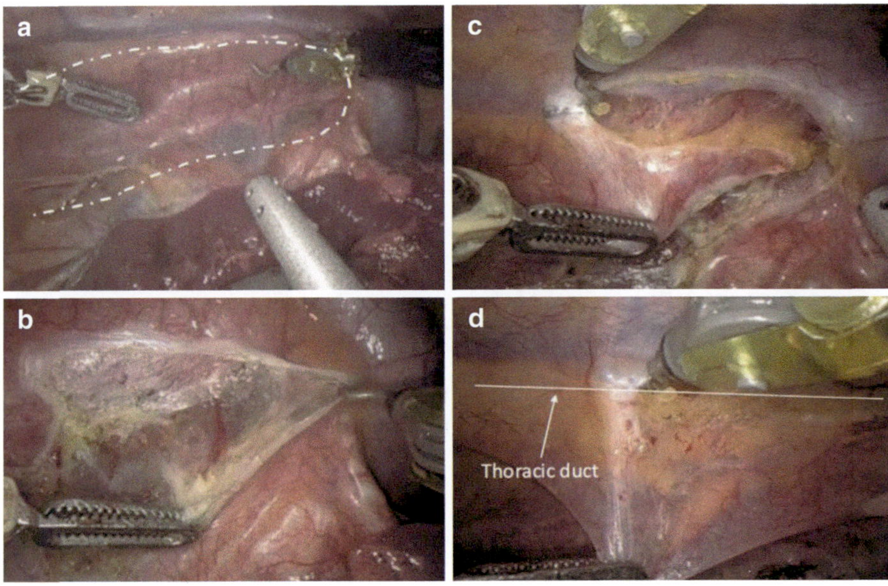

Fig. 14.6 Incision of the parietal pleura. (**a**) The interrupted line demonstrates the dissection plane of the parietal pleural. (**b**) The dissection of the pleura below the azygos arch and the esophagus. (**c**) The completion of the pleural dissection below the azygos arch. (**d**) The caudal plane with visualization of the thoracic duct

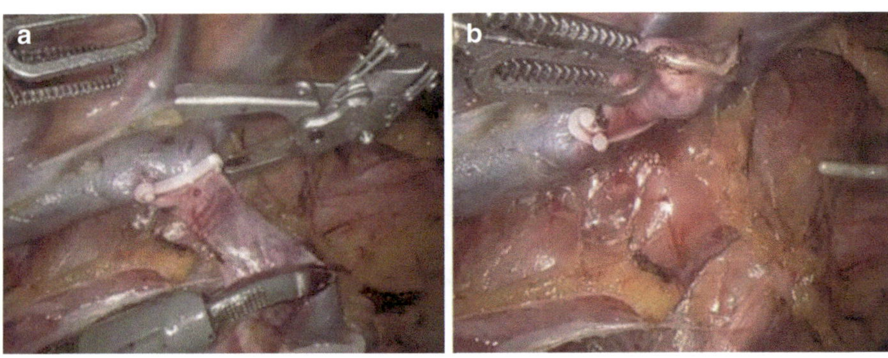

Fig. 14.7 The dissection of the azygos vein. (**a**) After clipping of the distal part. (**b**) The stump can be used to facilitate a better visualization of the underlying tissue (the traction through T1 fenestrated tip-up grasper should be at the 12th hour of your screen)

The use of ICG can be helpful, but the medium should be injected into the inguinal lymph nodes before the abdominal part or into the jejunal lymph nodes during the abdominal part (as shown in Fig. 14.9).

When mobilizing the esophagus, try to identify small arteries coming from the aorta, the left and right pulmonary veins, the left and right bronchus and the trachea. When attempting to retrieve lymph nodes in the vicinity of important structures

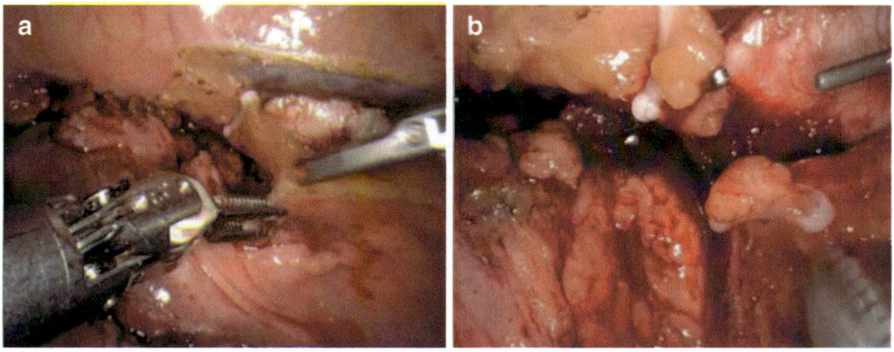

Fig. 14.8 The dissection of the thoracic duct. (**a**) The preparation and clipping of the distal part. (**b**) The dissected thoracic duct after clipping the proximal part

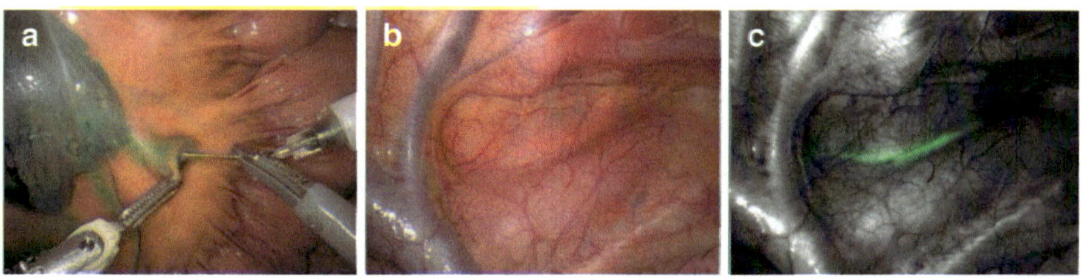

Fig. 14.9 ICG visualization of the thoracic duct. (**a**) The medium is injected in the lymph nodes of the jejunum during the abdominal phase. (**b**) The thoracic duct view in normal mode. (**c**) The thoracic duct (green) after enabling the Firefly™ mode of the da Vinci platform

such as those mentioned above, try to reduce the maximum current applied to the tissue to avoid thermal damage to the airways. If possible, the vagus nerve should be transected in relation to the cardiac branches. During this step, the T1 tip-up grasper should be used to provide countertraction (12th hour of your screen). If necessary, the assistant should apply traction to the 6th hour of your screen. The next step is to prepare the subcarinal lymph nodes so that they can be retrieved *en bloc* with the specimen. The assistant should gently compress the bronchial system with an atraumatic instrument to facilitate better visualization of the fatty tissue borders of the region (Fig. 14.10).

The posterior mediastinal and supradiaphragmatic lymph nodes are also retrieved *en bloc* with the specimen (damage to the airway should be avoided at this stage, even if this means that the lymph nodes from this station have to be removed separately from the specimen). After mobilizing the distal part of the intrathoracic esophagus from the diaphragm (and the crura, if not completely done during the abdominal phase), the full mobilization of the esophagus is achieved. Subsequently,

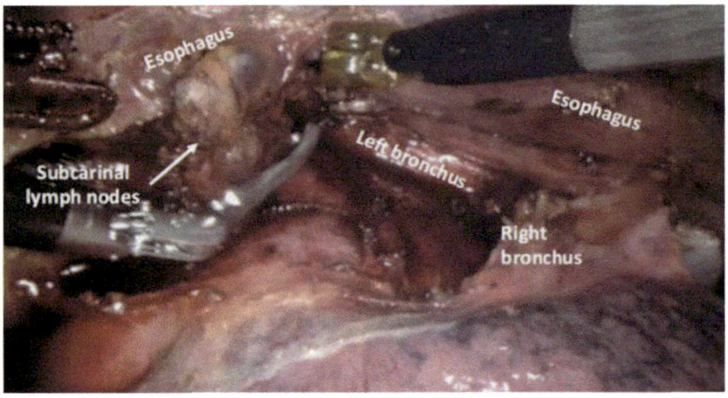

Fig. 14.10 The dissection of the subcarinal lymph nodes

the dissection of the specimen at the level of the azygos vein can be performed. The esophageal wall can be opened using monopolar scissors or hooks. After completing a purse string suture of the proximal end, externalize both suture ends via T5. Secure the distal esophageal opening through T5 with a grasper. Attempt to ascend the conduit into the thoracic cavity using gentle traction, maintaining contact with the vessel end at all times. At this point, we will describe the end-to-side circular anastomotic technique used in our clinic. As there is still no consensus on the ideal anastomotic type for intrathoracic reconstruction, alternative anastomotic types such as a linear stapled or hand-sewn anastomosis can be used. The robotic instruments are retrieved and the trocars are undocked. T5 is removed and a mini-thoracotomy is performed 2–3 cm anterior and 2 cm posterior to the epicenter of T5. A wound protector is placed and the 25 or 28 mm anvil (CEEATM, Covidien, Mansfield, MA, USA) is passed through the mini-thoracotomy to the proximal end of the esophagus, and the purse string is tightened. The specimen is then externalized through the mini-thoracotomy and the right angulation of the conduit is checked (the stapler line along the lesser curvature should be opposite to the aorta). The specimen is then partially externalized, a small incision is made at the end of the lesser curvature at the stapler line, and the stapler shaft is inserted through the incision and brought into the thoracic cavity. The shaft pin of the stapler is exteriorized cranially near the greater curvature of the gastric conduit. The shaft and anvil are approximated under continuous visualization. Using a hand-held grasper through T2, the fatty tissue of the greater omentum is removed from the anastomotic fronts to avoid stapling this tissue into the anastomosis. The anastomosis is created and the stapler removed. The specimen is divided using a linear stapler (Fig. 14.11). Single interrupted monofilament sutures may be used to secure the anastomosis (alternatively a continuous barbed resorbable suture may be used). A pleural tent and the use of a 180–270° omental flap can be further created around the anastomosis. The trocars are removed and a chest tube is inserted through T1. Once the lung is fully expanded, the mini-thoracotomy and wound are closed.

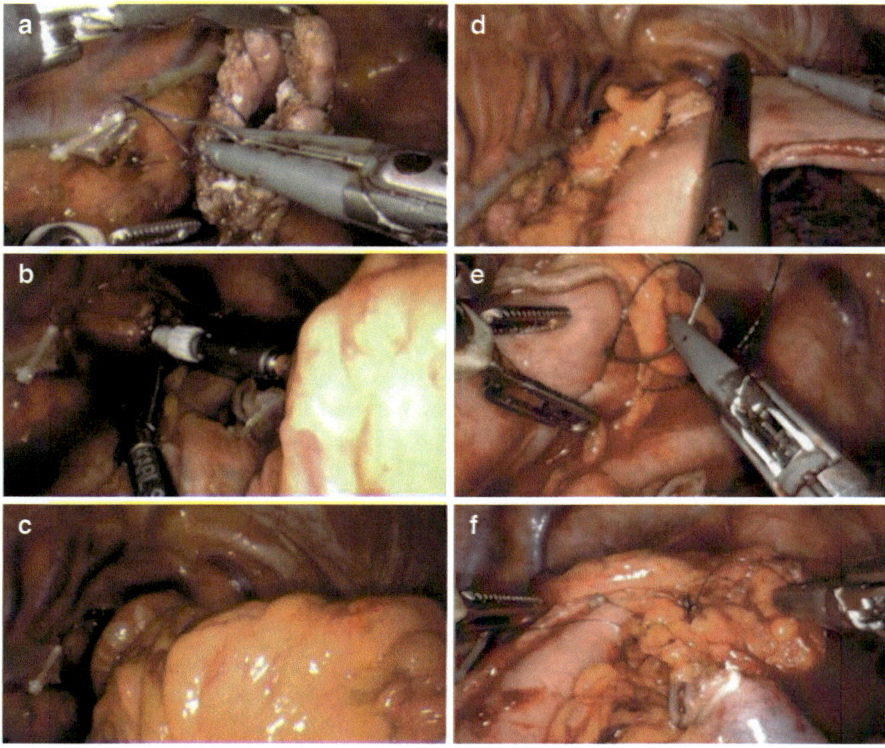

Fig. 14.11 The intrathoracic circular-stapled end-to-side esophagogastrostomy. (**a**) The purse string of the proximal end (esophagus) before the placement of the anvil. (**b**) The connection of the anvil (esophagus) with the spike (gastric conduit). (**c**) The approximation of both ends. (**d**) The dissection of the specimen via linear stapler. (**e**) A continuous barbed suture is placed at the anastomosis. (**f**) A pleural tent and a 270° omental flap are placed around the anastomosis

Robotic-Assisted McKeown Esophagectomy

The fully robotic minimally invasive "one surgeon–one assistant" 4-arm transabdominal, transthoracic, and transcervical esophagectomy with D2 lymph node dissection with gastric pull-up reconstruction is presented. The three phases—thoracic, abdominal, and cervical—are described. We recommend this procedure for tumors located in the upper or upper/middle esophagus.

Thoracic Phase

The thoracic phase is the first phase of the McKeown procedure. This phase shares many steps with the thoracic phase of the Ivor-Lewis procedure described above. If meticulous right and left recurrent laryngeal nerve (RLN) lymph node dissection is required, all trocars can be moved cranially in one intercostal space (9th, 7th, 5th, and 3rd for the four robotic arms). After complete mobilization of the esophagus below the azygos vein and completion of the lymphadenectomy in the middle and lower mediastinum, the operation continues in the upper mediastinum.

Instrument Placement
T1: Fenestrated bipolar forceps.
T2: Camera.
T3: Monopolar hook or scissors.
T4: Tip-up fenestrated grasper.

The lymph nodes of the RLN are dissected. The parietal pleura should be incised parallel to the right vagus nerve extending towards the right subclavian artery. This is the recurrent point for the right RLN. These lymph nodes should be dissected separately from the specimen.

Dissection of the left RLN is more difficult and requires good visualization of the left RLN. The trachea should be gently rotated clockwise. The tip-up grasper through T1 is used to retract the esophagus dorsally and the assistant will rotate the trachea. The soft tissues of the left paratracheal space are carefully dissected, leaving the left RLN untouched. The ventral lymph nodes are dissected first, followed by the dorsal lymph nodes. The esophagus can then be safely mobilized to the thoracic outlet. A thoracic tube is placed and the wounds are closed.

Abdominal and Cervical Phases

The abdominal phase described in the Ivor-Lewis section shares many similarities to the McKeown abdominal phase. The patient is placed in the supine position with the head slightly tilted to the right and the neck extended. To facilitate passage of the specimen through the posterior mediastinum to the neck, it is advisable to divide the specimen from the gastric conduit. The two ends can then be reattached with interrupted sutures (tip of the gastric conduit).

After creating the anastomosis in the cervical region (see below), the stomach should be retracted in the abdomen for a few centimeters and the pylorus should be close to the hiatus. This is the end of the abdominal phase.

It is clear that the cervical phase will begin before the end of the abdominal phase, and this step can be also performed by a second surgical team. An incision parallel and median to the medial border of the left sternocleidomastoid muscle (approximately 4 cm) should start from the jugulum and extend cranially. After dissecting the platysma, the dissection follows the layers to the thoracic inlet. At this point, the cervical esophagus should be identified. A loop may be used to encircle the esophagus for better traction. Once the cervical esophagus has been mobilized, the specimen and conduit can be advanced to the neck. The cervical esophagus is dissected and the specimen is retrieved. We perform a circular-stapled anastomosis, but other techniques can be used for reconstruction (linear or hand-sewn anastomosis). The anastomosis can be further secured with interrupted absorbable monofilament sutures. A small soft drainage is placed posterior to the anastomosis and the wounds are closed with interrupted sutures (platysma and skin). The cervical phase is complete.

Good teamwork is essential for a successful robotic operation. A clear role for each team member remains the cornerstone of a successful procedure. The use of the robotic assistance may lead to further surgical precision and facilitate more extended lymphadenectomies in the upper mediastinum. It is expected that the continuous technological development of the robotic systems as well as promising robotic processes such as RACE (robotic-assisted transhiatal and transcervical esophagectomy) could totally alter today standards.

References

1. Ferlay J, Colombet M, Soerjomataram I, Parkin DM, Pineros M, Znaor A, et al. Cancer statistics for the year 2020: an overview. Int J Cancer. 2021;1
2. Lepage C, Drouillard A, Jouve JL, Faivre J. Epidemiology and risk factors for oesophageal adenocarcinoma. Dig Liver Dis. 2013;45(8):625–9.
3. Cho S. Fistulas between the esophagus and adjacent vital organs in esophageal cancer. Korean J Thorac Cardiovasc Surg. 2020;53(4):211–6.
4. Zhong XQ, Li GX. Successful management of life-threatening aortoesophageal fistula: a case report and review of the literature. World J Clin Cases. 2022;10(12):3814–21.
5. He LR, Qiao W, Liao ZX, Komaki R, Ho L, Hofstetter WL, et al. Impact of comorbidities and use of common medications on cancer and non-cancer specific survival in esophageal carcinoma. BMC Cancer. 2015;15:1095.
6. Arends J, Bachmann P, Baracos V, Barthelemy N, Bertz H, Bozzetti F, et al. ESPEN guidelines on nutrition in cancer patients. Clin Nutr. 2017;36(1):11–48.
7. Valsangkar N, Salfity HVN, Timsina L, Ceppa DP, Ceppa EP, Birdas TJ. Operative time in esophagectomy: does it affect outcomes? Surgery. 2018;164(4):866–71.
8. Takahashi C, Shridhar R, Huston J, Meredith K. Esophagectomy from then to now. J Gastrointest Oncol. 2018;9(5):903–9.
9. Lai G, Guo N, Jiang Y, Lai J, Li Y, Lai R. Duration of one-lung ventilation as a risk factor for postoperative pulmonary complications after McKeown esophagectomy. Tumori. 2020;106(1):47–54.
10. Fabbi M, Hagens ERC, van Berge Henegouwen MI, Gisbertz SS. Anastomotic leakage after esophagectomy for esophageal cancer: definitions, diagnostics, and treatment. Dis Esophagus. 2021;34(1):1.
11. In H, Palis BE, Merkow RP, Posner MC, Ferguson MK, Winchester DP, et al. Doubling of 30-day mortality by 90 days after esophagectomy: a critical measure of outcomes for quality improvement. Ann Surg. 2016;263(2):286–91.
12. Low DE, Kuppusamy MK, Alderson D, Cecconello I, Chang AC, Darling G, et al. Benchmarking complications associated with esophagectomy. Ann Surg. 2019;269(2):291–8.
13. Haverkamp L, Seesing MF, Ruurda JP, Boone J, Hillegersberg RV. Worldwide trends in surgical techniques in the treatment of esophageal and gastroesophageal junction cancer. Dis Esophagus. 2017;30(1):1–7.
14. de Groot EM, Goense L, Kingma BF, Haverkamp L, Ruurda JP, van Hillegersberg R. Trends in surgical techniques for the treatment of esophageal and gastroesophageal junction cancer: the 2022 update. Dis Esophagus. 2023;36(7):doac099.
15. Mariette C, Markar SR, Dabakuyo-Yonli TS, Meunier B, Pezet D, Collet D, et al. Hybrid minimally invasive esophagectomy for esophageal cancer. N Engl J Med. 2019;380(2):152–62.

16. Biere SS, van Berge Henegouwen MI, Maas KW, Bonavina L, Rosman C, Garcia JR, et al. Minimally invasive versus open oesophagectomy for patients with oesophageal cancer: a multicentre, open-label, randomised controlled trial. Lancet. 2012;379(9829):1887–92.
17. van der Sluis PC, van der Horst S, May AM, Schippers C, Brosens LAA, Joore HCA, et al. Robot-assisted minimally invasive thoracolaparoscopic esophagectomy versus open transthoracic esophagectomy for resectable esophageal cancer: a randomized controlled trial. Ann Surg. 2019;269(4):621–30.
18. Yang Y, Li B, Yi J, Hua R, Chen H, Tan L, Li H, He Y, Guo X, Sun Y, Yu B, Li Z. Robot-assisted versus conventional minimally invasive esophagectomy for resectable esophageal squamous cell carcinoma: early results of a multicenter randomized controlled trial: the RAMIE Trial. Ann Surg. 2022;275(4):646–53.
19. Tagkalos E, van der Sluis PC, Berlth F, Poplawski A, Hadzijusufovic E, Lang H, van Berge Henegouwen MI, Gisbertz SS, Müller-Stich BP, Ruurda JP, Schiesser M, Schneider PM, van Hillegersberg R, Grimminger PP. Robot-assisted minimally invasive thoraco-laparoscopic esophagectomy versus minimally invasive esophagectomy for resectable esophageal adenocarcinoma, a randomized controlled trial (ROBOT-2 trial). BMC Cancer. 2021;21(1):1060.
20. Tagkalos E, Grimminger P, Gao X, Chiu CH, Uzun E, Lang H, Wen YW, Chao YK. Incidence and predictors of textbook outcome after minimally invasive esophagectomy for cancer: a two-center study. Cancers. 2024;16:1109.
21. Hernandez JM, Dimou F, Weber J, et al. Defining the learning curve for robotic-assisted esophagogastrectomy. J Gastrointest Surg. 2013;17:1346–51.
22. Sarkaria IS, Rizk NP, Grosser R, et al. Attaining proficiency in robotic-assisted minimally invasive esophagectomy while maximizing safety during procedure development. Innovations. 2016;11(4):268–73.
23. van der Sluis PC, Ruurda JP, van der Horst S, Goense L, van Hillegersberg R. Learning curve for robot-assisted minimally invasive thoracoscopic esophagectomy: results from 312 cases. Ann Thorac Surg. 2018;106(1):264–71.
24. Grimminger PP, Hadzijusufovic E, Babic B, van der Sluis PC, Lang H. Innovative fully robotic 4-arm Ivor Lewis esophagectomy for esophageal cancer (RAMIE4). Dis Esophagus. 2020;33(3):doz015.
25. Grimminger PP, Hadzijusufovic E, Ruurda JP, Lang H, van Hillegersberg R. The da Vinci Xi robotic four-arm approach for robotic-assisted minimally invasive esophagectomy. Thorac Cardiovasc Surg. 2018a;66(5):407–9. https://doi.org/10.1055/s-0038-1636933.
26. Grimminger PP, Hadzijusufovic E, Lang H. Robotic-Assisted Ivor Lewis Esophagectomy (RAMIE) with a standardized intrathoracic circular end-to-side stapled anastomosis and a team of two (surgeon and assistant only). Thorac Cardiovasc Surg. 2018b;66(5):404–6. https://doi.org/10.1055/s-0037-1606198.

15 Robot-Assisted Partial and Total Gastrectomy

Raj G. Vaghjiani

Introduction

On January 29, 1881, Theodor Billroth performed the first successful gastric resection at his Viennese clinic which included the eponymous gastroenteric reconstruction [1]. Although previous surgeons had attempted such a complex procedure, this was the first case of a technical success (the patient reportedly passed away months later from metastatic disease). Since this time, surgery of the stomach has advanced tremendously taking into account not only the complex physiology of nutrient digestion but also the mechanics of gastroenteric flow. Fast forward to over 100 years later in 1991, the first laparoscopic-assisted gastrectomy was described by Seigo Kitano's group [2]. Rapid advancements in both laparoscopic, and, more recently, robotic techniques, have allowed for the continued adoption of minimally invasive approaches to gastric resection.

This chapter will provide a brief synopsis of the indications for gastric resections as well as a technical guide to a breadth of robot-assisted gastric resections and the associated alimentary reconstructions. Although the majority of robot-assisted resections for GI malignancies in the United States are done with the Intuitive Surgical da Vinci platform, the descriptions provided will attempt to highlight technical aspects that could be easily translated to various platforms as well as upcoming iterations.

Indications

Gastric cancer remains a major source of worldwide cancer burden, accounting for the fifth most commonly diagnosed cancer as well as the fifth leading cause of cancer mortality [3]. As detailed investigations into the pathogenesis of gastric

R. G. Vaghjiani (✉)
University of Texas Medical Branch, Galveston, TX, USA
e-mail: rgvaghji@UTMB.EDU

S. Samreen et al. (eds.), *The SAGES Manual of Robotic Surgery*,
https://doi.org/10.1007/978-3-031-86927-3_15

adenocarcinoma have continued, the approach to management has simultaneously become more intricate, often entailing a multitude of therapies depending on the stage of the malignancy at discovery [4]. Additionally, the ideal extent of surgery as well as the associated lymphadenectomy continues to evolve, especially as different geographic cohorts are prone to variable incidence, detection, and surgical capabilities. Finally, although gastric adenocarcinoma is often a commonly discussed indication for robotic resections, the breadth of entities that may be appropriate for a robotic approach include gastrointestinal stromal tumors (GIST), neuroendocrine tumors, leiomyomas, sarcomas, polyps/adenomas, and benign peptic disease. Specific extent of resection is beyond the scope of this chapter; however, the application of the techniques would be for the most part identical.

Positioning and Port Placement

For the vast majority of gastric resections, the patient can be positioned supine with a 10–25 degree reverse Trendelenburg orientation. This can aid in upper gastrointestinal dissection, and thus the use of either a footboard or a split-leg table with footrests should be applied. The robotic platform is located to the left of the patient but with increasingly versatile systems, both a left-sided and right-sided approach can be used. If there is the possibility that the gastric resection may extend into the thorax and require an esophagogastrectomy, then a left-sided placement may allow for an easy transition for the thoracic/lateral portion of the operation (Fig. 15.1).

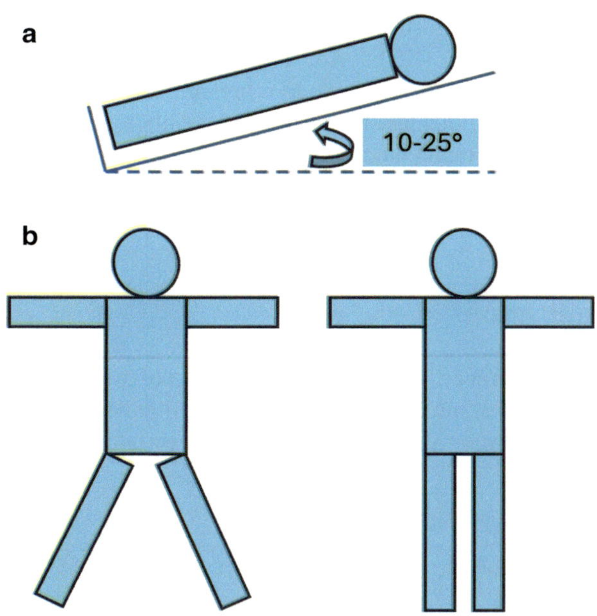

Fig. 15.1 (**a**) A reverse Trendelenburg position can aid in dissection of the upper abdominal space and hiatus. (**b**) Either a split leg with foot rests or a straight leg with footboard should be used to allow for the steep angle required. The robot can be positioned either to the left or right of the patient with the arms in extension

Port placement can vary depending on the extent of resection and/or lymphadenectomy required. Generally, a 4-port configuration with the addition of single assistant port is adequate for the most extensive gastric resections. Three 8 mm ports can be placed in a semi-lunar orientation in the supraumbilical/umbilical space, with one additional 12 mm port to allow for stapler introduction and specimen extraction. An additional fixed, liver retractor can also be used in the subxiphoid position.

Local Resection: "Wedge Gastrectomy"

For indications that do not require extensive margins nor lymphadenectomy, limited local resections may be appropriate. If a tumorous growth is the target, that is, GIST, then localization can be difficult if there is no extensive extraluminal component or high-fidelity tactile feedback. In these situations, intraoperative endoscopy plays a crucial role. Notably, there are situations in which the resistive ability of the pylorus is overcome by intraluminal air pressure, and an additional clamp on the proximal small bowel via the assistant port may aid in preventing excessive gaseous small bowel dilatation and consequent loss of operating domain. Alternatively, preoperative endoscopic tattooing may serve a similar function analogous to its use in the localization of colonic polyps.

Following patient positioning and port placement, a 30-degree videoscope is used to explore the abdomen and identify the lesion. For targets that are on the anterior surface of the stomach, a division of the gastrocolic ligament may be omitted. If the lesion is located in an amenable position, a wedge gastrectomy can be performed using either a robotic stapler or a hand-held equivalent. For locations such as the gastric fundus or the lesser curvature, the application of the stapler may not be possible because of physical restraints. Importantly, one must consider the anatomic sequelae of the resection as well; the use of the stapler on more precarious regions could lead to mechanical and functional issues with esophagogastric transit. In this situation, a more limited resection using a combination of sharp dissection and focal electrocautery may allow for a "closer" margin excision and preservation of gastric tissue in certain important territories. For this maneuver especially, the dexterity afforded by the robotic platform allows for a very tailored excision. The resultant defect can subsequently be closed with either a single- or dual-layer sutured approximation.

A completion upper endoscopy can be selectively applied to examine the closure. There are multiple adjuncts to ensuring the absence of a leak beyond visual examination. One method utilizes the instillation of saline into the upper abdominal region to inundate the now-closed defect while simultaneously instilling intragastric air. Air bubbles identified intra-abdominally would indicate an inadequate closure and need for additional maneuvers. Another method utilizes near-infrared fluoroscopy (either available inbuilt on certain robotic platforms or as a separate laparoscopic videoscope). Intragastric dilute indocyanine green (ICG) is used to pressurize the luminal space either via endoscope or orogastric tube, and then the extraluminal area is examined with the specialized camera to identify any extravasation of the ICG.

Lymphadenectomy

As mentioned, the indication for gastric resection may necessitate concomitant removal of draining lymph nodes. The lymphatic efferent of the stomach is anatomically varied, although for the most part predictable and described according to multiple standards. The Japanese gastric cancer treatment guidelines are one experience that provides a stat-driven outline to the gastric lymphadenectomy (Fig. 15.2) [5].

Lymphadenectomy of the immediate perigastric stations (1,2, 3, 4, 5, and 6) can be accomplished *en bloc* during the gastric dissection or as separate maneuvers as long as attention is paid to the anatomic envelopes where these stations reside. If taken *en bloc*, care must be taken to ensure that an overly aggressive skeletonization

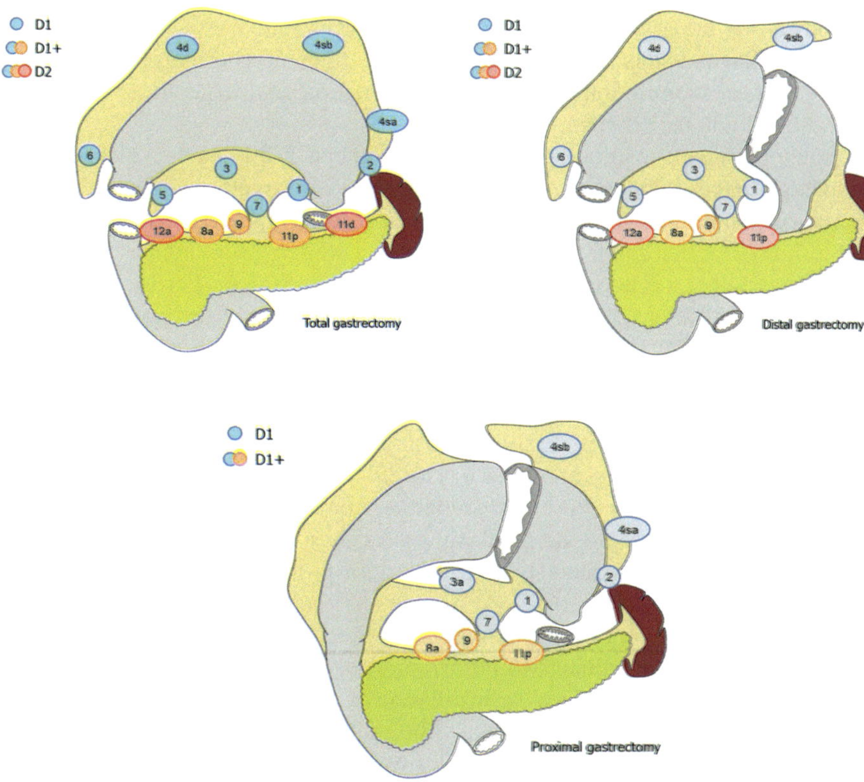

Fig. 15.2 The Japanese Gastric Treatment Guidelines 2021 delineation of relevant lymph node stations depending on the extent of gastrectomy and tumor location. Clockwise: Total gastrectomy, distal gastrectomy, and proximal gastrectomy. (Reproduced from Japanese Gastric Cancer Treatment Guidelines 2021, 6th edition, under the Creative Commons License CC BY 4.0)

of the stomach does not lead to retained or inadequate lymph node dissection. Particularly in overweight and obese patients, a larger amount of perigastric adipose tissue may need to be resected in order to achieve adequate harvest. This dissection can be accomplished with a bipolar sealer or with sharp/blunt dissection and clip placement, with the former technique being particularly useful in the rotund patient.

The additional stations (7, 8, 9, 10, 11, and 12) are where the robotic platform's manual dexterity can be extraordinarily advantageous. Access to these stations is accomplished with ventral retraction of the stomach body following completion of the retrogastric dissection. In resections where the left gastric artery is planned to be left in situ, we find that division of the coronal vein can aid in the mobilization of the station 7 lymph node packet.

There has been growing interest in novel approaches to aid lymph node dissection, particularly to increase yield. One such maneuver utilizes near-infrared imaging and ICG instillation into various locations (peritumoral, subserosal, submucosal, etc.). Although initial data is still evolving, the widespread adoption and long-term clinical outcomes of international patient cohorts are still awaited.

Proximal Gastrectomy

Proximal gastrectomy is begun with exposure of the gastrocolic ligament at the level of the transverse mesocolon. Once incised, the greater omentum can be freed from the transverse mesocolon using a bipolar sealer. Consequent exposure of the omental bursa and visualization of the posterior aspect of the stomach is a key maneuver. The greater curve of the stomach is thus dissected with a bipolar sealer. This maneuver should be undertaken with great care as a medial deviation can lead to inadequate lymph node harvest in addition to inadvertent partial transections of the gastroepiploic vessels. By maintaining a distance of anywhere from 2 to 4 cm away from the stomach, the dissection can be carried cephalad.

Once the left gastroepiploic artery and vein are encountered, the bipolar sealer or a stapling device is used to divide the bundle. A combination of ventral and caudad gastric retraction can aid in this portion of the dissection. Finally, the short gastric vessels will be encountered. Attention must be paid to vector of retraction applied to the stomach at this juncture as overzealous maneuvers will lead to inadvertent vascular avulsion or splenic damage. In most situations, the short gastric vessels can be divided with a bipolar sealer. Once completed, the ventral-most portion of the left diaphragmatic crus is exposed and will serve as the anatomic boundary of the lateral dissection. For some patients, this portion of the dissection can only be accomplished after freeing the posterior aspect of the stomach. The retrogastric dissection, including the division of any gastropancreatic attachments, is achieved using sharp dissection as this minimizes the chance of inadvertent thermal injury to the pancreatic parenchyma. Focal electrocautery can be applied for any small vessels encountered.

The right crus can then be dissected. This is begun by incising the lesser omentum and carrying this plane cephalad. Retraction of the esophagogastric junction toward the patient's left with simultaneous tension on the right crus will allow for ideal visualization so the distal-most esophagus can be dissected from the hiatus. A similar counter-maneuver can be applied circumferentially so that the left, anterior, and posterior portions of the junction are freed. A penrose drain about esophagogastric junction can also aid with these retractions.

Once these initial dissections are completed, then the point of transection on the stomach can be identified. Both arteriovenous arcades (gastroepiploic and right gastric) are separately identified and divided so as to allow for an uneventful gastric division. Sequential fires of either the handheld or robotic stapler are then used, and the proximal stomach (and attached omentum) can then be placed in the left upper quadrant. This exposes the left gastric artery and vein and allows access to any additional lymph node stations that require extirpation.

At this point, adequate mobilization of the distal esophagus can be confirmed. The vagal nerves are identified and divided, and division of the esophagus is done with a linear stapler device. Stay sutures may be utilized to fixate the dissected esophagus at an intrabdominal position at the crus. Depending on tumor location, consideration should be given to intraoperative pathology consultation to ensure adequate margins.

Distal Gastrectomy

The initial dissection for the distal gastrectomy is begun similar to the proximal gastrectomy. Accordingly, after division of the left gastroepiploic arcade, the dissection is then carried rightward along the greater curvature. Gentle cephalad and ventral stomach retraction will allow for a clear visualization of the investment that exists between the colonic mesocolon and the gastroepiploic arcade. This dissection is carried toward the liver, with the gallbladder serving as the anatomic border of the rightward dissection.

The retrogastric dissection is carried out as above; however, now a more inferior and rightward extent is required. In many patients, identification of the gastroduodenal artery (GDA) as it exits the inferior boarder of the pancreas is a key landmark. This annotates the fusion of the aforementioned investment as the GDA meets the gastroepiploic arcade and can be divided with the bipolar sealer or between clips to allow for a full dissection of the infrapyloric region. During this maneuver, a gastric band dissector can be used to create a retrovascular tunnel and thus allow for an easier *en bloc* dissection of the nodal tissue before the stapler/clip division.

The lesser omentum is then entered and the supra-pyloric dissection is accomplished after the right gastric artery is identified and ligated either with bipolar energy or between clips. The proximal duodenum is then divided with a stapling device, and the specimen can then be retracted cephalad and to the left to allow for any additional lymph node dissection required.

As described above for the distal transection site during a proximal gastrectomy, in this operation the proximal transection site is cleared identically and the stomach divided with sequential stapler fires. Again, intraoperative pathologic consultation can be a valuable adjunct to ensure margin status.

Total Gastrectomy

A total gastrectomy, for the sake of brevity, can be thought of as a functional combination of the proximal and distal gastrectomy; however, there are some sequential maneuvers that can make a total removal of the stomach a more efficient endeavor.

First, routine use of the fixed liver retractor will aid immensely in the hiatal dissection. The dissection of the greater curve begins toward the right analogous to the distal gastrectomy. This is the time at which an omentectomy can also be completed and kept with the specimen. Once the proximal duodenum is divided, any additional retrogastric lymph node dissection is completed and the remainder of the cephalad dissection is performed according to the proximal gastrectomy.

Reconstruction

The reestablishment of enteric flow is an oft-overlooked, yet critically important consideration after liberation of the stomach. Each method of reconstruction has its benefits and drawbacks and should be discussed with the patient in conjunction with their resection plan. The specifics of nutritional outcomes, subsequent quality of life, weight maintenance, and need for future revisional procedures is a topic worthy of its own discourse; however, the robotic gastrointestinal surgeon should have a familiarity with a majority of techniques so that they can be applied expeditiously as needed.

The confirmation of adequate blood flow to a newly created anastomosis can also be a point of great surgical ire, especially following extensive resection and perivascular lymph node harvest. The robotic and MIS platform is again well suited as intraoperative intravascular ICG and near-infrared fluoroscopy can not only reaffirm adequate flow, but potentially alter reconstruction choices if early malperfusion is detected.

Billroth I

A direct anastomosis between the divided duodenum and the remaining proximal stomach in the case of a distal gastrectomy can be achieved using a hand-sewn technique. The distal staple line is sharply excised as is the proximal staple line, and a two-layer hand-sewn gastro-duodenal anastomosis is fashioned. Alternatively, a circular stapler can also be used to achieve the same fusion.

Billroth II with Braun Enteroenterostomy

The transverse colon is retracted cephalad, and the ligament of Treitz is identified. A distance of approximately 20–30 cm is traced distally and will serve as the point of anastomosis. This loop of jejunum is brought cephalad in either an antero- or retro-colic fashion and apposed to the divided stomach. The posterior aspect of the stomach is preferred as a site of anastomosis to allow for physiologic emptying of the gastric reservoir. A dual-layer, hand-sewn gastro-jejunal anastomosis is then completed. Alternatively, a linear stapler can also be used to create the anastomosis with subsequent closure of the common gastro-jejunal enterotomies.

Following this, the afferent and efferent limbs of the newly apposed jejunal loop are approximated. A linear stapler is used to create a common channel with subsequent closure of the common enterotomies.

Roux-en-Y

A Roux-en-Y configuration for the re-establishment of continuity can be achieved in similar fashion. In this situation, the length of the Roux limb must be considered heavily. During the common application of the Roux-en-Y reconstruction during bariatric reconstruction, the long length of the Roux limb can portend a more significant weight loss; a metric that is not so desired when reconstructing the potential cancer patient.

When creating either the gastro-jejunal or esophago-jejunal anastomosis, a hand-sewn, two-layer anastomosis is fashioned. The hand-sewn method is also particularly useful in the setting of an esophagojejunostomy where the anatomic limitations of a linear stapler within the hiatus are magnified, although the use of an intraluminal anvil and circular stapler could also be used in this limited space.

Double-Tract Reconstruction

Following a proximal resection, the use of a double-tract reconstruction may also be used. This is begun by fashioning a Roux limb as described. Following the creation of the esophagojejunostomy, an end-to-side gastrojejunostomy between the Roux limb and the remaining stomach is created. This is accomplished with a sharp enterotomy on both viscera followed by a two-layer hand-sewn anastomosis. A variation of this can also be accomplished with a circular stapler.

Conclusion

The robotic platform is an immensely versatile and efficacious tool that can allow for increasingly complex surgical resections with improved recovery. Mastery of these techniques requires detailed surgical forethought, but once planned and executed, can lead to excellent patient outcomes.

Disclosures None.

References

1. Pappas TN. The first 40 years of Gastrojejunostomy: from Billroth to Murphy to Mayo. Ann Surg Open. 2022;3(3):e200. https://doi.org/10.1097/as9.0000000000000200.
2. Kitano S, Iso Y, Moriyama M, Sugimachi K. Laparoscopy-assisted Billroth I gastrectomy. Surg Laparosc Endosc. 1994;4(2):146–8.
3. Bray F, Laversanne M, Sung H, Ferlay J, Siegel RL, Soerjomataram I, Jemal A. Global cancer statistics 2022: GLOBOCAN estimates of incidence and mortality worldwide for 36 cancers in 185 countries. CA Cancer J Clin. 2024;74(3):229–63. https://doi.org/10.3322/caac.21834.
4. National Comprehensive Cancer Network, Gastric Cancer (Version 4.2024). https://www.nccn.org/professionals/physician_gls/pdf/gastric.pdf. Accessed Aug 2024.
5. Japanese Gastric Cancer Association. Japanese gastric cancer treatment guidelines 2021 (6th edition). Gastric Cancer. 2023;26(1):1–25. https://doi.org/10.1007/s10120-022-01331-8.

16 Robotic Sleeve Gastrectomy

Maria S. Altieri

Introduction

With the rise in the prevalence of obesity in the United States and around the world, the field of bariatric surgery is witnessing an increasing demand. Sleeve gastrectomy is a metabolic procedure that involves resection of approximately 60–70% of the greater curvature of the stomach. Due to its perceived safety profile and excellent weight loss, sleeve gastrectomy has surpassed the Roux-en-Y gastric bypass as the most commonly performed metabolic and bariatric surgery today in the United States [1].

The utilization of the robotic platform in the area of metabolic and bariatric surgery has been evolving since the late 1990s [2]. The robotic platform offers several theoretical advantages, including precision in tissue manipulation, greater dexterity due to the elimination of physiological tremor, and enhanced three-dimensional (3-D) imaging. Patients with body mass index (BMI) >50 kg/m^2 present a particular challenge to both surgery and anesthesia due to body habitus and comorbidities. There are several considerations, making conventional laparoscopy more difficult, mainly because of the limited space due to excessive hepatomegaly and intra-abdominal fat and thick abdominal wall, which may require excessive torque on the laparoscopic instruments and ports. Robot-assisted approaches have the potential to alleviate a number of these challenges, thus making the platform particularly useful [3, 4]. The main perceived limitations of the robot-assisted surgery are cost and time to set-up. However, with increased utilization, time to set-up has been improving and perceived intraoperative cost can be neutralized by lower rates of complications and shorter hospital time.

Studies have compared conventional laparoscopy and robot-assisted sleeve gastrectomy and have had mixed results. Nasser et al. compared patients undergoing robot-assisted sleeve gastrectomy versus laparoscopic sleeve gastrectomy between

M. S. Altieri (✉)
Department of Surgery, Hospital of the University of Pennsylvania, Philadelphia, PA, USA
e-mail: Maria.Altieri@pennmedicine.upenn.edu

S. Samreen et al. (eds.), *The SAGES Manual of Robotic Surgery*,
https://doi.org/10.1007/978-3-031-86927-3_16

2015 and 2017. The study compared 685 RSG versus 56,808 LSG cases. The RSG group had a longer operative time, longer hospital length of stay, and overall similar morbidity and mortality. After multivariable logistic regression, patients undergoing RSG had a higher risk for an organ space surgical site infection [5]. A systematic review in 2017 showed that robotic sleeve gastrectomy showed significantly higher mean operative time and increased length of hospital stay. Complications such as incidence of leak, wound infection, and bleeding were comparable [6]. Another recent study showed that the outcomes in robotic bariatric surgery were comparable with the laparoscopic approach despite longer operative times [7]. As higher BMI can lead to increased risk of complications [8], the robotic platform can help decrease that risk. In addition, while it may have longer operative time, robotic sleeve gastrectomy has a less-steep learning curve compared to laparoscopic sleeve gastrectomy [8, 9].

Some of the opponents of the utilization of the robotic platform have cited concerns about higher costs. Several studies have noted higher costs for robotic sleeve gastrectomy [10]. In a publication in 2019, cost analysis of robotic sleeve gastrectomy compared to laparoscopic sleeve gastrectomy revealed no substantive differences in surgery-associated costs. While operative costs were significantly higher, robotic sleeve gastrectomy had a shorter length of stay [11].

Operative Technique

The surgical team consists of a surgeon and bed-side assist. At teaching institutions, a teaching console may be present. As such, the trainee, either resident or fellow, can perform parts of the procedure, while the primary surgeon observes and directs, controls one of the arms, and has the ability to take over in certain instances. In smaller operating rooms, the bed may need to be positioned in a way to be able to dock the robotic platform.

Once anesthesia is induced, the patient is placed in a supine position. Both patient's arms can be extended. We usually do not place foleys as this procedure is relatively short. As most institutions have a Xi platform, the robot can be docked from either side of the patient. The robot is draped in a sterile fashion prior to the procedure start.

A nasogastric tube or a suction bougie is inserted to decompress the stomach. After the patient is being positioned and draped, entry into the abdomen is performed, dependent on surgeon's preferences. We prefer either a Veress at Palmer's point or an optical entry. The abdomen is insufflated to 15 mmHg. All ports are placed after obtaining pneumoperitoneum. The camera port is about 15–20 cm from the xiphoid slightly to the left of the midline. A 12 mm port is placed at least 8 cm lateral to that and 2 8-mm ports are placed to the left of the camera. It is important to note that in obese patients with insufflated abdomen, intra-abdominal distance is less than expected based on the location of the skin incisions. Thus, it is critical that all ports are placed at least 8 cm apart in order to prevent arm collision. A liver retractor is placed with care to have an adequate clearance while docking the robotic platform. We prefer a Nathanson liver retractor in the subxiphoid location, but others like a snake retractor on the patient's right side.

When docking, the robot must be in position such as that the angle between the robot column and the camera is at around 10°. The robotic platform is targeted toward the stomach. The patient is placed in reverse Trendelenburg position, usually at about 12°; however, if higher, BMI can go to 18–21°, in order to see the hiatus.

After positioning the robotic platform, the 30° camera is inserted first as the camera is 30° down (R2). The targeting setting is used to align the rest of the arms. The rest of the arms are attached. All the essential equipment is inserted into the abdomen under direct visualization. In our case, we use 2 Cadiere graspers (R1 and R4) and a vessel sealer (R3). We do not use an assistant port (Fig. 16.1).

The surgery begins by entering into the lesser sac by dividing the gastrocolic ligament (Fig. 16.2). If two surgeons are working, the first surgeon can control R1–R3, while the second surgeon can control R4 for retraction. The dissection is carried toward the angle of His. Posterior gastric adhesions must be completely divided in order to prevent inadvertent injury to the pancreas or rotation of the sleeved stomach.

As the dissection is carried cephalad, care must be taken as the fundus is mobilized away from the spleen by dividing the gastrosplenic ligament, so that there is no injury to the spleen. The goal is to be able to identify left crus and clear the posterior attachments of the fundus and mobilize the fat pad. Complete mobilization of the fundus is very important so that there is no injury to the esophagus or the spleen during firing of the staple, as well as being able to take the whole fundus. In

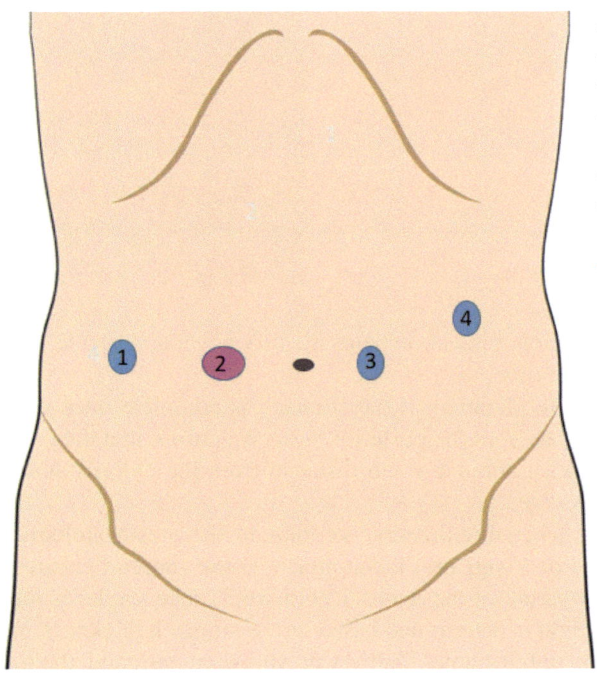

Fig. 16.1 Port position for robot-assisted sleeve gastrectomy

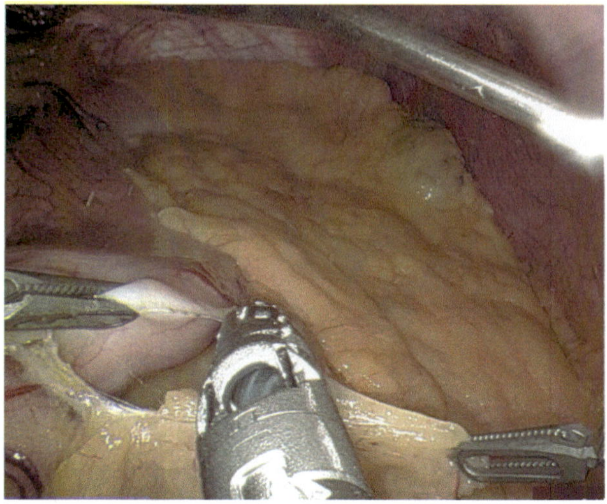

Fig. 16.2 Dissection of the gastrocolic ligament

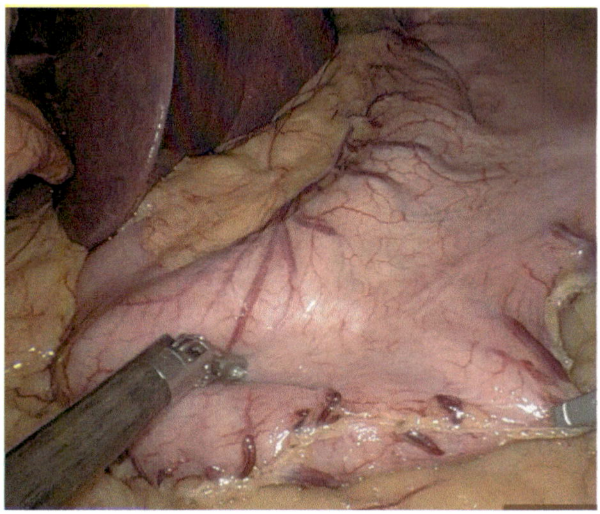

Fig. 16.3 Positioning of the bougie or Visigi

addition, dissection helps identify any hiatal hernia, which should be repaired at the same time.

Mobilization of the stomach is complete once the lesser curvature vessels are visible from the posterior view. We ensure that the gastrocolic ligament is dissected at least about 5–6 cm distance from the pylorus and all posterior attachments are dissected.

When mobilization is complete, the anesthesiologist is asked to advance the bougie or Visigi into the stomach as the surgeon ensures that it lies along the lesser curvature of the stomach (Fig. 16.3). The stapler is introduced via R1 as the staple height is determined based on the stomach thickness. We prefer to use green load as the initial stapler load. As previously mentioned, the first load is fired about 5–6 cm

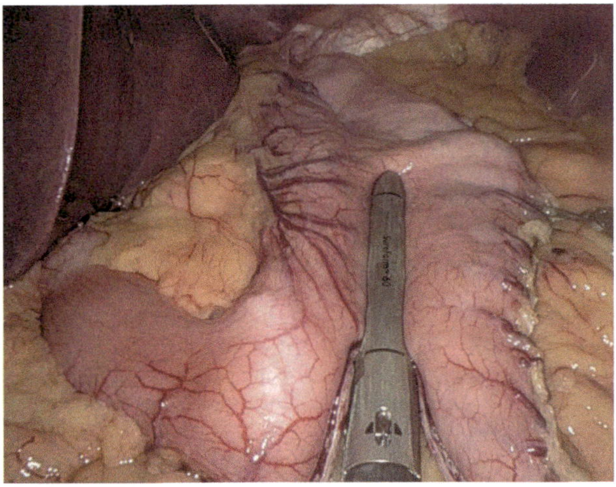

Fig. 16.4 Stapling the stomach

distance from the pylorus. Prior to the firing of the stapler, it is important to ensure that no other tubing is in the stomach in order not to incorporate it in the stapled stomach. If during the firing of the first load there is no resistance, we proceed with blue loads. Each staple is lined next to the bougie or Visigi with care not to constrict or leave too much stomach behind (Fig. 16.4). Also, the lateral retraction is important in order to ensure to grasp tissue in such a way so it does not cause twisting of the sleeved stomach. We are not using any buttressed reinforcements, but others can use stapled reinforcements or oversaw the staple line.

When the sleeve is complete, a leak test can be performed. Some surgeons prefer to do that with diluted methylene blue or indocyanine green (ICG) and/or air in order to detect leakage. In addition, performing an endoscopy can be done to evaluate for twisting, intraluminal bleeding, while at the same time performing a leak test. Then the robotic platform is undocked and the specimen removed. Tisseal can be applied, especially if no staple line reinforcement or no oversawing of the staple line is performed, although there is no literature if this helps lower leak or bleeding rates [12]. The 12 mm port is usually closed with a 0-Vicryl.

A great addition to the robotic platform is the ability to follow your trends on the My Intuitive app. Through this app, the surgeon can compare their times to other surgeons and see areas of improvement, such as instrument changes and time being active on the console. In addition, especially at a teaching institution, the surgeon can see how much is being done by the trainee, thus it can be used as a teaching tool.

Conclusion

The robotic platform appears beneficial in patients with super-obesity, although longer operative times can be noted. However, robotic assistance may help overcome the operative difficulties encountered in the patients with super-obesity. In addition, rapid reduction in operative times with growing experience can be achieved. While surgeon satisfaction and experience cannot be measured, the robotic platform can provide a better ergonomics and experience for surgeons.

References

1. Alsuhibani A, Thompson JR, Wigle PR, Guo JJ, Lin AC, Rao MB, Hincapie AL. Metabolic and bariatric surgery utilization trends in the United States: evidence from 2012 to 2021 National Electronic Medical Records Network. Ann Surg Open. 2023;4(4):e317.
2. Cadiere GB, Himpens J, Vertruyen M, Favretti F. The world's first obesity surgery performed by a surgeon at a distance. Obes Surg. 1999;9:206–9.
3. Cadière GB, Himpens J, Vertruyen M, Bruyns J, Germay O, Leman G, et al. Evaluation of telesurgical (robotic) NISSEN fundoplication. Surg Endosc. 2001;15:918–23.
4. Elli E, Gonzalez-Heredia R, SarvepalliS MM. Laparoscopic and robotic sleeve gastrectomy: short- and long-term results. Obes Surg. 2015;25:967–74.
5. Nasser H, Ivanics RRS, Leonard-Murali S, Genaw J. Perioperative outcomes of robotic versus laparoscopic sleeve gastrectomy in the super-obese. J Surg Res. 2020;249:34041.
6. Magouliotis D, Tasiopoulou VS, Sioka E, Sacharouis D. Robotic versus laparoscopic sleeve gastrectomy for morbid obesity: a systematic review and meta-analysis. Obes Surg. 2017;27(1):245–53.
7. Ho K, Hsu C, Maegawa F, et al. Operative time and 30-day outcome in bariatric surgery: comparison between robotic and laparoscopic approach: 4-year MBSAIP database analysis. J Am Coll Surg. 2022;235:1138–44.
8. Benedix F, Bwnwsix DD, Knoll C, et al. Are there risk factors that increased the rate of staple line leakage in patients undergoing primary sleeve gastrectomy for morbid obesity? Obes Surg. 2014;24:1610–6.
9. Surgery., Clinical Issues Committee of American Society for Metabolic and Bariatric. Sleeve gastrectomy as a bariatric procedure. Surg Obes Relat Dis. 2007;3:573–6.
10. Adair MJ, Alharthi S, Ortiz J, et al. Robotic surgery is more expensive with similar outcomes in sleeve gastrectomy: analysis of the NIS database. Am Surg. 2019;85(1):39045.
11. El Chaar M, Gacke J, Ringold S, Stoltzfus J. Cost analysis of robotic sleeve gastrectomy (R-SG) compared with laparoscopic sleeve gastrectomy (L-SG) in an single academic center: debunking a myth! Surg Obes Relat Dis. 2019;15(5):P675–9.
12. Aggarwal S, et al. Outcome of laparoscopic sleeve gastrectomy with and without staple line oversewing in morbidly obese patients: a randomized study. J Laparoendosc Adv Surg Tech A. 2013;23(11):895–9.

17 Robotic Roux-en-Y Gastric Bypass

Hany Takla

Abbreviations

ASMBS	American Society of Metabolic and Bariatric Surgery
BMI	Body Mass Index
BMP	Basic Metabolic Panel
CBC	Complete Blood Count
CCK	Cholecystokinin
DVT	Deep Venous Thrombosis
EWL	Excess Weight loss
FDA	Food and drug administration
GLP1	Glucagon like peptide 1
ICG	Indocyanine green
IFSO	International federation for the Surgery of Obesity and Metabolic Disorders
IV	Intravenous
JJ	Jejunojejunostomy
MBSAQIP	Metabolic and Bariatric surgery Accreditation and Quality improvement Program
MBS	Metabolic and Bariatric surgery
MIS	Minimally invasive surgery
NSAID	Non-Steroidal anti-inflammatory drugs
PYY	Peptide tyrosine tyrosine
SG	Sleeve gastrectomy
T2D	Type 2 Diabetes Mellitus
VTE	Venous Thromboembolism

Supplementary Information The online version contains supplementary material available at https://doi.org/10.1007/978-3-031-86927-3_17.

H. Takla (✉)
Bariatric and abdominal wall Surgery, Orlando Health Weight loss and Bariatric Surgery Institute, Orlando, Florida, USA

S. Samreen et al. (eds.), *The SAGES Manual of Robotic Surgery*,
https://doi.org/10.1007/978-3-031-86927-3_17

Introduction

Minimally invasive bariatric surgical procedures have been the standard practice for several decades. Laparoscopy is currently considered the standard of care as an approach for different bariatric procedures [1].

Robotic surgery as an approach for bariatric surgery has been a subject of debate for at least two decades since the platform passed FDA approval. One could argue that the exponential growth of robotics in surgery could end such a debate. The robotic platform offers several advantages that are always advertised, but in the morbidly obese population it offers an added advantage. The weight of the abdominal wall translates into a torque or force to resist in order to be able to move the instruments, which, in laparoscopy with a straight instrument, offers a challenge to the operating surgeon and assistant, and the visceral fat retraction and exposure of tight angles at the angle of His also adds to the challenge. All of these factors are dealt with by the operating surgeon and assistant in addition to the technical challenges of a demanding operation such as the gastric bypass. The robotic platform with all the technical and visual advantages takes these physical challenges out of the equation. It offers the operating surgeon physical comfort, superior three-dimensional vision, and seamless stable retraction to allow the focus to fall onto the technical steps of the operation [2].

There are several studies in the literature looking into this, and most concluded that robotic gastric bypass is certainly equivalent and, in some instances, superior to laparoscopy despite the longer operative times for novel surgeons [3] (Table 17.1).

Expert robotic surgeons will always argue that with experience comes shorter operative times and better outcomes like with any novel instrument or approach. The last argument is looking at the market share and growth of robotic gastric

Table 17.1 Review of contemporary role of robotics in bariatric surgery by Bindal et al. [3]

Study	*N*	Type	Operative time (min)	Overall morbidity (%)	Major morbidity (%)	Conversion (%)	Los (day)
Sanchez (5)	50	RCT	130.8	0	0	1	2.72
Ayloo (6)	90	CCT	207	2.2	1.1	0	2
Fourman (7)	1,750	Systematic review	192	7.9	NA	NA	2.72–3
Hagen (8)	143	CCT	NA	16.1	NA	1.4	7.4
Tieu (9)	1100	Case series	155	14	4.09	0	NA
Renaud (10)	154	Case series	141	33.1	11	2.6	NA
Ahmad (10)	172	CCT	155	NA	0	0	2.4
Smeenk (11)	100	CCT	117	5	3	0	2
Economopoulos (12)	5155	Meta-analysis	NA	NA	NA	NA	NA
Myers (13)	100	CCT	144	NA	12	NA	2.1
Benizri (14)	100	CCT	130	24	13	0	9.3
Nasser (4) (Revisional)	1230	RS	196.7	9.3%	NA	0.7	2.4

RCT randomized controlled trial, CCT clinical controlled trial, RS retrospective study, NA not available

bypass over the past 5–10 years. In this chapter, we will try to highlight the indications, preoperative preparation, technical steps, and postoperative instructions and outcomes for robotic traditional Roux-en-Y gastric bypass (RYGB).

RYGB was initially thought to result in weight loss both by a restrictive and malabsorptive mechanism. However, the mechanism in which the operation works is quite complex, including an increase in energy expenditure and alteration in the hormonal network, gut microbiota, and metabolic efficiency.

Ghrelin, also known as the hunger hormone, produces an orexigenic state and thus has been of great interest in obesity and bariatric surgery research. The production of this hormone is by cells located in the gastric fundus that is predominantly excluded in RYGB, postulating a decreased postsurgical circulating level. However, there have been inconsistencies in bariatric research, with some studies showing no change in levels of ghrelin after bariatric surgery, while some were showing an increase. Studies, including that by le Roux et al., report that concomitant vagotomy in RYGB patients may inhibit the effect of ghrelin on appetite stimulation [4]. An increase in anorexigenic hormones such as CCK, GLP-1, PYY, and amylin may be attributed to the decrease in meal sizes observed in these patients postoperatively. Furthermore, GLP-1, released by L-cells in the terminal ileum and colon, has many physiologic functions apart from increased satiety and decreased food intake—it not only stimulates insulin secretion but also increases insulin sensitivity. Postprandial increase in GLP-1 is reportedly seen as early as 1 week postoperative and is proposed to be essential in the resolution of diabetes mellitus after RYGB [5].

Indications

- Basic indications for bariatric surgery have evolved over the years. In this section, we will try to highlight important points to be discussed with the patient prior to choosing a gastric bypass. In October 2022, american society of metabolic and bariatric surgery (ASMBS) and international federation for the surgery of obesity and metabolic disorders (IFSO) published updated indications for metabolic and bariatric surgery, which includes individuals with a body mass index (BMI) ≥35 kg/m^2, regardless of the presence, absence, or severity of comorbidities. Metabolic and baritric surgery (MBS) should be considered for individuals with metabolic disease and BMI of 30–34.9 kg/m^2. BMI thresholds should be adjusted in the Asian population such that a BMI ≥25 kg/m^2 suggests clinical obesity, and individuals with BMI ≥27.5 kg/m^2 should be offered MBS.
- In clinical practice, we usually discuss the benefits and risks for each procedure and give the patient the choice to pick which procedure fits their weight and metabolic profile. Part of the informed decision about pursuing a gastric bypass is to utilize the available online calculators such as the MBSAQIP Bariatric Risk/Benefit Calculator as well as literature review support.
- Typically, from the weight loss standpoint RYGB offers 60–70% Excess Weight loss or equivalent to 30% of total body weight. Although gastric bypass compared with sleeve gastrectomy was associated with greater percentage excess weight loss at 5 years, the difference was not statistically significant [8].

- We advise all of our patients with regards to weight loss that the RYGB is able to achieve 60–70% excess weight loss (EWL). Our experience in our center has been more consistent toward the 70% range.
- From the metabolic standpoint, despite superior weight loss after RYGB, T2D remission rates did not differ significantly between RYGB and SG after 2 years. Long-term follow-up data are needed to define the role of SG in the treatment of patients with obesity and T2D [6, 7].
- Reflux disease has been a matter of debate; however, it is now well established that sleeve gastrectomy is a refluxogenic procedure and typically in practice we prefer to offer RYGB for patients who have severe symptomatic reflux despite medical therapy, patients who suffer from Barrett's esophagus, and patients with grade C and D esophagitis on preoperative endoscopy. This could be regarded as a more aggressive approach favoring RYGB in these patients. However, RYGB procedure has had the most success over the years despite some of the rare long-term potential complications such as marginal ulcers and internal hernias.
- We routinely use the MBSAQIP Bariatric Surgical Risk/Benefit Calculator with our patients to help them make an informed decision about the choice of their operation.
- It is also of additional benefit to have the patient answer a brief questionnaire about individual procedures to ensure they understand all aspects as well as long-term risks and follow-up necessary to avoid complications.

Contraindications

- Relative contraindications can include Crohn's disease and psychosocial disorders, including drug or alcohol use disorders. A high degree of patient understanding of risks and lifestyle implications of surgery needs to be proven, and hence patients with severe intellectual disability are unlikely to be successful candidates. Patients with epilepsy should have a review of their medications as the absorption is affected by bypass surgery. Hence, careful decision-making with the involvement of pharmacists and neurologists should be sought preoperatively [9].
- Absolute contraindications include pregnancy. Those with severe incapacitating systemic diseases, including end-stage renal disease, unstable coronary artery disease, severe heart failure, cirrhosis, portal hypertension, and/or active cancer, are not offered surgery [10].

Patient Preparation

- Preoperative preparation involves having a formal evaluation for bariatric surgery, which is not only an anatomical change but also a mindset change for the patient.
- Typically, our patients go through a behavioral modification class to assess and improve their ability to cope with the dietary and lifestyle modifications involved after bariatric surgery. In addition, we require our patients to follow a medically supervised diet guided by our dieticians for at least 3 months prior to surgery.

Obviously, insurance requirements vary, but as suggested by the ASMBS letter to insurance companies regarding mandatory pre-bariatric surgery diet regimens the longer patients wait before surgery the less successful and invested they become in the preoperative preparation phase without any improvement in outcomes or success rate [11].

- During the preparation phase, we also require all of our patients to have a formal psychological evaluation to assess for major psychologic or eating disorders that gives time for therapy if needed prior to surgery.
- Our patients are also assessed by our nurse practitioner to see if there is a specific medical workup that is required to optimize their medical condition for the procedure.
- In recent years and with progress in minimally invasive techniques and improvement of operative times with experience, the anesthetic risks for bariatric surgery are very minimal even for elderly patients and patients pursuing bariatric surgery as a bridge for organ transplant [12].
- After maximum medical optimization as well as patient readiness and full understanding of the procedure and lifestyle modification commitment, the patient is considered ready for surgery.

Operating Room Setup and Patient Positioning

In this section, we will try to highlight the operating room setup as well as patient positioning prior to starting the procedure and utilize visual illustrations more than text to give a better picture and understanding of the setup. This also in our experience helps novice surgeons have a better understanding of the procedural steps (Video 17.1).

- After anesthesia induction, the patient is positioned supine with both arms placed out on arm boards. We use a foot board to secure the patient while in reverse Trendelenburg position. Proper padding and positioning are confirmed (Fig. 17.1).

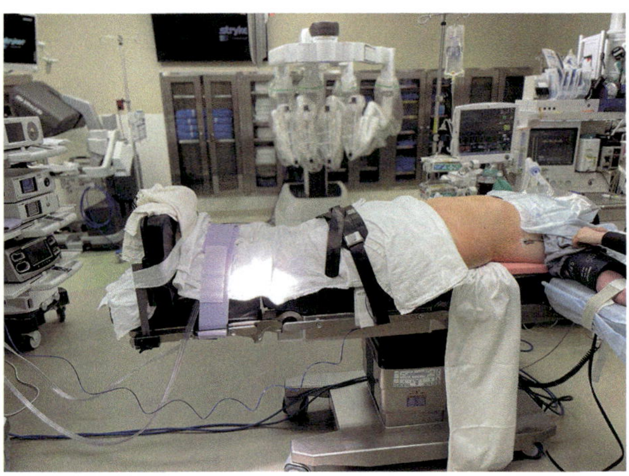

Fig. 17.1 Patient positioned supine with both arms out

Technique (Key Operative Steps)

- We usually gain access to the peritoneal cavity using a Veress needle in the left upper quadrant at Palmer's point.
- There are a variety of techniques, and we would recommend continuing to use the same method used in training or the method that the surgeon is most comfortable with.
- We then enter the abdominal cavity after insufflation to 15 mm Hg using an 8 mm optiview technique. This provides a cushion during trocar entry to minimize the risk of visceral injury.
- For Roux -en- Y Gastric bypass, our technique involves using four trocars, two 12 mm robotic trocars, and two 8 mm robotic trocars placed as shown in Fig. 17.2.
- We prefer using two 12 mm ports as it provides a more comfortable angle for the vertical staple line while creating the gastric pouch.
- The patient is then placed in reverse Trendelenburg position, and the robotic platform is docked (Figs. 17.3, 17.4, 17.5 and 17.6).
- The first step of the operation is to retract the left lobe of the liver. This is usually done using a standard Nathanson retractor or a barbed suture to create a liver Hammock. The following step is to dissect the phreno-esophageal ligament and separate the GE junction from the left crus of the diaphragm. This also allows for inspection for hiatal hernia (Figs. 17.7 and 17.8).

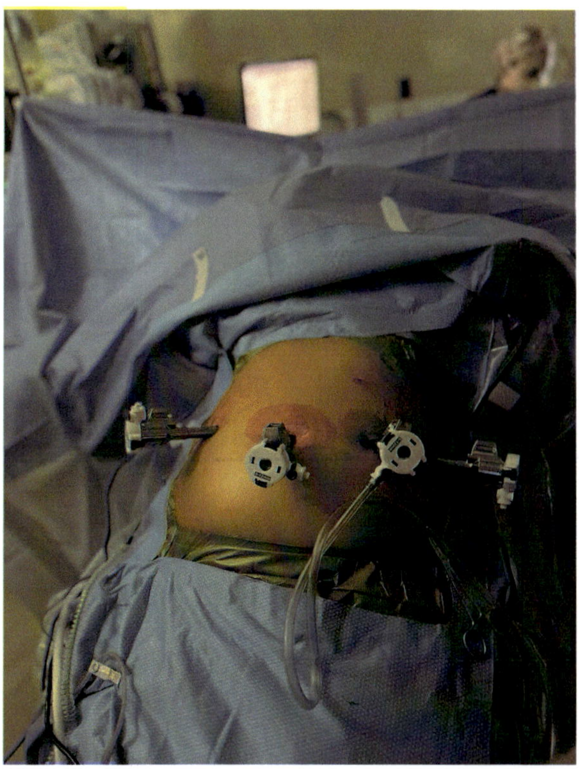

Fig. 17.2 Port placement

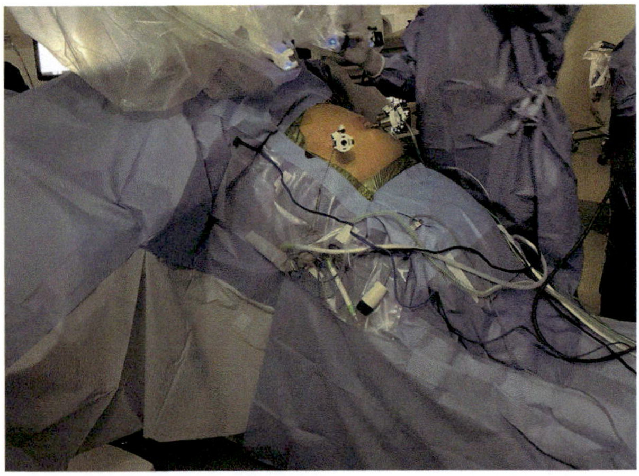

Fig. 17.3 Patient in reverse Trendelenburg position

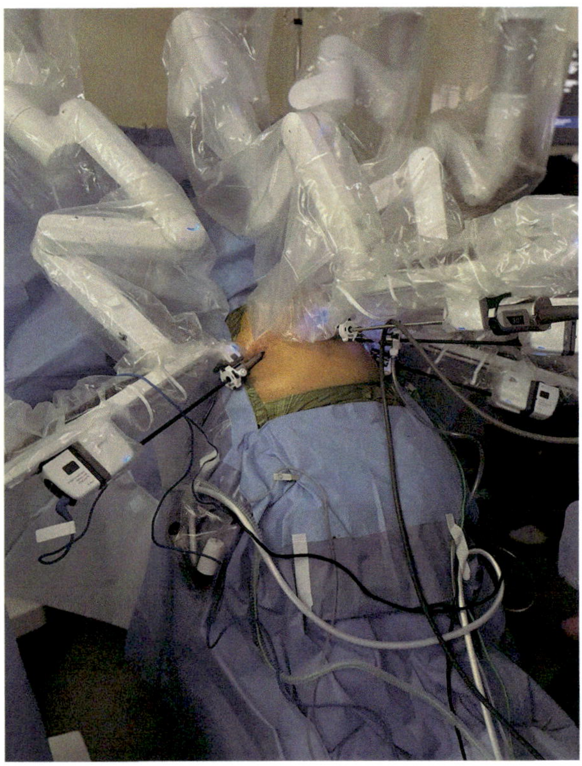

Fig. 17.4 Robotic arms docked

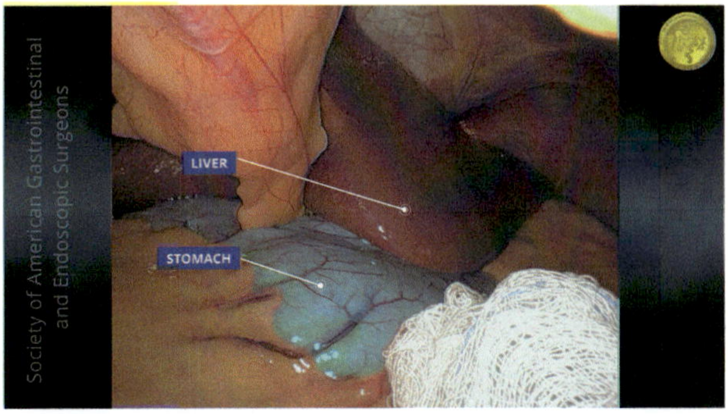

Fig. 17.5 Initial view of the abdomen

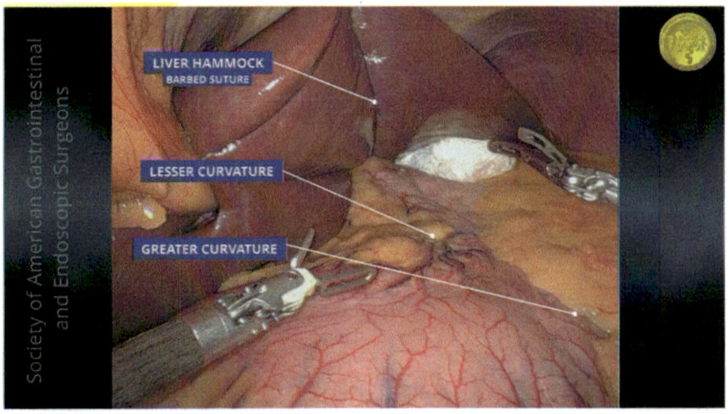

Fig. 17.6 Left lobe of the live retracted using a liver Hammock using barbed suture

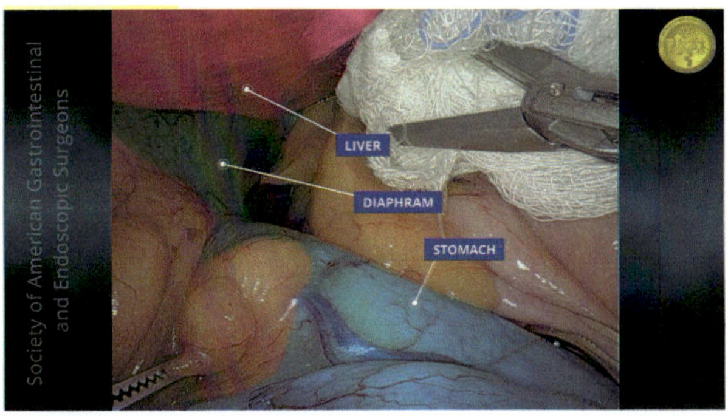

Fig. 17.7 Identification of landmarks at the GE junction

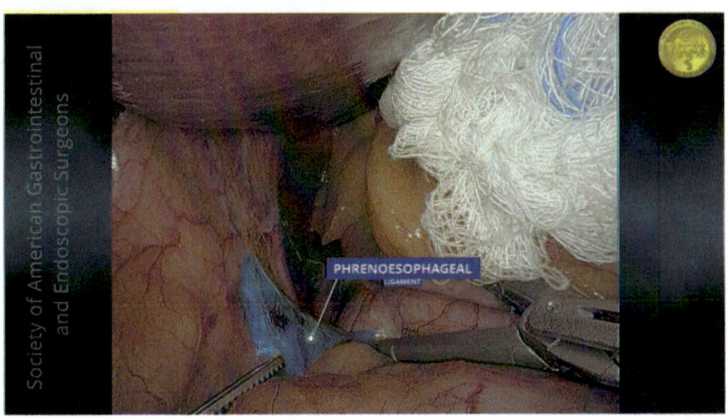

Fig. 17.8 Identifying the phreno-esophageal ligament and looking for a hiatal hernia

- The next step is to create the gastric pouch. We usually use a few landmarks to ensure creation of a properly sized gastric pouch. The first method is to measure about 5 cm vertically from the GE junction, which is the point where the transverse fire of the stapler is started to create the pouch transverse staple line. Another landmark that can be used is just above or at the second crossing vein seen on the anterior wall of the stomach (Fig. 17.9).
- There are a couple of techniques to dissect the lesser curve of the stomach and to be able to create the gastric pouch transverse staple line, either a perigastric dissection, which is the method preferred in our practice, versus division of lesser omentum including the left gastric vessels and nerve of Latarjet. We generally prefer the perigastric method as it theoretically preserves more blood supply to the pouch and nerve supply, which could potentially help with emptying. As shown by Van Wezenbeek et al. in 2016, the omental transection technique may also increase the risk of leaks, bleeding, and abscess formation (Figs. 17.10 and 17.11).
- Careful dissection is carried out along the lesser curve dividing all the medial and posterior vessels to the lesser curve of the stomach using a bipolar energy device. Hand-over-hand blunt dissection helps create a tunnel until reaching the lesser sac. Care should be taken in the presence of posterior adhesions between the posterior wall of the stomach and the retroperitoneal fat as this could potentially risk injury to the pancreas or splenic artery. Once the lesser sac is entered, the

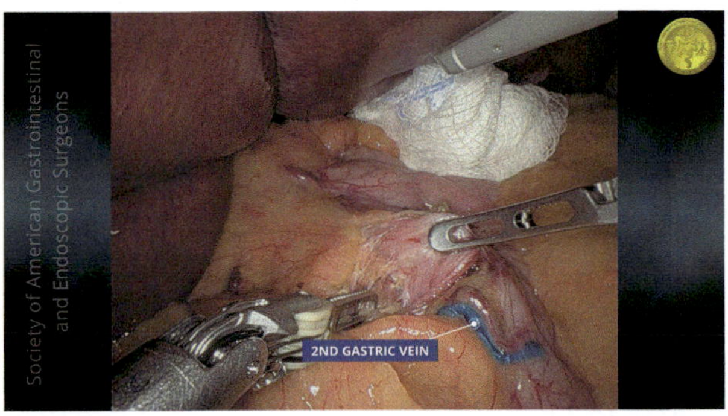

Fig. 17.9 Starting the perigastric dissection above or at the second crossing vein

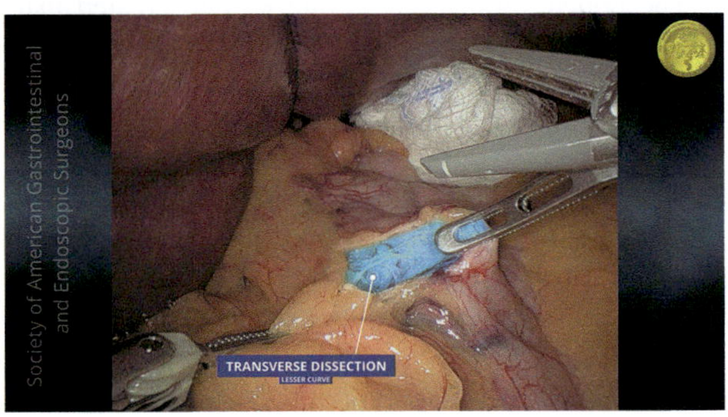

Fig. 17.10 Dividing all the small branches at the lesser curve

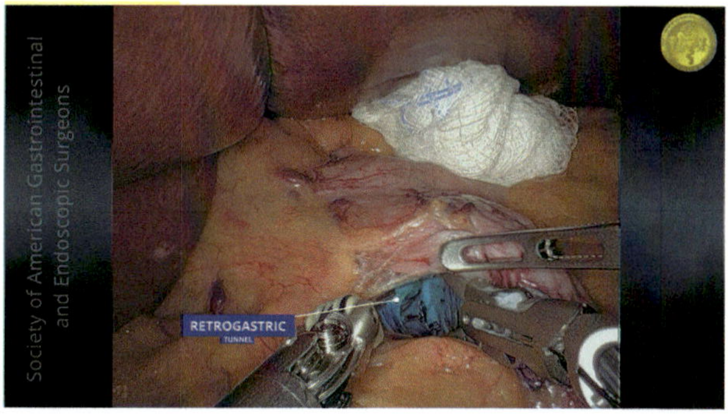

Fig. 17.11 Identifying the retrogastric tunnel into the lesser sac

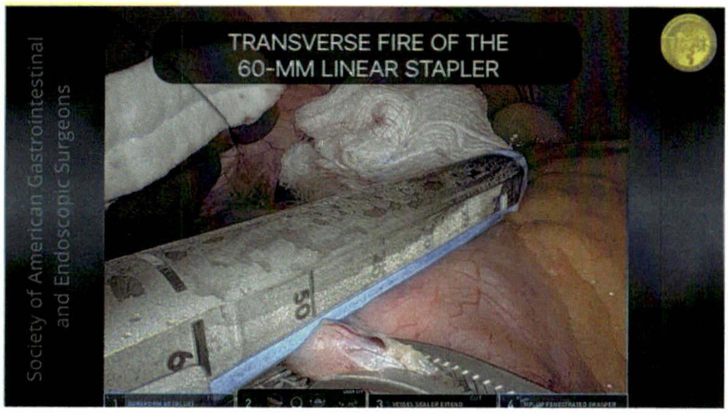

Fig. 17.12 Insertion of the stapler into the retrogastric tunnel

stapler is used to create a 50 mm transverse staple line to allow for a two-layered 18–20 mm anastomosis. The bougie is introduced by anesthesia and advanced to create a longer anterior wall of the pouch than the posterior wall to give room to create an anastomosis along the anterior wall of the gastric pouch (Figs. 17.12 and 17.13).

- Subsequently, the vertical retrogastric tunnel is created with a vertical trajectory toward the GE junction, careful division of retrogastric fat using a bipolar energy device is done taking care not to injure the pancreas, splenic artery and properly dividing the posterior short gastrics to avoid any traction injury to these vessels (Fig. 17.14).
- The pouch vertical staple line is then created usually using two firing of the 60 mm robotic stapler with blue or white loads depending on the thickness of the stomach tissue (Figs. 17.15, 17.16, 17.17 and 17.18).
- We routinely check the blood supply of the pouch by asking anesthesia to give 7.5 mg of Intravenous Indocyanine green. For the most part, pouches are usually well vascularized (Fig. 17.19); however, this becomes even more important in revisional procedures where some of the gastric blood supply may have been already interrupted previously.
- The next step is to create the gastrojejunal anastomosis. Our routine practice is to perform an antecolic antegastric two-layered hand-sewn gastrojejunostomy using the omega loop technique.

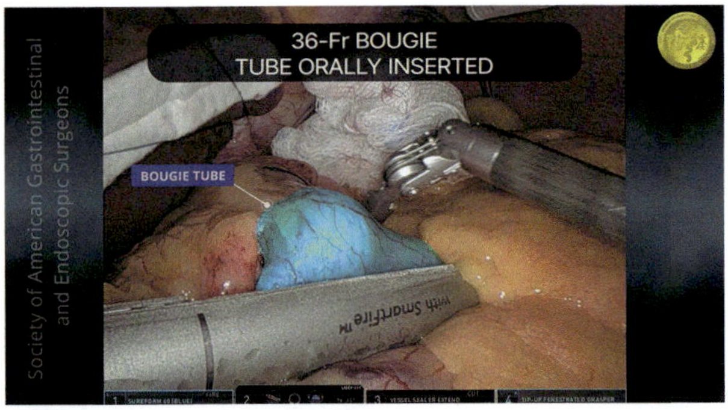

Fig. 17.13 Transverse staple fire to create the gastric pouch

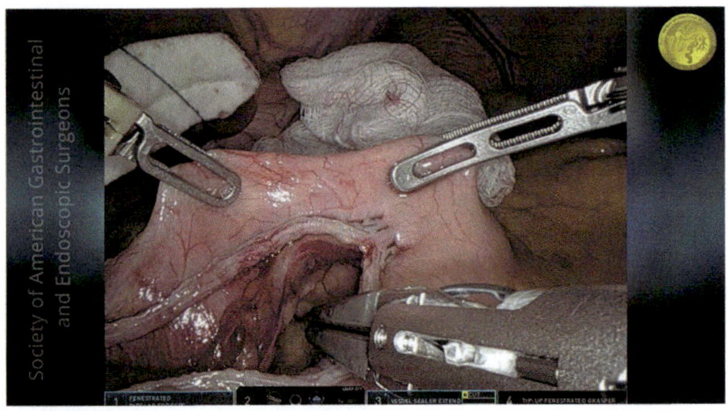

Fig. 17.14 Vertical retrogastric dissection

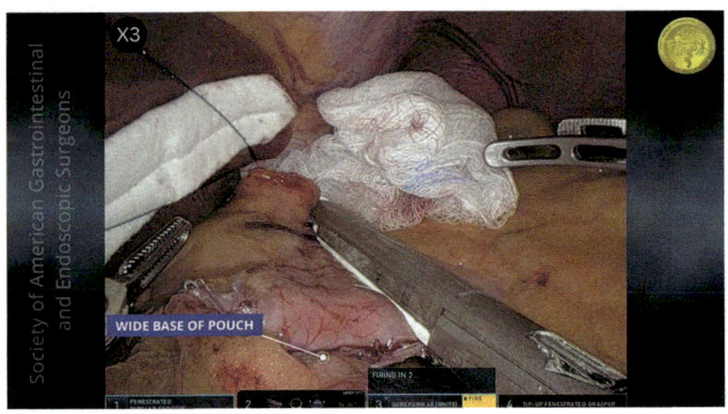

Fig. 17.15 Vertical staple fire to create the gastric pouch along the bougie

- The greater omentum is reflected cephalad, and we usually split the greater omentum until reaching the anti-mesenteric border of the transverse colon; this allows the Roux limb to reach the pouch in an antecolic-antegastric fashion without undue tension.
- Occasionally with shortened thick small bowel mesentery, a retrocolic-retrogastric Roux limb is necessary, but in our experience this is a rare occurrence.
- The ligament of Trietz is then identified, and then we use the tip up grasper robotic instrument to assist in counting 70–85 cm of biliopancreatic limb. As noted in several studies, the length of the BP limb is an important contributor to

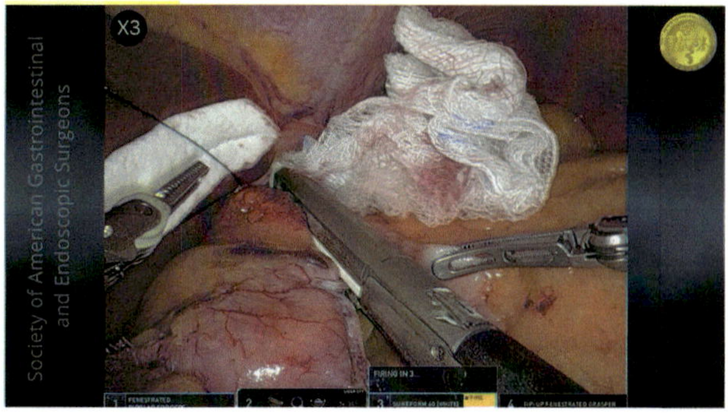

Fig. 17.16 Second vertical staple fire

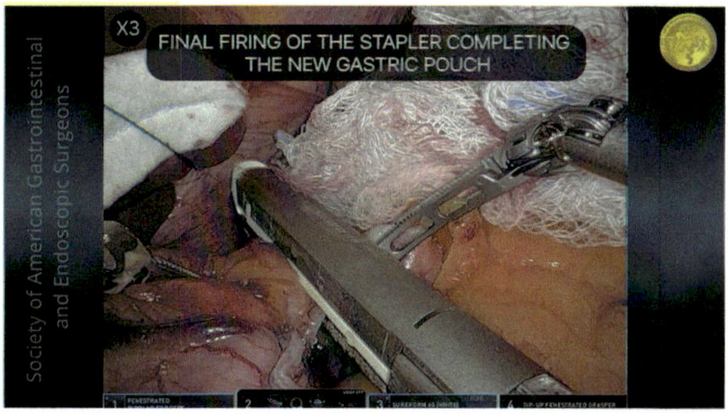

Fig. 17.17 Final staple fire to separate the gastric pouch from the gastric remnant

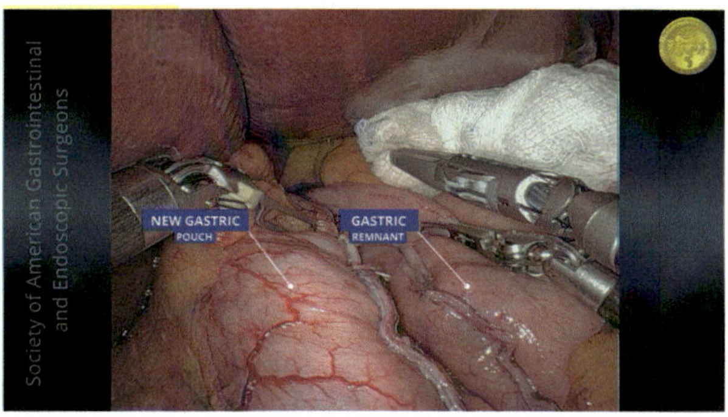

Fig. 17.18 Completed gastric pouch

the malabsorptive function of the procedure. In our practice, we do vary the BP limb length slightly based on BMI. One crucial step here is to ensure that the BP limb connecting to the ligament of Trietz stays on the right side of the screen (patient's left upper quadrant), especially when using the omega loop technique that we routinely use in our practice. This step ensures that a Roux en-O configuration does not occur (Figs. 17.20, 17.21, 17.22 and 17.23).

- The loop of jejunum is then brought up into the upper abdomen with the BP limb on the right side of the screen and the Roux limb on the left side of the screen; the loop is then attached to the transverse staple line of the pouch to create the outer (second) layer of the anastomosis. This is done using a 3/0 slowly

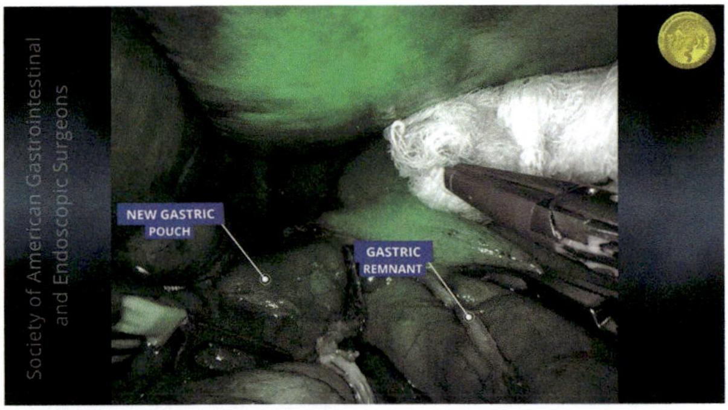

Fig. 17.19 ICG used to check the blood supply of the gastric pouch

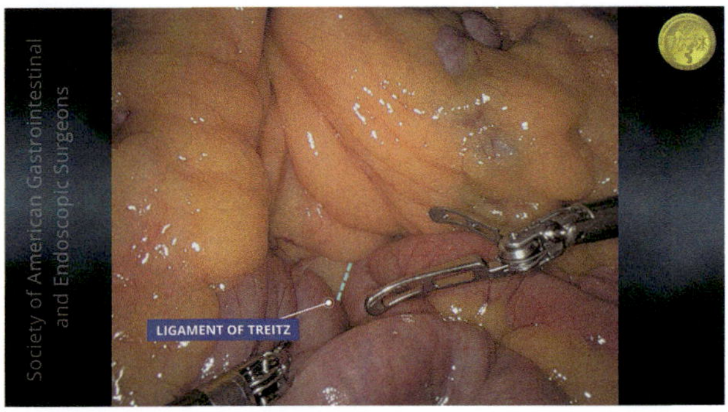

Fig. 17.20 Identifying the ligament of Treitz

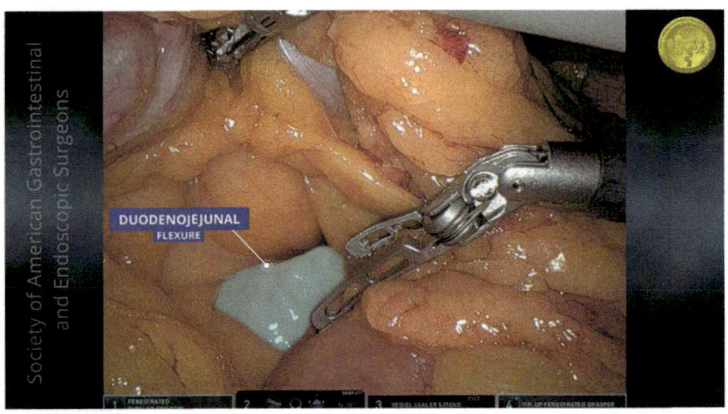

Fig. 17.21 Confirming the duodenojejunal junction

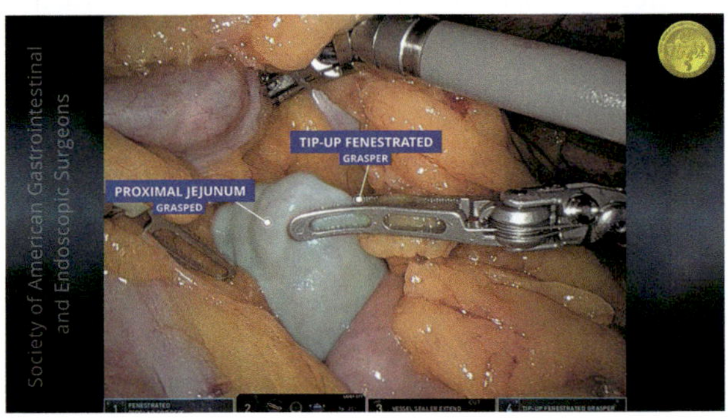

Fig. 17.22 Identifying the direction of the BP and Roux limbs to avoid Roux-en-O configuration

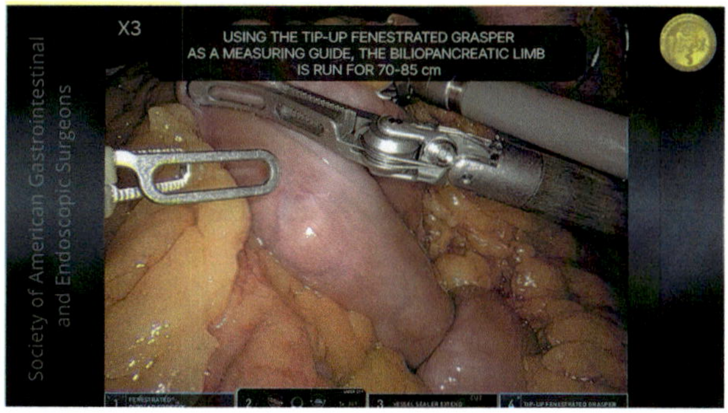

Fig. 17.23 Counting the BP limb length using the tip up grasper

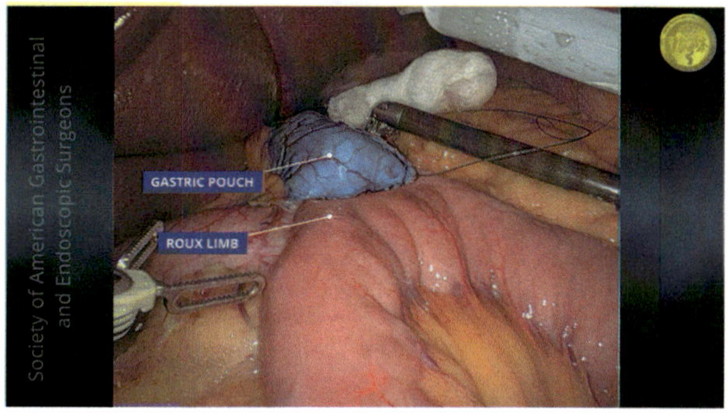

Fig. 17.24 Attaching the omega loop to the transverse pouch staple line using 3/0 absorbable suture

absorbable barbed suture. This is locked at the left corner of the pouch and left in place to be used for the anterior second layer (Fig. 17.24).

- A gastrotomy is then performed using the cut function on the monopolar scissors over the bougie. We try to measure the length of the gastrotomy and enterotomy, which is usually about 2 cm that allows sufficient anastomosis caliber and minimize the risk of stricture (Fig. 17.25).
- Once the gastrotomy and enterotomy are completed, we then start performing a hand-sewn anastomosis using a 3/0 slowly absorbable barbed suture starting at the left corner, then progressing to the posterior layer and the anterior layer. Subsequently, we then use the previous 3/0 suture to complete and anterior second layer moving from the left of the anastomosis to the right (Fig. 17.26).
- After the anastomosis is constructed, we then use the bougie to test for a leak; we usually have anesthesia move the bougie to mid pouch and inject 20 cc of water mixed with 7 cc of ICG to test for a leak, and we then follow that with 20 cc of air to ensure that the anastomosis is air tight as well. This fluid is then suctioned and the bougie is removed (Fig. 17.27).
- Next the biliopancreatic limb is divided using a 60 mm robotic stapler; the line of division is aligned with the vertical staple line of the pouch to avoid Candy Cane syndrome (Figs. 17.28, 17.29 and 17.30).
- The next step is to count the Roux limb, which we usually use 130–150 cm length Roux limb depending on the BMI. We usually use a ruler to count and ensure that the length is as accurate as possible (Fig. 17.31). The counting is

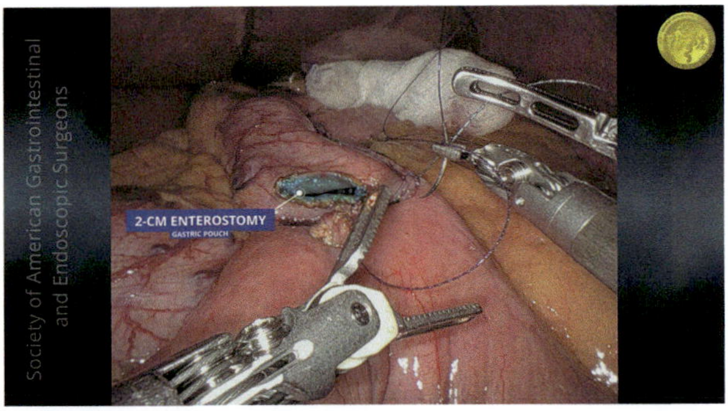

Fig. 17.25 2 cm gastrotomy and enterotomy are created

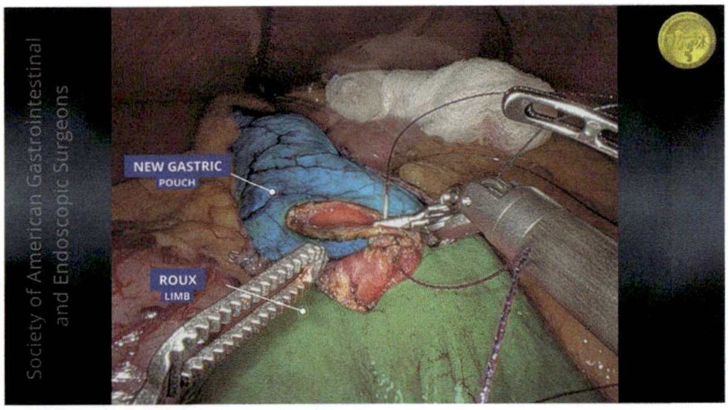

Fig. 17.26 Inner layer of the anastomosis is created using 3/0 absorbable suture

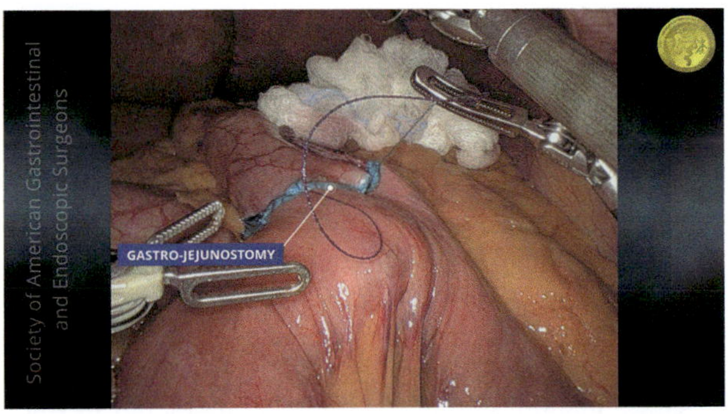

Fig. 17.27 Second anterior layer of the anastomosis is then placed

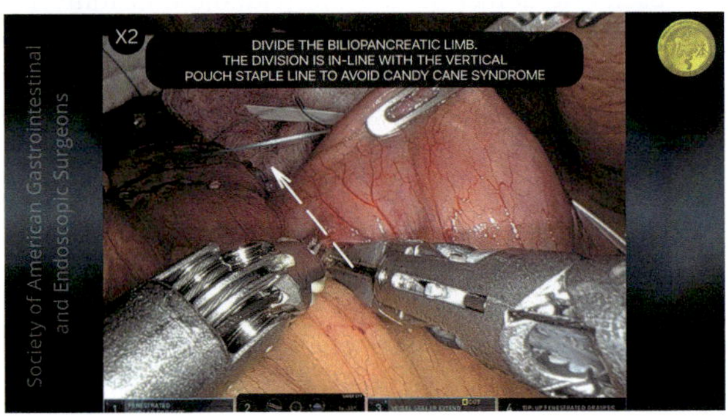

Fig. 17.28 A window created in mesentery of biliopancreatic limb

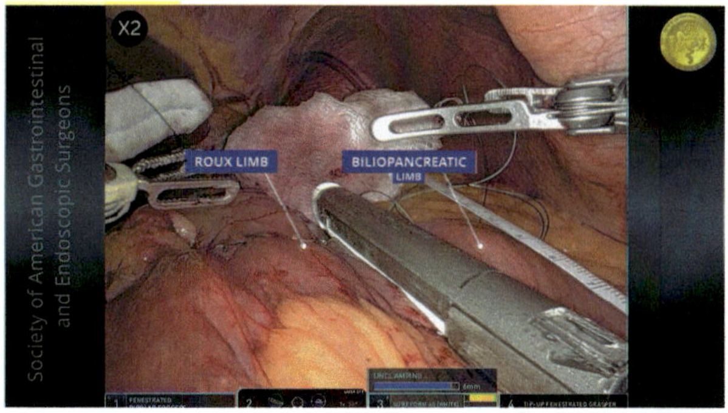

Fig. 17.29 BP limb divided using the robotic stapler

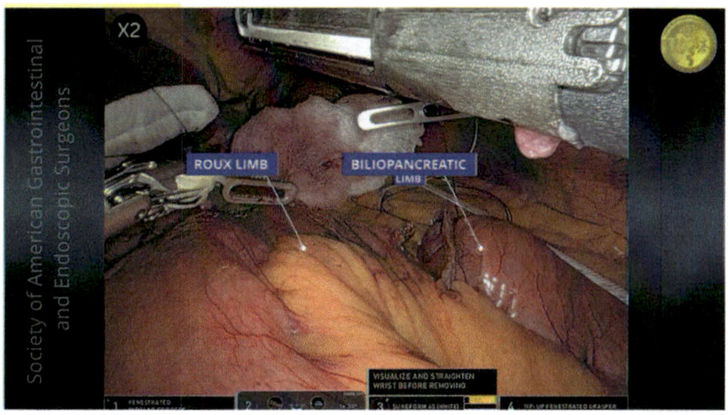

Fig. 17.30 Completed division of BP limb to separate the omega loop into alimentary and BP limbs

usually done in a counterclockwise fashion. After reaching the point where the Roux limb will be anastomosed to the BP limb, an enterotomy is made in the Roux limb, Another enterotomy is made in the BP limb just distal to the staple line; a side-to-side Jejunojejunostomy is then created using a 60 mm robotic stapler (Figs. 17.32, 17.33 and 17.34).

- We then place a simple interrupted suture at the posterior corner of the anastomosis to allow for traction on the anastomosis to distract the enterotomy to the right and allow easy closure of common enterotomy (Fig. 17.35).
- The common enterotomy channel is then closed using a running 3/0 slowly absorbable barbed suture in two layers (Fig. 17.36).
- Subsequently, the anastomosis is distracted to the left upper quadrant and the mesenteric defect behind the jejunojejunostomy is closed using a running 2/0 ethibond suture. Care should be taken to avoid excessive angulation of the Roux limb going into the jejunojejunostomy during this step (Figs. 17.37 and 17.38).
- The final step is to close the pseudo-Peterson space behind the Roux limb by suturing the mesentery of the Roux limb to the transverse mesocolon using a permanent suture as well (Figs. 17.39 and 17.40).
- We routinely perform upper endoscopy to ensure patency of the anastomosis and inspect for any bleeding in the gastric pouch or at the gastrojejunostomy (Fig. 17.41).
- The procedure is then concluded.

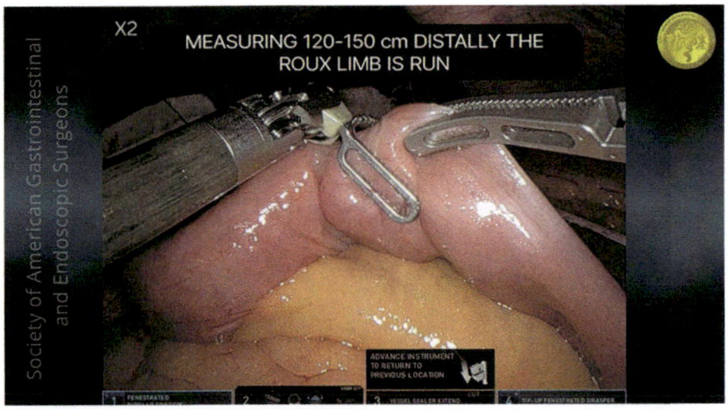

Fig. 17.31 The Roux limb is then counted

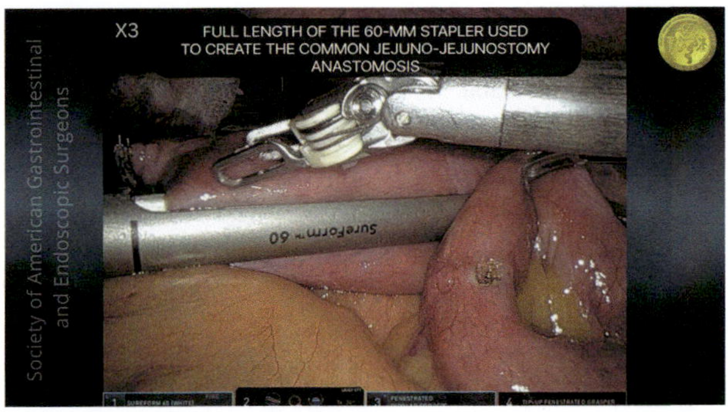

Fig. 17.32 After making enterotomies, a side-to-side jejunojejunostomy is created

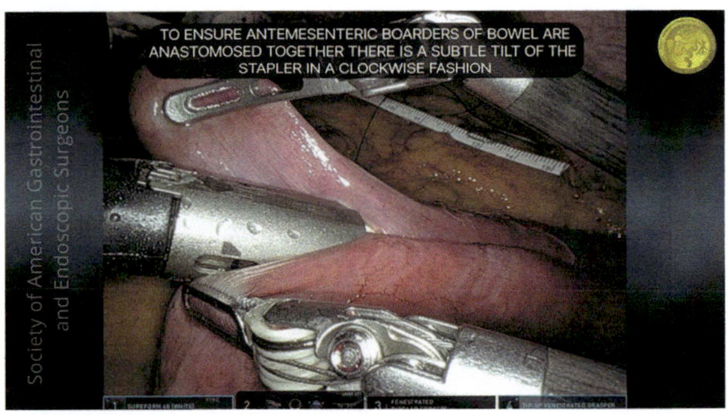

Fig. 17.33 The stapler is rotated slightly to allow antemesenteric borders of the bowel to be anastomosed

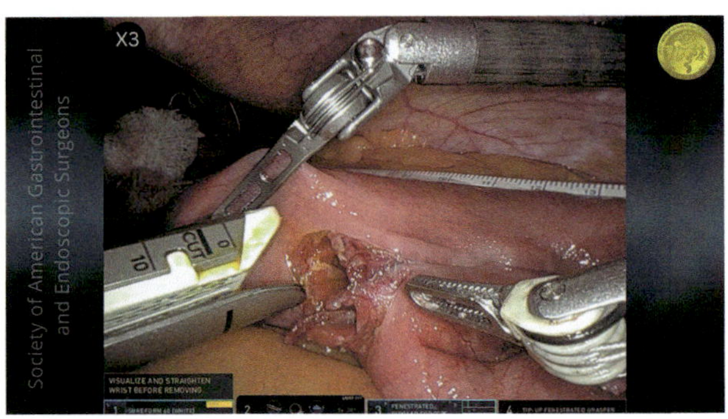

Fig. 17.34 The staple line is inspected for bleeding

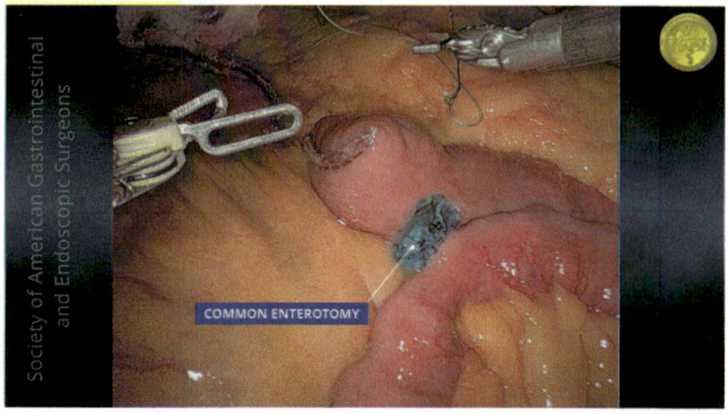

Fig. 17.35 The common enterotomy is positioned for closure

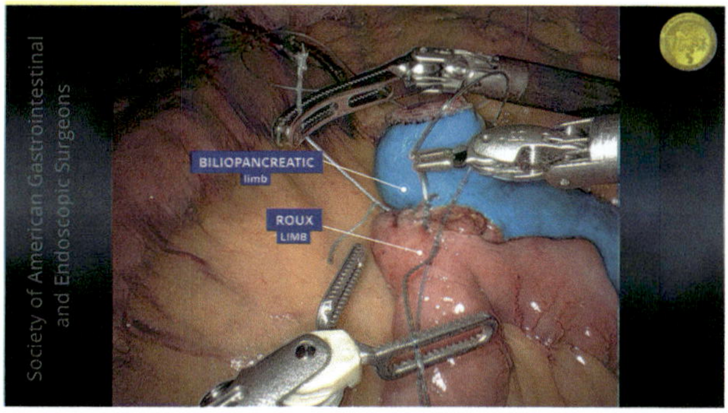

Fig. 17.36 The enterotomy is closed using a running 3/0 absorbable suture

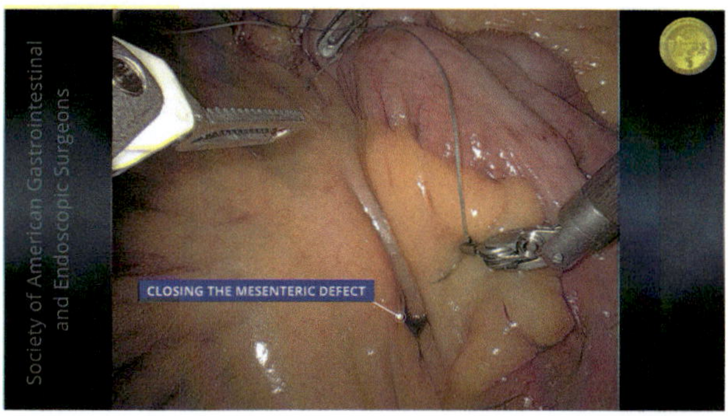

Fig. 17.37 Closure of mesenteric defect behind the jejunojejunostomy using 2/0 permanent suture

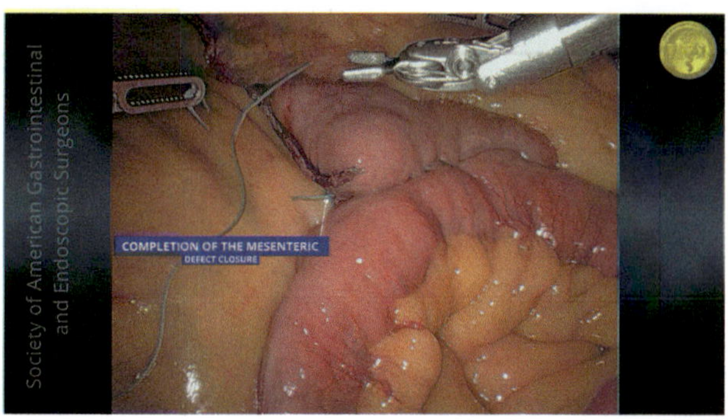

Fig. 17.38 Completed closure of mesenteric defect

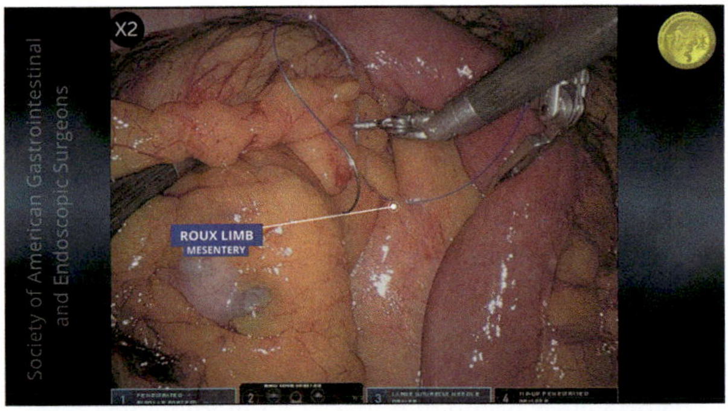

Fig. 17.39 Exposure of pseudo-Peterson space

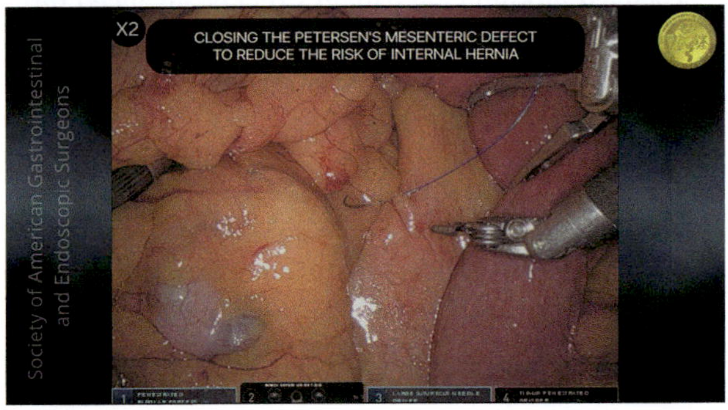

Fig. 17.40 Closure of pseudo-Peterson space using a nonabsorbable suture

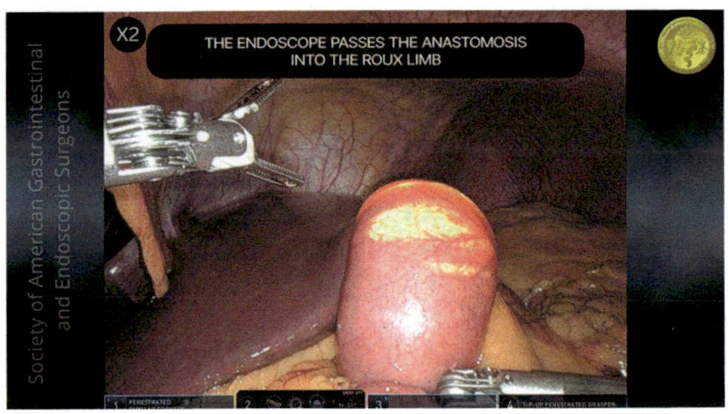

Fig. 17.41 Endoscopy to inspect the anastomosis

Postoperative Management and Instructions

- In our practice, all of our patients are admitted to the floor for observation for 24 h and most are discharged the next morning when they meet the criteria for discharge.
- We usually obtain a Hematocrit level 4 h postoperatively and a complete blood count (CBC) and basic metabolic panel (BMP) the next morning. This gives a baseline in case any postoperative bleeding issues are encountered.
- The main monitoring parameters we follow are signs of bleeding, early leaks that are very uncommon as well as venous thromboembolism (VTE) events. Some of

the signs are common between different parameters that include tachycardia, fever, increasing abdominal pain, peritoneal signs, and metabolic derangements. One should be diligent in investigating these signs as it may signify an underlying early complication. Failure of normal progression should keep the surgeon on alert to investigate the underlying etiology.

- We use prophylactic heparin routinely postoperatively unless the patient has a contraindication or a coagulopathy that would require a different type of deep venous thrombosis (DVT) prophylaxis.
- We usually start with a water trial in the recovery room once the patient is fully conscious, and then advance to a noncarbonated, nonconcentrated sweet low-calorie clear liquid diet in 3–4 oz increments.
- The next morning the patient's diet is advanced further to include protein shakes in 3–4 oz increments, and, if well tolerated, the patient is usually discharged home within 24 h of their procedure.
- We use scheduled Tylenol and IV NSAID for pain control while the patient is admitted with small narcotic doses as needed for breakthrough pain, which is infrequently needed.
- The patient is also placed on an oral proton pump inhibitor for 1 month postoperatively to theoretically reduce hyperacidity and risk marginal ulcers as well as allowing mucosal healing in the early postoperative period.
- The first postoperative visit is usually scheduled within 1–2 weeks postoperatively.

Complications

Early Complications

An anastomotic leak from the gastrojejunal anastomosis is a potentially fatal complication. It typically manifests within 24 h in a gastric bypass; however, it could manifest later. We quote our patients 0.5–1% risk in our practice, especially with the different intraoperative checks, including leak test using ICG, upper endoscopy, and checking blood supply at the anastomosis using ICG as well.

Hemorrhage from anastomoses and staple lines has a high chance of resolving spontaneously, but may require transfusion while awaiting resolution.

Bowel obstruction can occur early or late, the former due to Roux-en-O error, where the closed-loop obstruction is created by misidentification of Roux and BP limbs. Early bowel obstruction can also be due to iatrogenic stricture at the jejunojejunal anastomosis either due to a kink as the Roux limb enters the anastomosis or due to intraluminal bleeding, port site hernia, and small bowel volvulus. Early internal hernias are very uncommon. If any of these issues are identified, prompt surgical intervention is necessary to avoid further complications and avoid precipitation of a Gastrojejunal anastomotic leak.

Deep vein thrombosis or pulmonary embolism can be fatal after bariatric surgery, and so prevention is critical, with intermittent calf pumps intraoperatively, compression stockings, and postoperatively chemical prophylaxis.

Late Complications

Internal herniation can occur in gastric bypass in one of three ways. Peterson's hernia can occur following herniation of bowel through the defect created between the jejunal mesentery of the alimentary limb and the transverse mesocolon. The other two hernias can occur at the mesenteric defect created by the jejunojejunostomy (JJ) anastomosis and through the mesocolic defect if the Roux limb passes retrocolic. As weight is lost, the bowel anatomy changes and mesenteric defects can become accentuated or created. The presentation is often subacute, with postprandial pain or bloating; however, acute presentations with strangulation can also occur. Diagnostic laparoscopy is the investigation of choice, with a reduction of the hernia and closure of the mesenteric defect [13, 14].

Stricture at the gastrojejunal anastomosis can occur in up to 5% of patients. Contributing factors include excess tension, ischemia and technical aspects of methods used to create the anastomosis [15, 16].

Micronutrient deficiency can occur, and lifelong vitamin/mineral supplementation is essential for preventing these deficits caused by the loss of absorption at the duodenojejunal region of the bowel. Common deficiencies include thiamine, vitamin B12, folate, iron, zinc, and vitamin D.

Dumping syndrome can present as postprandial malaise precipitated by the rapid passage of food into the anastomosed jejunum at the GJ anastomosis. Management is typically conservative with advice on altering diet and decreasing the size of meals.

Outcomes and Conclusion

- Roux-en-Y gastric bypass has been standard in metabolic and bariatric surgery for several decades, and the outcomes and safety profile are well known and beyond the context of this chapter.
- Patients who undergo RGYB are typically reported to experience approximately 60–70% excess body weight loss, with over 75% control of comorbidities. In a study published in *NEJM* looking at 12-year weight and metabolic outcomes after gastric bypass, the adjusted mean change from baseline body weight in the surgical group was −45.0 kg, −36.3 kg, and – 35.0 kg at 2, 6, and 12 years, while that in the two nonsurgical groups (1: no surgery due to insurance reasons; 2: did not seek surgery) at 12 years was −2.9 kg and 0.0 kg, respectively. Similarly, higher rates of remission in the surgical group when evaluating preoperative comorbidities such as type 2 diabetes (51% at 12 years), hypertension, and hyperlipidemia [17].

- Roux-en-Y gastric bypass (RYGB) demonstrates high rates of type 2 diabetes mellitus (T2DM) remission, a phenomenon hypothesized to be mediated mainly by weight loss. Compared to procedures that do not bypass the proximal small intestines, such as sleeve gastrectomy (SG), RYGB exhibits weight-loss-independent intestinal mechanisms conducive to T2DM remission. In a retrospective review, Ghanem et al. showed that T2DM remission rates after RYGB are maintained despite weight recurrence, arguing for a concurrent weight-loss-independent metabolic benefit likely facilitated by bypassing the proximal small intestine [18].
- Furthermore, it was shown in a retrospective cohort review that patients with a recent history of T2DM who undergo early RYGB experience significantly higher and earlier T2DM remission compared to patients with a prolonged history of preoperative T2DM, suggesting potential benefit of early surgical intervention to manage patients with obesity and T2DM [19].
- It is, however, important to mention and explore if the shift in paradigm toward robotic bariatric surgery has contributed to improved surgical outcomes for these procedures.
- There are several studies as mentioned in the introduction that looked at this, and so far it has been demonstrated that the outcomes are comparable to the laparoscopic approach, especially after the surgeon moves past their learning curve.
- It is arguable that with the advanced ergonomics, superior visual tools, and wristed instruments, the robotic platform is superior in its offerings to the surgeon and enables a wider variety of surgeons with variable skill set to adopt MIS surgery, especially in the field of bariatric surgery.
- The gastric bypass is a technically demanding operation with a variety of steps that require superior technical skills and can be challenging for trainees and young surgeons. In our experience, the robotic platform allows easier adoption and teaching of these technically challenging steps.
- In addition, the marked increase in market share for robotic bariatric surgery is a sign that the technology is here to stay and is well sought by surgeons as well as patients.

References

1. Wittgrove AC, Clark GW, Tremblay LJ. Laparoscopic gastric bypass, Roux-en-Y: preliminary report of five cases. Obes Surg Incl Laparosc Allied Care. 1994;4(4):353–7.
2. Beckmann JH, Bernsmeier A, Kersebaum J-N, et al. The impact of robotics in learning Roux-en-Y gastric bypass: a retrospective analysis of 214 laparoscopic and robotic procedures. Obes Surg. 2020;30:2403.
3. Bindal V, Bhatia P, Dudeja U, Kalhan S, Khetan M, John S, Wadhera S. Review of contemporary role of robotics in bariatric surgery. J Minim Access Surg. 2015;11(1):16–21. https://doi.org/10.4103/0972-9941.147673. PMID: 25598594; PMCID: PMC4290112.
4. Park CW, Torquati A. Physiology of weight loss surgery. Surg Clin North Am. 2011;91(6):1149–61, vii.
5. Peterli R, Wölnerhanssen B, Peters T, Devaux N, Kern B, Christoffel-Courtin C, Drewe J, von Flüe M, Beglinger C. Improvement in glucose metabolism after bariatric surgery: comparison

of laparoscopic Roux-en-Y gastric bypass and laparoscopic sleeve gastrectomy: a prospective randomized trial. Ann Surg. 2009;250(2):234–41.

6. Aminian A. Bariatric procedure selection in patients with type 2 diabetes: choice between Roux-en-Y gastric bypass or sleeve gastrectomy. Surg Obes Relat Dis. 2020;16(2):332–9. https://doi.org/10.1016/j.soard.2019.11.013. Epub 2019 Dec 2
7. Wallenius V, Alaraj A, Björnfot N, Orrenius B, Kylebäck A, Björklund P, Werling M, Thorell A, Fändriks L, Maleckas A. Sleeve gastrectomy and Roux-en-Y gastric bypass in the treatment of type 2 diabetes. Two-year results from a Swedish multicenter randomized controlled trial. Surg Obes Relat Dis. 2020;16(8):1035–44. https://doi.org/10.1016/j.soard.2020.04.033. Epub 2020 May 5
8. Salminen P, Helmiö M, Ovaska J, Juuti A, Leivonen M, Peromaa-Haavisto P, Hurme S, Soinio M, Nuutila P, Victorzon M. Effect of laparoscopic sleeve gastrectomy vs laparoscopic Roux-en-Y gastric bypass on weight loss at 5 years among patients with morbid obesity: The SLEEVEPASS Randomized Clinical Trial. JAMA. 2018;319(3):241–54. https://doi.org/10.1001/jama.2017.20313. PMID: 29340676; PMCID: PMC5833550.
9. Angeles PC, Robertsen I, Seeberg LT, Krogstad V, Skattebu J, Sandbu R, Åsberg A, Hjelmesaeth J. The influence of bariatric surgery on oral drug bioavailability in patients with obesity: a systematic review. Obes Rev. 2019;20(9):1299–311.
10. O'Brien PE. Bariatric surgery: mechanisms, indications and outcomes. J Gastroenterol Hepatol. 2010;25(8):1358–65.
11. Jamal MK, DeMaria EJ, Johnson JM, Carmody BJ, Wolfe LG, Kellum JM, Meador JG. Insurance-mandated preoperative dietary counseling does not improve outcome and increases dropout rates in patients considering gastric bypass surgery for morbid obesity. Surg Obes Relat Dis. 2006;2(2):122–7. https://doi.org/10.1016/j.soard.2006.01.009.
12. Orandi BJ, Purvis JW, Cannon RM, Smith AB, Lewis CE, Terrault NA, Locke JE. Bariatric surgery to achieve transplant in end-stage organ disease patients: A systematic review and meta-analysis. Am J Surg. 2020;220(3):566–79. https://doi.org/10.1016/j.amjsurg.2020.04.041. Epub 2020 Jun 13. PMID: 32600846; PMCID: PMC7484004
13. Altieri MS, Carter J, Aminian A, Docimo S Jr, Hinojosa MW, Cheguevara A, Campos GM, Eisenberg D. Clinical Issues Committee of the American Society for Metabolic and Bariatric Surgery. American Society for Metabolic and Bariatric Surgery literature review on prevention, diagnosis, and management of internal hernias after Roux-en-Y gastric bypass. Surg Obes Relat Dis. 2023;19(7):763–71. https://doi.org/10.1016/j.soard.2023.03.019. Epub 2023 Apr 8
14. Stenberg E, Ottosson J, Magnuson A, et al. Long-term safety and efficacy of closure of mesenteric defects in laparoscopic gastric bypass surgery: a randomized clinical trial. JAMA Surg. 2023;158(7):709–17. https://doi.org/10.1001/jamasurg.2023.1042.
15. Carrodeguas L, Szomstein S, Zundel N, Lo Menzo E, Rosenthal R. Gastrojejunal anastomotic strictures following laparoscopic Roux-en-Y gastric bypass surgery: analysis of 1291 patients. Surg Obes Relat Dis. 2006;2:92–7.
16. Gonzalez R, Lin E, Venkatesh KR, Bowers SP, Smith CD. Gastrojejunostomy during laparoscopic gastric bypass: analysis of 3 techniques. Arch Surg. 2003;138:181–4.
17. Sarabu N. Weight and metabolic outcomes 12 years after gastric bypass. N Engl J Med. 2018;378(1):93–4.
18. Ghanem OM, Abi Mosleh K, Kerbage A, Lu L, Hage K, Abu Dayyeh BK. Continued diabetes remission despite weight recurrence: gastric bypass long-term metabolic benefit. J Am Coll Surg. 2024;238:862.
19. Hage K, Abi Mosleh K, Sample JW, Vierkant RA, Mundi MS, Spaniolas K, Abu Dayyeh BK, Ghanem OM. Preoperative duration of type 2 diabetes mellitus and remission after Roux-en-Y gastric bypass: A single center long-term cohort study. Int J Surg. 2024;110:6214.

18 DS/SADI

Paul Anthony Karam, Sarah Samreen, Andrew Lin, and Maher El Chaar

Introduction

Robotic-assisted (RA) surgery offers a unique set of advantages over traditional laparoscopic techniques, including enhanced precision, improved dexterity, and three-dimensional visualization [1]. Those advantages have resulted in an increased adoption rate in metabolic and bariatric surgery (MBS). In a recent manuscript by Bauerle et al., there was a nationwide increase in the utilization rate of RA approach in MBS between 2015 and 2020 according to the Metabolic and Bariatric Surgery Accreditation and Quality Improvement Project (MBSAQIP) data [2]. However, the use of the RA approach in MBS remains controversial for various reasons. To start, studies comparing the outcomes of RA-MBS to standard laparoscopic techniques based on MBSAQIP have shown conflicting results [3–6]. The conflicting results may be due to selection and exclusion criteria, matching processes, and differences in the definition of the outcome measures utilized in the studies [7]. In a recent study, we suggested the use of a standardized definition of outcome measures in comparing the RA approach to the standard laparoscopic approach using MBSAQIP data [8].

In addition, most studies have shown increased operation length and increased healthcare costs [3, 9].

In our center, however, we have shown that the application of the RA approach for the performance of MBS is not associated with increased healthcare costs compared to the standard laparoscopic approach [10, 11]. We have also shown that the standardization of the surgical approach can result in improved operating room efficiency as measured by operating room length, wheels in wheels out, and turnover time [12].

P. A. Karam · A. Lin · M. El Chaar (✉)
Bariatric Surgery Department, St Luke's University Health Network, Bethlehem, PA, USA

S. Samreen
Surgery, The University of Texas Medical Branch, Galveston, TX, USA

S. Samreen et al. (eds.), *The SAGES Manual of Robotic Surgery*,
https://doi.org/10.1007/978-3-031-86927-3_18

Therefore, standardization and experience can potentially improve operating room efficiency and lower healthcare costs irrespective of which surgical approach is utilized.

In terms of patient selection, currently, most health insurance payers follow the 1991 National Institutes of Health (NIH) guidelines for approval [13]. In 2022, the ASMBS/IFSO guidelines recommended MBS for individuals with a BMI>35, regardless of comorbidities, and patients with a BMI>30 with associated metabolic disease [14]. The choice of the appropriate MBS procedure depends on patient obesity-related health conditions, patient expectations, and preferences and surgeon expertise. The role of the surgeon is to provide all the information to help the patient make an informed decision [15].

Currently, the sleeve gastrectomy is the most performed MBS procedure followed by the Roux-en-Y gastric bypass (RYGB) [16]. Biliopancreatic diversion with duodenal switch (BPD-DS) and the single-anastomosis duodenoileal bypass with sleeve gastrectomy (SADI-S) are less commonly performed but are gaining popularity thanks to the RA approach. According to a recent study, up to 28% of BPD-DS are performed using an RA approach [2].

The first biliopancreatic diversion with duodenal switch (BPD-DS) that we know today was first performed in 1988 [17]. The advantage of BPD-DS over RYGB includes higher weight loss in patients with a BMI>50 and better diabetes remission rates [18]. However, given the complexity of this procedure and the increased adverse events compared to RYGB [19–21], BPD-DS is not commonly performed and constitutes less than 2% of the overall number of MBS cases performed in 2020 [16]. Variations in the lengths of the alimentary limb and common channel have been described, with observed increased vitamin absorption and decreased number of daily bowel movements in patients with a longer common channel [22, 23]. At our institution, we prefer a longer common channel (200 cm) over the standard 100 cm to avoid long-term nutritional deficiencies.

In 2007, a variant of the BPD-DS was introduced that involved creating a single anastomosis: the single-anastomosis duodenoileal bypass with sleeve gastrectomy (SADI-S) [24, 25]; by 2018, this procedure was established as a primary bariatric procedure.

SADI-S was shown to be associated with higher diabetes remission rates and similar weight loss results compared to RYGB [26]. Compared to BPD-DS, however, the results of SADI-S are suboptimal [27, 28]. Although SADI-S is technically less challenging than BPD-DS, it is associated with higher early postoperative complication rates compared to RYGB when performed as a primary procedure [29–31]. Interestingly, it has been shown to be as safe as RYGB when performed as a revisional procedure following sleeve gastrectomy [32].

At our institution, SADI-S is primarily offered as a revisional procedure to patients who have undergone previous sleeve gastrectomy and are suffering from weight recurrence, provided they do not have concomitant gastroesophageal reflux disease.

Patient Preparation

Patient preoperative workup includes nutritional and psychological assessment, complete history with physical examination, upper endoscopy with biopsies to evaluate for *H. pylori*, evaluation for obstructive sleep apnea, as well as cardiac evaluation. Revision patients may undergo upper gastrointestinal series, 24 h pH studies or wireless pH studies, and high-resolution manometry as indicated. Patients are also screened for any increased risk for VTE and/or PE.

We employ an enhanced recovery pathway for our MBS patients. Enhanced recovery pathways differ among institutions and involve preoperative, intraoperative, and postoperative protocols [33]:

Prior to surgery, patients are placed on a liquid high-protein diet for 2 weeks.

Although the benefits of preoperative carbohydrate loading remain unknown, we have our patients consume a carbohydrate drink the night before and the morning of surgery as part of our pathway.

On the day of surgery, patients are given a preoperative dose of intravenous fosaprepitant [34], intravenous acetaminophen, and oral celecoxib [35] with the aim of decreasing postoperative nausea and postoperative opiate use. Patients are also given DVT chemoprophylaxis and a single dose of intravenous antibiotics within 1 h of incision.

Surgical Technique

The initial setup applies to all our bariatric procedures. We place the patient in the supine position with the arms out and secured to arm boards with web rolls. This allows us to keep the arms from falling off when positioning the OR bed without risking too much constriction on the limbs. A footboard is also placed to avoid patient slippage.

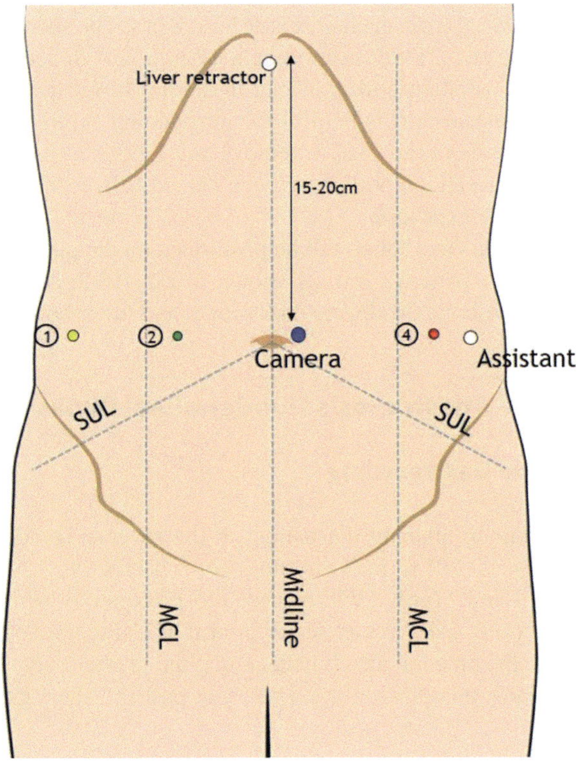

Fig. 18.1 Layout of robotic port placement

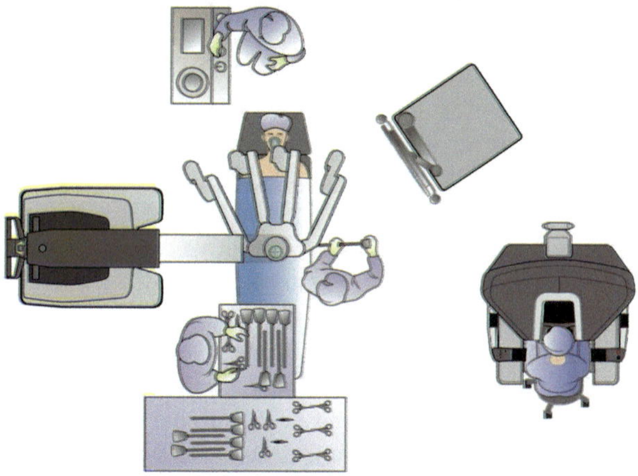

Fig. 18.2 Overhead view of operating room organization

Our usual port layout includes four robotic ports and one assistant port, as shown in Fig. 18.1. We start off by measuring approximately 15–20 cm caudally from the xiphoid and slightly to the left of midline for our first port, which will be our camera port. We then introduce a Veress needle through the incision to establish pneumoperitoneum. For the patients who have undergone prior abdominal surgeries, we introduce the Veress needle at Palmer's point.

Once a bilateral TAP block has been performed, we place our ports in a line perpendicular to the midline at the same level as our initial camera port, ensuring that the distance from each port is at least 8 cm. The second port from the patient's right (robotic arm 2) will need to be a 12 mm port to accommodate a robotic stapler. A 12 mm assistant port is placed in the left lower quadrant, lateral to robotic arm 4. The assistant port is helpful for introducing sutures and gauze into the abdominal cavity without the need to remove any robotic arms and can also assist with retraction. Once all the ports have been placed, a liver retractor is placed in the epigastric region for exposure.

The DaVinci robot will be positioned on the patient's right, and the assistant will be on the patient's left, as shown in Fig. 18.2. Automatic targeting is completed using a robotic 30-degree endoscope, and the robotic arms are docked.

Single Anastomosis Duodenolleal Bypass

Sleeve Gastrectomy

We start by placing the patient in the reverse Trendelenburg position at approximately 15–20° to perform our sleeve gastrectomy. A Cadiere forceps is placed in arms 1 and 2 (arm 2 will be used most frequently while arm 1 is used to assist with retraction) and a vessel sealer in arm 4. Using the vessel sealer, we start by taking down the omental attachments along the greater curve staying close to the stomach. We carry this dissection all the way past the short gastrics and to the left crus. In morbidly obese patients, freeing the fundus all the way to the angle of His can be quite challenging. It is important to have good retraction of the left lateral lobe of the liver, make good use of arm 1 for retraction of the stomach, and sometimes have the assistant retract the adipose tissue for better exposure. At this stage, if a hiatal hernia is identified, it is repaired.

Once the stomach is freed, we place a 36 Fr bougie down to the antrum ensuring that it is flush with the lesser curve of the stomach. The Cadiere forceps in arm 2 is substituted for a robotic stapler, and our sleeve gastrectomy is performed along the bougie. It is important to ensure that the incisura is not narrowed to avoid strictures. Different staple loads can be used depending on the tissue thickness and the surgeon's experience. We do not use buttressing material, though the staple line is imbricated with a running 2-0 Vicryl suture. It is important not to create a tight sleeve during stapling as oversewing can narrow the lumen further.

Bowel Measurement

Once the sleeve gastrectomy has been completed (refer to the robotic sleeve gastrectomy chapter), we place a Cadiere forceps in arms 2 and 4, leaving arm 1 empty, and the bed is flattened. The omentum and transverse colon are flipped cephalad to identify the terminal ileum. We then measure 250–300 cm of bowel distal to proximal, starting from the ileocecal valve. To improve precision, a ruler can be inserted into the abdomen and placed on the transverse colon while running the bowel. This will be the length of the common channel. We then tack this segment of bowel to the omentum at the level of the transverse colon with a 2-0 Vicryl suture.

Duodenal Dissection

We replace arm 4 with a vessel sealer and place the patient in the reverse Trendelenburg between 15° and 20°. We then carry out dissecting the greater omentum off the stomach distally beyond the sleeve staple line and approximately 2–3 cm past the pylorus. Dissection is kept in proximity to the gastric wall to avoid injuring the gastroepiploic vessels. This approach allows us to lift the stomach and dissect off the first portion of the duodenum under direct visualization in a retrogastric fashion. A window is then created in the gastrohepatic ligament close to the superior border of the duodenum. Dissection is carried out for 2–3 cm distal to the pylorus, care is taken to avoid injuring the gastroduodenal artery that can be visualized when lifting the duodenum. The perforating small branches supplying the duodenum posteriorly is our landmark to stop our dissection. We then place a robotic white-loaded stapler in arm 2 and fire across the first portion of the duodenum, ensuring that we are distal to the pylorus. This transection straightens out the stomach and allows for easier maneuverability for our duodenoileostomy. This maneuver also allows us to push the bougie further into the pylorus, which helps us create our anastomosis.

Duodenoileostomy

Our duodenoileostomy is performed entirely handsewn and in two layers. We place a SutureCut Needle Driver in arm 4 and Cadiere forceps in arms 1 and 2. We mainly use arm 2 to assist with suturing and arm 1 will help with retraction as needed. We start by creating a posterior layer with a running 2-0 absorbable V lock suture: suture bites will pass through the staple line on the duodenal side, and healthy seromuscular bites on the antimesenteric border of the ileum (Fig. 18.3). This layer runs the width of the duodenum. We then place monopolar scissors in arm 4 and make our duodenotomy approximately 1.5 cm over the bougie ensuring that the incision is approximately 0.5 cm away from our suture line. We then mirror those measurements for our enterotomy.

We switch out the scissors for a Suture cut in arm 4, and for our inner layer, we use two 2-0 Vicryl running sutures. We start by performing the inner layer with a 9-inch suture. We start from the corner on the patient's left, internalizing the knot by going in-to-out on the duodenum and out-to-in on the bowel (Fig. 18.4). We then complete the posterior inner layer in-to-out on the duodenum and out-to-in on the ileum while ensuring visualization of full-thickness bites of the duodenum and ileum (Fig. 18.5). We carry this running suture anteriorly and stop it midway with the suture on the duodenal side. We then run a 7-inch suture starting from the same corner externalizing the knot by going out-to-in on the duodenum and in-to-out on the bowel. We then complete the anterior inner layer out-to-in on the duodenum and in-to-out on the bowel, leaving the last few sutures loose. This allows passage of the bougie through the anastomosis with the purpose of avoiding any narrowing when tying out sutures. Once the bougie has been pushed through, we can sinch down on the loose sutures and tie our two running sutures together to close our inner layer (Fig. 18.6). It is important to ensure there are no air knots when anchoring the running sutures, as this can be a site for enteric leak. Keeping the bougie in place, we then complete our outer layer with a running 2-0 absorbable V lock in a horizontal mattress fashion. It is easy to take large bites while running a horizontal mattress. This can cause the anastomosis to narrow and should be avoided.

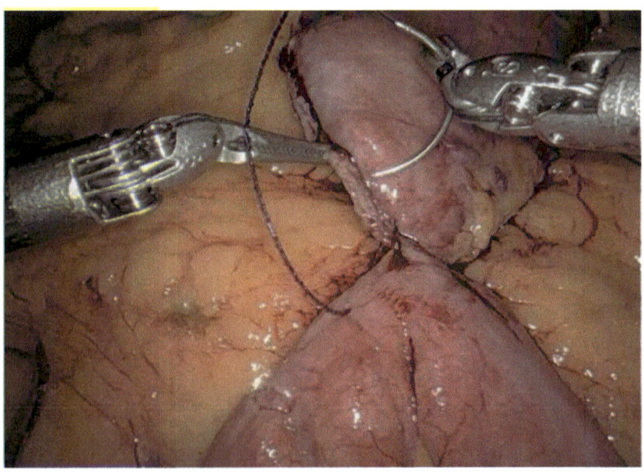

Fig. 18.3 Posterior outer layer of the duodenoileostomy

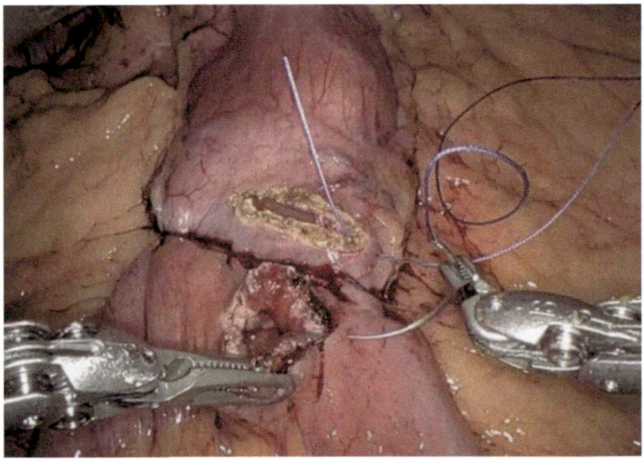

Fig. 18.4 Inner layer anchoring suture of the duodenoileostomy

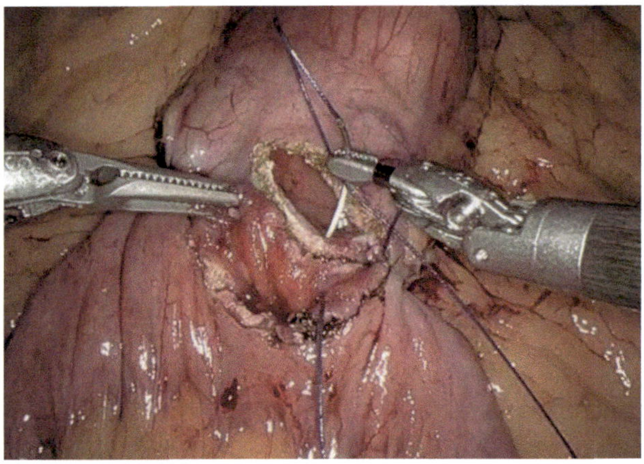

Fig. 18.5 Posterior inner layer of the duodenoileostomy

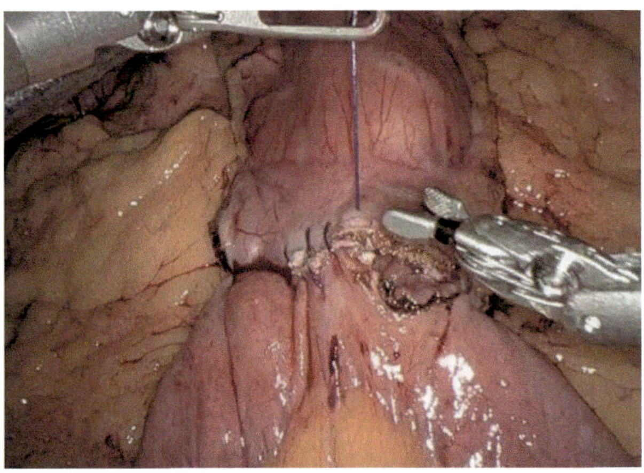

Fig. 18.6 Completing the inner layer of the duodenoileostomy

Leak Test and Closure

Once the anastomosis is completed, an intraoperative upper endoscopy is performed, as is a leak test. This is done by obstructing the afferent and efferent limbs for proper insufflation and irrigating the anastomosis to look for an air leak. Any area of leak should be closed with a 2-0 Vicryl suture.

Once the robot is undocked, our 12 mm port site is used to extract the specimen, which is subsequently closed using a 0-Vicryl on a suture passer. This port site can be dilated if extraction proves difficult. The skin is then closed with 4-0 Monocryl.

Biliopancreatic Diversion and Duodenal Switch

Bowel Measurement

Using the same robotic layout for the SADI, we start off with a sleeve gastrectomy (refer to the *sleeve gastrectomy* portion of the chapter). Then, we run the bowel distal to proximal from the ileocecal valve. We measure 200 cm, which will be the length of the common channel, and mark it with a 2-0 Vicryl suture. This can also be marked with a clip applier on the mesentery, which allows for marking the mesentery in the correct orientation in addition to the bowel itself. Different colored sutures may also be useful in this instance. From there, we measure an additional 100 cm, which will be the length of our alimentary limb. This is marked with a 2-0 Vicryl suture and tied to the omentum at the level of the transverse colon.

Enteroenterostomy

Once our duodenoileostomy is completed (refer to the *duodenal dissection and duodenoileostomy* portion of the chapter), we create a window in the mesentery of the afferent limb. It is important not to involve too much of the mesentery to avoid devascularizing the alimentary or biliopancreatic limb. The mesenteric division can be extended if additional mobilization is needed. The premarked 200 cm loop of bowel is then brought up to the biliopancreatic limb, and the assistant uses a grasper to hold the two loops in place to line them up for an isoperistaltic anastomosis. Using a Cadiere forceps in arm 4 and monopolar scissors in arm 2, we perform an enterotomy in the common channel and the biliopancreatic limb on the antimesenteric border. It is important to perform an enterotomy at least 0.5 cm from the staple line of the BP limb. This approach will provide room for closure of the common enterotomy. We then use a white staple load in arm 2, placing the larger limb of the stapler in the BP limb, to create our anastomosis. During this step, the assistant is helpful in positioning the bowel for easy positioning of the stapler.

We then place a SutureCut in arm 4 and use the Cadiere forceps in arm 1 to close the common enterotomy. This layer is closed in two layers using two running 2-0 Vicryl sutures.

We then use a nonabsorbable 2-0 V lock to close enteroenterostomy mesenteric defect. We also close the pseudo-Peterson's defect in a similar fashion. It is important not to take deep bites on the mesentery to avoid inadvertently injuring a blood vessel, which can lead to hematomas. We start at the root of the mesentery and run it up, stopping just shy of the bowel wall.

We then perform an intraoperative upper endoscopy with a leak test, undock the robot, remove the specimen, and close.

Postoperative Care

Postoperative care is standardized for all bariatric patients. Heart rates and oxygen saturation are monitored in all postoperative patients. Patients who have obstructive sleep apnea are instructed to bring their CPAP machines with them.

Unless they have issues ambulating, all patients are instructed to walk within a few hours following surgery and instructed to walk regularly.

Patients are started on a clear liquid diet 6 h after surgery, starting with 30 cc (medicine cups) of water every 15 min, and document their progress.

They are placed on DVT chemoprophylaxis postoperatively and have sequential compression devices placed when not ambulating. Patients are not routinely placed on extended VTE chemoprophylaxis at discharge, although some factors may lead to its prescription, such as a prior history of VTE/PE and/or minimally ambulating patients [36].

Antiglycemics, antihypertensive agents, and diuretics are held postoperatively, and patients are instructed to follow up with their PCPs at discharge to evaluate whether these medications need to be resumed. If patients are on multiple medications, an inpatient consultation to internal medicine can be helpful in calibrating what needs to be resumed or held in the immediate postoperative period.

On postoperative day 1, we obtain a morning complete blood count (CBC) and basic metabolic panel (BMP), and patients are started on a full liquid diet. We do not routinely order an upper GI following these procedures.

If patients are clinically stable, laboratory values are within normal limits and are tolerating a liquid diet, they are discharged on postoperative day 1.

It is important to closely follow patients in the outpatient setting to monitor their progress and obtain routine nutritional lab work. Given the nature of the surgery, patients are at risk for vitamin deficiencies that need to be repleted.

References

1. Moorthy K, Munz Y, Dosis A, et al. Dexterity enhancement with robotic surgery. Surg Endosc. 2004;18(5):790–5.
2. Bauerle WB, Mody P, Estep A, et al. Current trends in the utilization of a robotic approach in the field of bariatric surgery. Obes Surg. 2023;33(2):482–91.

3. Acevedo E, Mazzei M, Zhao H, et al. Outcomes in conventional laparoscopic versus robotic-assisted primary bariatric surgery: a retrospective, case-controlled study of the MBSAQIP database. Surg Endosc. 2020;34(3):1353–65.
4. Clapp B, Liggett E, Jones R, et al. Comparison of robotic revisional weight loss surgery and laparoscopic reviosnal weight loss surgery using the MBSAQIP database. Surg Obes Relat Dis. 2019;15(6):909–19.
5. Lundberg PW, Stoltzfus J, Chaar ME. 30-day outcomes of robot-assisted versus conventional laparoscopic sleeve gastrectomy: first analysis based on MBSAQIP. Surg Obes Relat Dis. 2019;15(1):1–7.
6. Nasser H, Munie S, Kindel TL, et al. Comparative analysis of robotic versus laparoscopic revisional bariatric surgery: perioperative outcomes from the MBSAQIP database. Surg Obes Relat Dis. 2020;16(3):397–405.
7. Petrick AT, Rosenthal R, Wood C. Understanding the causes of conflicting outcomes reported using the same cohorts from the MBSAQIP PUF data registry. Surg Obes Relat Dis. 2021;17(9):e42–5.
8. Chaar ME, Petrick A, Clapp B, et al. Outcomes of robotic-assisted bariatric surgery compared to standard laparoscopic approach using a standardized defintion: first look at the 2020 Metabolic and Bariatric Surgery Accreditation Quality Improvement Project (MBSAQIP) data. Obes Surg. 2023;33(7):2025–39.
9. Dudash M, Kuhn J, Dove J, et al. The longitudinal efficiency of robotic surgery: an MBSAQIP propensity matched 4-year Comparision of robotic and laparoscopic bariatric surgery. Obes Surg. 2020;30(10):3706–13.
10. Chaar ME, Gacke J, Ringold S, et al. Cost analysis of robotic sleeve gastrectomy (R-SG) compared with laparoscopic sleeve gastrectomy (L-SG) in a single academic center: debunking a myth! Surg Obes Relat Dis. 2019;15(5):675–9.
11. King K, Galvez A, Stoltzfus J, et al. Cost analysis of robotic roux-en-Y gastric bypass in a single academic center: how expensive is expensive? Obes Surg. 2020;30(12):4860–6.
12. Chaar ME, Michaud A, Stoltzfus J, et al. Improving operating room efficiency of robotic-assisted metabolic and bariatric surgery through standardization. Obes Surg. 2023;33(11):3411–21.
13. NIH conference. Gastrointestinal surgery for severe obesity. Consensus development conference panel. Consens Statement. 1991;9(1):1–20.
14. Eisenberg D, Shikora S, Aarts E, et al. 2022 American Society for Metabolic and Bariatric Surgery (ASMBS) and International Federation for the Surgery of Obesity and Metabolic Disorders (IFSO): indications for metabolic and bariatric surgery. Surg Obes Relat Dis. 2022;18(12):1345–56.
15. Lee YC, Wu WL. Shared decision making and choice for bariatric surgery. Int J Environ Res Public Health. 2019;16(24):4966.
16. Clapp B, Ponce J, DeMaria E, et al. American Society for Metabolic and Bariatric Surgery 2020 estimate of metabolic and bariatric procedures performed in the United States. Surg Obes Relat Dis. 2022;18(9):1134–40.
17. Hess DS, Hess DW. Biliopancreatic diversion with a duodenal switch. Obes Surg. 1998;8(3):267–82.
18. Sovik TT, Taha O, Aasheim ET, Engstrom M, Kristinsson J, Bjorkman S, et al. Randomized clinical trial of laparoscopic gastric bypass versus laparoscopic duodenal switch for superobesity. Br J Surg. 2010;97(2):160–6.
19. Sudan R, Maciejewski ML, Wilk AR, Nguyen NT, Ponce J, Morton JM. Comparative effectiveness of primary bariatric operations in the United States. Surg Obes Relat Dis. 2017;13(5):826–34.
20. Risstad H, Sovik T, Engstrom M, et al. Five-year outcomes after laparoscopic gastric bypass and laparoscopic duodenal switch in patients with body mass index of 50 to 60 a randomized clinical trial. JAMA Surg. 2015;150(4):352–61.
21. Moller F, Hedberg J, Skogar M, et al. Long-term follow-up 15 years after duodenal Swithc or gastric bypass for super obesity: a randomized controlled trial. Obes Sur. 2023;33(10):2981–90.

22. Lebel S, Dion G, Marceau S, et al. Clinical outcomes of duodenal switch with a 200-cm common channel: a matched, controlled trial. Surg Obes Relat Dis. 2016;12(5):1014–20.
23. Malo FC, Marion A, Rioux A, et al. Long alimentary limb duodenal switch (LADS): an exploratory randomized trial, results at 2 years. Obes Surg. 2020;30(12):5047–58.
24. Sanchez-Pernaute A, Rubio Herrera MA, Perez-Aguirre E, et al. Proximal duodenal-ileal end-to-side bypass with sleeve gastrectomy: proposed technique. Obes Surg. 2007;17(12):1614–8.
25. Mitzman B, Cottam D, Goriparthi R, et al. Stomach intestinal pylorus sparing (SIPS) surgery for morbid obesity: retrospective analyses of our preliminary experience. Obes Surg. 2016;26(9):2098–104.
26. Cottam A, Cottam D, Zaveri H, et al. An analysis of mid-term complications, weight loss, and type 2 diabetes resolution of stomach intestinal pylorus-sparing surgery (SIPS) versus Roux-En-Y Gastric Bypass (RYGB) with three-year follow-up. Obes Surg. 2018;28:2894–902.
27. Gebelli JP, Lazzara C, de Gordejuela AGR, et al. Duodenal switch vs single-anastomosis duodenal switch (SADI-S) for the treatment of grade IV obesity: 5-year outcomes of a multicenter prospective cohort comparative study. Obes Surg. 2022;32(12):3839–46.
28. Yashkov Y, Bordan N, Torres A, et al. SADI-S 250 vs roux-en-Y duodenal switch (RY-DS): results of 5-year observational study. Obes Surg. 2021;31(2):570–9.
29. Verhoeff K, Mocanu V, Jogiat U, et al. Patient selection and 30-day outcomes of SADI-S compared to RYGB: a retrospective cohort study of 47,375 patients. Obes Surg. 2022;32(7):1–8.
30. Balamurugan G, Sagaya JL, Subbiah TS, et al. Comparison of efficacy and safety between roux-en-Y gastric bypass (RYGB) vs one anastomosis gastric bypass (OAGB) vs single anastomosis Dudeno-ileal bypass with sleeve gastrectomy (SADI-S): a systematic review of bariatric and metabolic surgery. Obes Surg. 2023;33(7):2194–209.
31. Chao GF, Canner J, Hamid S, et al. Outcomes of SADI and OAGB compared to RYGB from the metabolic and bariatric surgery quality improvement program: the North American Experience. Obes Surg. 2024;34:337. https://doi.org/10.1007/S11695-023-07019.
32. Ceha CMM, van Wezenbeek MR, Versteegden DPA, et al. Matched short-term results of SADI versus GBP after sleeve gastrectomy. Obes Surg. 2018;28(12):3809–14.
33. Stenberg E, Dos Reis Falcao LF, O'Kane M, et al. Guidelines for perioperative care in bariatric surgery: Enhanced Recovery After Surgery (ERAS) society recommendations: a 2021 update. World J Surg. 2022;46(4):729–51.
34. Aghazarian G, Lind R, Motola D, et al. Impact of emend on perioperative bariatric surgery antiemetic utilization, patient satisfaction, and costs. Surg Laparosc Endosc Percutan Tech. 2023;33(3):265–9.
35. Monte S, Rafi E, Cantie S, et al. Reduction in opiate use, pain, nausea, and length of stay after implementation of a bariatric enhanced recovery after surgery protocol. Obes Surg. 2021;31(7):2896–905.
36. American Society for M, Bariatric Surgery Clinical Issues C. ASMBS updated position statement on prophylactic measures to reduce the risk of venous thromboembolism in bariatric surgery patients. Surg Obes Relat Dis. 2013;9(4):493–7.

19 Revisional Foregut and Bariatric Surgery

Michelle Nessen and Carlos A. Galvani

Introduction

Since their introduction in the early- to mid-1990s, laparoscopic antireflux surgery and laparoscopic bariatric surgery gained collective interest and quickly became the gold standard for the treatment of GERD and severe obesity [1, 2]. The widespread adoption of laparoscopy was due mainly to its well-known advantages compared to open surgery. Curiously, these two surgical modalities share few similarities and differences. For example, despite remarkably low morbidity and mortality rates, the operations are underused due to the perception of long-term side effects and fear of failure, which impacts referral patterns. Unfortunately, the definition of surgical success varies substantially for both modalities. Although antireflux and bariatric surgery have consistently shown to be effective with very high success rates, revisional surgery is necessary in up to 3–6% of patients after antireflux surgery and up to 16.7% of patients after bariatric surgery [1, 3, 4].

Revisional procedures include a broad spectrum of surgeries that are meant to benefit patients who have either recurrent or persistent disease or patients who have complications of the index procedure. It is widely recognized that the results of revisional operations for persistent or recurrent disease are sometimes less satisfactory than the results obtained following the primary procedure. This is especially true after multiple surgical attempts. However, when the indication is appropriate and addressed by appropriate surgical technique, many patients can benefit from a

M. Nessen
Clinical Instructor of Surgery, Department of Minimally Invasive and Bariatric Surgery, Tulane University, New Orleans, LA, USA
e-mail: mnessen@tulane.edu

C. A. Galvani (✉)
Department of Minimally Invasive and Bariatric Surgery, Louisiana State University, Baton Rouge, LA, USA
e-mail: cgalva@lsuhsc.edu

S. Samreen et al. (eds.), *The SAGES Manual of Robotic Surgery*,
https://doi.org/10.1007/978-3-031-86927-3_19

reoperation. Logically, revisional procedures are associated with increased operative times and morbidity. Several reports in the literature have underscored the feasibility and safety of laparoscopic revisional procedures [5, 6]. Furthermore, the Society of American Gastrointestinal and Endoscopic Surgeons (SAGES) has published independent guidelines addressing revisional antireflux and bariatric surgery [7–9]. When considered together, these guidelines have significant similarities and they offer a word of caution to surgeons considering embarking on these complex procedures; "Laparoscopic revisional procedures may be performed safely only by experienced surgeons, but with more complications than primary procedures; therefore, the relative risks and benefits of laparoscopy should be considered on a case-by-case basis."

Robotic surgery has been proposed as an alternative to surmount some of the technical challenges associated with revisional procedures [10]. Even though the application of robotics in revisional foregut and bariatric surgery is emerging, it is not yet widespread. Some series have demonstrated its feasibility and safety, although recent advances in robotic technology can potentially improve upon those outcomes and demonstrate clear advantages favoring the routine use of robotics. Herein, we describe our evaluation and treatment of patients requiring reoperative foregut and bariatric surgery and the potential benefits of robotic surgery.

Part I: Revisional Foregut Surgery

Introduction

Even though antireflux surgery is very effective and surgery failure is uncommon, it is estimated that 10–20% of patients will experience symptoms recurrence after antireflux surgery` [11].

The evaluation and management of patients with recurrent, persistent, or new symptoms after antireflux surgery, the identification of the cause of failure, and the selection of patients who need revisional surgery remains a challenge [12]. Nonetheless, it is clear that patients who present with symptoms after antireflux surgery must be systematically evaluated to identify the cause of failure, and treatment must be tailored to the patient.

Numerous reports have suggested that only surgeons with substantial experience in foregut and minimally invasive surgery should attempt laparoscopic revisional antireflux surgery [13]. The nature of revisional surgery poses a distinctive challenge for the surgeon due to its morbid anatomy (adhesions, distorted anatomy, etc.) and the many procedural steps described to obtain optimal results. In addition, patient factors such as age >70, obesity, comorbidities, and previous surgeries play a significant role in the incidence of postoperative complications and must be considered preoperatively. It is also recognized that revisions take longer, have longer hospital stays, and more complications compared to primary antireflux surgery [14].

The introduction of robotic technology in primary foregut surgery has not demonstrated significant clinical advantages [15]. Although not widely reported in the literature, the application of robotics in revisional surgery has shown decreased conversion rates, shorter hospital stay, and minimal morbidity compared to laparoscopy [16, 17]. The technology available to the robotic surgeon offers increased autonomy due to the self-assisting feature and self-driving of the robotic camera. Other advantages of the robotic platform are mainly attributed to the improved visualization, exposure, and enhanced dissection.

Indications for Revision

Indications for reoperation should be based primarily on the patient's physiological state, the severity of symptoms, and the response to conservative therapy. Patients should undergo an extensive workup, including barium swallow, esophageal manometry, upper endoscopy, pH study, and gastric emptying study if necessary [11]. A strong correlation between the symptoms, preoperative workup and the patterns of failure could potentially help select the most appropriate treatment for the patient [12, 17].

- Surgical intervention should be considered in patients who have persistent, recurrent, or new foregut symptoms (heartburn, dysphagia, chest pain, regurgitation, asthma, hoarseness, chronic cough, or laryngitis).

And

- Confirmed physiologic abnormalities (objective evidence of failure).

Or

- Definable anatomic defect.

Options for Revision

The choice of reoperative procedure must be personalized to the patient, taking into account several factors: patterns of failure, the presence of a recurrent hiatal hernia, esophageal length, Barrett's esophagus, number of previous antireflux procedures, presence of obesity, and the viability of the gastric fundus after fundoplication takedown.

In many instances, the final decision is made intraoperatively based on the patient's anatomy. As mentioned, the surgical plan should be tailored to each patient's specific needs and may include palliative options (gastropexy and/or gastrostomy tube placement), and/or takedown of the fundoplication.

Options include.

- Redo-fundoplication (partial or total) with or without hiatal hernia repair if present
  - First time redo, normal BMI, normal esophageal motility

  - With/wo pyloroplasty (if confirmed gastroparesis)
- Conversion to RYGB anatomy
  - Obesity and/or severe obesity in patients willing to undergo the surgery. Non-obese patients with more than 2 prior failed fundoplications
  - A large hiatal hernia
  - Gastroparesis
  - Esophageal dysmotility or dilation
  - Fundus not suitable for fundoplication
  - Nonobese patients with a clear anatomic reason for failure (i.e., wrap disruption, slipped fundoplication)
- Collis gastroplasty (patients with foreshortened esophagus after extensive mediastinal dissection)

Operative Principles: Robotic Revisional Foregut Surgery

The general principles of revisional procedures are similar regardless of the antireflux procedure of choice:

- Access
- Adhesiolysis
  - Between the left lobe of the liver and stomach, between the liver and the fundoplication, around the hiatus and the GE junction, and finally mobilization of the fundoplication.
- Crural dissection (taking down the crural repair or not)
- Circumferential dissection of the esophagus in the mediastinum
- Take down the prior fundoplication
- Perform crural closure (mesh vs no mesh)
- Choice of antireflux procedure

Presurgical Care: Optimization/Prehabilitation

The preoperative physical status of the patient, the risk of surgery and anesthesia are important for preoperative risk mitigation [18]. Consideration of comorbid conditions is equally important as the diagnosis is frequently made in older debilitated patients and preoperative evaluation is essential for assessing the operative risk in the individual patient. Special emphasis should be placed on smoking cessation and alcohol, adjusting antihypertensive and antidiabetic treatment, incentive spirometry for improving breathing capacity, treating anemias, and improving exercise tolerance [19]. Another modifiable risk factor that could increase the risk for postoperative complications is the patient's nutritional status. It is well known that many patients suffer from severe dysphagia, nausea, and vomiting from secondary gastroparesis before reoperative antireflux surgery. Depending on the urgency of the procedure as well as the procedure selection, the surgical team should decide whether to defer the surgery to minimize postoperative risk.

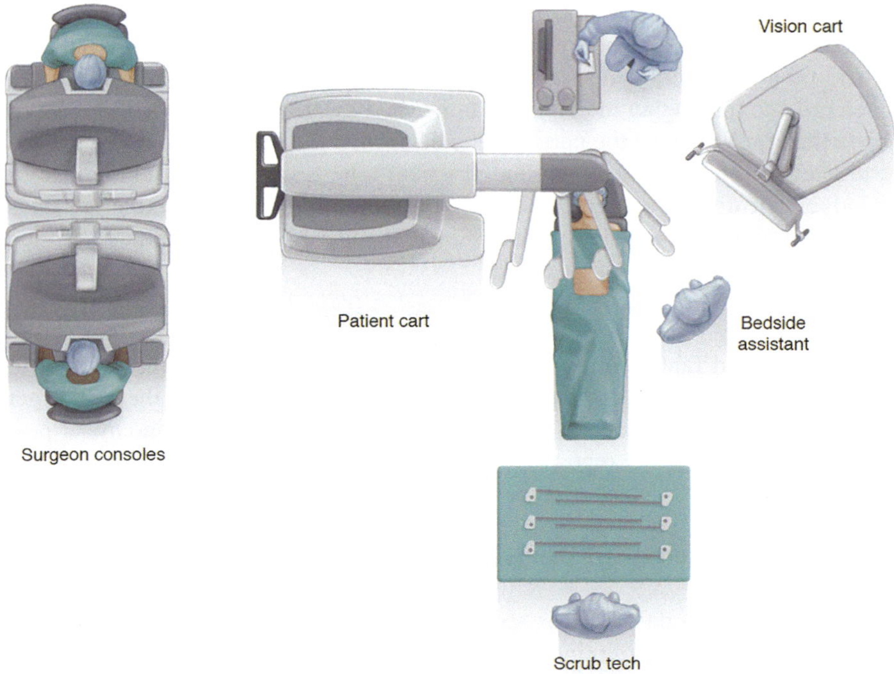

Fig. 19.1 Operating room layout. Typical setup for bariatric and foregut robotic cases. The vision cart is typically opposite to the patient cart and scrub tech with instruments at the foot of the bed

Operating Room Setup

A large operating room is preferable when performing robotic surgery. Larger operating rooms allow the robot components to be stored in the room and allow the operating room personnel to more freely around the room. The room should also facilitate docking of the system depending on the type of surgery to be performed. Preferably, the room will be a dedicated room with an integration system to allow for flat panel monitors mounted from the ceiling, $CO2$ gas is piped directly into the room for insufflation, and ceiling-mounted equipment booms can house insufflators, electrosurgical units, laparoscopic camera equipment, and lights sources. The operating table is placed directly under the room lights. Anesthesia equipment is located at the head of the operating table. The advent of the new da Vinci Xi offers some advantages with respect to the da Vinci Si providing streamlined setup and port placement.

- An overview of the operating room layout is shown in Fig. 19.1.

Patient Positioning

The patient is placed in a supine position with the arms kept open and properly padded. The patient is then secured to the bed around the legs using a safety strap. Pneumatic compression devices are placed on the lower legs prior to induction of anesthesia. Following successful endotracheal intubation, an orogastric tube is placed to decompress the stomach. Preoperative antibiotics are given prior to making an incision. An upper body warming device is then placed above the nipples. Once the patient is positioned, a face protection donut is used to protect the patient's face and endotracheal tube from inadvertent damage or dislodgement during movement of the robotic endoscope. Once this is established, the abdomen and lower chest are prepped widely with iodine and then sterile drapes.

Troubleshooting

- The Integrated Table Motion feature of the da Vinci Xi allows for the OR table to pair with the system. The surgeon can reposition the table during the case to get optimal exposure and access to the target anatomy, increase autonomy, or provide immediate patient repositioning.

Access/Port Placement/Liver Retraction

The port placement described is specific to the da Vinci Xi System. Entry into the abdominal cavity is obtained using an optical technique in the periumbilical area, just to the left of the midline, using an 8 mm robotic optical trocar. However, if history of open surgery, the entry to the abdominal cavity will migrate to the left upper quadrant, right upper quadrant, and sometimes periumbilical using a Hassan technique (upper midline incision, hernia repair, etc.). If optical technique is used, a 5 mm 0/30 degree laparoscope is used for access and port placement. The first port is placed in the left mid-abdomen two fingerbreadths lateral to the umbilicus and one palm-width inferior to the left costal margin. This port is used for the robotic camera (arm #2). Insufflation is started to 15 mmHg. Three 8-mm trocars are then placed at the same level of the camera port: 8-mm port on the right midclavicular line (arm #1), one on the left midclavicular line (arm #3), and one in the left anterior axillary line (arm #4). A 5-mm subxiphoid incision is used for the placement of the Nathanson liver retractor. Finally, an assistant port (8 mm) is inserted in between arms #2 and #3 (Fig. 19.2). At this point, the robotic surgical cart is approximated into position and the arms are attached to the four specific trocars. The da Vinci Xi Surgical System can be docked from the patient's right or left side.

Troubleshooting

- If the liver retractor cannot be placed at the beginning of the case due to adhesions, we still dock the robot to expedite the adhesiolysis. Once this is completed, the left lobe of the liver can be retracted using an internal liver retractor such as a liver sling (Fig. 19.3). This could be done with barbed sutures between the diaphragm and the abdominal wall.

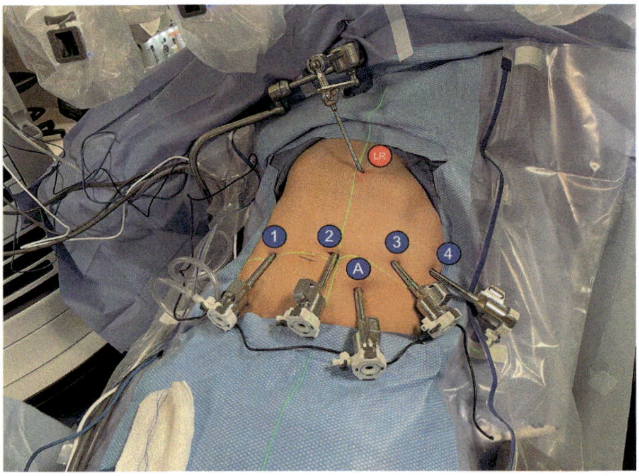

Fig. 19.2 Port placement. 1. 12 mm right midclavicular line. 2. 8 mm (camera port) left and cephalad to umbilicus. 3. 8 mm left midclavicular. 4. 8 mm left anterior axillary line. A. Assist port inferior and between 2 and 3 (or 1 and 2). LR. Liver retractor subxiphoid

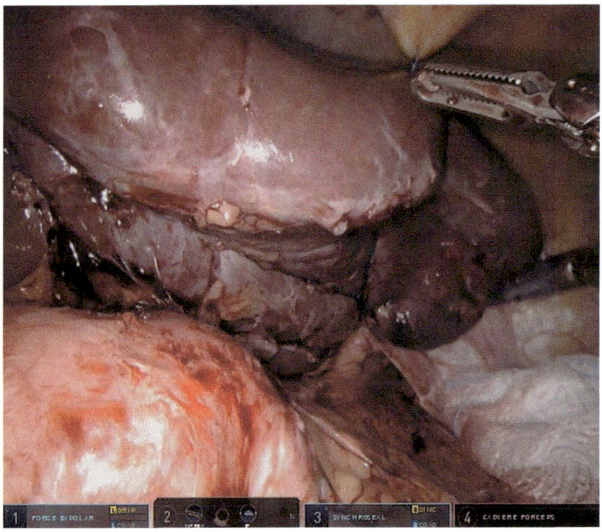

Fig. 19.3 Liver retraction using barbed suture

Adhesiolysis, Crural Dissection, and Circumferential Dissection of the Esophagus

Depending on whether the previous procedure was done open or laparoscopic, the adhesions could form around the midline incision, and most frequently between the liver and the stomach. The main goal is to clear the anterior stomach/fundoplication/GE junction if possible.

Early docking of the robot is key to facilitate exposure and visualization while taking down adhesions. Adhesions are usually taken down with a combination of blunt maneuvers and robotic scissors. The advantages of the articulated monopolar scissors in this stage are related to extended reach and precision taking down adhesions in tight spaces to separate the liver from the diaphragm, from the stomach and many times to separate the right crura/stomach from the inferior vena cava (IVC) or the stomach from the splenic area. The next step is the release of the fundoplication from hiatal structures. If the fundoplication is observed herniated through a tight opening at the hiatus, taking down the previous crural repair is advised to prevent gastric injuries. Dense adhesions are usually found between the posterior fundoplication and the previous crural repair. This could also be complicated by the presence of a previously implanted mesh or more nonabsorbable frequently pledgets. Once both crura are cleared, and a posterior esophageal window is observed, a Penrose drain is placed around the lower esophagus and circumferential dissection of the esophagus is started. The lower esophagus is then retracted by arm #4. This is a key step of this lengthy procedure. Depending on the previous surgery (e.g., paraesophageal hernia repair), extensive lysis of adhesions and mediastinal dissection will be required.

Careful separation of the mediastinal pleura, aorta, and pericardium from the esophagus can be challenging. The extensive use of scissors in this situation can potentially increase bleeding of the operative field. Transhiatal dissection of the esophagus is continued in a cephalad direction. The goal of the dissection is to get to a virgin area within the mediastinum likely proximal to the previous surgery. The articulated vessel sealer/synchroseal device and the force bipolar are used during this step and are key in this tight space (Fig. 19.4). Mobilization of the esophagus can typically be accomplished using blunt dissection of relatively thin alveolar tissue by exercising traction and countertraction maneuvers always dissecting away from the esophagus. The progression of the dissection is as follows: right side of the esophagus, posterior, left side of the esophagus and anterior.

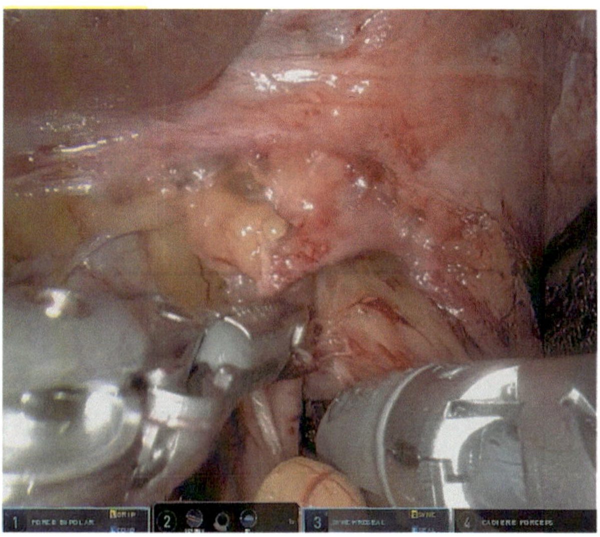

Fig. 19.4 Anterior mediastinal dissection. Sweeping blunt movements with Arms #1 and #3 used to dissected mediastinum

Troubleshooting

- The "scope flip" feature of the Xi system allows to perform a better esophageal mobilization due to the direct visualization of the mediastinal structures.
- The mediastinal dissection is facilitated by self-driving of the scope and the extensive use of the fourth arm.
- Pleural injury or tear is not an uncommon complication due to the previous dissection. Although intraoperative capnothorax may develop after the opening of the mediastinal pleura, its consequences for the patient are negligible since CO_2 is quickly reabsorbed and the lung is rarely involved. It is extremely important for the operating surgeon to communicate with the anesthesiologist if pleural injury ensues. Adequate monitoring of end-tidal carbon dioxide levels (EtCO2) and airway pressures will facilitate early diagnosis. Positive end-expiratory pressure (PEEP) application is an effective way of managing pneumothorax secondary to the passage of gas into the pleural space. In our experience, decreasing the intra-abdominal pressure (10 mmHg) has helped stop CO_2 diffusion into the pleural cavity. We prefer not sealing pleural injury to prevent tension pneumothorax.

Fundoplication Takedown

This step of the procedure entails taking down the prior wrap and bringing the fundus of the stomach to its original position in the left upper quadrant. This is primarily done with robotic scissors. Identifying the previously the gastro-gastro or gastroesophageal stitches in the anterior esophagus facilitates this step. We prefer to start with the right side of the fundoplication and carefully dissecting the right half of the wrap off the lower esophagus. (Fig. 19.5) After this is accomplished, the dissection continues outer side of the wrap. Then the dissection moves to the left side by dissecting of the wrap from the left side of the esophagus. Any remaining hernia

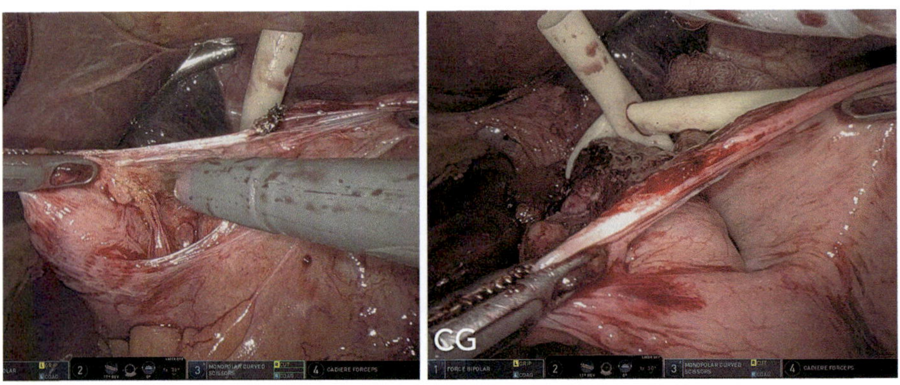

Fig. 19.5 Takedown of fundoplication. Both right and left side portion of the prior fundoplication must be freed

sac should be removed. Upper endoscopy usually confirms that the fundoplication was completely undone. Endoscopy will also confirm the indemnity of the esophagus before the crural repair. The surgeon should also confirm the viability of the fundus of the stomach if a redo-fundoplication is planned.

Crural Repair

The esophagus is retracted anteriorly and to the left by arm #4, and the vessel sealer is replaced with a suture cut needle driver. Closure of the diaphragmatic defect is started at the junction of the right and left crus to decrease tension on every stitch and is carried out anteriorly. The closure is performed using running nonabsorbable barbed suture (2-0). We routinely place multiple running loose bites tightened sequentially ("pulley system") advancing toward the esophagus (Fig. 19.6).

A 54-56Fr taper tip bougie is passed down the esophagus to tailor the closure and avoid postoperative dysphagia. However, the bougie is not left in place during the closure since it will compromise exposure and could also result on injury to the esophagus.

Troubleshooting

- It is paramount for the surgeon to monitor the advancement of the bougie by the anesthesia team to prevent esophageal perforations.
- If excessive tension is observed during the crural repair, additional tactics should be used to decrease radial forces, such as decreasing the pneumoperitoneum pressure to 8–10 mmHg and loosening the liver retraction. Even though less frequent relaxing incisions are a suitable alternative.

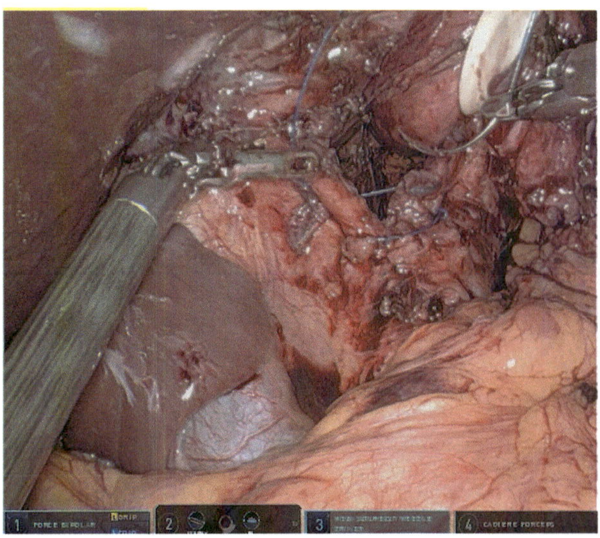

Fig. 19.6 Posterior crural repair with barbed suture. The "pulley system" used to sequentially tighten posterior crura to reduce tension

- If undue tearing of the right crus is observed, consideration to a relaxing incision of the should be given. In this case, the goal is to first perform a right relaxing incision, and if this approach were not sufficient to guarantee a tensionless repair, a left relaxing incision should be performed.

Mesh Reinforcement

The crural defect must be closed prior to mesh placement. Bridging of the diaphragmatic defect is not recommended. A ruler is introduced in order to tailor the mesh to the patient. Furthermore, a "U-shaped" or "reverse C"-shaped bioabsorbable mesh is cut to size to reinforce the closure of the diaphragmatic defect (Fig. 19.7). Our preference is a "reverse C" mesh for both posterior and anterior coverage. The mesh is placed onlay and secured in place to the edge of the right and left crura and at the bottom of the repair with nonabsorbable interrupted stitches. It is our practice to place the hiatal fixation stitches at 1, 4, 8, and 11 o'clock around the circumference of the hiatus. Mesh reinforcement is considered useful to prevent early recurrences (6–12 months).

The ideal mesh characteristics are

- Slow absorbable
- Low profile, easy to use (introduce, position, fixate)
- Decrease risk for erosion
- Does not preclude reoperation

It is our practice to routinely use mesh in the following situations:

- Large hiatal hernias (>5 cm)
- Closure under tension
  – Observed tearing of the R crus

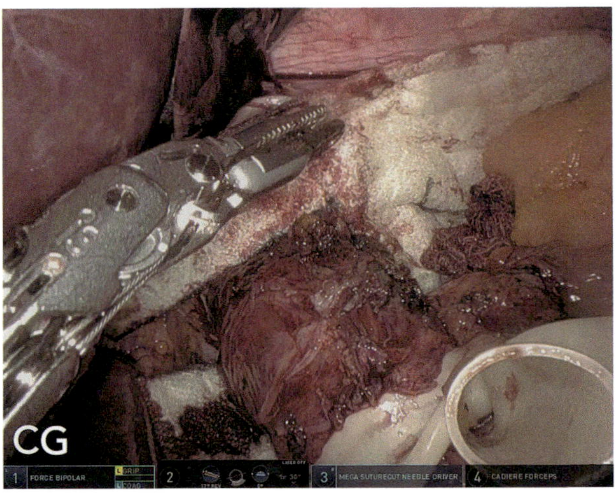

Fig. 19.7 Mesh placement. Mesh configured in "reverse C" orientation to ensure anterior and posterior coverage

- Redo operations
- Relaxing incisions
- Patients with obesity with large hiatal hernias

Antireflux Procedure

- *Redo-Fundoplication*

When a redo-fundoplication is indicated, our preferred procedure is a Toupet fundoplication gauged over a bougie. A "shoeshine" maneuver is performed to make sure the right and left sides of the fundoplication are symmetric (Fig. 19.8). The right and left graspers then bring toward the anterior esophagus. The bougie is inserted after the stomach is passed behind the esophagus. At this time, arm # 4 holds the right side of the wrap in place while swapping to arm #1 for placement of the first stitch of the fundoplication. A total of three 2-0 silk stitches are used to fix the wrap to the right side of the esophagus; the most proximal stitch was used to secure the wrap to the esophagus and the right crura. This followed by three 2-0 silk stitches between the wrap and the left side of the esophagus; the most proximal stitch is used to secure the wrap to the esophagus and the left crura (Fig. 19.9). At the completion of the procedure, the bougie is carefully removed.

Upper endoscopy is routinely performed at the completion of the case to check the indemnity of the esophagus, stomach, and the adequacy and patency of the fundoplication (Fig. 19.10).

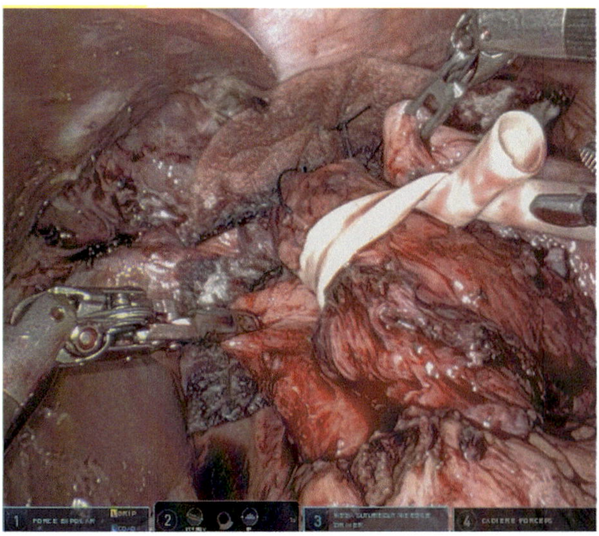

Fig. 19.8 Creation of posterior Toupen fundoplication. "Shoeshine" technique employed to ensure symmetry

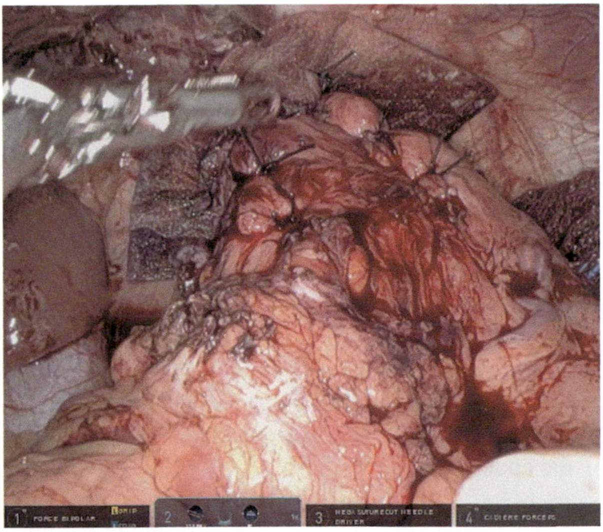

Fig. 19.9 Completed Toupen fundoplication. Silk sutures used to fix fundus to the crura and esophagus

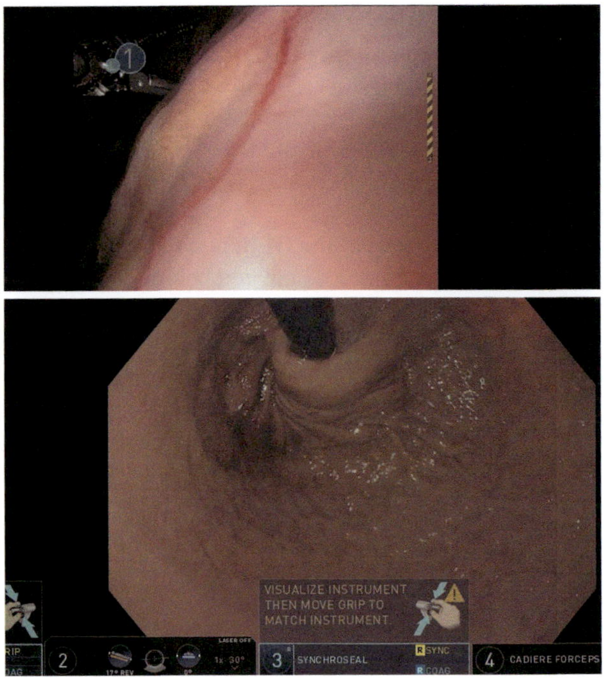

Fig. 19.10 Upper endoscopy after completion of wrap. After completion of the wrap, upper endoscopy is used to visualize the "omega" shape wrap in retroflexion

Troubleshooting

- The fundoplication prevents reflux and acts to anchor the stomach in the abdomen.
- Insertion of the bougie by the anesthesia team should be closely monitored by the operating surgeon. Frequent verbal communication is key. Gentle anterior traction of the Penrose drain by the surgeon straightens up the esophagus to facilitate the entrance of the bougie into the abdominal esophagus.
- We routinely use 56 F bougie; however, in smaller patients, a smaller bougie size is used to prevent mucosal tearing.
- Construction of the fundoplication should be with the fundus of the stomach and not with the body of the stomach to avoid redundant gastric tissue posterior to the esophagus. Retroflex view on postoperative endoscopy should demonstrate proper position and configuration of the wrap [20]. Endoscopy also decreases the incidence of postoperative dysphagia by assessing resistance to the passage of the endoscope.

- *Conversion to a Roux-en-Y Near Esophago-jejunostomy*

When the decision is to proceed with an acid diverting procedure, a Roux-en-Y near esophago-jejunostomy is our preferred procedure [21]. This is performed in very specific situation such as severe damage to the fundus, the presence of gastroparesis, multiple previous fundoplications, or obesity the patient should be consented and adequately counseled in advance since this procedure involves additional risks. If the patient is agreeable, this is our preferred procedure instead of a "wedge gastroplasty."

After identification of the GE junction, the angle of His, and the lesser curvature of the stomach, a window is created behind the stomach just below the first hepatic branch. Then, the stomach is divided with linear robotic stapler (blue load) with one fire horizontal and 1 1/2 fires vertical towards the angle of His with buttress material to create a small gastric pouch. This is followed by the creation of an "omega loop" with a 50–75 cm bilio-pancreatic limb and a 75–120 Roux limb. Then the small bowel is divided just to the left of the gastric pouch to separate the biliary limb form the Roux limb. A stapled side-to-side jejuno-jejunostomy was created with a robotic linear stapler 60 mm (white load). All defects are closed with nonabsorbable barbed sutures. A "hand-sewn" gastrojejunostomy is performed in two layers with running absorbable 3-0 absorbable barbed sutures. Once this is completed, the Roux limb is clamped distally and the upper abdomen is filled with water to perform an air leak test. The gastroscope was inserted into the patient's esophagus insufflating along the way. The gastric pouch is entered and the anastomosis is traversed while insufflating. If no air leak is noted, the procedure is completed.

Troubleshooting

- Port placement for this procedure is slightly different than the one used for redo-fundoplication, and the surgeon should plan accordingly. Specifically, trocars are placed lower to allow access to the inframesocolic space like our bariatric procedures.

- Complete takedown of the fundoplication is a key step of this procedure to allow identification of the GE junction and prevent firing the stapler across the wrap.

- *Wedge Gastroplasty*

A wedge gastroplasty is rarely performed in our practice, but it is sometimes necessary if one cannot obtain at least 2–3 cm of intra-abdominal esophagus with no tension. For this procedure, the same port placement is utilized as for the redo-fundoplication; however, a 12 mm trocar is placed in the left upper quadrant (arm #3) for the robotic stapler. We use the original technique described in 2004 [22].

A 54/6-French taper tip bougie is passed down the esophagus and kept close to the lesser curve of the stomach. The stomach is marked about 3 cm from the angle of His parallel to the bougie. Starting at the greater curvature the robotic linear stapler 60 (blue load) is fired until the 3 cm mark is reached. Subsequent fires are directed vertical toward the angle of His parallel to the bougie (Fig. 19.11). The fundoplication is placed as close as possible to the native gastroesophageal junction. A partial posterior fundoplication is preferred.

Troubleshooting

- Placing fundoplication as close as possible to the native gastroesophageal junction keeps the staple line of the neo-esophagus covered by the fundoplication.
- Careful inspection of the stomach to ensure adequate perfusion is paramount and can be achieved with the use of Firefly with ICG-green.

Outcomes

At least two systematic reviews and meta-analysis of laparoscopic revisional antireflux surgery have demonstrated increased conversion rates (7–8.7%), with an overall complications rate of 14–15.6%, reaffirming that laparoscopic reoperative antireflux surgery has significantly higher morbidity than primary antireflux surgery [13, 23] In addition, the long-term outcomes of revisional procedures are generally less satisfactory than primary surgery. This is potentially related to the intrinsic

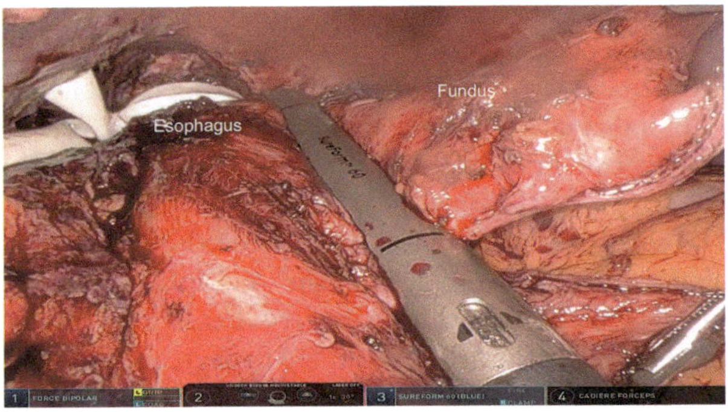

Fig. 19.11 Wedge gastroplasty. Stapler firing toward angle of His during wedge gastroplasty

technical difficulties due to dense adhesions and distortion of the anatomy from the previous surgery.

On the other hand, robotic surgery offers camera stability for long periods of time, articulated instruments, and self-retraction. These features offer increased precision, dexterity, improved exposure, control, and improved ergonomics that make the surgery less mentally stressful and less physically taxing. The clinical value observed while using this technology is validated by decreased operative times, conversions, morbidity, pain, and hospital stay. Robotic foregut surgery has demonstrated favorable short-term outcomes compared to the laparoscopic approach despite the increased incidence of higher incidence of reoperative cases in the robotic group [24, 25]. Another advantage several authors have reported is decreased use of esophageal lengthening procedures [25]. Furthermore, a very high complete or partial resolution of symptoms has been reported and the majority of patients no longer requiring daily PPIs [16].

In summary, the use of robotics in revisional foregut surgery may result in significant improvements in perioperative outcomes for these challenging procedures.

Part II: Revisional Bariatric Surgery

Introduction

Due to an ever-increasing number of bariatric procedures performed and length of follow-up, the number of patients who need revisional surgery is climbing [4]. The number of revision procedures performed has observed a 311% increase since 2011 [26].

The rate of revisional surgery varies in different bariatric procedures. It could be as high as 40% after AGB, 10–20% after RYGB, and 5.5% after sleeve gastrectomy (SG) [27]. There are various reasons for revision of an index procedure. They can be categorized into two main groups: (1) complications after primary bariatric surgery, not including immediate postoperative complications, and (2) patients who have insufficient weight loss or weight regain after primary bariatric surgery (5).

Revisional bariatric procedures can also be classified as

- Conversion. Procedures that change from an index procedure to a different type of procedure.
- Corrective. Procedures addressing complications or incomplete treatment effect of a previous bariatric operation.
- Reversal. Procedures that restore original anatomy.

The complication rate after laparoscopic revisional surgery is 15–31% and is highly dependent on the specific revisional procedure [28]. The application of robotics in primary bariatric surgery is emerging but not yet widespread. In primary surgeries, it has been demonstrated to decrease anastomotic leaks, reoperations, and decreased length of hospital stay when compared to laparoscopy [29, 30].

As it pertains to revisional bariatric surgery, some series have demonstrated its feasibility and safety, although recent advances in robotic technology can potentially improve upon those outcomes and demonstrate clear advantages favoring the routine use of robotics [31]. Here, we describe our evaluation and treatment of patients requiring reoperative bariatric surgery and the potential benefits of robotic-assisted surgery.

Preoperative Assessment

The first step for patients being evaluated for revisional surgery is to perform a detailed history and physical examination. It is important to obtain the operative reports from previous operations to better understand the surgical technique used in the initial surgery. One should also investigate patients' dietary habits, percentage of initial weight loss, and subsequent weight regain, symptoms such as dysphagia, GERD, food regurgitation, and postprandial abdominal pain. These symptoms could be a sign of anatomical issues such as stenosis at the anastomosis, hiatal hernia, marginal ulcer, pouch dilation, gastro-gastric fistula in patients with a history of gastric bypass, or inadequate removal of gastric fundus in initial SG.

An upper gastrointestinal endoscopy and barium swallow are initial tests that are helpful in understanding surgical anatomy and diagnosis of some of the above conditions. The endoscopy can detect sequel of GERD such as esophagitis, stricture and Barrett's esophagus, hiatal hernia, marginal ulcer or anastomotic stenosis, bleeding, and gastro-gastric fistula. A barium swallow is a complementary study to better understand the altered surgical anatomy. It can also delineate anatomical and functional stenosis, obstruction, or fistula. If a patient has dysphagia without obvious mechanical reasons, esophageal manometry or gastric emptying study can be beneficial to rule out functional issues.

Reviewing the operative report(s) from previous surgeries is always valuable in understanding the surgical technique used in the primary operation. For example, in the case of RYGB, it is useful to know how the bypass was reconstructed (retrocolic vs. antecolic, etc.) or whether the mesenteric defects were closed. In the case of an SG, it is important to know what size bougie was used to construct the sleeve and whether a hiatal hernia was identified and repaired. This will allow the surgeon to appropriately prepare preoperatively.

Patient Selection for Robotic Revisional Bariatric Surgery

The decision to perform revisional surgery should be based on the index procedure:

1. Complications after primary bariatric surgery, not including immediate postoperative complications.
   (a) Laparoscopic adjustable gastric band (LAGB): Postoperative complications after LAGB are band slippage, erosion, stenosis, band intolerance, esophageal dilation, severe GERD, and port-related problems.

(b) Nonadjustable gastric band (NAGB): Most complications post NAGB are nausea, vomiting, severe GERD, malnutrition, band erosion, and esophageal dilation.
(c) Roux-en-Y gastric bypass (RYGB): Marginal ulcer, bleeding, anastomotic stricture, dilated gastric pouch, and gastro-gastric fistula are common after RYGB.
(d) Laparoscopic sleeve gastrectomy (LSG): Severe GERD is the most common cause for revisional surgery after SG. Patients can also suffer from sleeve dilation and strictures.
(e) Duodenal switch (DS): Malnutrition is one of the most common complications of DS. Because of the SG associated to the DS, GERD is a possible complication of the DS.
(f) Vertical banded gastroplasty: Patients with VBG most common complains are severe GERD, band erosion, stricture, dysphagia, and disruption of the staple line.

2. Patients who have insufficient weight loss, weight regain, or recurrence of obesity-related medical conditions after primary bariatric surgery. Prior to any revisional surgery, all patients with weight regain or insufficient weight loss should go for consultation with the program psychologist and dietician.

Figure 19.12 shows a decisional flowchart according to the index procedure and the indication for RRBS.

Technical Aspects of Robotic Revisional Bariatric Surgery

- *Access*
- *Adhesiolysis*
  - *Identification of the surgical anatomy (upper endoscopy)*
  - *Identification of the right crus*
- *Hiatal hernia repair*
- *Anatomy*
  - *Takedown*
  - *Reconstruction*
    Gastric/intestinal stapling (staple size, stomach anatomy, wall thickness)
    GI reconstruction (hand-sewn anastomosis)
- *Leak test (upper endoscopy)*

Setup

Four robotic trocars, a liver retractor, and assist port are utilized in revisional cases. Setup and port placement for revisional cases are generally similar to the setup for RYGB. It is recommended to use an assistant port for easy access to bedside suctioning and insertion and removal of sponges/sutures.

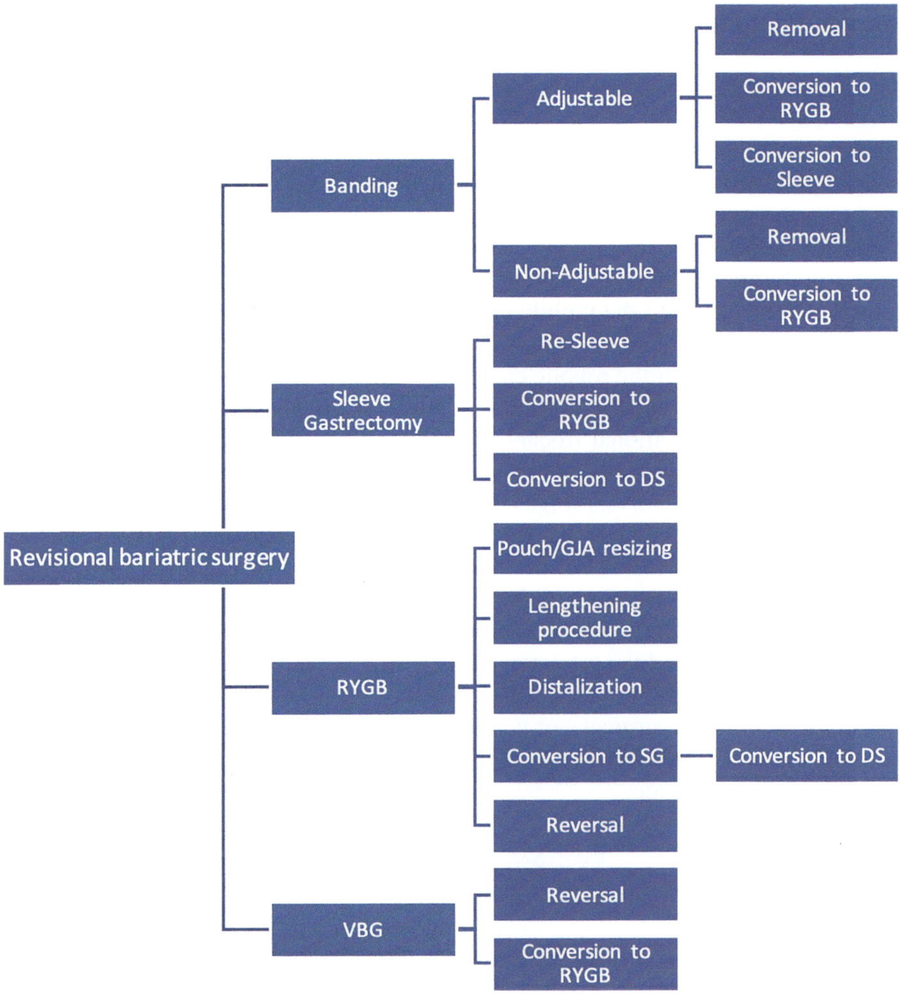

Fig. 19.12 Decisional flowchart for revisional surgery. Goals and decisions based on index operation and patient-specific factors

- Arm #1: fenestrated bipolar; stapler
- Arm #2: 3DHD endoscope
- Arm #3: vessel sealer (or SynchroSeal); monopolar scissor; suture cut needle driver
- Arm #4: Cadiere (or Tip-Up)

Access/Port Placement/Liver Retraction

The port placement described it is specific for the da Vinci Xi System. Entry into the abdominal cavity is obtained through a gasless optical technique in the periumbilical area, just to the left of the midline, using an 8 mm robotic optical trocar. However, if history of open surgery, the entry to the abdominal cavity will migrate to the left upper quadrant, right upper quadrant, and sometimes periumbilical using a Hassan technique. If gasless technique is used, a 5 mm 0/30 degree laparoscope is used for access and port placement. The first port is placed in the left mid-abdomen two fingerbreadths lateral to the umbilicus and one palm-width inferior to the left costal margin.

This port is used for the robotic camera (arm #2). If previous open surgery (midline incision, hernia repair, etc.), the first entry port is placed left subcostal. From this position, 2–3 additional trocars are placed along the left midclavicular line. Depending on the complexity of the adhesions, the robot can be docked to facilitate and expedite the adhesiolysis (Fig. 19.13).

Insufflation is started to 15 mmHg. Two 8-mm trocars and one 12-mm trocar are then placed at the same level of the camera port: 12-mm port on the right midclavicular line (arm #1), one on the left midclavicular line (arm #3), and one in the left anterior axillary line (arm #4). A 5-mm subxiphoid incision is used for the placement of the Nathanson liver retractor. Finally, an assistant port (8 mm) is inserted in between arms #2 and #3 or between #1 and #2 (see Fig. 19.2, post placement). At this point, the robotic surgical cart was approximated into position and the arms are attached to the four specific trocars. The da Vinci Xi System can be docked from the patient's right or left side.

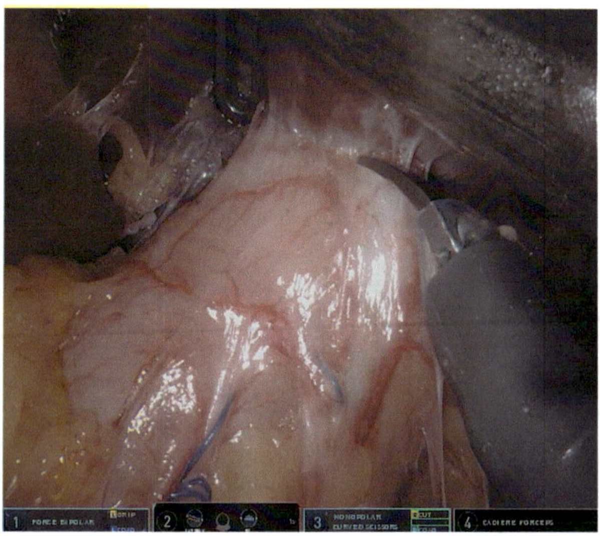

Fig. 19.13 Adhesiolysis. Early docking of the robot to facilitate adhesiolysis, as seen here between pouch and liver

Troubleshooting

- If the liver retractor cannot be placed at the beginning of the case due to adhesions, we still dock the robot to expedite the adhesiolysis. Once this is completed, the left lobe of the liver can be retracted using an internal liver retractor such as a liver sling (see Fig. 19.3). This could be done with barbed sutures between the diaphragm and the abdominal wall.

Surgical Technique

Regardless of the indication for index procedure, robotic-assisted gastric bypass is the most common revisional procedure in our practice. The most common revisional bariatric procedures are either conversions from LAGB, NAGB, LSG, VBG, or corrective of the RYGB anatomy due to either pouch/anastomosis dilations or strictures. Since the specific surgical revision is dependent on the index procedure for the purpose of this chapter, we will describe general technical aspects that can be applied in several circumstances. Revisional procedures are performed in one stage whenever possible.

1. *Adhesiolysis*

One of the most challenging aspects of bariatric revisional surgery is adhesiolysis. Depending on whether the previous procedure was done open or laparoscopic, the adhesions could form around the midline incision, and most frequently between the stomach and liver. Other common areas for adhesions are at the angle of His and around the hiatus and also to retrogastric structures such as the pancreas. In our experience, the adhesiolysis can be started laparoscopically in order to create enough space for the insertion of the robotic trocars and docking of the robotic system. However, we try to dock the robot as early as possible to facilitate the adhesiolysis and shorten operative time. Sometimes this can represent starting with two working arms.

Once the robotic system is docked, the adhesiolysis continues with monopolar scissors in arm #3 and a fenestrated bipolar instrument in arm #1. The main advantages of the robotic system at this stage of the revisional procedure are self-assisting, better exposure/visualization of structures, and the articulated energy device. These benefits decrease the incidence of iatrogenic perforations and bleeding. While separating the left lobe of the liver from the anterior stomach, the identification of the right crus is our main anatomic landmark and will facilitate the recognition of the anatomy of the hiatus, identification of hiatal hernias, and prevent injuries to vascular structures such as the inferior vena cava (IVC). This portion of the procedure could be relatively bloody and for that reason the utilization of two energy sources (arms #1/#3) is a significant progress from laparoscopic surgery.

- The fourth robotic arm gives the console surgeon greater autonomy during robotic-revisional bariatric surgery by providing tireless self-retraction and improved exposure.
- The purpose of the bedside assistant is to be able to suction, retract, and insert/remove sponges and sutures throughout the duration of the case. The assistant will also help with changing the robotic instruments as needed.

2. *Hiatal Hernia Repair*

After identifying the right crus, its dissected carefully off the esophagus. This dissection is typically carried out from anterior to posterior along the right crus starting at the right side of the phrenoesophageal membrane until fully exposing the right crus. After complete exposure of the right crus, a retroesophageal window is created and extended exposing the confluence of the crura. At this point, the Penrose drain is passed behind the esophagus and used to encircle the esophagus and vagus nerves. Then attention is focused on the left crura, typically the dissection starts from posterior to anterior, and is continued in a circular manner around the rim of the hiatus with complete takedown of the phrenoesophageal membrane. The dissection is continued with a combination of blunt dissection and the vessel sealer until complete exposure of the left crus is achieved. Transhiatal dissection of the esophagus is started and continued in a cephalad direction. The articulated vessel sealer device and the fenestrated bipolar grasper are used for the circumferential dissection of the esophagus. Mobilization of the esophagus can typically be accomplished using blunt dissection of relatively thin alveolar tissue by exercising traction and countertraction maneuvers always dissecting away from the esophagus. The esophageal mobilization is completed only after 2–3 cm of intra–abdominal esophagus are observed to be well into the abdomen without tension. The esophagus is retracted anteriorly and to the left by arm #4, and the vessel sealer is replaced with a suture cut needle driver. Closure of the diaphragmatic defect is started at the junction of the right and left crus to decrease tension on every stitch and is carried out anteriorly. The closure is performed using running nonabsorbable barbed suture. We routinely utilize a "shoe lacing technique" in order to decrease tension of the repair (see Fig. 19.6).

- The incidence of hiatal hernias during reoperative surgery is much higher than reported for after primary bariatric surgery. Simultaneous repair of hiatal hernias during reoperative surgery is warranted.

3. *Identification of the Surgical Anatomy (Upper Endoscopy/Tilepro)*

At any point during the procedure if the anatomy cannot be defined, upper endoscopy is used. The TilePro™ feature is used to project intraoperative endoscopic images onto the console screen. The upper endoscopy can be performed by the bedside assistant.

- TilePro is a multi-image video display mode of the da Vinci Xi that allows the surgeon to simultaneously view up to two additional images, such as intraoperative endoscopy, as a picture-on-picture on the three-dimensional console screen and assistant monitors (Fig. 19.14).

4. *Anatomy Take-Down/Reconstruction*

After the adhesiolysis is completed and anatomy of the previous surgery is outlined, the previous anatomy is taken down according to the surgical plan. The risk of leak after revisional surgery is higher than primary surgery likely due to the less predictable tissue thickness. For that reason, when using staplers for resection of previous anastomosis, distal stomach, first portion of the duodenum, devascularized stomach, or thickened small bowel, one should use a staple load with proper height due to chronic inflammation and edema scarring. This point deserves special consideration when using staple line reinforcement. It is also important to be cognizant of previous staple lines, suture materials, clips, and silastic/mesh banding that could cause the stapler to jam and cause a misfire and damage the tissue. Irrespective of the index procedure, it is critical to identify and preserve in the left gastric artery unless an esophago-jejunostomy is the plan procedure. The Firefly feature of the robotic system can facilitate the identification of the vascular supply after intravenous injection of indocyanine green (Fig. 19.15).

Our preference is to use the robotic linear stapler (SureForm60™) with stapler line reinforcement to decrease bleeding and potentially leaks. The stapler comes with white, blue, green, and black reloads that can be selected according to the tissue thickness. This stapler also offers a 120-degree cone of articulation that allows for less tissue pulling and improved tissue transection. In addition, the increased articulation of the stapler could decrease the need for two 12 mm trocars in the field. An additional feature of the robotic stapler that is also practical in revisional cases is the "ForceFire" option. This option becomes available mainly after the tissues are clamped unsuccessfully due to increased thickness. At this time, the system

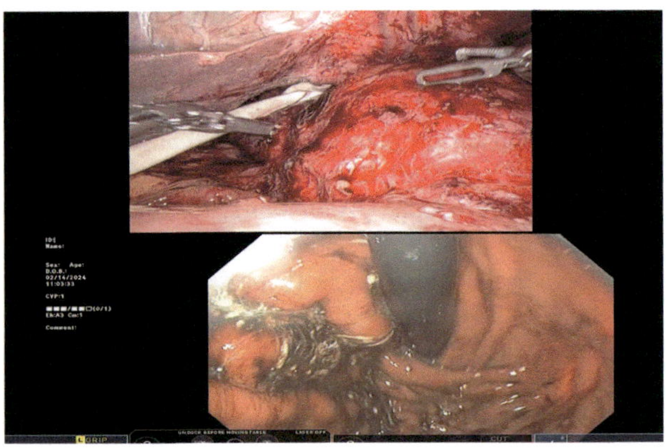

Fig. 19.14 Intraoperative endoscopy. The TilePro™ function can be used to help delineate anatomy, such as the location of the GE junction and to confirm full reduction of hiatal hernia

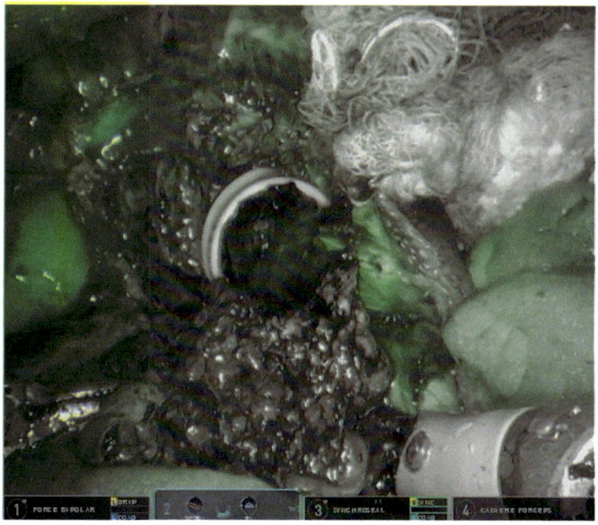

Fig. 19.15 Evaluation of perfusion. Indocyanine green administered intravenously can be used to evaluate perfusion of gastric pouch after revision via the FireFly function of the robot

provides feedback by giving a message that the "Tissue too thick to fire." The console surgeon chooses whether to abort the fire or override and complete the fire. It is worth mentioning this feature is only available with black reloads.

- Nonadjustable gastric band (NAGB): Extensive lysis of adhesions is usually required during this case since these cases were routinely performed in an open fashion. Finding and removing the band from the perigastric position is an essential step of the procedure. If the band cannot be removed due to adhesions, then excision of the stomach proximal and distal of the band should be performed. Alternatively, if the band is eroded into the gastric lumen, transgastric removal of the band can be attempted. Reconstruction will most likely be in the shape of a gastric bypass.
- Laparoscopic adjustable gastric band (LAGB): Excision of the perigastric capsule created by the band is essential to prevent staple misfiring (Fig. 19.16). Common conversion procedures post LAGB removal are SG and gastric bypass. Usual stapler reloads for either gastric bypass or sleeve conversion are blue, green, or black depending on tissue thickness.
- LSG—conversion to gastric bypass: Adhesiolysis is performed from the antrum of the stomach progressing in a cephalad direction until the angle of His. If a neofundus is present, it should be complete freed and excised during the creation of the gastric pouch. Usual stapler reloads for pouch creation are either blue or green. Care must be taken to identify clips on the staple line from the index procedure. If the intention is to preserve the sleeve and conversion to duodenal switch, dissection of the inferior aspect of the sleeve is performed until the first portion of the duodenum (2–3 cm distal to the pylorus). In patients with chronic sleeve fistulas, conversion to esophagojejunostomy must be considered (Fig. 19.17).

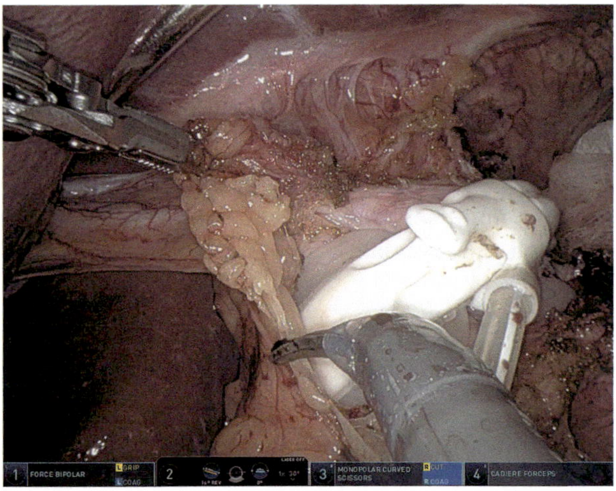

Fig. 19.16 AGB removal. Adhesions around the band and excision of the capsule are facilitated by the robotic platform

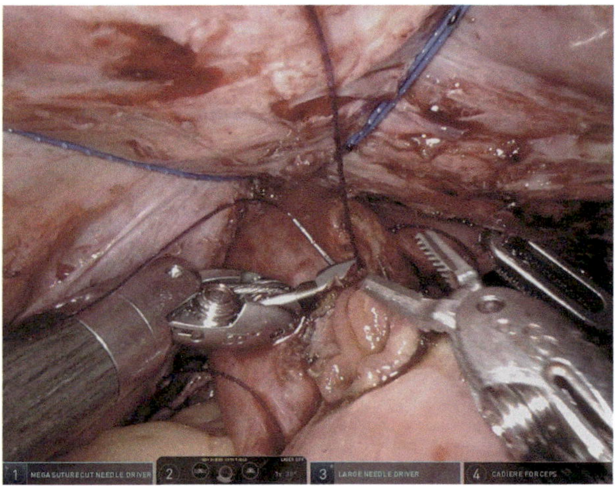

Fig. 19.17 Conversion of SG to esophagojejunostomy. Hand-sewn esophagojejunostomy performed with robotic platform safe and feasible

- Vertical banded gastroplasty (VBG): Conversion to gastric bypass; the gastric pouch must be created proximal to the ostoma and medial to the gastro-gastric staple line of the VBG. It is our practice to excise the fundus and most of the body of the stomach that includes the previous staple line. For this purpose, the short gastric vessels are taken down with vessel sealer. Stapler reloads for the gastric resection are usually black or green.
- RYGB: It is crucial to delineate the anatomy of the gastric bypass at the beginning of the procedure. The remnant stomach is dissected off the gastric pouch with robotic monopolar scissors. Then the posterior aspect of the GJA and the proximal alimentary limb are also dissected off. If the gastric bypass reconstruction was done, retro-colic/retro-gastric further dissection may be necessary to be able to perform the reconstruction with no tension. Also, if a

banded bypass was performed the previous nonadjustable band must be removed. Once the anastomosis is freed (Fig. 19.18), the gastric pouch is transected proximal to the GJA with linear stapler with either blue or green reload. The proximal jejunum is also transected with a white reload along with the mesentery of the small bowel. There are multiple options for revision of a gastric bypass, including revision of the GJA anastomosis, pouch trimming, distalization, lengthening procedure, and conversion to duodenal switch and reversal.

5. *GI Reconstruction*

Commonly, the GI reconstruction is carried out in the form of gastric bypass (gastrojejunostomy). However, a hand-sewn anastomosis (HSA) can be performed during reversal/conversion procedures such as gastro-gastrostomy, duodeno-ileostomy, or esophago-jejunostomy. Our HSA preferred technique is a continuous double-layered anastomosis constructed with barbed sutures and almost identical in every situation (Fig. 19.19). Whenever possible, our preference is for an antecolic-antegastric anastomosis. For the purpose of this chapter, we will describe our GJA technique (32). The ligament of Treitz is identified and the small bowel is run distal to the ligament, and a loop was chosen that will be able to reach the upper abdomen (100 cm). Then the small bowel loop was attached to the proximal stomach with a running 3-0 absorbable barbed suture to create the omega loop. A gastrotomy and jejunotomy are created with monopolar scissors. To create the gastrotomy, the anesthesia team will advance the bougie slowly to create tenting of the anterior wall of the stomach; at this time, the gastrotomy is carried out with cautery against the bougie. Then a 1.5–2 cm gastrojejunostomy was "hand-sewn" in two layers using two needle drivers and absorbable 6-inch barbed sutures (x3). Starting from lateral to medial, an inner posterior layer of running 3-0 absorbable barbed suture is created with full-thickness bites between the stomach and jejunum. Once the posterior layer is completed, the bougie is advanced into the jejunum to stent the anastomosis. Finally, two anterior layers of running seromuscular (Lembert sutures) absorbable 6-inch 3-0 barbed sutures are

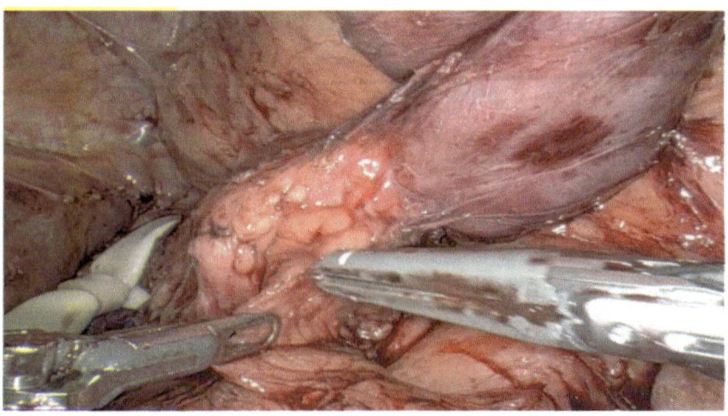

Fig. 19.18 Mobilization and resection of gastrojejunal anastomosis. Revision of gastric bypass may include recreation of gastrojejunal anastomosis. Here the old anastomosis including proximal alimentary limb is being resected with plan for reconstruction

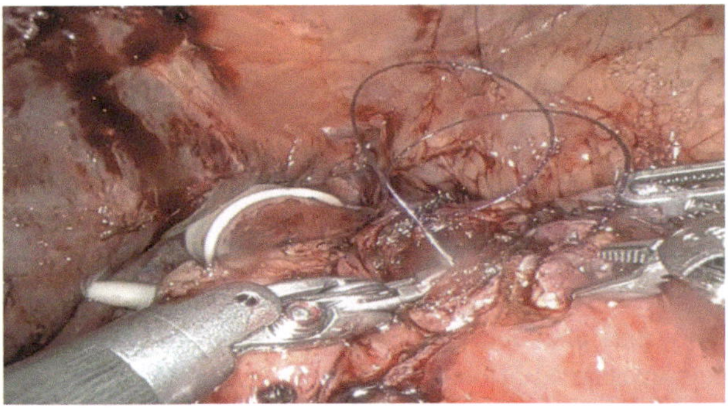

Fig. 19.19 Hand-sewn anastomosis. A two-layered hand-sewn anastomosis is created with running barbed 3-0 absorbable suture

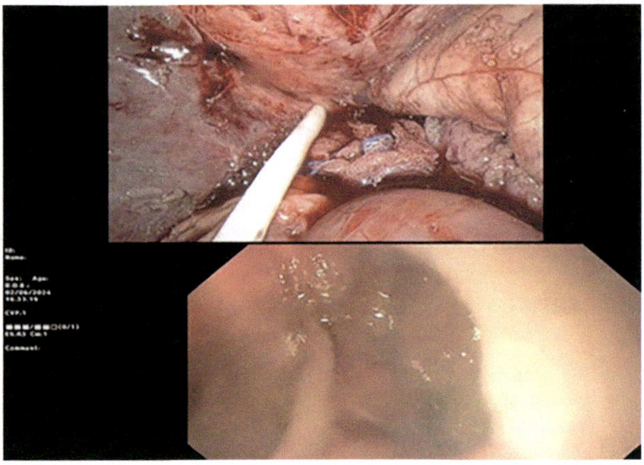

Fig. 19.20 Leak test. Positive leak test with bubbles constantly seen coming from anastomosis submerged in saline

used. Once this is completed, the alimentary limb is clamped distally and the upper abdomen was filled with water to perform an air leak test. The robotic image is switched to TilePro™ that enables the endoscopic view to be incorporated into the surgical field of view within the console. The gastroscope is inserted into the patient's esophagus insufflating along the way. The gastric pouch is entered, and the anastomosis is traversed. If no air leak is observed, the procedure is completed. If there is a positive leak, further investigation is warranted (Fig. 19.20).

(a) If needed and depending on the type of revisional procedure to be performed, the entire length of the small should be counted.
(b) The HSA has the advantages of allowing for direct examination of the anastomosis, reducing the risk of bleeding, and can be used in situations where the use of stapler would be contraindicated like such us poor quality or thicker tissue. In addition, it has decreased long-term complications such as strictures.
(c) The most notable advantages of the use of robotics for the HSA are the surgeon's autonomy, decreased variability, and reproducibility that lead to better quality anastomosis.

Outcomes

It was common knowledge that revisional bariatric surgery is complex and has an increased rate of complications. Yet, the implementation of robotic-assisted revisional bariatric surgery has shown to be safe and effective whether it is performed in the presence of complications or insufficient weight loss or weight regain after the primary procedure [28, 33–35]. Several case series have reported shorter length of stay and decreased readmission and anastomotic complications. In addition, the robot may also decrease conversion rates to open surgery [36]. Reported outcomes demonstrate additional weight loss and resolution of associated medical conditions. Increased costs associated with robotic surgery have consistently been described as pitfalls to its implementation. Streamlining of technique and instrumentation costs can be potentially mitigated.

For patients who are considered candidates for robotic revisional bariatric surgery, an extensive workup is justified to delineate the anatomy of the index procedure. Even though robotics offers a good safety profile to revisional surgery, it is critical for the operating surgeon to have substantial experience not only with primary bariatric surgery but robotic surgery to prevent complications.

References

1. Dallemagne B, Weerts J, Markiewicz S, Dewandre JM, Wahlen C, Monami B, et al. Clinical results of laparoscopic fundoplication at ten years after surgery. Surg Endosc. 2006;20(1):159–65.
2. Wittgrove AC, Clark GW, Tremblay LJ. Laparoscopic gastric bypass, roux-en-Y: preliminary report of five cases. Obes Surg Incl Laparosc Allied Care. 1994;4(4):353–7.
3. Grant AM, Boachie C, Cotton SC, Faria R, Bojke L, Epstein DM, et al. Clinical and economic evaluation of laparoscopic surgery compared with medical management for gastro-oesophageal reflux disease: 5-year follow-up of multicentre randomised trial (the REFLUX trial). Health Technol Assess. 2013;17(22):1–167.
4. Clapp B, Ponce J, DeMaria E, Ghanem O, Hutter M, Kothari S, LaMasters T, Kurian M, English W. American Society for Metabolic and Bariatric Surgery 2020 estimate of metabolic and bariatric procedures performed in the United States. Surg Obes Relat Dis. 2022;18(9):1134–40.
5. Oelschlager BK, Lal DR, Jensen E, Cahill M, Quiroga E, Pellegrini CA. Mediumand long-term outcome of laparoscopic redo fundoplication. Surg Endosc. 2006;20:1817–23.
6. Brethauer SA, Kothari S, Sudan R, et al. Systematic review on reoperative bariatric surgery American Society for Metabolic and Bariatric Surgery Revision Task Force. Surg Obes Relat Dis. 2014;10(5):952–72.
7. SAGES Guidelines Committee. SAGES guideline for clinical application of laparoscopic bariatric surgery. Surg Endosc. 2008;22(10):2281–300.
8. Slater BJ, Dirks RC, McKinley SK, Ansari MT, Kohn GP, Thosani N, Qumseya B, Billmeier S, Daly S, Crawford C, Ehlers AP, Hollands C, Palazzo F, Rodriguez N, Train A, Wassenaar E, Walsh D, Pryor AD, Stefanidis D. SAGES guidelines for the surgical treatment of gastroesophageal reflux (GERD). Surg Endosc. 2021;35(9):4903–17.
9. Kohn GP, Price RR, DeMeester SR, Zehetner J, Muensterer OJ, Awad Z, Mittal SK, Richardson WS, Stefanidis D, Fanelli RD, SAGES Guidelines Committee. Guidelines for the management of hiatal hernia. Surg Endosc. 2013;27(12):4409–28.

10. Dreifuss NH, Mangano A, Hassan C, Masrur MA. Robotic Revisional bariatric surgery: a high-volume center experience. Obes Surg. 2021;31(4):1656–63.
11. Patti MG, Allaix ME, Fisichella PM. Analysis of the causes of failed Antireflux surgery and the principles of treatment: A review. JAMA Surg. 2015;150(6):585–90.
12. Smith CD, McClusky DA, Rajad MA, Lederman AB, Hunter JG. When fundoplication fails: redo? Ann Surg. 2005;241(6):861–9; discussion 869–71.
13. Furnee EJB, Draaisma WA, Broeders IA, Gooszen HG. Surgical reintervention after failed antireflux surgery: a systematic review of the literature. J Gastrointest Surg. 2009;13:1539–49.
14. Owen B, Simorov A, Siref A, et al. How does robotic anti-reflux surgery compare with traditional open and laparoscopic techniques: a cost and outcomes analysis. Surg Endosc. 2014;28:1686–90.
15. Tolboom RC, Draaisma WA, Broeders IAMJ. Evaluation of conventional laparoscopic versus robot-assisted laparoscopicredo hiatal hernia and antireflux surgery: a cohort study. J Robot Surg. 2016;10:33–9.
16. Elmously A, Gray KD, Ullmann TM, Fahey TJ 3rd, Afaneh C, Zarnegar R. Robotic Reoperative anti-reflux surgery: low perioperative morbidity and high symptom resolution. World J Surg. 2018;42(12):4014–21.
17. Carbo AI, Kim RH, Gates T, D'Agostino HR. Imaging findings of successful and failed fundoplication. Radiographics. 2014;34(7):1873–84.
18. Vetter TR, Bader AM. Continued evolution of perioperative medicine: realizing its full potential. Anesth Analg. 2020;130:804–7.
19. Jindal P, Patil V, Pradhan R, Mahajan HC, Rani A, Pabba UG. Update on preoperative evaluation and optimisation. Indian J Anaesth. 2023;67(1):39–47.
20. Jobe BA, Kahrilas PJ, Vernon AH, et al. Endoscopic appraisal of the gastroesophageal valve after antireflux surgery. Am J Gastroenterol. 2004;99(2):233–43.
21. Awais O, Luketich JD, Tam J, Irshad K, Schuchert MJ, Landreneau RJ, Pennathur A. Roux-en-Y near esophagojejunostomy for intractable gastroesophageal reflux after antireflux surgery. Ann Thorac Surg. 2008;85(6):1954–9. discussion 1959–61
22. Terry ML, Vernon A, Hunter JG. Stapled-wedge Collis gastroplasty for the shortened esophagus. Am J Surg. 2004;188:195–9.
23. Symons NRA, Purkayastha S, Dillemans B, et al. Laparoscopic revision of failed antireflux surgery: a systematic review. Am J Surg. 2011;202:336–43.
24. Soliman BG, Nguyen DT, Chan EY, Chihara RK, Meisenbach LM, Graviss EA, Kim MP. Robot-assisted hiatal hernia repair demonstrates favorable short-term outcomes compared to laparoscopic hiatal hernia repair. Surg Endosc. 2020;34(6):2495–502.
25. Gerull WD, Cho D, Arefanian S, Kushner BS, Awad MM. Favorable peri-operative outcomes observed in paraesophageal hernia repair with robotic approach. Surg Endosc. 2021;35(6):3085–9.
26. English WJ, DeMaria EJ, Hutter MM, et al. American Society for Metabolic and Bariatric Surgery 2018 estimate of metabolic and bariatric procedures performed in the United States. Surg Obes Relat Dis. 2020;16(4):457–63.
27. Park JY, Kim YJ. Revisional bariatric surgery. In: Choi SH, Kasama K, editors. Bariatric and metabolic surgery. Berlin/Heidelberg: Springer-Verlag; 2014.
28. Snyder B, Wilson T, Woodruff V, Wilson E. Robotically assisted revision of bariatric surgeries is safe and effective to achieve further weight loss. World J Surg. 2013;37(11):2569–73.
29. Economopoulos KP, Theocharidis V, McKenzie TJ, et al. Robotic vs. Laparoscopic Roux-En-Y Gastric bypass: a systematic review and meta-analysis. Obes Surg. 2015;25(11):2180–9.
30. El Chaar M, King K, Pastrana M, Galvez A, Stoltzfus J. Outcomes of robotic surgery in revisional bariatric cases: a propensity score-matched analysis of the MBSAQIP registry. J Robot Surg. 2021;15(2):235–9.
31. Cheng YL, Elli EF. Role of robotic surgery in complex Revisional bariatric procedures. Obes Surg. 2021;31(6):2583–9.

32. Galvani CA. Robotic Roux-En-Y Gastric Bypass (RA-RYGB). In: Gharagozloo F, Patel VR, Giulianotti PC, Poston R, Gruessner R, Meyer M, editors. Robotic surgery. Cham: Springer; 2021. https://doi.org/10.1007/978-3-030-53594-0_59.
33. Inabnet WB, Belle SH, Bessler M, et al. Comparison of 30-day outcomes after non LapBand primary and revisional bariatric surgical procedures from the longitudinal assessment of bariatric surgery study. Surg Obes Relat Dis. 2010;6(1):22–30.
34. Bindal V, Gonzalez-Heredia R, Elli EF. Outcomes of robot-assisted roux-en-Y gastric bypass as a Reoperative bariatric procedure. Obes Surg. 2015;25:1810.
35. Gray KD, Moore MD, Elmously A, et al. Obes Surg. 2018;28:1852.
36. Buchs NC, Pugin F, Azagury DE, et al. Robotic revisional bariatric surgery: a comparative study with laparoscopic and open surgery. Int J Med Robot. 2014;10(2):213–7.

20 Robotic Transabdominal Preperitoneal (TAPP) Inguinal Hernia Repair

Samuel Guba and Richard Lu

Introduction

More than 20 million inguinal hernia repairs are performed annually worldwide. In the United States, it is among the top five most common major outpatient operations performed in males over 18 years of age [1]. There has been a shift toward minimally invasive inguinal hernia repair (MI IHR) from open techniques, particularly with recent rapid adoption of robotic technology. MI IHR has been associated with decreased early postoperative pain, earlier return to daily activities, and decreased analgesic use compared to open repair [2].

A systematic review and meta-analysis demonstrated the overall recurrence rate after MI IHR was 1.2%, with other studies demonstrating risk of chronic pain being around 2.1%, risk for seroma/hematoma around 4.1%, and risk of skin/soft tissue infection at 2.9% [3–5]. It is important to note that negative consequences from inguinal hernia repair can be devastating, thus highlighting the importance of having a solid foundation of inguinal anatomy and sound operative techniques.

Preoperative Evaluation

The workup for an inguinal hernia begins with a thorough history and physical examination. Most inguinal hernias can be diagnosed with exam alone; however, equivocal exam findings with a high suspicion for inguinal hernia disease warrants further evaluation. Additional imaging with either ultrasound or CT can be obtained. This can provide valuable information in diagnosing an occult hernia, contralateral disease, or elucidating complex anatomy such as in the setting of recurrence or scrotal involvement. Modifiable risk factors such as diabetes, smoking, chronic

S. Guba · R. Lu (✉)
Department of Surgery, University of Texas Medical Branch, Galveston, TX, USA
e-mail: rllu@utmb.edu

S. Samreen et al. (eds.), *The SAGES Manual of Robotic Surgery*,
https://doi.org/10.1007/978-3-031-86927-3_20

cough, COPD, and obesity should be optimized. There is substantial literature that highlights elective hernia repair should be deferred in patients with an A1c greater than 8%. In our practice, we further recommend smoking cessation and reaching a BMI of less than 35 prior to elective hernia repair. Patients should be counseled on the risks of the procedure which are discussed later in the chapter. Furthermore, the finding of a contralateral hernia should be discussed with the patient as these are found in 10–25% of patients [6].

Multiple operative techniques for inguinal hernia repair exist and can be categorized by anterior versus posterior approaches, each with mesh and non-mesh options. MI IHR is typically synonymous with posterior mesh approaches and has demonstrated advantages over open repair techniques including decreased postoperative and chronic pain as well as quicker return to normal activities [7]. MI IHR has been suggested as the preferred approach in primary unilateral groin hernias in males, bilateral inguinal hernias, femoral hernias, and women given their high incidence of femoral hernias [8]. As MI IHR typically refers to a posterior mesh approach, it is the method of choice for managing inguinal hernia recurrences following an open anterior approach. The most common types of MI IHR include the transabdominal preperitoneal (TAPP) and the totally extraperitoneal (TEP) approaches. The TAPP approach typically has a shorter learning curve than TEP and has other advantages such as the ability to rapidly assess the contralateral groin for a concomitant hernia and visualization of structure both above and below the peritoneal flap to prevent injury to underlying intra-abdominal viscera. Advantages for the TEP approach include the ability to avoid the intraperitoneal space and obviating the need for peritoneal flap closure. However, TEP can be cumbersome due to limited working space and closely placed trocars. This can be further complicated with docking of the robotic platform. In addition, the ease of robotic suturing lessens the advantage of minimal suturing in TEP versus TAPP. Contraindications to MI IHR include inability to tolerate general anesthesia or pneumoperitoneum, severe ascites, strangulated hernia with concurrent sepsis, and extensive intra-abdominal adhesions. History of previous pelvic surgery such as prostatectomy may also deter one from selective minimally invasive approach.

Robotic TAPP

Patient Positioning and Preparation

The patient is placed on the operating room table in the supine position with both arms tucked and pressure points padded. The patient's hips should be positioned over the break of the bed in case flexion is needed. This expands the distance between the anterior superior iliac spine (ASIS) and the costal margins to facilitate port placement. We routinely do not place a Foley catheter unless the patient has a significant history of urinary problems or if the bladder is suspected to be involved in the hernia. Hair removal is completed with clippers, as this has a lower incidence of SSI than shaving. Routine usage of antibiotic prophylaxis in elective inguinal hernia repair with mesh placement remains a controversial topic. The European Hernia Society does not recommend routine prophylaxis in the setting of elective inguinal hernia repairs using mesh in low-risk patients. However, antibiotic prophylaxis may be considered in certain high-risk scenarios such as in the setting of immunosuppression, recurrence, old age, long surgery duration, or in facilities with high SSI rates >4–5% [9].

Instrumentation

The authors predominantly use three main instruments during robotic TAPP: monopolar curved scissors, fenestrated bipolar forceps, and the Mega SutureCut™ needle driver (Intuitive Surgical, Sunnyvale, CA). Should more robust grasping strength be necessary, a ProGrasp™ forceps or force bipolar are useful options; however, care should be used when manipulating delicate tissue such as viscera. A Cadiere forceps or Tip-Up fenestrated grasper can be useful instruments for retraction via a fourth assistant port if necessary.

Trocar Placement and Docking

Pneumoperitoneum should be established with the surgeon's preferred technique. In our practice, we typically establish pneumoperitoneum using a Veress needle at Palmer's point. An optical trocar is then placed in the midline at least 15 cm away from symphysis pubis and the Veress needle is removed under direct visualization. Two additional working ports are placed directly lateral to the initial trocar with a minimum distance of 8 cm from each other. A fourth assistant port may be placed for retraction in challenging cases. The operating table is then placed in Trendelenburg to at least 15° and rotated away from the side of the hernia, to slide intra-abdominal viscera away from the operative field. It is important to evaluate for a contralateral inguinal hernia. For operative efficiency, mesh and suture can be placed into the abdomen at this time. The robot is then docked and the robotic instruments are deployed into the field.

Dissection

The peritoneal incision is started at least 4 cm away from the defect with the flap extending from the ASIS to the median umbilical fold targeting the preperitoneal space. If performing bilateral hernia repair, extension of the peritoneal incision across the midline to the contralateral ASIS can be completed or another peritoneal incision can be made depending on surgeon's preference.

Recently, the critical view of the myopectineal orifice (CV of the MPO) was developed using best practices to standardize the dissection performed during MI IHR [10]. The following steps must be achieved but may be performed in any order:

1. The pubic tubercle must be identified and dissected beyond midline. For large direct hernias, it is recommended to dissect to the contralateral Cooper's ligament (CL).

   All adipose tissue should be cleared from Hesselbach's triangle, and a direct inguinal hernia should be ruled out (Fig. 20.1).
2. The bladder must be dissected 2 cm below CL to facilitate mesh placement in the space of Retzius and to prevent mesh displacement from bladder distension (Fig. 20.2).
3. A femoral hernia should be ruled out by dissecting between CL and the iliac vein to identify the femoral orifice (Fig. 20.3).
4. The cord elements (vas deferens and gonadal vessels) should be parietalized such that they lay flat. The psoas muscle should be visualized, and upward traction of the peritoneum should not trigger movement of the cord elements (Fig. 20.4).
5. Cord lipomas should be reduced, which are typically lateral to the cord elements. These lipomas can typically be reduced and placed over the mesh. However, large cord lipomas may need to be excised to avoid mesh disruption (Fig. 20.5).
6. The peritoneum should be dissected laterally beyond the ASIS and swept inferiorly well behind the inferior border of the mesh.
7. Perform the dissection, provide mesh coverage, and ensure that mesh and any fixation is placed 2 cm above an imaginary line between the internal ring and the ASIS.
8. Mesh should be placed once complete dissection and hemostasis are achieved (Fig. 20.6). The mesh should be at least 15 × 10 cm, but a larger mesh may be necessary for larger defects. One should choose a mesh that adapts to the contour of the space and the cord structures. The mesh should lay flush against the wall without creases or folds. Splitting of the mesh for pass-through of cord structures should be avoided. It is critical to ensure that the mesh does not "clamshell" during deflation.

The dissection should be relatively avascular if the correct planes are achieved and maintained. It is critical to understand the location of significant neurovascular structures and protect them from injury. The "triangle of doom" contains the iliac vessels and is bounded by the vas deferens, gonadal vessels, and the peritoneal fold.

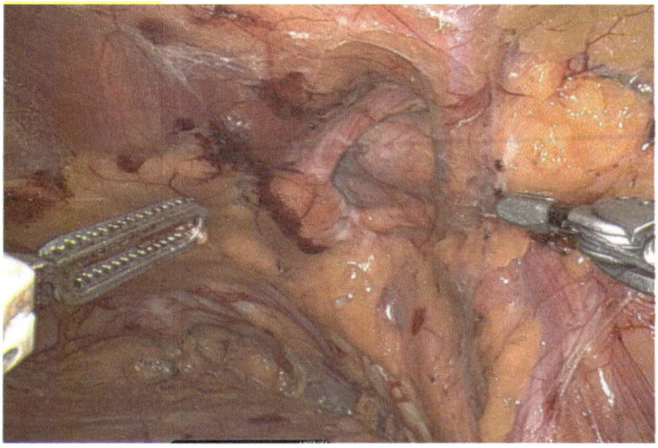

Fig. 20.1 Dissection of Hesselbach's triangle. In this patient, a right direct inguinal hernia is present

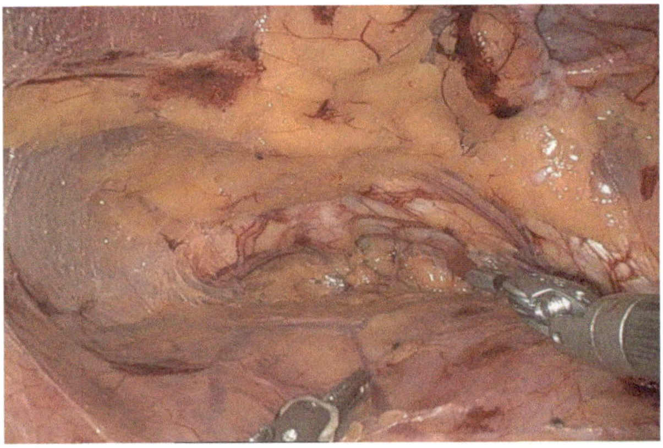

Fig. 20.2 Development of the space of Retzius. Adequate space must be established to prevent mesh displacement with bladder distension

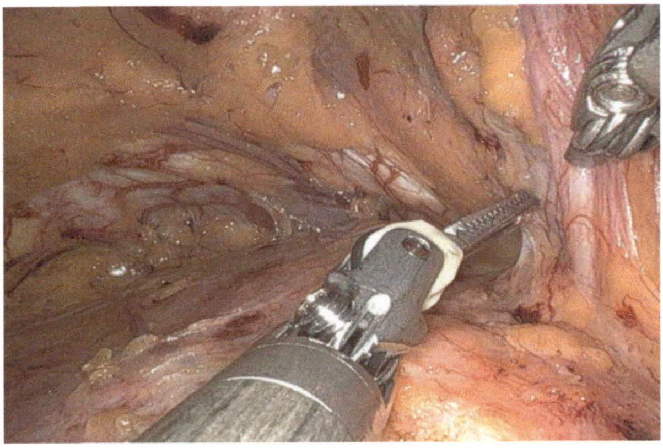

Fig. 20.3 Identification of the right external iliac vein

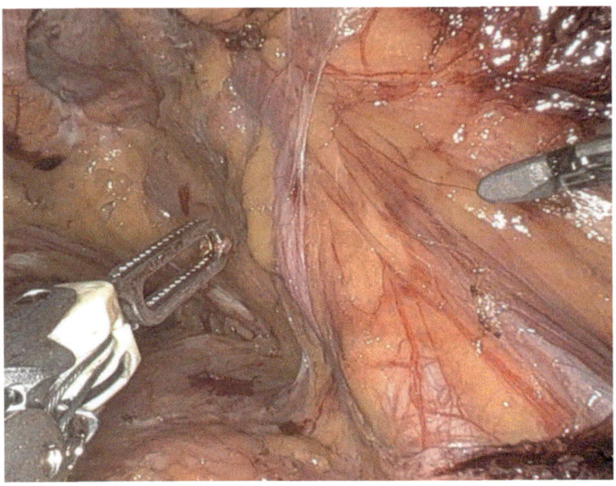

Fig. 20.4 Parietalization of the cord structures. Upward traction of the peritoneal flap should not cause movement of the cord structures

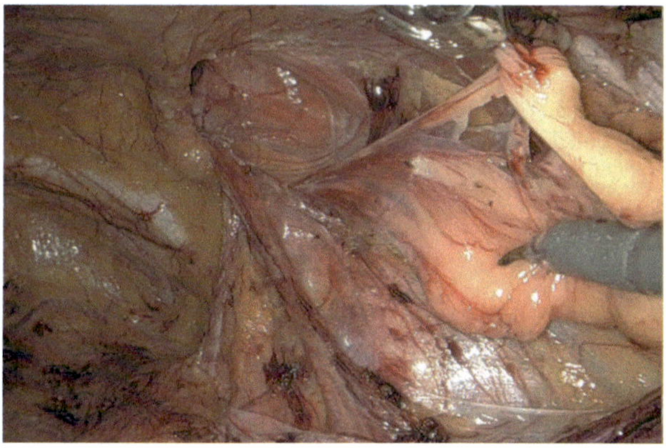

Fig. 20.5 A large cord lipoma encountered during a right inguinal hernia repair. The cord lipoma is a piece of retroperitoneal fat that originates from the lateral wall and passes through the deep inguinal ring. Care is taken to dissect the gonadal vessels away medially

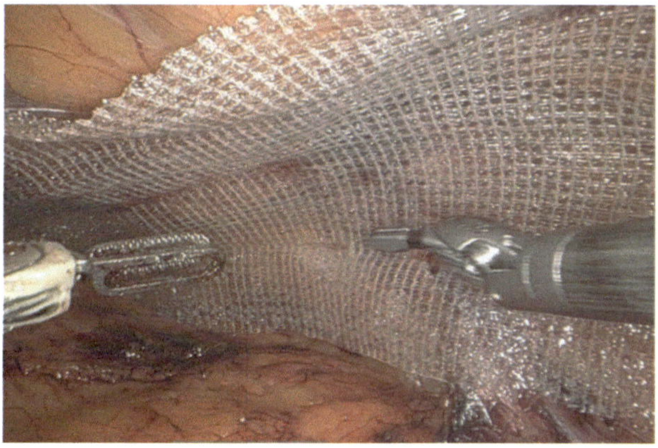

Fig. 20.6 Placement of self-gripping mesh

Aggressive dissection in this area, particularly step 5 of the CV of the MPO, may potentially cause injury to these structures. The "triangle of pain" is found laterally, bounded by the iliopubic tract, gonadal vessels, and peritoneal fold. This area contains branches of the genitofemoral nerve and lateral femoral cutaneous nerves. Aggressive dissection should be avoided in this region with care to leave the transversalis fascia on the side wall. Exposing bare muscle on the lateral wall may lead to nerve injury. Approximately 40–50% of patients will have an anatomic variance of vessels connecting the obturator and epigastric vessels known as the corona mortis or "crown of death." Care should be given to avoid injury to these vessels while dissecting within the retropubic space of Rezius and exposing the femoral space [11].

Mesh

As mentioned, at least a 10 cm × 15 cm mesh should be utilized to ensure adequate coverage of the MPO with the goal of 3–4 cm of mesh overlap for any defect(s). There are many options for mesh that are suitable for MI

IHR. Differences in mesh include material, porosity, weight, and flat versus anatomic. The authors typically use a self-gripping polyester mesh. Given that the mesh is in an extraperitoneal position, a composite mesh is not necessary. For bilateral inguinal hernias, two meshes with adequate medial overlap are used.

The type of mesh fixation, if utilized, is typically selected based on surgeon's preference. Our general preference is to not fixate the mesh as there is evidence supporting overall equal recurrence rates when comparing fixation to non-fixation and potential for increased acute and chronic pain with fixation. However, fixation is recommended for large direct defects [7, 12]. Some literature suggests that atraumatic mesh fixation techniques such as with cyanoacrylate may reduce early postoperative pain [12]. No fixation should be placed at or below the iliopubic tract to avoid injury to neurovascular structures.

Closure

After verifying correct mesh placement and hemostasis, the peritoneal flap is then closed. It is important to address any fenestrations that may cause an intraparietal hernia. Redundant hernia sacs should be excised or oversewn to prevent intraparietal hernias. The authors use a 3-0 absorbable barbed suture for closure. Once the peritoneal flap is closed, the robot is undocked. In our practice, we insert a 5 mm laparoscopic suction cannula into the peritoneal flap to deflate the space (Fig. 20.7). Gentle pressure is applied over the patient's groin to evacuate additional CO_2 within the scrotum. Pneumoperitoneum is then released under direct visualization to ensure that the mesh stays flat along the abdominal wall. Should the mesh fold, pneumoperitoneum should be reestablished, and the mesh repositioned accordingly. If a 10 mm or greater-sized trocar was used, the fascial defect should be closed.

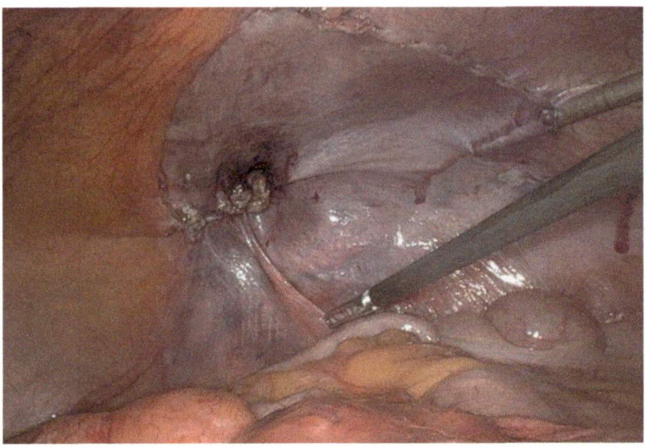

Fig. 20.7 Deflation of the preperitoneal space. The mesh can be seen with good apposition to the abdominal wall

Special Cases

Acute Presentation

Although not an absolute contraindication to robotic repair, acutely incarcerated and strangulated hernias present challenges to this approach and should be performed by experienced surgeons. Preoperative reduction of hernia contents should be attempted to facilitate minimally invasive dissection and manipulation of herniated structures. The operation is completed in the same manner as detailed earlier in the chapter. In the setting of a large, incarcerated hernia, a releasing incision may be made on the transversalis sling to increase the working space to assist with reduction of the sac. Furthermore, the ring can be enlarged with an anteromedial incision for direct hernias and with an anterolateral incision for indirect hernias. Additionally, the bedside assistant can provide external pressure to aid in reduction. If these attempts remain unsuccessful, a hybrid approach may be completed that combines the posterior approach with an open approach to reduce the contents of the sac [13].

In the setting of a strangulated hernia where ischemic bowel is identified intraoperatively, the contents should be observed and a decision made regarding bowel viability. Indocyanine green may be a useful adjunct in these cases to assess viability. If bowel resection is needed, we recommend against proceeding with mesh repair and a tissue repair should be performed either posteriorly or anteriorly.

Inguinoscrotal Hernias and Loss of Domain

There is an increased risk of recurrence with larger hernias, especially with large direct defects. It is recommended a larger mesh be used rather than the standard recommended size of 10 cm × 15 cm. Medial overlap of mesh with fixation to Cooper's ligament is critical when managing large direct hernias.

Giant inguinoscrotal hernias with loss of domain pose significant challenges in reduction of herniated contents. Intra-abdominal hypertension or abdominal compartment syndrome may occur due to the disproportion between the domain of the abdominal cavity and the herniated contents, increasing the chances of perioperative complications. Botulinum toxin injection or progressive pneumoperitoneum (PPP) may be useful adjuncts in these cases. Injection of botulinum toxin into the muscle can cause temporary muscle paralysis that can assist with elongation of the abdominal muscles to increase the intra-abdominal space. This generally is completed with injection spanning from 6 to 45 days preoperatively. This method, however, is costly and associated with prolonged hospital stay. PPP involves gradual insufflation of CO_2 into the peritoneal cavity for 1–2 weeks preoperatively to increase intra-abdominal domain and may be combined with botulinum toxin injection. Although this is another measure that can improve overall outcomes in the management of giant inguinoscrotal hernias, it is associated with increased hospital stays and potential for infection [14]. In extreme cases, visceral reduction has been described. This can add the potential for significant morbidity such as anastomotic leaks, mesh infection, and cardiopulmonary compromise after reduction.

Concomitant Inguinal Hernia Repair and Robotic-Assisted Radical Prostatectomy

Inguinal hernias and prostate cancer are commonly seen together in the older population. Prior studies have indicated a rate of 13–33% of concomitant inguinal hernias during prostatectomy [15]. Multiple studies demonstrate that robot-assisted radical prostatectomy with concomitant inguinal hernia repair is safe and does not increase mesh-related complications [16].

Common Complications

Hematomas and Seromas

Seroma and hematoma formation remains a relatively common post-operative complication of MI IHR. This is due to fluid or blood collecting in the dead space that persists after repair. Some surgeons preferentially leave drains to prevent these fluid collections. However, in our practice, we reserve drain placement for large inguinoscrotal or complex inguinal hernias. The decision for drain placement must be balanced with having a foreign body adjacent to the mesh, which theoretically may increase the chance for infection. In a recent systematic review and meta-analysis, placement of a closed suction drain in the preperitoneal space demonstrated significantly lower incidence of seroma formation [17]. Most small seromas and hematomas may be managed conservatively with observation, however, those that are large and symptomatic should be drained. One should have a low threshold to explore and evacuate early large postoperative hematomas as they can cause significant discomfort and mesh displacement. Postoperative hematomas after TAPP can be evacuated laparoscopically (Figs. 20.8 and 20.9). Hematomas that cause hemodynamic instability, are rapidly expanding, or have active contrast extravasation on CT imaging should undergo urgent exploration.

Chronic Pain

Chronic pain is pain that persists over 3 months after surgery. This is a significant postoperative complication that can have major impacts on the patient's quality of life. Minimally invasive surgery has a lower incidence of chronic pain when compared to open repairs [18]. There are some preoperative patient-related risk factors for chronic pain, such as young age, female sex, preoperative pain, and chronic pain in other locations [19]. For minimally invasive posterior approaches, extensive dissection and mesh fixation should be avoided below the iliopubic tract to avoid nerve

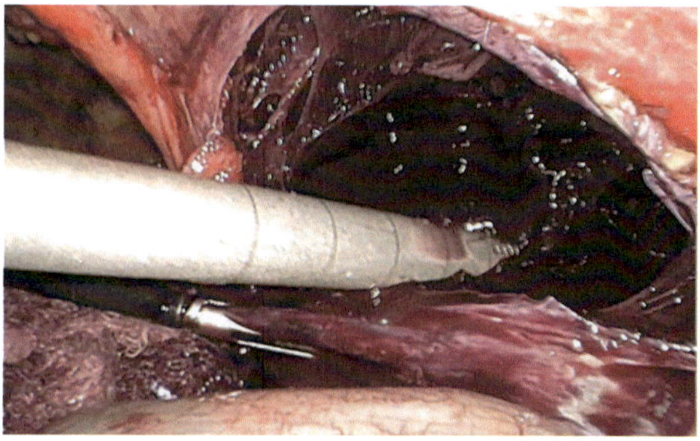

Fig. 20.8 Laparoscopic hematoma evacuation following TAPP

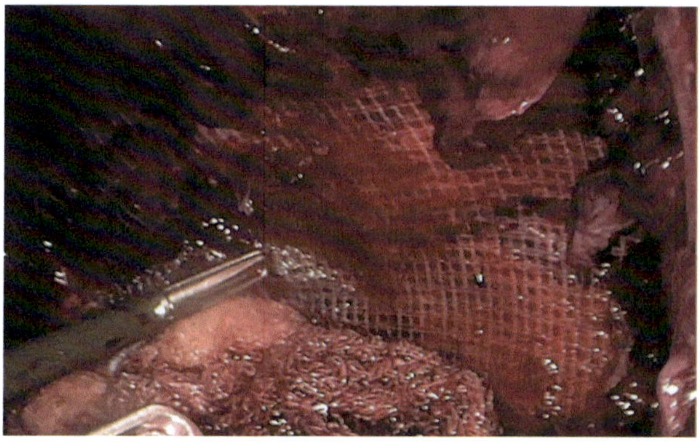

Fig. 20.9 The previously placed mesh can be seen after clot is removed

injury. Management of chronic pain begins with conservative measures such as rest and over-the-counter anti-inflammatory medications. Neuropathic pain may be treated with GABA modulators. Cases refractory to conservative management may warrant nerve blocks or surgical neurectomy. Treatment adjuncts include physical therapy and massage. A multidisciplinary approach to chronic pain patients is paramount.

Recurrence

Recurrence rates of robotic approaches to MI IHR remain similar to open repairs [20]. Conditions that chronically increase intra-abdominal pressure (i.e., chronic cough, benign prostatic hyperplasia), connective tissue disorders, and infection can increase risk for recurrence. Hernia recurrence after an anterior inguinal hernia repair should be approached posteriorly. Recurrences with mesh plugs or other three-dimensional mesh constructs may require partial mesh excision for satisfactory preperitoneal mesh placement (Fig. 20.10). If recurrence is encountered after a posterior repair, an anterior open approach is recommended. The previously placed mesh is typically left in place unless there is a compelling reason for explantation

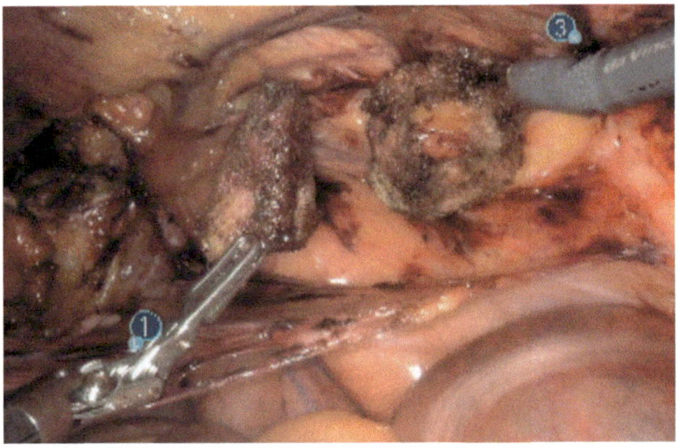

Fig. 20.10 Excised mesh plug. The plug would have hindered appropriate mesh placement

such as nerve entrapment. Should mesh excision be warranted, a new mesh is not typically placed in the same setting as it may confound postoperative results.

Testicular Ischemia

Although a rare complication, injury to the spermatic vessels can lead to ischemic orchitis. Mindfulness of the cord structures particularly while repairing large inguinoscrotal hernias with extensive sac dissection decreases the risk of injury. Primary abandonment of the hernia sac for large scrotal hernias has been shown to be an effective technique to prevent this complication [21, 22].

Mesh Infection

Mesh infection can be a devastating complication. It is important to distinguish from a superficial surgical site infection, as mesh infections tend to present in a delayed fashion and necessitate mesh removal. Conservative treatment may be initiated first, with mesh removal being performed at least 3 months after onset of infection. The uninfected part of mesh will continue incorporation, and infected part will further separate from tissue secondary to exudate, making mesh removal easier. If prior posterior repair was completed, the mesh is typically removed in similar fashion, leaving the anterior anatomy intact for future repair [23].

Conclusion

Inguinal hernia repairs are among the most common major outpatient operations performed, with a shift occurring toward minimally invasive approaches. This has been associated with decreased early postoperative pain, earlier return to daily activities, and decreased analgesic use compared to open repair. Furthermore, the robotic platform proves to be a valuable tool in the posterior repair of inguinal hernias, allowing for improved ergonomics for the surgeon.

References

1. McDermott KW, Liang L. Overview of major ambulatory surgeries performed in hospital-owned facilities, 2019; 2006.
2. Chen LS, Chen WC, Kang YN, Wu CC, Tsai LW, Liu MZ. Effects of transabdominal preperitoneal and totally extraperitoneal inguinal hernia repair: an update systematic review and meta-analysis of randomized controlled trials. Surg Endosc. 2019;33(2):418. https://doi.org/10.1007/s00464-018-6314-x.
3. Solaini L, Cavaliere D, Avanzolini A, Rocco G, Ercolani G. Robotic versus laparoscopic inguinal hernia repair: an updated systematic review and meta-analysis. J Robot Surg. 2022;16(4):775. https://doi.org/10.1007/s11701-021-01312-6.
4. Charles EJ, Mehaffey JH, Tache-Leon CA, Hallowell PT, Sawyer RG, Yang Z. Inguinal hernia repair: is there a benefit to using the robot? Surg Endosc. 2018;32(4):2131. https://doi.org/10.1007/s00464-017-5911-4.
5. Aiolfi A, Cavalli M, Micheletto G, et al. Robotic inguinal hernia repair: is technology taking over? Systematic review and meta-analysis. Hernia. 2019;23(3):509. https://doi.org/10.1007/s10029-019-01965-1.
6. Bittner R, Montgomery MA, Arregui E, et al. Update of guidelines on laparoscopic (TAPP) and endoscopic (TEP) treatment of inguinal hernia (international Endohernia society). Surg Endosc. 2015;29(2):289. https://doi.org/10.1007/s00464-014-3917-8.
7. Elmessiry MM, Gebaly AA. Laparoscopic versus open mesh repair of bilateral primary inguinal hernia: a three-armed randomized controlled trial. Ann Med Surg. 2020;59 https://doi.org/10.1016/j.amsu.2020.08.055.
8. Poulose BK, Chen DC, Poulose BK. Clinical guidelines synopsis of groin hernia management. JAMA Surg. 2020;155(10):980. https://doi.org/10.1001/jamasurg.2020.2608.
9. Zamkowski MT, Makarewicz W, Ropel J, Bobowicz M, Kąkol M, Smietański M. Antibiotic prophylaxis in open inguinal hernia repair: a literature review and summary of current knowledge. Wideochirurgia I Inne Techniki Maloinwazyjne. 2016;11(3):127. https://doi.org/10.5114/wiitm.2016.62800.
10. Daes J, Felix E. Critical view of the myopectineal orifice. Ann Surg. 2017;266(1):e1. https://doi.org/10.1097/SLA.0000000000002104.
11. Noussios G, Galanis N, Chatzis I, et al. The anatomical characteristics of Corona mortis: a systematic review of the literature and its clinical importance in hernia repair. J Clin Med Res. 2020;12(2):108. https://doi.org/10.14740/jocmr4062.
12. HerniaSurge Group. International guidelines for groin hernia management. Hernia Published online. 2018.
13. Gupta RK, Lomanto D. Laparo-endoscopic approach to complex inguinal hernia [inguinoscrotal hernias: sliding hernias]. In: Mastering endo-laparoscopic and thoracoscopic surgery; 2023. https://doi.org/10.1007/978-981-19-3755-2_58.
14. El Shamarka AH, Zidan MH, Youssef MS, El Banna AH, Mourad M. A case of giant inguino-scrotal hernia managed by preoperative pneumoperitoneum with an unforeseen complication and outcome: a case report and review of literature. Hernia. 2023;27(6) https://doi.org/10.1007/s10029-023-02870-4.
15. Bedir F, Altay MS, Kocatürk H, Bedir B, Hamidi N, Canda AE. Concurrent inguinal hernia repair during robot-assisted transperitoneal radical prostatectomy: single center experience. Robot Surg. 2021;8:39. https://doi.org/10.2147/rsrr.s339892.
16. Jaber AR, Moschovas MC, Rogers T, et al. Simultaneous hernia repair following robotic-assisted radical prostatectomy is safe with low rates of mesh-related complications. J Robot Surg. 2023;17(4):1653. https://doi.org/10.1007/s11701-023-01574-2.

17. Ng TP, Loo BYK, Chia CLK. Seroma-prevention strategies in minimally invasive inguinal hernia repair: a systematic review and meta-analysis. Int J Abdomin Wall Hernia Surgery. 2023;6(1):14. https://doi.org/10.4103/ijawhs.ijawhs_5_23.
18. Haladu N, Alabi A, Brazzelli M, et al. Open versus laparoscopic repair of inguinal hernia: an overview of systematic reviews of randomised controlled trials. Surg Endosc. 2022;36(7):4685. https://doi.org/10.1007/s00464-022-09161-6.
19. Olsson A, Sandblom G, Franneby U, Sondén A, Gunnarsson U, Dahlstrand U. Do postoperative complications correlate to chronic pain following inguinal hernia repair? A prospective cohort study from the Swedish Hernia Register. Hernia. 2023;27(1) https://doi.org/10.1007/s10029-021-02545-y.
20. Rodrigues-Gonçalves V, Verdaguer-Tremolosa M, Martínez-López P, Fernandes N, Bel R, López-Cano M. Open vs. robot-assisted preperitoneal inguinal hernia repair. Are they truly clinically different? Hernia. 2024;28(4):1355–63. https://doi.org/10.1007/s10029-024-03050-8.
21. Nikolian VC, Pereira X, Arias-Espinosa L, et al. Primary abandonment of the sac in the management of scrotal hernias: a dual-institution experience of short-term outcomes. Hernia. Published online. 2024. https://doi.org/10.1007/s10029-024-03009-9.
22. Claus C, Malcher F, Trauczynski P, et al. Primary abandon of hernia sac for inguinoscrotal hernias: a safe way to cut corners. Surg Endosc. 2023;37(11):8421. https://doi.org/10.1007/s00464-023-10416-z.
23. Zou Z, Cao J, Zhu Y, Ma Q, Chen J. Treatment of mesh infection after inguinal hernia repair: 3-year experience with 120 patients. Hernia. 2023;27(4) https://doi.org/10.1007/s10029-022-02702-x.

21 Robotic Transabdominal Preperitoneal (r-TAPP) and Intraperitoneal Onlay Mesh (r-IPOM) Hernia Repairs for Ventral Hernias

Rachel Reed, Savannah Smith, Eli Mlaver, and S. Scott Davis Jr.

Introduction

Ventral hernias are being seen with increasing frequency throughout the United States, with an average of 610,000 repairs performed annually [1]. This number has doubled since 2006. Over the past decade, there has been a steady movement toward robotic surgery with up to 32% of the repairs being performed robotically [1, 2]. Robotic techniques, many of which are adapted from concepts used in both open and laparoscopic ventral hernia repairs, continue to evolve. This includes a recent trend to make efforts to place the mesh in extraperitoneal locations. When translated to the robot, ergonomic difficulties associated with laparoscopic instruments are lessened and visualization is improved. In this chapter, we will discuss both the robotic-assisted transabdominal preperitoneal (r-TAPP) and the intraperitoneal onlay mesh (r-IPOM) hernia repairs for ventral hernias, both of which are important techniques for general surgeons to have in their armamentarium.

Preoperative Considerations

Preoperative considerations for robotic ventral hernia repairs do not differ greatly from those used in both laparoscopic and open repairs. For all cases, thorough history and physical examination should be completed, including pertinent past histories such as smoking status, diabetes, use of immunosuppressants, and obesity.

Supplementary Information The online version contains supplementary material available at https://doi.org/10.1007/978-3-031-86927-3_21.

R. Reed · S. Smith · E. Mlaver · S. Scott Davis Jr. (✉)
Department of Surgery, General and GI Surgery, Emory University School of Medicine, Atlanta, GA, USA
e-mail: sdavisj@emory.edu

S. Samreen et al. (eds.), *The SAGES Manual of Robotic Surgery*,
https://doi.org/10.1007/978-3-031-86927-3_21

Furthermore, it is important to delineate past surgical history, specifically previous abdominal wall surgeries. Physical examination is vital to assess for defect size, abdominal compliance, presence of diastasis recti, prior surgical scars (to correlate to reported surgical history), presence of central obesity or visceral adiposity, and integrity of the overlying skin envelope. For those with a more complex abdominal wall surgical history or concerning hernia examination, cross-sectional imaging should be obtained to assist in further surgical planning.

A detailed preoperative discussion of the patient's goals is critical to planning a successful plan of care. The goals of one patient may be different from those of another and these goals must be matched to the patient condition with consideration of physical presentations which may include signs of frailty, other concurrent medical conditions, the patient's activities of daily living, and local home environment. Preoperative discussion regarding different techniques is also important.

A strong knowledge of the layers of the abdominal wall is crucial prior to any hernia operation. Operative choices are not "one size fits all," and a tailored approach is necessary. The main goals of any hernia surgery include reduction of the hernia, closure of the primary defect if feasible, and developing a space where a 5 cm or more overlap of the mesh can be achieved [3]. Larger defects may be increasingly likely to require bridged repair or need for myofascial releases to achieve closure of the fascial defects, and in defects >10 cm, an open approach robotic would be recommended [4]. In return for a more complicated dissection (facilitated by robotic advantages for most surgeons), r-TAPP allows for the mesh to be placed in an extraperitoneal location, theoretically decreasing the risk of adhesions or mesh-related complications. It also allows for closure of the fascia that has been dissected off the hernia sac, and decreased requirement for fixation which can be associated with increased postoperative pain. If the surgeon is unable to create an adequate peritoneal flap or the patient is found to have multiple small ventral hernias ("Swiss cheese hernia"), then r-IPOM is preferred. Other considerations while creating the flap include the increased robotic difficulty of a dissection in incisional defects when compared to primary defects as well as in larger defects as the peritoneum becomes less robust as the dissection moves further off the midline.

Intraoperative Considerations

Positioning and Preparation

Patients should be prepared robotic using agreed-upon enhanced recovery protocols employed increasingly and now considered standard of care. They should be administered the appropriate preoperative antibiotics, SCDs should be in place, and abdominal hair should be clipped. Patient preparation and positioning are similar for both techniques and the same port orientation can be used.

The patient is positioned supine. A Foley catheter is considered depending on surgeon discretion but is not required in most cases. Once the surgeon has determined port laterality (further discussed below), the surgeon can choose to position the arms in several ways. Both arms can be tucked, the ipsilateral arm is tucked with a loose sling to allow the arm to drop posteriorly to ensure full range of motion of the robotic arms with the contralateral arm extended, or both arms can be extended on arm boards. We have found the benefit of increasing the domain for the port locations by positioning the patient over the break in the bed and flexing 10–15 degrees to increase the space between the subcostal margin and the iliac crest. The patient should be strapped securely to the table in case table repositioning is needed during the operation. The abdomen should be prepped from the xiphoid to the pubis and as far lateral as possible, especially on the side designated for port placement.

Port Placement and Robotic Docking

Similar to the ports placed in conventional laparoscopic ventral hernia repair, the ports are placed laterally so the hernia defect can be triangulated by the three robotic arms needed for the case. Abdominal access is often gained via OptiView or Veress needle entry. This site can be influenced by previous surgeries, hernia location, and preoperative imaging findings. Access is most often obtained at Palmer's point, on the left side at the midclavicular line approximately 2–3 cm from the costal margin. If there is any concern regarding the safety of obtaining access at Palmer's point, an alternative entry point or open cutdown should be chosen.

Once pneumoperitoneum has been established, robotic port placement can begin. We typically use pneumoperitoneum pressures of 15 mm Hg, but after docking can consider decreasing the pressure if the abdominal domain will allow as this allows for easier defect closure and flatter prosthetic placement. If pneumoperitoneum is decreased during the case, remote centers should be reconfirmed as this can affect the depth of the trocars. Under direct visualization using the 5 mm laparoscopic trocar, two robotic ports are placed. The middle 8 mm port will be for the camera and should be as lateral as possible to allow more room for the working ports. Ideally, this port is approximately 15 cm from the hernia defect to facilitate visualization and dissection of the edge of the defect closest to the ports. In the lower quadrant, another 8 mm robotic trocar is placed slightly more medial to the camera port and superior to the iliac crest. This port should be assessed for potential conflict with the patient's thigh prior to starting the operation. If the trocar at Palmer's point can be used for the surgery, the port should be upsized to an 8 mm robotic trocar. If not, a third robotic 8 mm trocar should be placed cranial and just medial to the camera port. The three ports along the lateral abdomen should be in an arc and approximately 8 cm apart from one another. Care is taken during port placement to mentally visualize the arcs of the surgical arms and to anticipate arm conflicts which will be most apparent at the extreme ends of the proposed peritoneal flap closure. If the ports are placed too medial, the flap creation and subsequent closure will be more difficult. Facile bedside support familiar with robotic ergonomics and adjustment of robotic arms can also avoid significant frustration and difficulties during the case.

After the robotic trocars have been placed, the robot can be docked. The robot should be brought toward the patient laterally from the side opposite the ports.

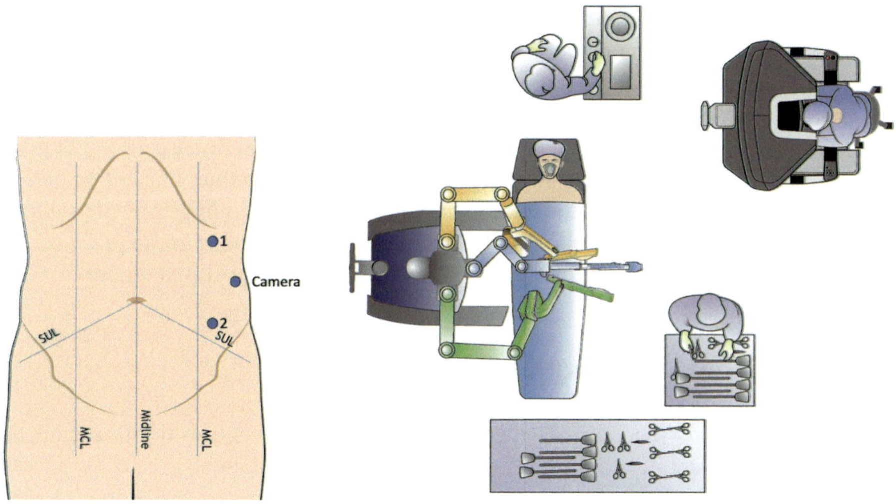

Fig. 21.1 Robotic ventral hernia repair port placement and operating room setup

Initial instruments include a grasping instrument (e.g., fenestrated bipolar or Prograsp) and monopolar scissors (Fig. 21.1).

R-TAPP

Similar to laparoscopic ventral hernia repair, the abdominal wall must be cleared of adhesions. If the hernia cannot be reduced preoperatively, it should be carefully reduced at this time or it will interfere with later attempts to reduce the sac. This can be facilitated by gentle external pressure from the bedside assistant if needed. The surgeon must be careful to avoid injury to any bowel involved with the hernia or surrounding adhesions and to preserve the peritoneum, which is essential to the repair. Once this has been completed, the surgeon will create the preperitoneal flap.

The preperitoneal flap should be started using monopolar scissors several centimeters lateral from the hernia defect on the side closest to the ports. In general, a larger overlap is better, and we try to start 10 cm from the defect when possible. A rule of thumb is to place a prosthetic that would cover the original defect by 5 cm in all directions, thus guiding the size for the flap. For example, a 2 cm defect warrants a 12 cm mesh (2 cm defect +5 cm overlap on each side), and a 6 cm defect would warrant a 16 cm prosthetic. This highlights how increasingly larger defects require larger dissections for an optimal repair and why larger defects may be better treated with other techniques.

The flap is then further developed via sharp and blunt dissection (sparing electrocautery use) such that there is adequate space circumferentially around the hernia for mesh placement and adequate overlap. In most cases, we endeavor to reduce the peritoneal sac as part of the peritoneal flap, and this is more difficult in incisional cases. Defects in this portion of the flap are more frequent in incisional cases and can usually be repaired later in the case. If an adequate flap cannot be developed given multiple ventral hernias or poor-quality peritoneum resulting in a flap with multiple defects, the surgeon should elect to transition to r-IPOM.

After an adequate preperitoneal flap has been created, the hernia defect should be closed primarily with long-term absorbable or permanent suture; barbed suture is preferred to facilitate this closure. This should be done using a running stitch that incorporates tissue from the hernia sac, if not reduced, to help close this space and reduce the risk of seroma formation. Incorporating subcutaneous tissue in this closure is not effective and may lead to puckering of the skin.

Following primary closure of the hernia defect, an appropriately sized uncoated mesh is introduced into the abdominal cavity and placed within the preperitoneal flap. Depending on the hernia and patient characteristics, we typically decide between self-fixating prosthetic which is lighter weight and standard flat sheet light/midweight polypropylene mesh. The latter requires sentinel fixation of the mesh while self-fixating meshes may not require further fixation. The mesh should be centered over the closed hernia defect. Once the mesh is appropriately placed, the peritoneal flap is closed with a running absorbable suture and any flap defects are subsequently closed primarily.

IPOM

IPOM is the most common current surgical approach for minimally invasive ventral hernia repair and the procedure for which there is the most long-term data about efficacy. Robotic hernia repair with intraperitoneal onlay mesh is indicated in patients with "Swiss cheese" defects, lateral hernia defects, and in patients without a peritoneal layer sufficient to create a preperitoneal flap [5].

The initial steps are similar to those of r-TAPP: clearing off the anterior abdominal wall by reducing the hernia and removing fatty tissue and adhesions and closing the primary defect with barbed absorbable suture if possible. The abdominal wall should be measured to select a composite mesh with an anti-adhesion barrier that will allow for adequate overlap circumferentially. Again, mesh size is chosen as described above and ideally based on original defect size plus 5 cm overlap in all directions. Defects are closed whenever possible which can be facilitated by decreasing pneumoperitoneum or placement of trans-facial sutures with a suture passer to help distribute the tension. After defect closure, the middle of the mesh should be marked, and two absorbable barbed sutures should be placed at what will be the cranial and caudal aspects of the mesh. The prepared mesh is rolled and introduced into the abdomen via a lateral port site. After unrolling the mesh, it is imperative to identify the uncoated and coated sides. The uncoated side is placed against the peritoneum, while the coated side faces the intraperitoneal contents. The technique for securing the mesh is surgeon dependent. Most commonly, a chandelier stitch is placed through the center of the incision to help position the mesh appropriately. The suture is then used to secure the edge of the mesh to the abdominal wall in a running fashion. A dolphin suturing technique is used most often. This involves small bites with minimal travel on the mesh and larger bites and travel on the tissue, minimizing the exposure of the barbed sutures to the abdominal viscera. Alternatively, monofilament sutures may be used if there is concern about the use of barbed sutures. Of note, in cases that require larger meshes (larger than 15 cm x 20 cm), we have noted more difficulty in using the robotic platform due to limitations caused by robotic arm collisions during the extremes of mesh fixation.

Conclusion

The significant increase in the number of ventral hernias requiring repair each year in the United States highlights the importance of the development and continuous evolution of surgical techniques for repair, including robot TAPP and IPOM. The outcomes including early readmission, urinary retention, hematoma, and seroma in these robotic-assisted repairs are similar to those seen in laparoscopic techniques [6]. Long-term outcomes including quality of life and recurrence favor robotic and laparoscopic repair, respectively [7]. While the learning curve is steep, requiring at least 46 cases to become proficient and optimize operative time, the shift toward robotic repair highlights the substantial advantages, including improved visibility and ergonomics [8]. As the rate of ventral hernias continues to increase in the United States, there will inevitably be continued refinement of these robotic techniques and development of further technologies to reduce recurrence and postoperative complications.

References

1. Schlosser KA, Renshaw SM, Tamer RM, Strassels SA, Poulose BK. Ventral hernia repair: an increasing burden affecting abdominal core health. Hernia. 2023;27(2):415–21. https://doi.org/10.1007/s10029-022-02707-6. Epub 2022 Dec 26. PMID: 36571666.
2. Sheetz KH, Claflin J, Dimick JB. Trends in the adoption of robotic surgery for common surgical procedures. JAMA Netw Open. 2020;3(1):e1918911. https://doi.org/10.1001/jamanetworkopen.2019.18911.
3. LeBlanc K. Proper mesh overlap is a key determinant in hernia recurrence following laparoscopic ventral and incisional hernia repair. Hernia. 2016;20(1):85–99. https://doi.org/10.1007/s10029-015-1399-9. Epub 2015 Jul 5. PMID: 26143072.
4. Earle D, Roth JS, Saber A, et al. SAGES guidelines for laparoscopic ventral hernia repair. Surg Endosc. 2016;30:3163–83. https://doi.org/10.1007/s00464-016-5072-x.
5. Sharma A, Berger D. The current role of laparoscopic IPOM repair in abdominal wall reconstruction. Hernia. 2018;22:739–41. https://doi.org/10.1007/s10029-018-1820-2.
6. Kennedy M, Barrera K, Akcelik A, Constable Y, Smith M, Chung P, Sugiyama G. Robotic TAPP ventral hernia repair: early lessons learned at an Inner City Safety Net Hospital. JSLS. 2018;22(1):e2017.00070. https://doi.org/10.4293/JSLS.2017.00070. PMID: 29472756; PMCID: PMC5802768.
7. Petro C, Thomas J, Tu C, Krpata D, Beffa L, Rosen M, Prabhu A. Robotic vs laparoscopic ventral hernia repair with intraperitoneal mesh: 1-year exploratory outcomes of the PROVE-IT

randomized clinical trial. J Am Coll Surg. 2022;234(6):1160–5. https://doi.org/10.1097/XCS.0000000000000171.

8. Kudsi OY, Gokcal F, Bou-Ayash N, Crawford AS, Chung SK, Chang K, Litwin D. Learning curve in robotic transabdominal preperitoneal (rTAPP) ventral hernia repair: a cumulative sum (CUSUM) analysis. Hernia. 2021;25(3):755–64. https://doi.org/10.1007/s10029-020-02228-0. Epub 2020 Jun 3. PMID: 32495055; PMCID: PMC7268975.

22 Complex Robotic Abdominal Wall Reconstruction

Cigdem Benlice, Bilgi Baca, and Omar Yusef Kudsi

Background

The evolution of ventral hernia repair techniques over the past several decades reflects a dynamic landscape in surgical approaches. When addressing complex ventral hernias requiring abdominal wall reconstruction (AWR), the substantiated evidence underscores the efficacy of achieving a durable repair through meticulous placement of mesh in the retromuscular position, coupled with the implementation of transversus abdominis release (TAR) techniques [1, 2]. Despite the historical preference for an open surgical approach in AWR, especially for addressing large and complex ventral hernias, the landscape is evolving with the growing popularity of robotic platforms, challenging traditional paradigms. Over the past decade, there has been a swift adoption of robotic surgical techniques, with a notable surge in their utilization within the realm of hernia repair, even in the absence of abundant high-level evidence [3].

The progressive integration of minimally invasive approaches by general surgeons, driven by advancements in surgical technology, has become a hallmark of contemporary surgical practice. LeBlanc and Booth first introduced laparoscopic ventral hernia repair (LVHR) in 1993 [4]. This minimally invasive approach, characterized by smaller incisions and gentler tissue handling, is associated with decreased postoperative pain, shorter recovery times, reduced hospital length of stay, and fewer wound complications when compared to open ventral hernia repair [5, 6]. Although laparoscopy has become standard in routine ventral hernia repairs, its application in the context of more intricate AWR procedures has been hampered

C. Benlice · B. Baca
Department of General Surgery, Acibadem Mehmet Ali Aydinlar University School of Medicine, Istanbul, Turkey

O. Y. Kudsi (✉)
Department of Surgery, Brigham and Women's Hospital, Harvard Medical School, Boston, MA, USA

S. Samreen et al. (eds.), *The SAGES Manual of Robotic Surgery*,
https://doi.org/10.1007/978-3-031-86927-3_22

by ergonomic challenges, particularly in accessing the retromuscular plane and executing intracorporeal suturing [7, 8]. As a consequence, open repairs have traditionally been perceived as the only viable approach for addressing large and complex defects. While proponents of robotic surgery emphasize the inherent benefits of a minimally invasive approach and underscore the perceived ergonomic advantages of the robotic console, critics express reservations regarding the associated increase in costs, extended operating room times, and a lack of clear-cut advantages over existing techniques. Despite the absence of high-quality evidence, the escalating interest in integrating robotic surgery into ventral hernia repairs prompts a pivotal inquiry into the tangible clinical benefits that may arise from this innovative approach [9].

As minimally invasive techniques gain widespread acceptance, an escalating number of studies have delved into exploring the outcomes of hernia repairs employing various approaches. In this setting, we provide an in-depth analysis of the complex robotic abdominal wall reconstruction technique and a summary of the present status of the existing evidence.

Definition of the Complex Abdominal Wall

The term "complex abdominal wall" encompasses various scenarios, generally referring to a patient's abdomen presenting with a ventral or incisional hernia or defect along with one or more of the following characteristics [10, 11]:

(a) History of previous mesh/related wound infection: A history of, or an ongoing, mesh or wound infection.
(b) Loss of domain: Instances where there is a reduction in the functional capacity or volume of the abdominal cavity, known as loss of domain.
(c) Recurrent hernia: One or more recurrences of the hernia.
(d) Large-sized defect: A large-sized defect, often defined as exceeding 10 cm in diameter.
(e) Enterocutaneous fistula: The presence of an enterocutaneous fistula.
(f) Extensive damage to the abdominal wall tissues, which may result from trauma, infection, or complications from prior surgeries.

Patients with complex abdominal walls often seek surgical repair for various reasons. This complexity can arise due to various factors, including the presence of large or recurrent hernias, extensive tissue damage, or complications from previous surgeries. A surgeon intending to approach the repair of a complex abdominal wall should be trained and prepared to employ a range of techniques as needed to achieve a favorable outcome. The management of a complex abdominal wall requires a thorough assessment of the patient's medical history, physical examination, and often advanced imaging studies. Surgical planning for complex abdominal wall repairs may involve specialized techniques, including component separation, mesh reinforcement, or even advanced technologies like robotic-assisted procedures.

Overall, the term "complex abdominal wall" underscores the challenges and intricacies involved in addressing specific conditions affecting the abdominal wall, necessitating a tailored and often multidisciplinary approach to achieve optimal outcomes [11].

The revised classification system developed by the Modified Ventral Hernia Working Group (mVHWG) stratifies hernia patients into different grades according to wound cleanliness and related risk factors: Grade 1 pertains to wounds that are clean with minimal risk of complications, grade 2 involves clean wounds with concurrent comorbidities or previous infections, and grade 3 encompasses clean contaminated to dirty wounds [12]. Acknowledging the limitations of the mVHWG in addressing hernia size considerations, the 2018 Dutch guideline on incisional hernias proposed a shift toward adopting the Hernia Patient Wound (HPW) classification [13]. This classification, similar to TNM staging, is designed to predict postoperative outcomes based solely on preoperative characteristics. Hernia width (H) is categorized as grade 1 (0–9.9 cm), grade 2 (10–19.9 cm), or grade 3 (>20.0 cm), while patient (P) comorbidities are noted as absent (0) or present (1) for instances of a BMI >35 kg/m2, current nicotine use, diabetes, or immunosuppression. Wound (W) or surgical field cleanliness is assessed as clean (0) or contaminated (1). When addressing complex hernias, robotic TAR at HPW stage II–IV emerges as the primary repair method, often favored by experienced robotic hernia surgeons [14].

A recent Delphi study conducted by the European Hernia Society (EHS) identified factors crucial to defining a complex incisional hernia [15]. Eighteen factors pertaining to the hernia and abdominal wall, the potential for concurrent infection in the surgical site, and patient comorbidities were incorporated into the definition. A hernia width exceeding 10 cm was deemed a significant threshold for complexity. While a first-time recurrent incisional hernia did not achieve consensus, consensus was reached for cases involving two or more previous repairs with subsequent recurrence. Various factors associated with prior abdominal surgeries, tissue manipulation, tissue removal, and previous use of component separation techniques also attained consensus, highlighting the influence of past surgeries on future hernia repairs. Only two patient-related factors deemed essential by the experts for defining a complex incisional hernia were a body mass index of at least 40 kg/m^2 and cirrhosis with ascites. These factors had previously been identified as independent risk factors for unfavorable postoperative outcomes [16].

Rationality and Adaption of Robotic Surgery

The rationality and adaptability of robotic surgery in ventral hernia repair are well supported by findings in the literature. Research studies, such as those by Belyansky et al., have shed light on the rational use of robotic platforms in complex abdominal wall reconstructions, especially for patients with large hernias requiring sophisticated techniques like TAR [17]. These studies demonstrate that robotic-assisted approaches can provide comparable operative times and clinical outcomes to traditional open methods while offering advantages such as reduced hospital stays and potentially lower overall costs [6]. The adaptability of robotic surgery is evident in its application to ventral hernia repairs, providing surgeons with enhanced precision and maneuverability in challenging anatomical scenarios. As the literature consistently highlights, the rational incorporation and adaptive nature of robotic surgery contribute to improved patient outcomes and represent a valuable tool in the evolving landscape of ventral hernia repair.

The emergence of robotic technology has brought about a transformative shift in the field of complex AWR, providing a novel solution that facilitates a minimally invasive approach. The substantial rise in the yearly estimated robotic cases for general surgeons, escalating from 10,000 to 246,000 between 2010 and 2017, reflects the swift and widespread adoption of this advanced technology. Notably, in the context of ventral hernia repairs, the use of robotic surgery has experienced a remarkable surge, witnessing a 44.8-fold increase between 2012 and 2018. This surge signifies a growing recognition and acceptance of robotic-assisted approaches within the surgical community, underlining the technology's potential benefits and applications in the specific domain of ventral hernia repairs [3, 18]. Robotic surgery is acclaimed for its purported enhancements in dexterity, precision, three-dimensional optics, and surgeon ergonomics. These advancements, including improved maneuverability and increased degrees of freedom, hold the potential to facilitate the repair of large or complex hernias that necessitate component separation techniques such as TAR [19]. However, this innovative approach comes with certain drawbacks, including elevated costs, reduced accessibility, and extended operative times in comparison to alternative methods. The ongoing debate revolves around whether the perceived benefits of robotic surgery can be justified in light of these associated costs and considerations.

Comparison of Different Surgical Approaches

In recent years, there has been a notable surge in interest in robotic surgery, driven by its potential to provide enhanced dexterity, precision, three-dimensional optics, and improved surgeon ergonomics. This research endeavors to assess whether these anticipated advantages result in measurable changes in both clinical and economic outcomes in ventral hernia repair. The focal points of evaluation include hospital length of stay and the recurrence of hernias, serving as primary indicators to gauge the impact of robotic surgery on patient outcomes and the overall economic landscape [20, 21].

In the realm of complex hernia surgery and abdominal wall reconstruction, open ventral hernia repair remains the conventional approach adopted by most surgeons [22]. Component separation techniques, such as TAR, prove beneficial in the repair of large and intricate hernias [23–25]. Mobilizing muscle and fascial layers during component separation facilitates a tension-free closure of the hernia defect, leading to enhanced abdominal wall function, particularly in cases involving loss of domain. However, the laparoscopic application of component separation is infrequently conducted due to ergonomic constraints. Robotic ventral hernia repair (RVHR) presents a compelling alternative, combining the benefits of minimally invasive surgery with improved access to anatomical planes that might be restricted in laparoscopic approaches [26]. Sub-analyses comparing robotic TAR (R-TAR) and open TAR (O-TAR) reveal that R-TAR is associated with a reduced hospital length of stay and a lower 30-day readmission rate, albeit at the expense of a longer operative time. Notably, intraoperative and wound complications did not exhibit significant differences between the two approaches. It is essential to acknowledge the limitations of these sub-analyses, which are constrained by the relatively low number of available studies, with fewer than 10 investigations exploring the role of robotic surgery in ventral hernia repair involving TAR. The majority of studies consistently highlight that RVHR is associated with higher costs and longer operative times in comparison to other surgical approaches, notably surpassing LVHR. The elevated costs attributed to RVHR include expenses related to robotic systems, software, equipment, and maintenance, outweighing the costs associated with both laparoscopic and open surgery [25, 27–29]. The financial considerations related to robotic surgery may be partially offset by potential reductions in hospital costs linked to shorter hospital length of stay and fewer complications. However, it's important to note that the validity of cost analyses is compromised by variations in reported cost calculations among different studies. Furthermore, the economic landscape is likely to differ between countries and economies, contributing to the complexity of assessing the true economic impact of RVHR. To enhance the reliability of future cost analyses, researchers may consider adopting shared and specific criteria for comparing both total and constituent costs. This approach could provide a more comprehensive understanding of the economic implications of RVHR and facilitate the development of strategies to mitigate associated costs. Additionally, exploring alternatives such as the use of recyclable or reusable equipment, as opposed to disposable items, may contribute to cost reduction in the equipment-related aspect of robotic surgery. Considering the evolving nature of the market, the emergence of new competitors offers the potential for increased affordability of robotic systems in the future. This aspect underscores the importance of ongoing research and exploration of cost-effective strategies to enhance the accessibility and feasibility of RVHR.

RVHR is notably associated with a significant increase in operative time compared to both LVHR and OVHR [23]. This extended operative duration in RVHR can be attributed to additional steps involved in docking/undocking equipment and the learning curve for operators [6, 27].

The increased operative time in RVHR may be influenced by factors such as the unique steps contributing to the prolonged duration, including setup and calibration of robotic equipment. It is foreseeable that with enhanced training, increased operator experience, and advancements in equipment setup, operative times and corresponding costs would likely decrease. As operators become more proficient and efficient in the use of robotic systems, the learning curve impact could diminish. Investigating specific factors that contribute to the prolonged operative time in RVHR could provide valuable insights. Understanding the nuances of each step and identifying areas for improvement may contribute to streamlining the surgical process and ultimately reducing the associated costs. As the field continues to evolve, research into these specific factors and ongoing advancements in technology and training may play a pivotal role in enhancing the efficiency and cost-effectiveness of RVHR procedures.

The management of hernia in individuals with obesity necessitates a multidisciplinary strategy. Obese patients experience notably higher perioperative complications and recurrence rates. For those at a low risk of hernia complications, undergoing a bariatric procedure prior to hernia repair might be considered. The outcomes of laparoscopic hernia repair in overweight patients have been enhanced through the adoption of robotic techniques, resulting in a high success rate in closing gaps and implanting mesh extraperitoneally [30]. The investigation into perioperative outcomes in patients undergoing RVHR has previously overlooked retrospectively a comparison between those with a BMI above 35 kg/m^2 and those below this threshold by our group. Despite this gap, our findings suggest that individuals with a BMI of 35 kg/m^2 or higher experience similar advantages from RVHR as their counterparts with a lower BMI [31]. Surprisingly, our study did not uncover any discernible differences between these two groups regarding postoperative morbidity and serious surgical events. This unexpected result challenges our initial hypothesis, indicating that BMI $\geq$ 35 kg/m^2 does not exert a significant influence on the short-term postoperative outcomes of RVHR. Moreover, the absence of notable perioperative morbidity, the avoidance of conversions to conventional surgeries, and the lack of perioperative mortality collectively underscore the safety and efficacy of RVHR in patients classified as class II and class III obese. These outcomes provide compelling support for the utilization of RVHR as a viable surgical option in this demographic. Our previous research marks a significant milestone as the pioneering exploration of RVHR in individuals classified as morbidly obese. Our findings provide robust evidence supporting the safety and feasibility of implementing RVHR in this challenging patient demographic. Notably, we identified several key factors—such as elevated BMI, the extent of adhesiolysis, prolonged off-console time during surgery, and the placement of intraperitoneal mesh—that correlated with heightened complication rates, particularly concerning early postoperative pain and discomfort [32]. Moving forward, it is imperative that further prospective studies are undertaken to delve deeper into the nuanced role of robotic surgery in the management of hernias in morbidly obese patients. These forthcoming investigations will play a pivotal role in not only refining surgical techniques but also in optimizing patient outcomes within this specific subset of the population. Further development of interdisciplinary protocols is required to facilitate a personalized approach. Subsequent research endeavors will continue to refine the advantages of robotic surgery and offer guidance for optimal customization.

Perioperative management presents a complex challenge, especially for patients reliant on antiplatelets and anticoagulants due to severe comorbidities like atrial fibrillation and coronary artery disease. Discontinuing these medications to mitigate the risk of excessive bleeding during surgery may elevate the risk of thrombotic events both during and after the procedure. While previous studies have explored this dilemma, they predominantly predate the era of minimally invasive surgery. We conducted a previous study to investigate the impact of antithrombotic medication on the postoperative trajectory of patients undergoing robotic ventral hernia repair [33]. Our findings revealed that patients receiving antithrombotic therapy exhibited an inherent predisposition to bleeding-related events, notably a higher incidence of postoperative hematomas. Additionally, these patients experienced a higher frequency of higher-grade complications and morbidity scores. Specifically, anticoagulants like warfarin and NOACs correlated with an elevated risk of bleeding-related complications, ranging from mild ecchymoses to severe gastrointestinal bleeding. This aligns with prior research indicating that anticoagulated patients undergoing surgery face an increased susceptibility to thromboembolic events and perioperative bleeding. Furthermore, the combination of advancing age and anticoagulant therapy significantly escalated the risk of postoperative bleeding and thromboembolic events. For instance, patients over 80 years old exhibited an almost threefold increase in the incidence rate of major hemorrhage compared to those under 60 years old. Interestingly, antiplatelet therapy, which remained uninterrupted for all patients in our cohort, did not demonstrate a significant association with increased bleeding-related events.

As the field continues to evolve, future studies could play a pivotal role in further delineating the precise role of robotic surgery in the context of large and complex hernia repair and abdominal wall reconstruction.

Preoperative Planning

Conducting a comprehensive history and physical examination is essential for deciding an effective operative plan. In particular, the presence of comorbidities such as diabetes, obesity, smoking, and collagen vascular disease can significantly impact the strategic approach to the operation. The inclusion of a computerized tomography scan for the abdomen and pelvis is crucial in preoperative planning, serving as the gold standard imaging test. This imaging modality allows for the identification of key details, including the size and location of the hernia defect, the contents of the hernia sac, and potentially the position of previously implanted mesh. By combining a thorough medical history with imaging results, surgeons can establish a risk/benefit ratio. This scale can then be presented to patients, enabling them to make well-informed decisions regarding the most suitable approach for addressing their specific hernia condition.

As a component of the preoperative preparation for hernia surgery, patients undergo a series of measures aimed at optimizing the surgical environment and patient safety. Mechanical bowel preparation is conducted to clear the bowel of its contents, reducing the risk of contamination during the procedure. To establish an optimal concentration from the outset, preoperative broad-spectrum intravenous antibiotics are administered within 30–60 minutes of the scheduled incision time. Deep venous prophylaxis is implemented using sequential compression devices to prevent venous thromboembolism, complemented by chemical prophylaxis through the administration of preoperative heparin. In standard practice, a Foley catheter and intraoperative orogastric tube are routinely placed in all cases to facilitate urinary drainage and prevent gastric distension, respectively. These comprehensive preoperative measures collectively contribute to creating a controlled and safe operative environment for hernia surgery, minimizing the risk of complications and ensuring patient well-being throughout the procedure.

The rectus to defect ratio (RDR) was developed to aid in preoperative surgical decision-making, serving as a valuable tool for predicting fascial closure during open incisional hernia repair with bilateral rectus myofascial release and placement of retromuscular mesh. This metric offers an objective measure that can be easily replicated using basic CT imaging. However, concerns arise regarding the applicability of RDR in robotic repairs, given the requirement for pneumo-insufflation during the procedure, which may affect its predictability as initially described for open repairs. The findings of this study affirm that RDR remains valid for robotic repair, albeit with a notable shift toward higher ratios. Specifically, an RDR exceeding 2.5 indicates a 94.2% likelihood of achieving fascial closure in robotic enhanced view total extraperitoneal (eTEP) repairs utilizing bilateral rectus myofascial release alone [34]. This underscores the utility of RDR as a simple, cost-effective, readily available, and reproducible method for anticipating the necessity of lateral myofascial release to achieve fascial closure following retromuscular dissection, applicable to both open and robotic approaches. The incorporation of RDR into surgical planning not only facilitates patient informed consent but also informs clinicians about the potential requirement for referral for specialized complex abdominal wall reconstruction procedures.

Botox Injection

In certain clinical contexts involving loss of domain due to muscle retraction and large defects exceeding 20 cm in width, the strategic application of botulinum toxin A (Botox®) has demonstrated efficacy in optimizing preoperative planning. Botox is utilized to induce temporary paralysis, resulting in elongation of the lateral abdominal wall muscles by an average of 4 cm. The procedure involves administering 200–300 units of Botox, appropriately diluted in 30 ml of saline, via six targeted injections meticulously delivered into both the external and internal oblique muscles, guided by ultrasound visualization. Patients typically undergo follow-up within 4 weeks, including a repeat CT scan to assess hernia volume before definitive robotic hernia repair as a predictor of complications. However, relying solely on absolute measurements may lead to unreliable outcomes due to variations in total abdominal volume among patients. To establish a more standardized measure across individuals, expressing hernia volume as a ratio or percentage of the total volume may be necessary. Additionally, defining intra-abdominal volume could vary depending on whether retroperitoneal organs are included or excluded from measurement [35].

Patient Selection

Regarding for the indications and contraindications for robotic TAR are not clearly determined in the literature as of now. Patients with an elevated risk of wound complications, such as those with diabetes, chronic obstructive pulmonary disease, or obesity, are likely to derive benefits from this minimally invasive approach. Individuals exhibiting poor skin condition, including extensive scars from prior wound issues or skin grafts, are not suitable candidates for robotic TAR. Caution is warranted when approaching hernias exceeding 20 cm, as closing such substantial defects can be challenging even in open approach. The decision on whether to proceed with robotic approach in these cases relies on the surgeon's judgment, experience, and the patient's abdominal wall compliance upon physical examination. Successful application of the robotic approach has been demonstrated for the closure of defects measuring 20 cm and beyond. On the other hand, patients with hernias, less than 10 cm, typically do not necessitate extensive myofascial release for defect reapproximation. Defects of this size are commonly repaired using variations of robotic ventral hernia repair, either through preperitoneal mesh placement or a single-dock approach that avoids TAR [6, 36].

Operative Procedure

Patient Positioning

The appropriate positioning of the patient is a critical aspect of surgical preparation, tailored to the specific characteristics of the abdominal wall defect. For midline abdominal wall defects located between the semilunar lines, the patient is placed in a supine position.

In contrast, for flank and lateral abdominal wall defects, a lateral decubitus position could be employed. This position involves the use of arm board and bean bag or other appropriate positioning devices to achieve optimal alignment (Fig. 22.1). These meticulous patient positioning strategies ensure accessibility and precision during hernia surgery while prioritizing patient safety and comfort.

Port Placement and Docking

Trocars are strategically positioned in the lateral abdominal wall, with the camera trocar placed midway between the costal margin and iliac crest, positioned near the midaxillary line. The working trocars are then placed slightly off the costal margin in the superior aspect and near the iliac crest in the inferior aspect, aligning with the anterior axillary line. This meticulous placement ensures optimal access and visualization during the surgical procedure (Fig. 22.2).

Intra-abdominal access is established through a 10 mm Optiview trocar at Palmer's point, typically located in the left upper quadrant. This step may involve

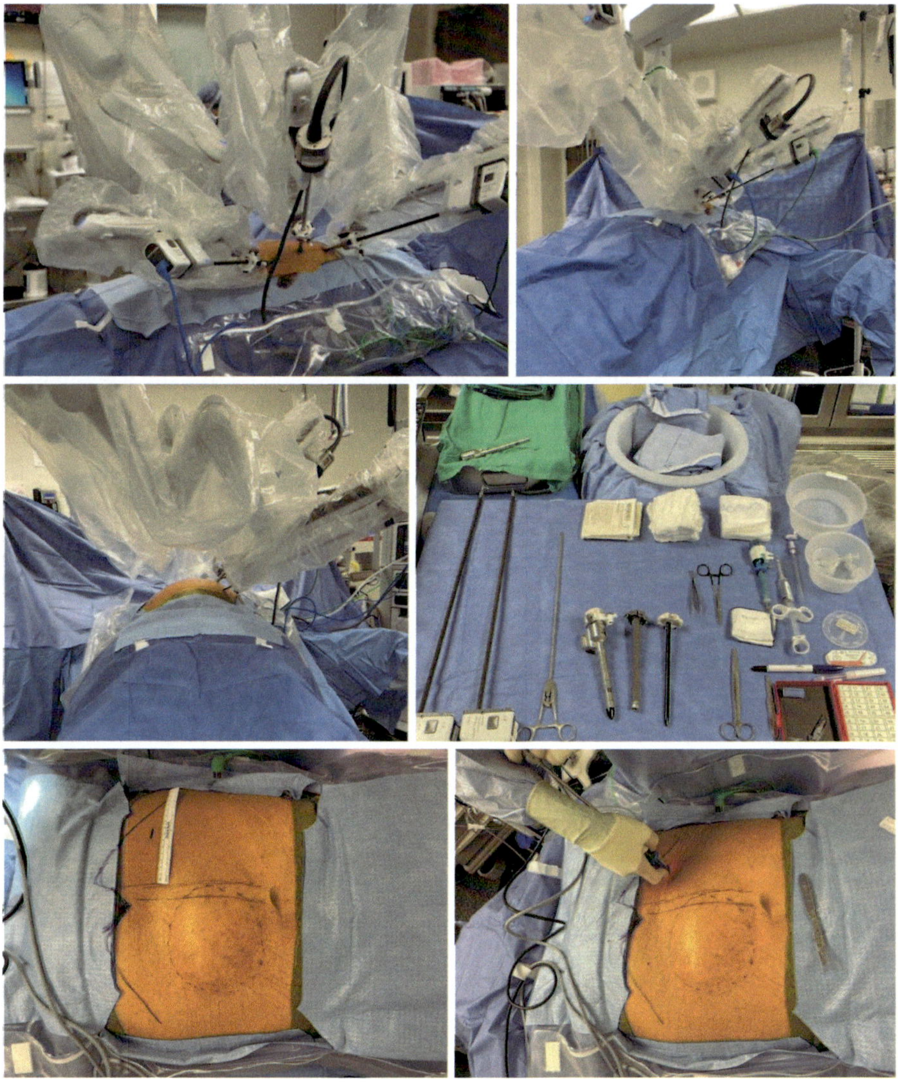

Fig. 22.1 Patient positioning

Veress insufflation, although it is also feasible without it. Following this, pneumoperitoneum is created with a pressure of 15 mmHg. To facilitate robotic-assisted surgery, an 8 mm robotic port is strategically positioned under laparoscopic visualization in the mid-lateral abdomen, maintaining a minimum distance of 15 cm from the hernia defect. Concurrently, an 8 mm port is introduced in the left or right lower quadrant. The initial 10 mm Optiview port is then exchanged for an 8 mm robotic port, enhancing the surgical field and enabling precise execution of the procedure. This meticulous placement of ports optimizes access and visualization for

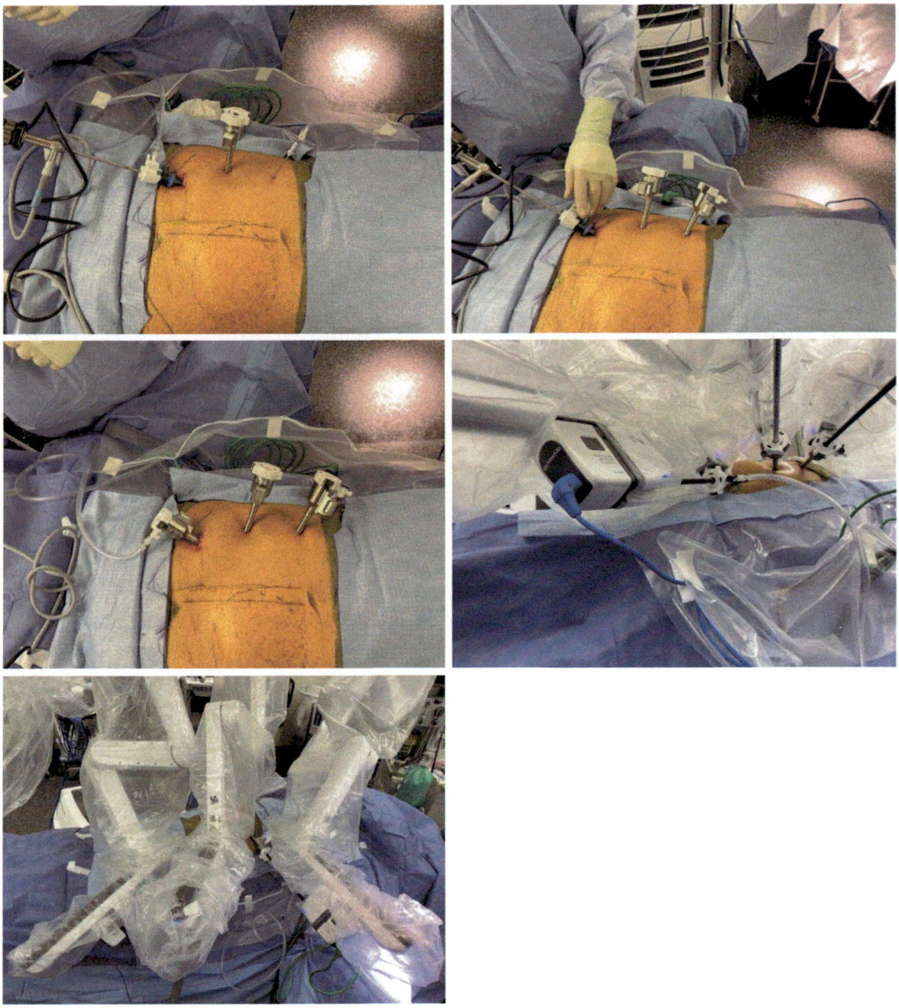

Fig. 22.2 Port placement and docking

subsequent steps in robotic ventral hernia repair, ensuring effective maneuverability and instrument utilization during the surgical process. On the contralateral side, the robotic system is docked in alignment with previously positioned ports. Utilizing a 30° scope initially facing upward, dissection of the ipsilateral abdominal wall is initiated. To improve preperitoneal dissection on the contralateral side, there is flexibility in adjusting the scope orientation. Specifically, the scope can be modified to a 0° position or a downward-facing 30° angle, facilitating optimal visualization and maneuverability during critical stages of the procedure. This adaptability in scope positioning ensures the surgical team can navigate anatomical structures efficiently, contributing to the precision and thoroughness of the robotic ventral hernia repair.

After docking the da Vinci patient cart as described, the arms are arranged according to Fig. 22.2. Monopolar curved scissors (da Vinci® Surgical System, Intuitive Surgical, Sunnyvale, CA) are inserted through the port just right side of the camera port. A bipolar grasper (double fenestrated) (da Vinci® Surgical System, Intuitive Surgical, Sunnyvale, CA) is inserted through the port just left side of the camera port.

Technique

The procedural sequence for robotic retromuscular ventral hernia repair with transversus abdominis release unfolds as follows:

After the initial careful incision of the posterior sheath lateral to the linea alba, followed by blunt dissection to separate the sheath from the rectus muscle and extend the dissection laterally to the semilunar line, critical landmarks, such as the intercostal neurovascular bundles and the thicker fascial condensation, are identified during this process. Continuing the dissection, the posterior sheath is retracted downward, revealing vertical stretch fibers along the linea semilunaris. This retromuscular dissection extends both above and below the hernia defect, ensuring sufficient preparation of the operative field. The peritoneum is strategically incised at the superior and inferior borders of the hernia, creating a continuous space between the preperitoneal and retromuscular compartments (Figs. 22.3 and 22.4). Initiating TAR involves incising the posterior lamella of the internal oblique and dividing the transversus abdominis muscle, entering either the preperitoneal or pretransversal space. This dissection proceeds laterally until the posterior flap lies flat across the viscera, typically reaching the level of the midaxillary line. The procedural sequence continues with the placement of three new trocars in the dissected space, and meticulous measurements of the hernia defect and dissected space guide the customization of the mesh. Mesh fixation is achieved by rolling and securing it lateral to the newly placed trocars. The robotic system is then redocked on the contralateral side, completing retromuscular dissection and TAR, bringing the initially placed trocars into the preperitoneal space. Closure of the posterior sheath is performed using absorbable, self-fixating sutures. The mesh is retrieved and deployed across the closed posterior sheath, securely fixated on the far side. Subsequently, the hernia defect is closed with absorbable, self-fixating sutures, ensuring comprehensive reinforcement. This step-by-step description highlights the precision and thoroughness of the robotic retromuscular VHR with TAR, emphasizing key anatomical landmarks and meticulous techniques employed throughout the procedure.

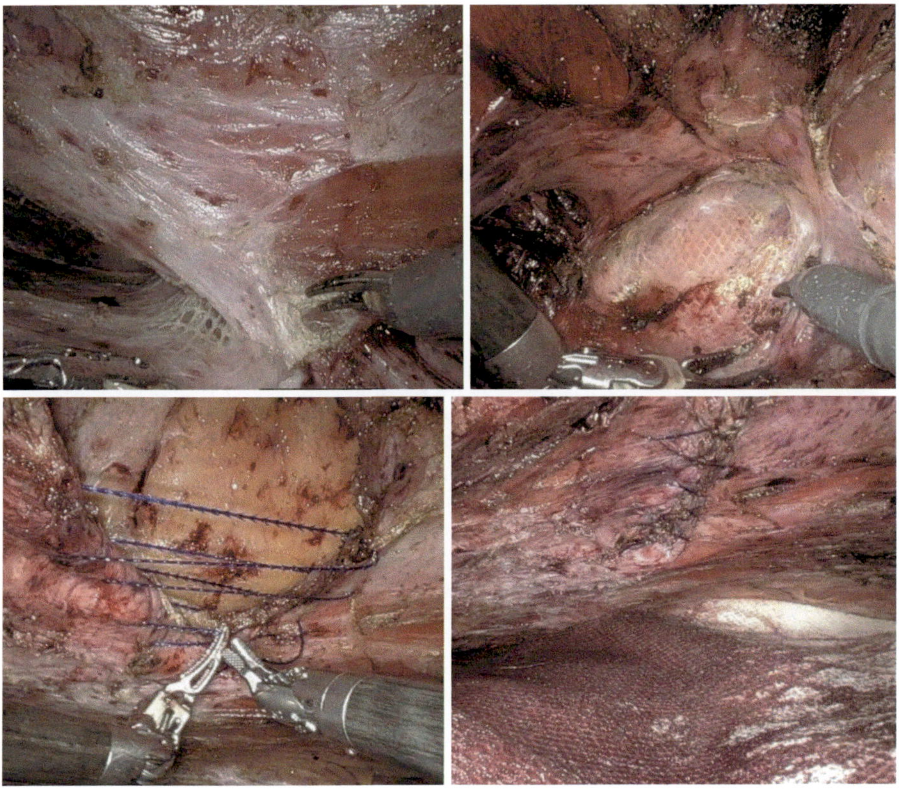

Fig. 22.3 Dissection in the retromuscular space reveals the previous mesh integrated within the posterior layer following recurrence from a prior retromuscular repair followed by defect closure and placement of new mesh

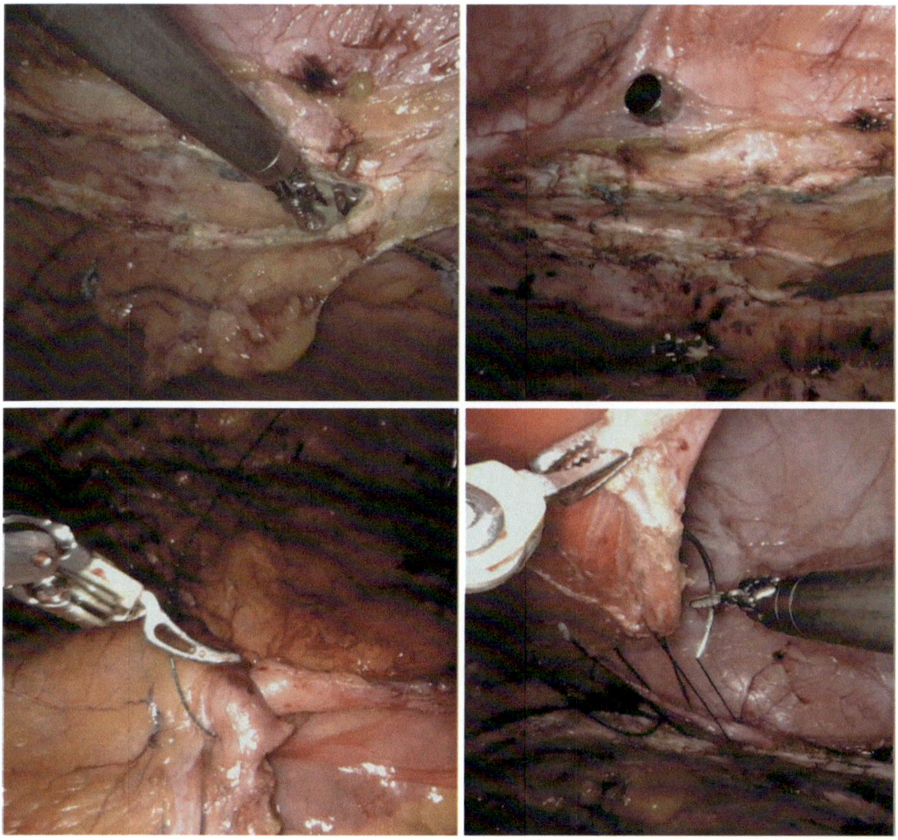

Fig. 22.4 Images of recurrent incisional hernia after prior rectus abdominus flap. Highlighting the integrated previous mesh, large defect width of 20 cm and the absence of rectus muscle

Hybrid Robotic Ventral Hernia Repair

The hybrid approach has become a preferred method for managing the complexities associated with recurrent incisional hernias, particularly those presenting challenges such as closing massive hernia defects in various clinical scenarios, including recurrence after rectus abdominis muscle flap, retrorectus repair, TAR, and in conjunction with excision of massive skin and soft tissue necrosis (Figs. 22.5 and 22.6). Additionally, it optimizes operative times, particularly in prolonged procedures involving extensive enterolysis and mesh removal. This hybrid approach combines the precision of robotic dissection and component separation with the efficacy of open fascial defect closure and mesh deployment. Comparative studies with open repair have shown that hybrid robotic ventral hernia repair results in a shorter length of hospital stay while maintaining similar rates of complication and wound morbidity.

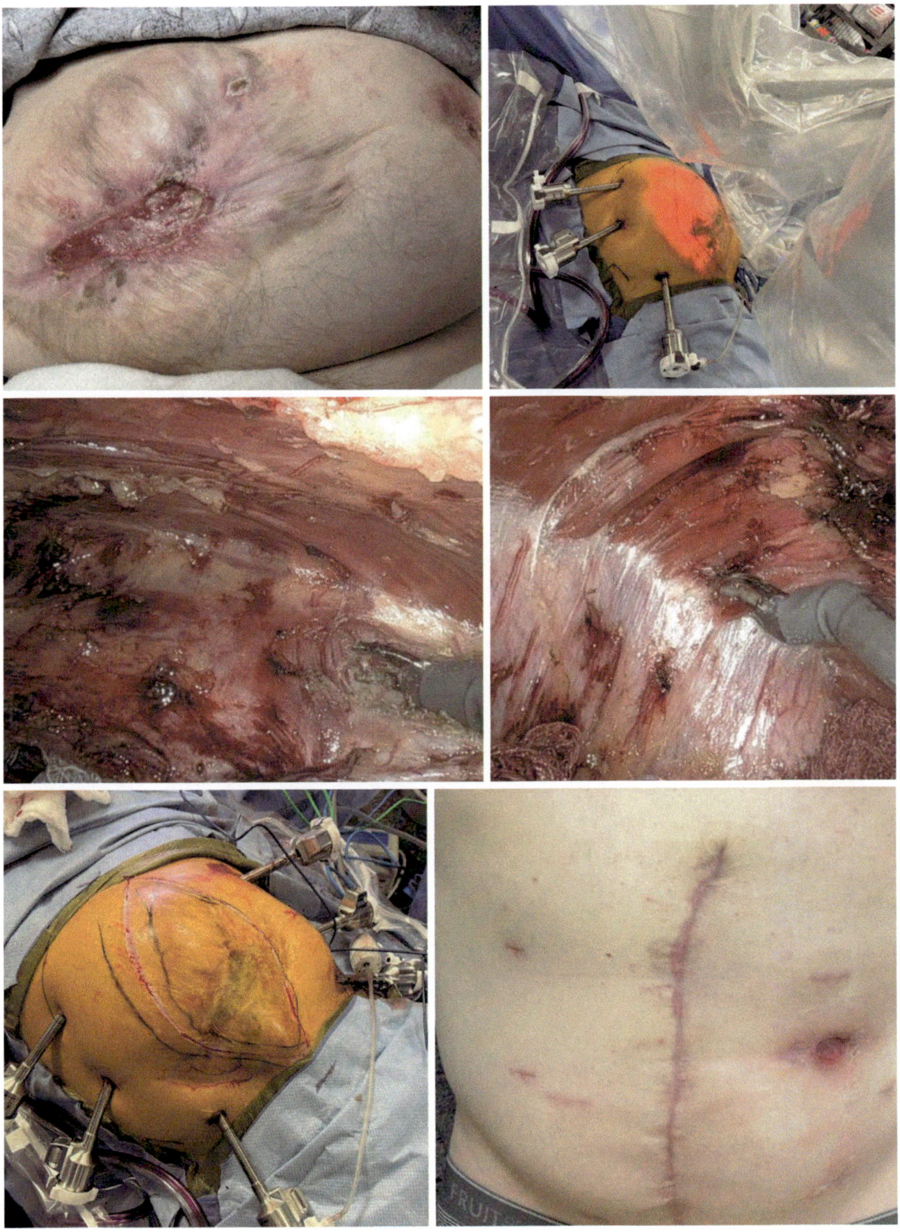

Fig. 22.5 Pre, intra, and post images of hybrid TAR for a complex incisional hernia after an open abdomen and hernia defect width of 24 cm

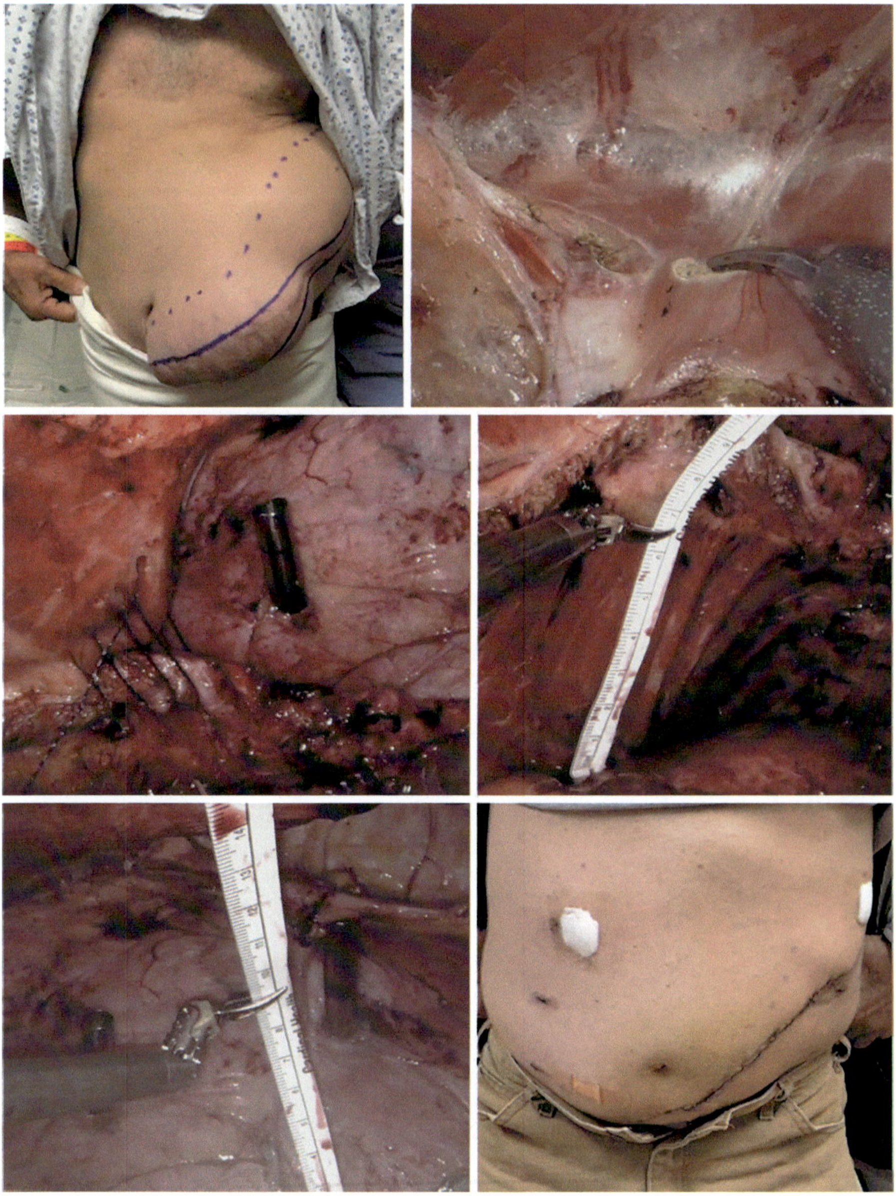

Fig. 22.6 Pre- and postoperative images of hybrid robotic TAR for lateral incisional hernia

Conclusion

The utilization of robotic technology in retromuscular ventral hernia repair, with or without the incorporation of transversus abdominis release, offers a distinctive advantage in restoring the functional integrity of the abdominal wall. This advanced surgical approach allows for the precise reestablishment of the anatomical structure, ensuring a robust closure. A key component of this procedure involves strategically placing mesh in an extraperitoneal sublay position. By reinforcing the abdominal wall in this manner, the mesh provides essential support and stability, contributing to the long-term durability of the repair. The robotic platform, with its enhanced dexterity and three-dimensional optics, facilitates meticulous execution of these steps, enabling surgeons to achieve a comprehensive restoration of the abdominal wall's functional anatomy. The integration of a comprehensive robotic approach in the management of complex ventral hernia surgery aims to tackle technical challenges while enhancing ergonomics. The distinctive feature of the fully robotic approach lies in overcoming technical difficulties, resulting in a streamlined surgical process and empowering surgeons to navigate the intricacies of complex abdominal wall anatomy with heightened precision. The superior ergonomics offered by robotic systems alleviate physical strain on the surgeon, ensuring sustained focus and dexterity throughout the procedure. As the realm of surgical innovation progresses, continuous scientific exploration is expected to unveil further insights into the advantages of such advancements. Despite inherent limitations concerning cost and potential operative time, optimism surrounds the potential of complex ventral hernia surgery. Ongoing learning and refinement within the field are anticipated to effectively address these challenges.

Conflicts of Interest and Source of Funding Dr. Kudsi have received consultancy fees from Intuitive Surgical and W.L. Gore outside the submitted work. Dr. Benlice and Dr. Baca have no conflicts of interest including relevant financial interests, activities, relationships, and affiliations.

References

1. Holihan JL, Nguyen DH, Nguyen MT, Mo J, Kao LS, Liang MK. Mesh location in open ventral hernia repair: a systematic review and network meta-analysis. World J Surg. 2016;40:89–99.
2. Appleton ND, Anderson KD, Hancock K, Scott MH, Walsh CJ. Initial UK experience with transversus abdominis muscle release for posterior components separation in abdominal wall reconstruction of large or complex ventral hernias: a combined approach by general and plastic surgeons. Ann R Coll Surg England. 2017;99(4):265–70.
3. Sheetz KH, Claflin J, Dimick JB. Trends in the adoption of robotic surgery for common surgical procedures. JAMA Netw Open. 2020;3(1):e1918911.
4. LeBlanc KA, Booth WV. Laparoscopic repair of incisional abdominal hernias using expanded polytetrafluoroethylene: preliminary findings. Surg Laparosc Endosc Percutan Tech. 1993;3(1):39–41.
5. Love MW, Carbonell AM. Robotic transversus abdominis release: A paradigm shift in complex abdominal wall surgery? Cir Esp. 2023;101:S28.
6. Tran E, Sun J, Gundara J. Systematic review of robotic ventral hernia repair with meta-analysis. ANZ J Surg. 2023;94:37.
7. Kelley WE Jr. The evolution of laparoscopy and the revolution in surgery in the decade of the 1990s. JSLS. 2008;12(4):351.
8. Madion M, Goldblatt MI, Gould JC, Higgins RM. Ten-year trends in minimally invasive hernia repair: a NSQIP database review. Surg Endosc. 2021;1–9:7200.
9. Maskal S, Beffa L. The role of robotics in abdominal wall reconstruction. Surg Clin. 2023;103(5):977–91.

10. Slater NJ, Montgomery A, Berrevoet F, Carbonell AM, Chang A, Franklin M, et al. Criteria for definition of a complex abdominal wall hernia. Hernia. 2014;18:7–17.
11. Piccoli M, Agresta F, Attinà GM, Amabile D, Marchi D. "Complex abdominal wall" management: evidence-based guidelines of the Italian Consensus Conference. Updat Surg. 2019;71:255–72.
12. Kanters AE, Krpata DM, Blatnik JA, Novitsky YM, Rosen MJ. Modified hernia grading scale to stratify surgical site occurrence after open ventral hernia repairs. J Am Coll Surg. 2012;215(6):787–93.
13. Working group Incisional Hernias. National Guideline for Treatment of Incisional Ventral Hernias. 2018.
14. Parker SG, Halligan S, Liang MK, Muysoms FE, Adrales GL, Boutall A, et al. Definitions for loss of domain: an international Delphi consensus of expert surgeons. World J Surg. 2020;44:1070–8.
15. Capoccia Giovannini S, Podda M, Ribas S, Montori G, Botteri E, Agresta F, et al. What defines an incisional hernia as 'complex': results from a Delphi consensus endorsed by the European Hernia Society (EHS). Br J Surg. 2024;111(1):znad346.
16. Park H, de Virgilio C, Kim DY, Shover AL, Moazzez A. Effects of smoking and different BMI cutoff points on surgical site infection after elective open ventral hernia repair. Hernia. 2021;25:337–43.
17. Belyansky I, Weltz AS, Sibia US, Turcotte JJ, Taylor H, Zahiri HR, et al. The trend toward minimally invasive complex abdominal wall reconstruction: is it worth it? Surg Endosc. 2018;32:1701–7.
18. Childers CP, Maggard-Gibbons M. Estimation of the acquisition and operating costs for robotic surgery. JAMA. 2018;320(8):835–6.
19. De Rosa M, Bugiantella W, Arteritano F, Mariani L, Ermili F, Ceccarelli G. The evolution of minimally invasive robotic surgery in the last 20 years. Robotic Surgery of Colon and Rectum. 2023;3–10.
20. Dhanani NH, Olavarria OA, Holihan JL, Shah SK, Wilson TD, Loor MM, et al. Robotic versus laparoscopic ventral hernia repair: one-year results from a prospective, multicenter, blinded randomized controlled trial. Ann Surg. 2021;273(6):1076–80.
21. Olavarria OA, Bernardi K, Shah SK, Wilson TD, Wei S, Pedroza C, et al. Robotic versus laparoscopic ventral hernia repair: multicenter, blinded randomized controlled trial. BMJ. 2020:370.
22. Coakley KM, Sims SM, Prasad T, Lincourt AE, Augenstein VA, Sing RF, et al. A nationwide evaluation of robotic ventral hernia surgery. Am J Surg. 2017;214(6):1158–63.
23. Nguyen B, David B, Shiozaki T, Gosch K, Sorensen GB. Comparisons of abdominal wall reconstruction for ventral hernia repairs, open versus robotic. Sci Rep. 2021;11(1):8086.
24. Roberts SH, Rodman CP, Meara MP. Short-Term Outcomes of Robotic vs Open Transversus Abdominus Release. J Am Coll Surg. 2019;229(4):e128.
25. Reeves J, Mehta S, Prabha RD, Salama Y, Mittal A. Robotic versus open transversus abdominis release and incisional hernia repair: a case-control study. Laparosc Endosc Robot Surg. 2020;3(3):59–62.
26. Halka JT, Vasyluk A, DeMare AM, Janczyk RJ, Iacco AA. Robotic and hybrid robotic transversus abdominis release may be performed with low length of stay and wound morbidity. Am J Surg. 2018;215(3):462–5.
27. Bracale U, Corcione F, Neola D, Castiglioni S, Cavallaro G, Stabilini C, et al. Transversus abdominis release (TAR) for ventral hernia repair: open or robotic? Short-term outcomes from a systematic review with meta-analysis. Hernia. 2021;1–10:1471.
28. Bittner JG, Alrefai S, Vy M, Mabe M, Del Prado PAR, Clingempeel NL. Comparative analysis of open and robotic transversus abdominis release for ventral hernia repair. Surg Endosc. 2018;32:727–34.
29. Kudsi OY, Gokcal F, Bou-Ayash N, Chang K. Comparison of midterm outcomes between open and robotic emergent ventral hernia repair. Surg Innov. 2021;28(4):449–57.
30. Dietz UA, Kudsi OY, Gokcal F, Bou-Ayash N, Pfefferkorn U, Rudofsky G, et al. Excess body weight and abdominal hernia. Visc Med. 2021;37(4):246–53.

31. Kudsi OY, Gokcal F, Chang K. Propensity score matching analysis of short-term outcomes in robotic ventral hernia repair for patients with a body mass index above and below 35 kg/m 2. Hernia. 2021;25:115–23.
32. Gokcal F, Morrison S, Kudsi OY. Robotic ventral hernia repair in morbidly obese patients: perioperative and mid-term outcomes. Surg Endosc. 2020;34:3540–9.
33. Kudsi OY, Kaoukabani G, Bou-Ayash N, Gokcal F. Do antiplatelets and anticoagulants have an impact on the clinical outcomes of robotic ventral hernia repair? Am J Surg. 2023;226:213.
34. Love MW, Davis S, Blackhurst D, Cobb W, Carbonell A, Warren J. Rectus to defect ratio for estimating the complexity of ventral hernia repair: Is it reliable for robotic surgery? Am J Surg. 2023;226(6):917–20.
35. Sabbagh C, Dumont F, Robert B, Badaoui R, Verhaeghe P, Regimbeau JM. Peritoneal volume is predictive of tension-free fascia closure of large incisional hernias with loss of domain: a prospective study. Hernia. 2011;15:559–65.
36. Zolin SJ, Fafaj A, Krpata DM. Transversus abdominis release (TAR): what are the real indications and where is the limit? Hernia. 2020;24:333–40.

23 Robotic Cholecystectomy

Samuel Cass, Jennifer Moffett, and Sarah Samreen

Introduction

Cholecystectomy repeatedly ranks as one of the most common procedures performed by general surgeons annually. With the evolution of robotic platforms, cholecystectomy has similarly risen as one of the most common robotic-assisted surgeries performed by both trainees and surgeons in the United States [1–3]. The advent of minimally invasive cholecystectomy began in the late 1980s with Mühe's description of the laparoscopic approach [4]. While initially met with hesitance, laparoscopic cholecystectomy gained traction over the next decade, supported by studies showing a reduction in postoperative pain, length of hospital stay, and shorter recovery time, and ultimately became the standard of care approach [5, 6]. In the same way, robotic cholecystectomy has been increasingly adopted over the past two decades following FDA approval in 2000 and the rapid evolution of robotic platforms since this time.

As with other surgeries described in this manual, the high-definition 3-D optics and wristed dexterity of robotic instruments aid dissection in patients with challenging biliary anatomy. Fluorescence cholangiography can additionally be utilized to assist in visualization of the biliary tree in complex cases. Multiport robotic cholecystectomy (MPRC) has been shown to be safe, and when compared to the laparoscopic approach, it has demonstrated similar short-term surgical outcomes, as well as similar operative times and hospital length of stay [7–10]. In a recent, widely circulated retrospective study from 2010 to 2019, the robotic approach was found to be associated with a slightly higher rate of bile duct injury compared to the laparoscopic approach (0.7% vs 0.2%, RR 3.2) [11]. However, this study had several limitations including an inability to account for surgical complexity as well as the surgeon learning curve. As the experience with robotic cholecystectomy increases

S. Cass · J. Moffett · S. Samreen (✉)
Department of Surgery, University of Texas Medical Branch, Galveston, TX, USA
e-mail: sasamree@UTMB.EDU

S. Samreen et al. (eds.), *The SAGES Manual of Robotic Surgery*,
https://doi.org/10.1007/978-3-031-86927-3_23

over time, prospective analyses of short- and long-term outcomes as well as cost-effectiveness analyses will be needed.

This chapter serves to describe the perioperative management and intraoperative techniques required for the safe application of multiport robotic cholecystectomy for biliary disease.

Indications

Overall, indications for cholecystectomy include symptomatic cholelithiasis, both calculous and acalculous cholecystitis, biliary dyskinesia, symptomatic gallbladder polyp greater than 1 cm, and gallstones >3 cm. Additionally, complicated biliary diseases including gallstone pancreatitis and choledocholithiasis warrant cholecystectomy with intraoperative cholangiography [12]. Ultimately, robotic systems and laparoscopic equipment are tools used to assist with cholecystectomy, and therefore, both approaches can be utilized for similar indications. However, many favor the robotic platform for patients with complex surgical or biliary anatomy due to the benefits of increased visualization and the use of fluorescence cholangiography. Contraindications are few and relative but include significant right upper quadrant abdominal surgery, end-stage cirrhosis, and complex cholecystoenteric fistula. For single-port surgery, relative contraindications include BMI > 50, need for cholangiography, or complex biliary pathology.

Robotic Equipment and the Operative Team

The most utilized robotic systems are the da Vinci Xi and Si surgical systems (Intuitive Surgical Inc., Sunnyvale, Ca) and will serve as the focus of the technical descriptions herein. However, the details from this chapter can be extrapolated for application of other systems that are either available or are currently in development.

The sterile component of the da Vinci system is the patient-side cart (PC) which is draped in sterile fashion and docked at the operating table. The PSC has four articulating robotic arms which control the endoscope and surgical instruments that are docked to the ports. Away from the operating table, the surgeon console (SC) serves as the working hub for the surgeon, equipped with high-definition, three-dimensional visualization and the technical controls for surgical equipment on the operative field. The visual cart (VC) is the processing center communicating between consoles, supporting hardware and software such as the optical light source, electrosurgical unit, and optical integration.

A coordinated operating room team is needed for efficient and safe robotic cholecystectomy. Reasonable docking and anesthesia times are achieved when operating teams consist of organized, well-trained personnel. In the OR, a circulating nurse and scrub nurse who are trained in robotic systems assist with setup, robotic docking, instrument exchange, and bedside assistance. Additionally, robotic equipment technicians assist with setup, troubleshooting, and locating robotic equipment, while a charge nurse assists with supervising and coordinating cases between multiple robotic ORs.

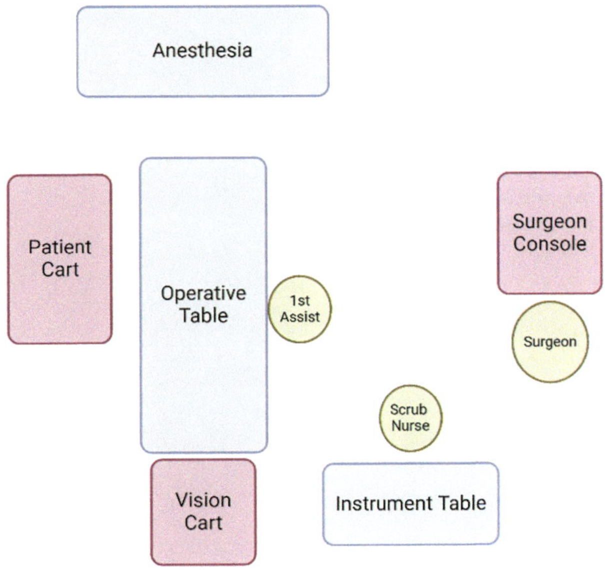

Fig. 23.1 Room layout

Room Setup and Patient Positioning

Patients are placed on the operating table in a supine position with all pressure points padded. The instrument table and scrub nurse are at the feet, opposite of the PC. For the da Vinci Xi, the rotating boom allows more freedom for the PC to be positioned on either side of the patient. The patient's arm on the side of the PC may be tucked. The location of the SC and VC depends on the OR layout; however, we recommend that SC placement allows for easy and direct visualization of the operative field (Fig. 23.1).

Port Placement and Robotic Docking

As with any minimally invasive case, the strategy for peritoneal entry depends on patient factors including body habitus and prior surgical history. Generally, it is our practice to obtain pneumoperitoneum with a Veress needle at Palmer's point. The abdomen is insufflated to as low as 8 mmHg, though standard pressure (12–15 mmHg) can be used if improved visualization is needed, and the patient's hemodynamics can tolerate the pressure. Next, we insert an 8 mm robotic trocar in the supraumbilical region under direct visualization with a laparoscope. Note, we ensure to place this port 15 cm from the operative field in the upper right quadrant. Alternatively, entry can be achieved through an open technique or the Veress technique at this supraumbilical site. Two 8 mm ports are placed in the upper right quadrant at the midclavicular and anterior axillary line. One 8 mm port is placed in the upper left quadrant at the midclavicular line, at the same level or slightly cephalad to the right-sided ports. We measure 8 cm between ports to avoid instrument collision (Fig. 23.2).

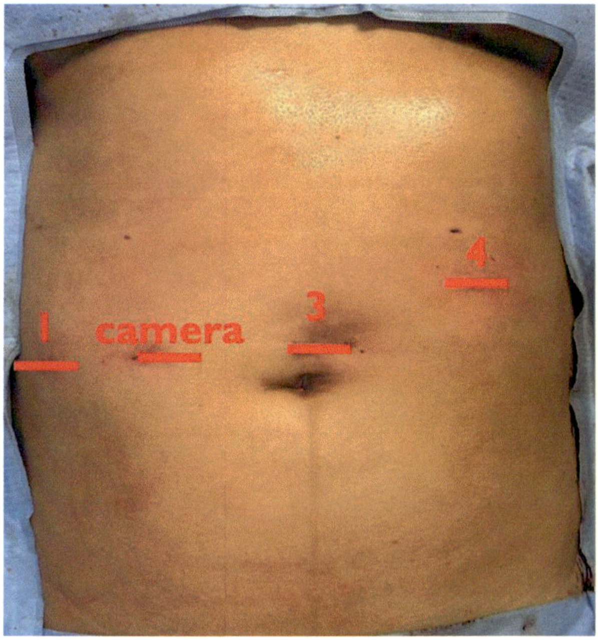

Fig. 23.2 Port placement for cholecystectomy. The camera is introduced into arm 2, a ProGrasp is used in arm 4 for gallbladder retraction, and arms 1 and 3 are used for dissection of the critical view with a fenestrated bipolar and hook

The patient is placed in the reverse Trendelenburg position (10–15 degrees) and tilted to the left side (3–5 degrees). After the pneumoperitoneum has been achieved and robotic ports placed, the PC is driven to the patient and docked to the supraumbilical port. A 30 degree, downward-facing endoscope is introduced in arm 3 and PC is targeted to the gallbladder. The remaining 8 mm ports are docked with appropriate spacing and clearance to prevent arm collision and patient injury.

We typically use the following instruments: bipolar in the right lateral arm, camera in the mid-right port, permanent cautery hook at the umbilical port, ProGrasp in the left upper quadrant, and a large clip applier exchanged at the umbilicus when clipping the cystic duct and artery. A Maryland bipolar forceps can be added if finer, blunt dissection is required. Monopolar curved scissors can be used for the sharp division of adhesions or cystic structures if needed. A suction irrigator can be utilized for bleeding and gallbladder spillage.

Robotic Dissection

After identifying the gallbladder, the fundus is grasped and retracted cephalad over the liver (ProGrasp). If any adhesions are encountered, these can be lysed with hook cautery. The infundibulum of the gallbladder is then retracted laterally (f). In doing so, the triangle of Calot is splayed open for better visualization of cystic structures. Active manipulation of the infundibulum throughout the case provides dynamic exposure and tension throughout the dissection.

We begin the dissection by opening the peritoneum over the junction of the infundibulum with the cystic duct with hook cautery. The peritoneum reflections medial and lateral to the gallbladder are opened to provide better mobility and exposure, which facilitates a safer dissection. Once identified, the cystic duct and artery are dissected clear with a combination of blunt dissection and electrocautery. Complete dissection of the triangle of Calot is carefully performed until the critical view of safety is achieved before clipping any structure (Fig. 23.3).

Fluorescence cholangiography can additionally assist with delineating complex biliary anatomy. Indocyanine green (ICG) is a tricarbocynanine dye that is excreted through the biliary system, allowing for intraoperative visualization of biliary structures when visualized under infrared light (da Vinci Firefly). ICG can be a tool for visualizing biliary structures in complex cases (Fig. 23.4).

Once this view is achieved, hook cautery is replaced with the large clip applier. The cystic duct and artery are clipped twice. These structures are divided close to the gallbladder with scissors or hook cautery. When using hook cautery, the structures should be under adequate tension and are divided using a cutting current with the tip of the hook instrument. The gallbladder is then dissected off the hepatic fossa with hook cautery. The gallbladder is typically removed through the umbilical site in an endoscopic retrieval bag. Note, this incision may need to be extended to remove the specimen and, therefore, is closed with 0-Vicryl on a suture passer.

If an intraoperative cholangiogram (IOC) is indicated to visualize biliary anatomy or fluoroscopy is needed to perform transcystic common bile duct exploration, a C-arm can be brought in from either side of the patient and positioned between the robotic arms (Fig. 23.5). The cystic duct is ligated proximally with a clip and a cystic ductotomy is made just distal. A 4-French cholangiocatheter is introduced into the abdomen through a 14-gauge angiocatheter placed in the right upper quadrant. The catheter is positioned into the cystic duct and secured with an 0-Vicryl tie. Following completion of the IOC, the Vicryl is removed and two clips are placed distal to the ductotomy prior to dividing.

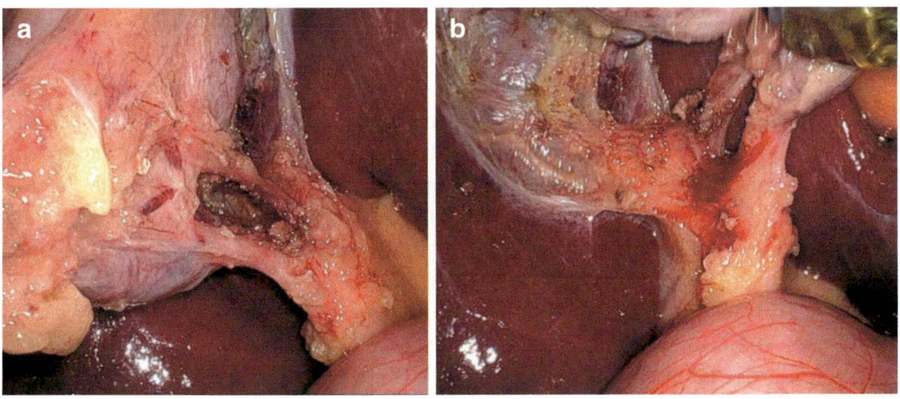

Fig. 23.3 Critical view of safety shown from the medial (**a**) and lateral (**b**) view of the hepatocystic triangle

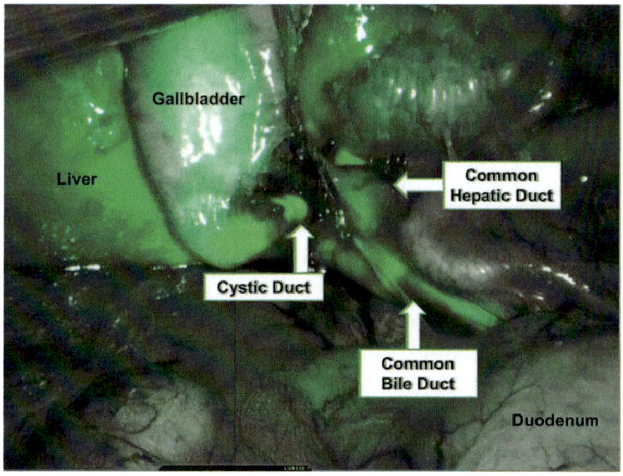

Fig. 23.4 Visualization of biliary structures using Firefly

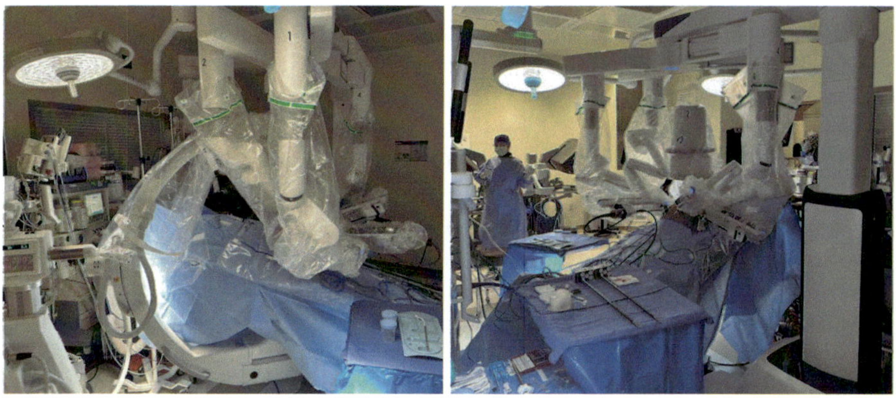

Fig. 23.5 C-arm positioning during fluoroscopy. The robotic arms are flexed out laterally and the C-arm is placed between arms 2 and 3

With the ability to detect common bile duct stones with intraoperative cholangiogram and fluorescence cholangiography, robotic approaches to common duct explorations have been described and have been shown to be feasible and safe [13, 14]. For complex biliary disease, both transcystic and transcholedochal approaches with balloon sphincteroplasty and cholangioscopy have been described. The robotic benefits of added dexterity may allow for improved surgeon comfort with instrumentation and closure of the common bile duct, which with time may result in lower rates of conversion to open procedures for complex biliary disease, though further studies are needed to substantiate this. Additionally, the single-stage robotic approach to choledocholithiasis with cholecystectomy and concomitant common bile duct exploration has equivalent clearance rates to ERCP while decreasing total hospital length of stay when compared to traditional two-stage management with cholecystectomy and ERCP [14].

Single-Port Robotic Cholecystectomy

To reduce the trauma of multiport placement, single-port robotic cholecystectomy (SPRC) was developed in 2011 and shown to be feasible [15, 16]. While its adoption has been limited due to the inherent ergonomic and technical challenges associated with single-site surgery, the safety of SPRC has been demonstrated.

A 2–3 cm horizontal umbilical incision is made and deepened with cautery to fascia. The fascia is opened horizontally and the peritoneum is entered. The da Vinci single-site port is introduced; this system has five openings for the camera, insufflation tubing, two robotic instruments, and an assistant port. The 8 mm camera trocar is introduced following insufflation and the PC is docked. Two robotic trocars are introduced. Although these cross at the level of the fascia in order to provide triangulation of the gallbladder, the da Vinci software compensates by associating the instrument tips with the ipsilateral surgeon controls. We use a fenestrated bipolar in arm 1 and hook cautery in arm 2. The assistant port is placed and a grasper can be introduced to lift the fundus of the gallbladder cephalad. Dissection is carried out in similar fashion as with laparoscopic or multiport robotic cholecystectomy.

References

1. Sheetz KH, Claflin J, Dimick JB. Trends in the adoption of robotic surgery for common surgical procedures. JAMA Netw Open. 2020;3(1):e1918911.
2. Stewart CL, et al. Common components of general surgery robotic educational programs. J Surg Educ. 2023;80(11):1717–22.
3. Vidovszky TJ, et al. Robotic cholecystectomy: learning curve, advantages, and limitations. J Surg Res. 2006;136(2):172–8.
4. Reynolds W. The first laparoscopic cholecystectomy. JSLS. 2001;5(1):89–94.
5. Lujan JA, et al. Laparoscopic cholecystectomy vs open cholecystectomy in the treatment of acute cholecystitis: a prospective study. Arch Surg. 1998;133(2):173–5.
6. Mannam R, et al. Laparoscopic cholecystectomy versus open cholecystectomy in acute cholecystitis: a literature review. Cureus. 2023;15(9):e45704.
7. Kane WJ, et al. Robotic compared with laparoscopic cholecystectomy: a propensity matched analysis. Surgery. 2020;167(2):432–5.
8. Breitenstein S, et al. Robotic-assisted versus laparoscopic cholecystectomy: outcome and cost analyses of a case-matched control study. Ann Surg. 2008;247(6):987–93.
9. Baek NH, et al. Short-term surgical outcomes and experience with 925 patients undergoing robotic cholecystectomy during a 4-year period at a single institution. Hepato-Gastroenterology. 2015;62(139):573–6.
10. Straatman J, et al. Assessment of patient-reported outcome measures in the surgical treatment of patients with gastric cancer. Surg Endosc. 2016;30(5):1920–9.
11. Kalata S, et al. Comparative safety of robotic-assisted vs laparoscopic cholecystectomy. JAMA Surg. 2023;158(12):1303–10.
12. Townsend CM, et al. Sabiston textbook of surgery: the biological basis of modern surgical practice. 20th ed. 2017; Philadelphia: Elsevier/Saunders. xxv, 2146 pages.
13. Latif J, et al. Robotic assisted common bile duct exploration for management of complex gallstone disease. Int J Surg. 2024;
14. DeJesus J, Horani K, Brahmbhatt K, Mesa CF, Samreen S, Moffett JM. Conquering the common bile duct: outcomes in minimally invasive transcystic common bile duct exploration

versus ERCP. Surg Endosc. 2024. https://doi.org/10.1007/s00464-024-11228-5. Epub ahead of print. PMID: 39289226.
15. Hernandez, J.M., et al., Laparoendoscopic single site cholecystectomy: the first 100 patients. Am Surg. 2009;75(8): 681–5; discussion 685–6.
16. Hong TH, et al. Transumbilical single-port laparoscopic appendectomy (TUSPLA): scarless intracorporeal appendectomy. J Laparoendosc Adv Surg Tech A. 2009;19(1):75–8.

24 Liver Resection and Biliary Reconstruction

Yee Lee Cheah and Caroline J. Simon

Introduction

Laparoscopic liver surgery has been performed since the 1990s, but an expansion of laparoscopic techniques, particularly in major hepatectomy procedures, has been restricted by limitations of the platform, including inadequate visualization, restricted range of motion of laparoscopic instruments, and concerns regarding intraoperative hemostasis during parenchymal transection [1, 2]. After the introduction of more sophisticated versions of the robotic platforms in the late 2000s, robotic surgery has been gaining popularity as an alternative minimally invasive technique for complex hepatobiliary and pancreatic surgery.

Robotic Liver Resection

Since the first reported robotic liver resection in 2003, multiple centers with specialized programs have reported growing numbers of robotic hepatectomy [3]. Advantages of the robotic platform include wristed instrumentation, 3-D visualization, simultaneous multi-image display, and real-time indocyanine green (ICG) fluorescence to guide resection [4]. These benefits allow meticulous dissection of the liver hilum and application of hemostatic techniques familiar to an open liver surgeon.

Supplementary Information The online version contains supplementary material available at https://doi.org/10.1007/978-3-031-86927-3_24.

Y. L. Cheah (✉) · C. J. Simon
JC Walter Jr Transplant Center, Sherrie and Alan Conover Center for Liver Disease and Transplantation, Houston Methodist Hospital, Houston, TX, USA

Department of Surgery, Houston Methodist Hospital, Houston, TX, USA
e-mail: ycheah@houstonmethodist.org

S. Samreen et al. (eds.), *The SAGES Manual of Robotic Surgery*,
https://doi.org/10.1007/978-3-031-86927-3_24

The largest multicenter study comparing robotic to open liver resection for hepatocellular carcinoma with propensity score matching reported that patients who underwent robotic surgery reported longer operative time but shorter hospital length of stay and fewer admissions to the intensive care unit. There was no difference in the overall and recurrence-related survival between the robotic and open groups, but the robotic group had lower incidence of post-hepatectomy liver failure [5]. In terms of oncological outcomes, robotic liver resection showed similar pathological outcomes, 3-year disease-free survival, and overall survival when compared to open liver resection for hepatocellular carcinoma [6].

A worldwide meta-analysis of robotic liver resection outcomes comparing robotic to laparoscopic or open liver resections revealed that overall robotic operative times were longer than laparoscopic or open cases. Overall complication rates were also comparable between robotic and laparoscopic liver resections with shorter length of hospital stays after robotic compared to open hepatectomy [7].

Patient Selection

There are no differences in the pathological indications for robotic versus open liver resection. The preoperative workup includes the clinical assessment, cross-sectional imaging (CT or MRI), and standard laboratory analysis, particularly liver biochemistry and function. Resectability and type of resection are determined by assessment of liver function, liver quality (presence of damage from cirrhosis, metabolic dysfunction-associated fatty liver disease (MAFLD), or chemotherapy effect), local tumor extent, and size of the future liver remnant. Occasionally, a focal liver biopsy of an indeterminate mass may be necessary if it influences treatment decisions, and a non-focal biopsy may be necessary to rule out underlying liver disease or damage.

A decision to use a robotic approach should depend on the surgical team's experience with the platform. It may be prudent to start with resection of the anterior and lateral segments during the early part of a surgeon's learning curve in robotic liver surgery and progress to major hepatectomy and resection of the superior-posterior segments after adequate experience is gained and good outcomes are achieved [8]. Patient factors such as previous laparotomy (particularly in the upper abdomen) or previous liver resection may complicate a robotic approach but can be attempted once competency with the platform is achieved [9]. Liver anesthesia management with low central venous pressure is standard for both open and robotic approaches [10]. Enhanced recovery protocols should be affected in appropriate patients when indicated [11].

General Patient Positioning and Port Placement for Liver and Biliary Surgery

Positioning

Patients are placed in a split-leg position to enable the bedside surgeon to stand between the patient's legs (Fig. 24.1). All pressure points are padded. Arm(s) may be abducted to enable access by anesthesiologist to intra-arterial and intravenous

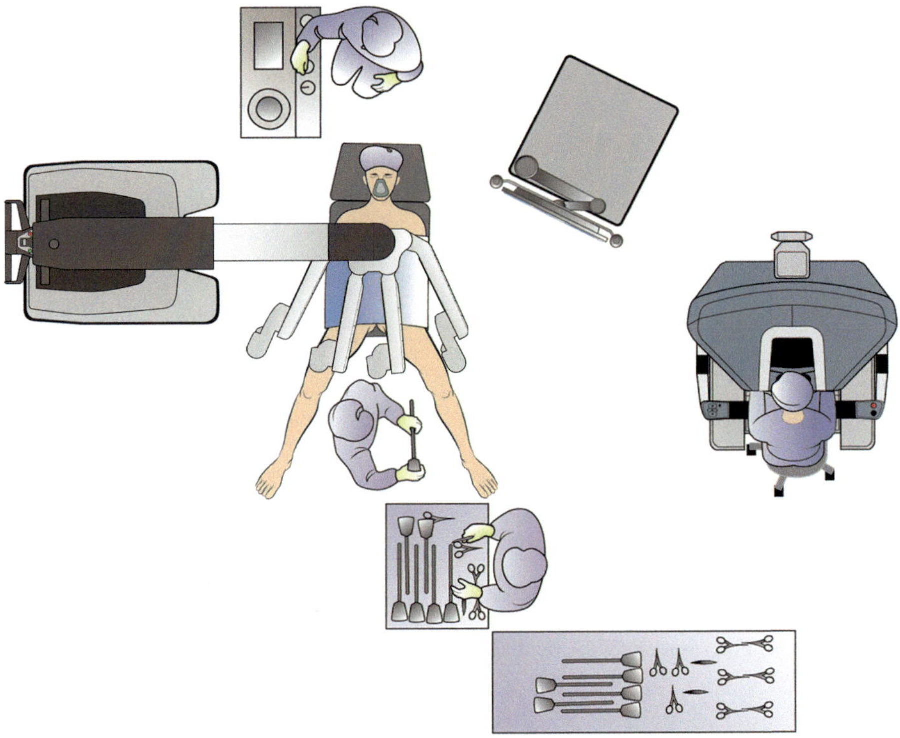

Fig. 24.1 Robotic operating room setup

cannulas during the procedure. The patient is secured to the operating table at the upper chest and hip levels. Both legs are secured to the leg extensions and footrests are used to prevent slippage during positioning.

Port Placement

Figure 24.2 depicts the usual port placements for right-sided versus left-sided liver resection, respectively. Both of these port positions work well for biliary surgery as well. The placement of the camera provides adequate visualization of the right or left side of the liver hilum as needed. The third arm is used for retraction and placed as a right-handed instrument. Two laparoscopic assistant ports are placed in the lower abdomen (12 mm and 5 mm). The liver specimen is usually extracted via a Pfannenstiel incision whereas a choledochal cyst or bile duct segment may be extracted via the 12 mm laparoscopic port. Pneumoperitoneum insufflation pressure is kept at or below 12 mm Hg to reduce the risk of air embolism through the hepatic veins.

Standard Robotic Instruments

1. Maryland bipolar (+ electrocautery).
2. Camera.

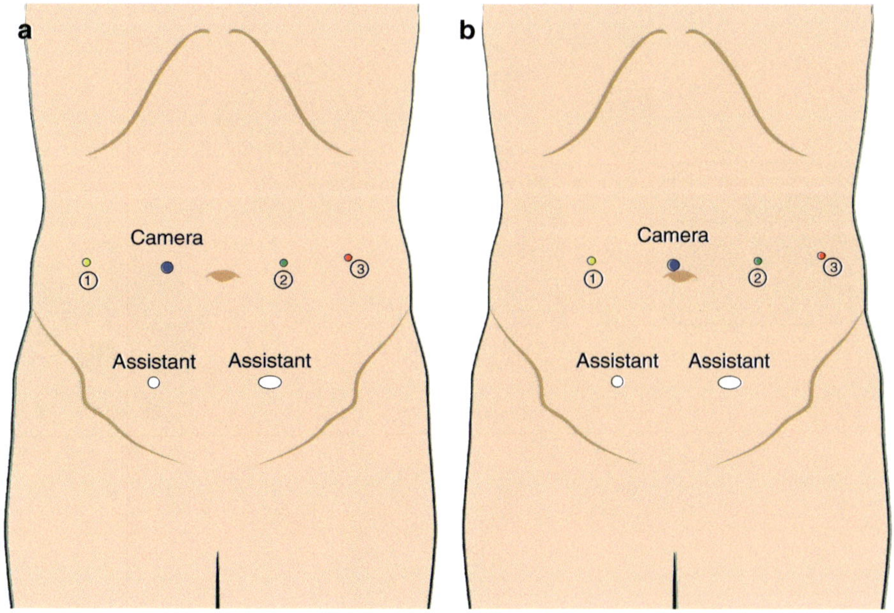

Fig. 24.2 (**a**) Port positioning for right-sided liver resection. (**b**) Port positioning for left-sided liver resection

3. Scissors (+ electrocautery).
4. Cadiere or Prograsp forceps.
5. Large needle driver.
6. Harmonic scalpel.
7. Small, medium, and large clip appliers.
8. Vessel sealer.

The detailed technique for two common types of major hepatectomy are described below. All other minor and major hepatectomies should follow the basic principles of hepatectomy, including inflow +/− outflow control followed by parenchymal transection. Pertinent tips on other types of hepatectomy are provided at the end of the liver resection section.

Right Hepatectomy (see Video 1)

Falciform Dissection

The ligamentum teres and falciform ligamentum are divided with robotic scissors using electrocautery up to the level of the hepatic vein-IVC confluence. The peritoneal covering of the hepatic vein confluence is incised, exposing the three hepatic veins. For a standard right hepatectomy, the superior extent of the future transection line is marked on the liver surface with electrocautery between the right and middle hepatic veins (Fig. 24.3).

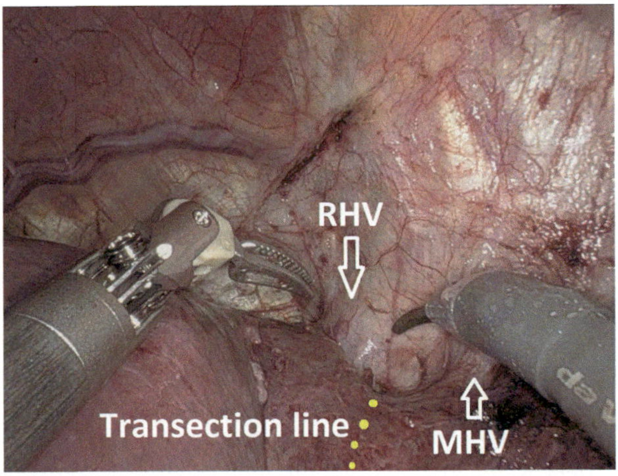

Fig. 24.3 Confluence of the hepatic veins and superior extent of transection line (dotted) between right (RHV) and middle (MHV) hepatic veins

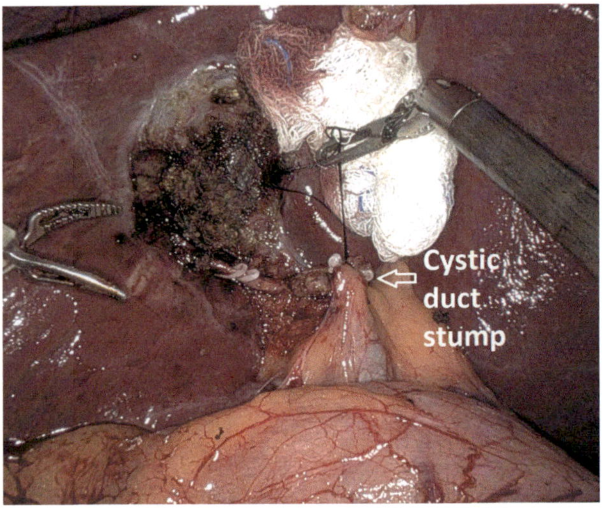

Fig. 24.4 Using the third arm to retract segment 4 and cystic duct stump exposing posterior aspect of common bile duct

Hilar Dissection

The third arm is used to retract segment 4B and gallbladder anterosuperiorly; a gauze is placed between the tip and elbow of the Cadiere/Prograsp to prevent injury to the liver surface. The laparoscopic assistant retracts the duodenum inferiorly with blunt-tipped instrument or suction device exposing the liver hilum. A standard cholecystectomy is performed, and the gallbladder specimen is placed in Morrison's pouch for later removal. The clipped cystic duct stump is now ligated with a 3/0 Vicryl tie or suture-ligated with a 3/0 Vicryl suture with tails left long. The tails are then grasped by the Cadiere/Prograsp positioned at segment 4B, and using the forceps as a pulley, the cystic duct is retracted anteriorly and slightly to the patient's left, exposing the lateral and right posterior aspect of the common hepatic duct (CHD) (Fig. 24.4).

Dissection of Right Hepatic Artery

The pulsation of a standard right hepatic artery (RHA) should be visible immediately behind the CHD at this stage. The lymphatic and nerve tissue lateral and posterior to the CHD are slowly dissected until the lateral wall of the artery is visualized. If the artery is not found in this manner, a second method follows the clipped cystic artery to its origin, which is usually the main or a branch of the right hepatic artery.

The posterior aspect of the standard RHA is loosely adherent to the anterior surface of the portal vein (PV) and the artery will need to be gently dissected off of the PV (Fig. 24.5). Once the anterior, lateral, and posterior walls of the artery are cleared, the tissues at the medial aspect of the RHA can be gently pushed away from the arterial wall and the artery may be encircled with a vessel loop. Care is taken not to injure the CHD and common bile duct (CBD), either via traction or cautery burn.

Alternatively, a replaced RHA from the superior mesenteric artery is usually found lying posterior-laterally along the course CBD and CHD. In this position, the artery is covered by a lymph node (Station 12b) that commonly stretches the right lateral length of the bile duct. This node will need to be excised or displaced inferiorly to gain access to the replaced RHA. The main difference in dissection of a replaced compared to a standard RHA is the close association of the length of the artery to the portal vein posteriorly and CBD anterolaterally. The encircled RHA can be divided between clips or ligatures.

Dissection of Right Portal Vein

Division of the RHA will expose the anterior surface of the RPV, enabling access to the portal vein bifurcation (Fig. 24.6). The plane between the CHD and anterior surface of the PV is gently developed by pushing the portal vein posteriorly off the attachments to the duct and RHA. Dissection proceeds cephalad until the bifurcation is encountered. Clear identification of the bifurcation is confirmed by visualization of the right, left, and main portal veins. The RPV anterosuperior surface is then carefully

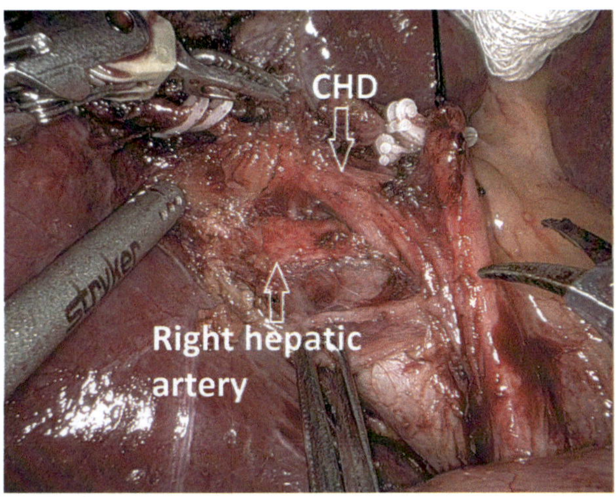

Fig. 24.5 Right hepatic artery noted between the common hepatic duct (CHD) and portal vein

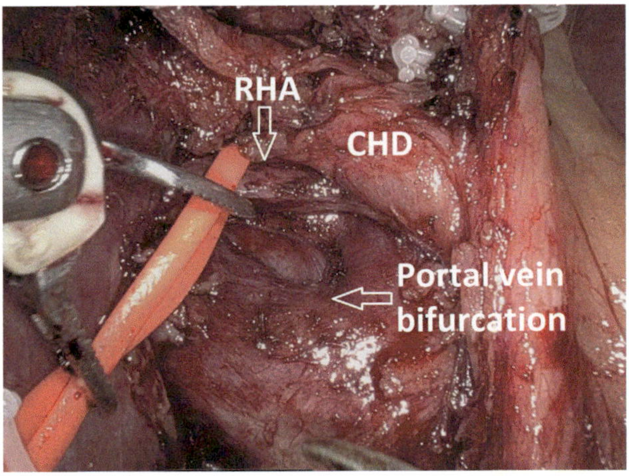

Fig. 24.6 Dissection of the portal vein bifurcation posterior to right hepatic artery (RHA) and common hepatic duct (CHD)

teased off the hilar plate by gently pressing the RPV posteriorly with the Maryland in the left hand and sweeping the tissues off the vein with the scissors in the right hand.

Attention is then moved to the dissection of the posterior aspect of the RPV. The peritoneal lining the posterior aspect of the RPV is divided and retracted posterior-inferiorly by the laparoscopic assistant. The posterior wall of the portal vein is dissected free from the peritoneum surface until the caudate branches are visualized and dissected free. The PV side of these branches are always ligated to avoid clips on the PV, hampering future clipping or stapling of the RPV, while the caudate side may be clipped.

Once all caudate branches are divided, the posterior RPV is then dissected off the hilar plate, moving cephalad until the dissection plane is met from the anterior side. Once this space is developed, the RPV is encircled with a vessel loop (Fig. 24.7). The RPV may be divided between large plastic clips or stapler at this stage. If the RPV is particularly short, the proximal RPV inflow can be clipped without division, in which case the completion of this process is performed later in the procedure (transection of the parenchyma and right hepatic duct increases the space around the RPV, which will enable placement of additional clips or a stapler prior to division).

Indocyanine Green Injection and Firefly™

Demarcation of right versus left liver lobes is enhanced by indocyanine green (ICG) dye injection (Fig. 24.8). We use a 2.5 mg dose of ICG given after inflow to the relevant lobe has been ligated. The line of demarcation is marked on the liver surface using electrocautery. Injecting the dye at this stage will also allow enough time for biliary excretion, which will assist in identification of the relevant-sided hepatic duct during parenchymal transection.

Mobilization of the Right Lobe

The third arm is moved to the inferior aspect of segments 5 and 6 and used to retract these segments superior-anteriorly, exposing the inferior layer of the right coronary and right triangular ligaments. These ligaments are divided using the scissors or vessel sealer, taking care not to injure the diaphragm. As more of the bare area is

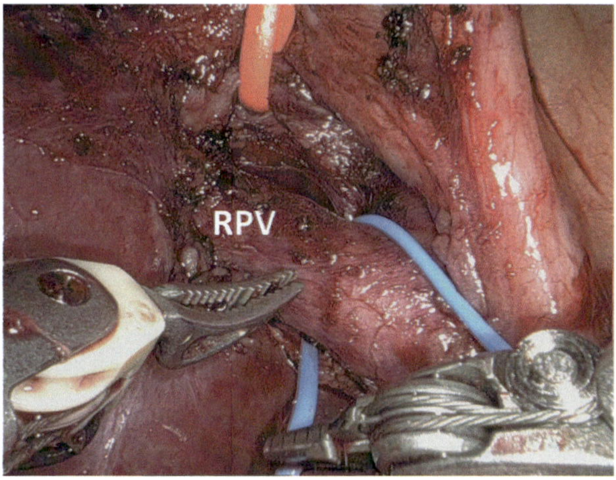

Fig. 24.7 Right portal vein (RPV) encircled with a blue vessel loop

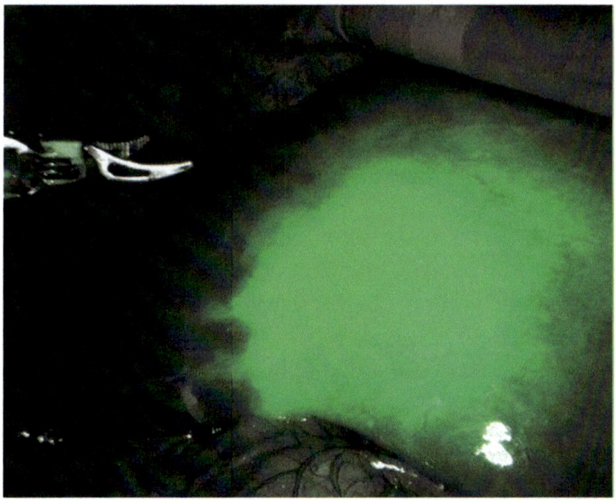

Fig. 24.8 Enhancement of right vs left lobe demarcation using ICG fluorescence

exposed, the third arm is moved sequentially superiorly and posteriorly to provide more retraction. The right adrenal gland is mobilized from the posterior surface of the liver. Once most of the bare area has been mobilized, we turn our attention medially toward the retrohepatic inferior vena cava (IVC).

The peritoneal lining between the caudate and IVC is divided, and the short caudate and hepatic veins draining directly to the IVC are serially divided between clips or with a vessel sealer (Fig. 24.9). Dissection continues in a cephalad direction on the anterior surface of the retrohepatic IVC, mobilizing the liver from the IVC. Caudate lobe division at this point helps cephalad dissection of the IVC. Laterally, the hepatocaval ligament will be encountered and can be left intact at this stage as division of this ligament is easier after parenchymal transection. The liver is carefully mobilized from the IVC until the area between the right and middle hepatic veins is reached. This completes the right lobe mobilization.

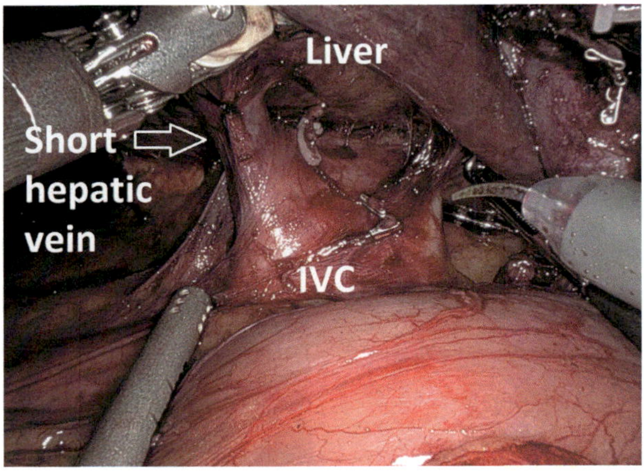

Fig. 24.9 Retrohepatic inferior vena cava (IVC) dissection showing a short hepatic vein branch

Parenchymal Transection and Bile Duct Division

Intraoperative Ultrasound

An ultrasound is performed to delineate the anatomy of the liver mass and rule out unsuspected liver metastasis prior to parenchymal transection. This examination also ensures that transection margins are accurately marked. Location of major pedicles and segmental draining hepatic veins which will be encountered during transection can also be detected on ultrasound and marked on the liver surface. Ultrasound images can be visualized in conjunction with the operative view on the console using the multi-display system (Fig. 24.10).

Retraction of the Liver Using "Rubber Band" Technique

One rubber band is secured to the liver edges at each side of transection plane with 3/0 Vicryl sutures [12]. Each rubber band is then externalized on the skin of the corresponding right and left upper abdomen and clamped to the drapes. This technique provides constant retraction of the transection plane without having to use any of the robotic or laparoscopic arms or a liver retractor (Fig. 24.11).

Parenchymal Transection

The third arm is used to gently lift the inferior surface of the liver off the hilum. Parenchymal transection is performed with harmonic scalpel and Maryland bipolar forceps (Fig. 24.12). Small intervening vessels and oozing from the parenchyma are controlled with bipolar electrocautery. Larger vessels including segmental veins may be clipped and divided with the harmonic device. As more of the parenchyma is transected, the liver edges are continually retracted due to the elasticity of the rubber bands.

An alternative technique is to deploy the laparoscopic Cavitron Ultrasonic Surgical Aspirator (CUSA, Integra Lifesciences, Princeton, NJ, USA) via one of the assistant ports to transect the parenchyma. The utility of this technique is dependent on the availability of a bedside surgeon who is facile in using the laparoscopic

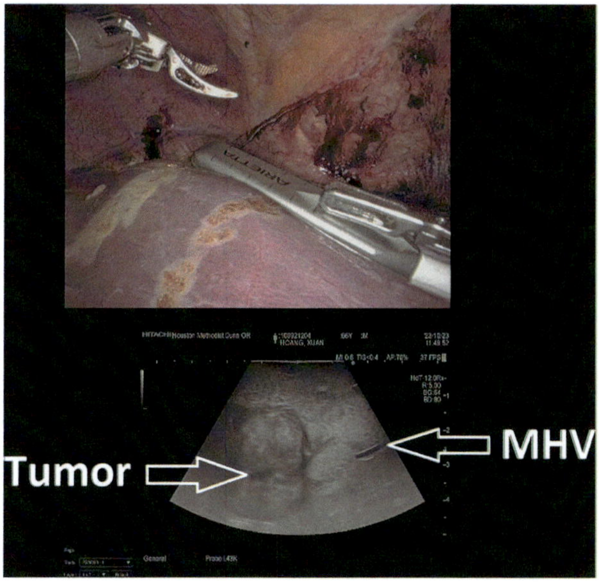

Fig. 24.10 Multiview display of ultrasound showing tumor and middle hepatic vein (MHV) location and operative view

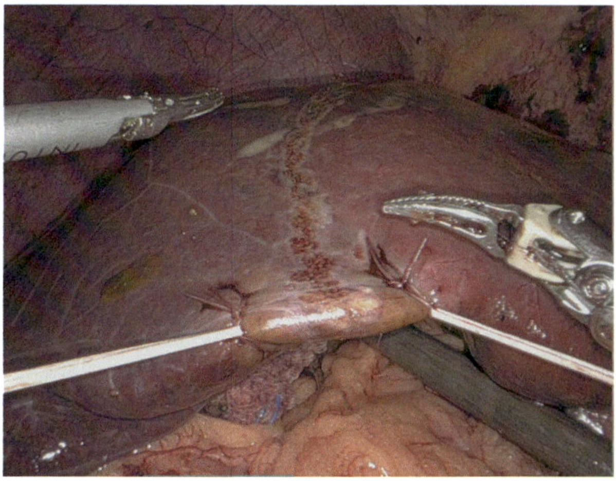

Fig. 24.11 Rubber band retraction technique

CUSA. When the majority of the parenchyma has been transected (leaving only a 1–2 cm strip of liver anterior to the IVC), the right hepatic duct (RHD) is divided.

Division of Right Hepatic Duct

ICG cholangiogram offers visualization of the bile ducts and biliary bifurcation using Firefly™. The location of RHD division is chosen based on the surgeon's interpretation of the cholangiogram. The RHD with surrounding hilar plate should be encircled with an umbilical tape. The duct is then divided between clips. The distal duct should be doubly clipped if there is enough length; if not, the stump should be suture-ligated above a single clip.

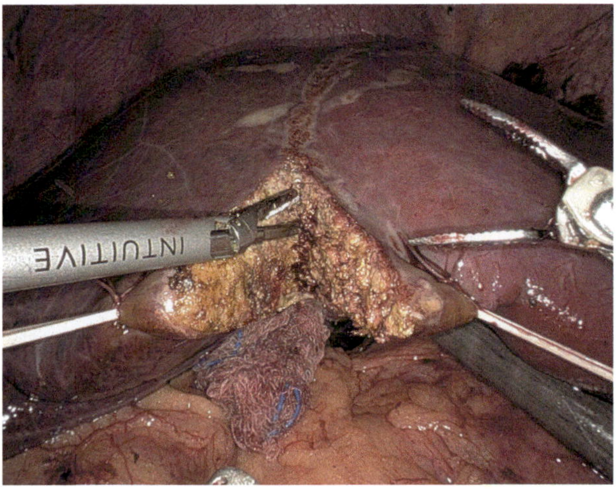

Fig. 24.12 Parenchymal transection with harmonic scalpel and bipolar Maryland forceps

Final Portion of Parenchymal Transection

Once the RHD is transected, the laparoscopic assistant inserts a grasper or suction catheter into the space previously created between the liver and retrohepatic IVC, which is used to lift the liver away from the IVC. This portion of the parenchyma is transected, heading cephalad toward the hepatic venous confluence. Finally, the grasper is inserted into the space between the right and middle hepatic vein, and the last portion of the parenchymal transection is completed.

Division of the Right Hepatic Vein and Hepatocaval Ligament, and Specimen Retrieval

The Maryland forceps is used to encircle the right hepatic vein (RHV) with an umbilical tape from within the transection plane (Fig. 24.13). The RHV is transected with a stapler. The hepatocaval ligament is also transected with a separate firing of the stapler. The right lobe is then placed into a plastic retrieval bag, which is removed via a Pfannenstiel incision. Final check for hemostasis and bile leak is performed and a drain is placed adjacent to the cut surface and externalized through one of the ports.

Left Hepatectomy

Falciform Dissection and Mobilization of the Left Lobe

Falciform dissection is similar to right hepatectomy. Additionally, the left triangular ligament is divided to mobilize the left lobe from its diaphragmatic attachments. The left lateral segment is retracted toward the patient's right abdomen using the third arm, exposing the gastrohepatic ligament, which is divided up to the level of the left hepatic vein. The Arantius ligament courses along the groove between the left lateral segment and caudate lobe from the left portal vein to the left/middle hepatic veins. It is divided at the superior pole of the caudate lobe, providing access

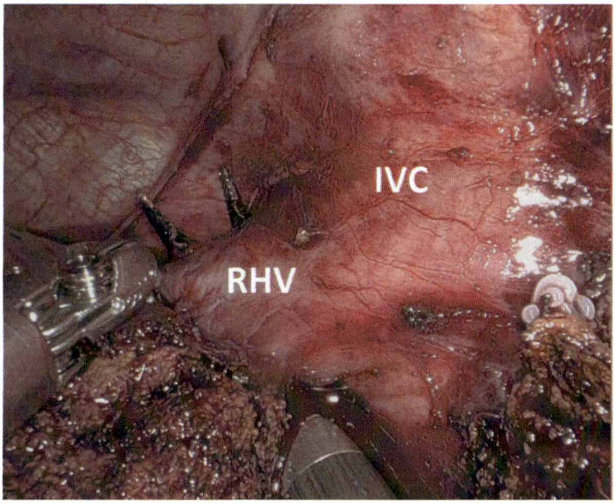

Fig. 24.13 Right hepatic vein (RHV) encircled with Maryland forceps after completion of parenchymal transection

to the posterior aspect of the left hepatic vein. Careful dissection in this area can enable encirclement of the middle and left hepatic veins; these veins can be divided with a stapler after the inflow is taken. If encirclement is difficult, the veins can be stapled at the end of parenchymal transection.

If the caudate lobe is to be resected as well, Spiegel's lobe is retracted with the tip of the third arm. It is mobilized from the IVC by incision of the peritoneal attachments and division of the hepatocaval ligament and the short hepatic veins draining the caudate directly to the IVC.

Hilar Dissection

Since the left-sided hilar structures are not covered anteriorly by the CBD, cholecystectomy may be performed at this stage, or after completion of the liver resection. The third arm is used with a gauze pad to retract segment 4B.

Dissection of the Left Hepatic Artery

The peritoneum over the left side of the hilum is opened and pulsation of the left hepatic artery (LHA) is located. This artery usually courses along the left side of the hilar base to the umbilical fissure and it is common for the LHA to be short, as it may divide early into the segment 4 and segment 2/3 branches. All lymphatic and nerve tissues are dissected away from the LHA, including the station 12a node, which is usually adherent to the left side of both the LHA and left portal vein (LPV). The LHA is encircled and divided between clips or ties.

If there is a replaced or accessory left hepatic artery, this is usually a branch of the left gastric artery and can be located during division of the gastrohepatic ligament. The branch is ligated and divided in this location.

Dissection of the Left Portal Vein

Division of the LHA will expose the anterior surface of the LPV. The plane between the left hepatic duct or hilar plate and superior-anterior surface of the LPV is gently developed by pushing the portal vein posteriorly and inferiorly off the attachments. Dissection proceeds transversely along the base of segment 4B from the portal vein bifurcation until the umbilical fissure. Several small segment 4B branches from the LPV are divided in a similar manner to the caudate branches.

Attention is then moved to the dissection of the posterior LPV. The peritoneal lining the posterior aspect of the LPV is divided and retracted posterior-inferiorly by the laparoscopic assistant. The caudate branches are divided after ligation in a similar manner as the right-sided caudate branches.

Once all caudate branches are divided, the posterior LPV is then dissected off the hilar plate, moving cephalad until the dissection is met from the anterior side. Once this space is developed, the LPV is encircled and is usually long enough to be divided between large plastic clips or a stapler.

Lobe Demarcation and Parenchymal Transection

ICG is used to demarcate the left lobe similar to the technique described with a right hepatectomy. Once the transection line is marked, the rubber band retraction technique is used here as described above. Parenchymal transection is performed as previously described. Intervening segmental veins are encircled and divided between clips or with energy device (Fig. 24.14). The caudate is transected from the right lobe if it is to be included in the specimen. If the caudate can be preserved, the transection line will change to a horizontal plane at the level of the hilum to separate the left lobe from the anterior of the caudate lobe. Once the left hepatic duct (LHD) has been divided (see below), the final part of the parenchymal transection is completed. If the middle and left hepatic veins have not been ligated prior to parenchymal transection, this step can be performed now with a stapling device.

Division of Left Hepatic Duct

The LHD is similarly identified using ICG cholangiogram (Fig. 24.15). If the bile duct margin is not relevant, the LHD is usually divided adjacent to the umbilical fissure to avoid injury to aberrant right hepatic duct branches.

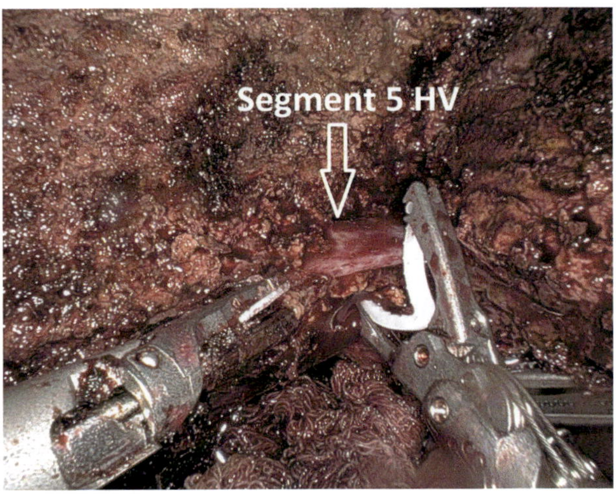

Fig. 24.14 Segment 5 hepatic vein (HV) clipped during parenchymal transection

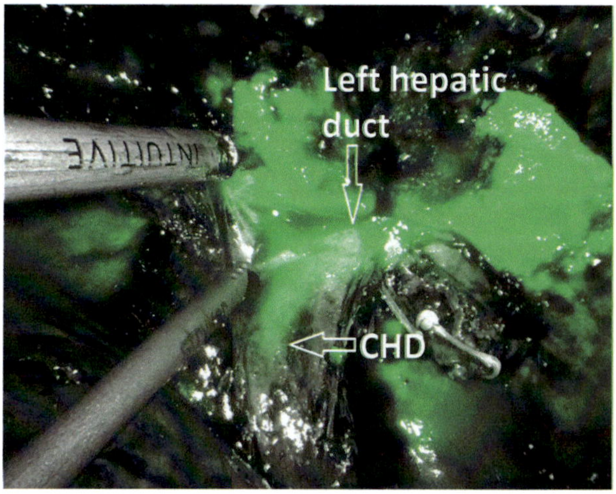

Fig. 24.15 ICG cholangiogram demonstrating common hepatic duct (CHD), biliary bifurcation, and site of division of left hepatic duct

Pringle Maneuver

An intermittent Pringle maneuver is useful when inflow control cannot be obtained prior to parenchymal transection or to reduce bleeding during parenchymal transection [13]. Most reports of the Pringle maneuver for minimally invasive liver surgery involve extracorporeal control of the tourniquet. In this technique, control of the Pringle maneuver in robotic surgery is in the hands of the bedside laparoscopic assistant surgeon. One end of a long moistened umbilical tape is inserted via a 5 mm laparoscopic port, leaving the other end outside the abdomen. The position of this port is usually on the opposite side of the lobe to be resected, i.e., the port is placed in the left abdomen in a right hepatic resection and vice versa. The tape is slung around the liver hilum and the end is externalized via the same port. The laparoscopic trocar is then removed and a small-bore chest tube or silastic catheter is slid over both strings, with the ends remaining extracorporeal. The bedside surgeon can then control the Pringle application in the style of a Rumel tourniquet.

Alternatively, intracorporeal Pringle maneuvers have been described, including applying a laparoscopic Satinsky clamp across the hilum, or leaving the ends of the tapes intracorporeal and cinching the tourniquet by inserting a large occluding clip. The Huang's loop is another intracorporeal technique, which uses a foreshortened urinary catheter, forming a loop by pulling the tail through the side hole [14]. The loop is cinched to apply the tourniquet and then secured with a clip.

Pertinent Technical Notes for Other Types of Hepatectomy

Left Lateral Sectionectomy

Port positions are similar to left hepatectomy. Parenchymal transection is usually performed to the left of the umbilical fissure and falciform ligament. Inflow control utilizes a Glissonian technique by division of the pedicles to segments 2 and 3 during parenchymal transection. The left hepatic vein can be divided between clips or with a stapler at the end of parenchymal transection (Video 2).

Right Posterior Sectionectomy

Port positions are moved slightly more to the right compared to a right hepatectomy. The patient should be positioned with right side up at 10–15 degrees. The falciform ligament can be looped with a suture, which is then externalized in the left abdomen and clamped to the drapes. The suture is used to retract the liver toward the patient's left side. The right posterior pedicle is found in Rouviere's sulcus in 70% of cases, which should be confirmed on preoperative imaging [15]. Inflow control is obtained using a Glissonian technique, with dissection in this area and transection of the pedicle using a stapling device. Demarcation with ICG can be performed to confirm isolation of the correct pedicle prior to division. The transection plane of a right posterior sectionectomy is rather long and should be in the direction of the right hepatic vein. The outflow can be taken from within the parenchyma during transection.

Segment 7 Resection

Port positions and retraction of falciform ligament are similar to right posterior sectionectomy. The patient may be rotated with the right side slightly up or even in a left semi-decubitus position. The patient's right hip may need to be lowered to prevent restriction of movement of the robotic arms. The third arm is used on segment 6 to retract the right lobe toward the left.

Segment 8 Resection

Port positions are similar to right posterior sectionectomy but may need to be placed more cephalad on the abdomen. Falciform ligament retraction toward the patient's left lower abdomen can help access to segment 8. For anatomical segment 8 resection, the confluence of the right and middle hepatic veins should be clearly visualized and accessible.

Central Hepatectomy (Segments 4a and 4b +/− 5 and 8)

These types of resections involve two parenchymal transection planes, which will prolong operative time. Port positions are similar to right hepatic resection. Pedicles to segment 4 are taken on the right side of the umbilical fissure during parenchymal transection. The right anterior pedicles in segments 5 and 8 resection can be isolated using the Glissonian technique prior to parenchymal transection or located during parenchymal transection. If the tumor is not close to the hilar area, it is best to avoid transecting down to the hilum (as long as margins are adequate) to prevent injury to the bifurcation of the bile duct or portal vein.

Robotic Biliary Reconstruction

Biliary reconstruction, particularly anastomosis of the intra- or extrahepatic bile ducts to the gastrointestinal tract, is commonly indicated in resection of choledochal cysts, repair of bile duct injury, resection of bile duct tumors, and palliative bypass.

Flexibility of the robotic platform enables anastomosis of even small segmental ducts to the jejunum. ICG cholangiogram on Firefly™ mode can be used to highlight the biliary anatomy. One of the largest series of robotic choledochal cyst excision in adults demonstrated that robotic surgery had longer operative times but lower complications compared to laparoscopic approaches [16]. Similarly for biliary reconstruction after bile duct injury, the robotic approach was associated with comparable morbidity to laparoscopic surgery but a higher primary patency rate of the hepaticojejunostomy anastomosis, though this did not reach statistical significance [17].

Patient Positioning, Port Placement, and Robotic Instruments

Positioning, port placement, and instrumentation are described above throughout the hepatectomy section. ICG is injected intravenously in the preoperative setting at least 30 minutes prior to incision to enable drainage into the biliary tract by the time cholangiogram is performed.

Delineation of Anatomy and Resection or Division of Bile Duct

The third arm is used with a gauze pad to retract segment 4B exposing the hilum.

Choledochal Cyst

For excision of the choledochal cyst, the right and left margins of the cyst are dissected from the hilar tissues proceeding toward the duodenum. In the majority of cases, the inferior extent of the cyst usually lies within the pancreatic head. This part is carefully dissected to avoid injury to the pancreatic parenchyma; small vessels are transected with an energy device. Once the inferior extent of the cyst is reached, it is transected between clips or with a staple. The inferior end is then retracted superiorly, and the posterior wall of the cyst is mobilized. The RHA is visualized crossing posterior to the CHD (conventional anatomy) and preserved. The gallbladder is taken down from the liver bed and cystic artery divided between clips. The gallbladder can be left attached to the cyst via the cystic duct. The common hepatic duct is divided and the specimen is retrieved with a plastic bag at the end of the procedure.

Bile Duct Injury

In-depth discussion of the type and timing of bile duct repair is beyond the scope of this chapter. Principles of operative repair of bile duct injury are (1) delineation of anatomy of the biliary and vascular system (both pre- and intraoperatively), (2) drainage of biloma, (3) debridement to healthy bile duct tissue, and (4) biliary reconstruction.

At the beginning of these cases, lysis of adhesions is commonly required, and any bile collections are drained. ICG cholangiogram is performed to confirm the anatomy of bile duct injury. This can be supplemented by conventional catheter cholangiogram. The technique to perform a catheter cholangiogram with the robot docked involves creating a space between the robotic arms for the C-arm machine. This space is made by increasing the gap between robotic arms 2 and 3 and introducing the C-arm here from the patient's right shoulder.

The type of biliary reconstruction is dependent on the type and location of the bile duct injury but will usually involve formation of a roux limb for anastomosis between the bile ducts and jejunum. The injured bile duct stump(s) should be debrided until healthy tissue is reached.

Resection of Hilar Cholangiocarcinoma or Palliative Biliary Bypass

Upon completion of the resection of hilar cholangiocarcinoma, the extrahepatic bile duct is removed en bloc with the hepatectomy specimen. The stump of the bile duct to the remnant is prepared for anastomosis.

For palliative biliary bypass, the bile duct proximal to the malignant obstruction is divided and the distal stump is closed with clips, staples, or suture-ligature. The proximal stump is then prepared for anastomosis.

Roux-en-Y Hepaticojejunostomy

The ligament of Treitz is located and a suitable location of the proximal jejunum is chosen where that the bowel can be brought up to the hilum without tension. The jejunum and the mesentery are transected at this area, and the distal jejunum is run for 40 cm (this will be the roux limb). This site is then anastomosed to the proximal jejunum using a stapled anastomosis and the enterostomy is sutured closed in two layers. The stump of the roux limb is brought up to the hilum in an antecolic fashion.

The bile duct stump is anastomosed end to side to an enterostomy in the roux limb using interrupted 5/0 or 6/0 polydioxanone (PDS) (Fig. 24.16). For large bile ducts, the posterior wall of the anastomosis can be performed with a continuous

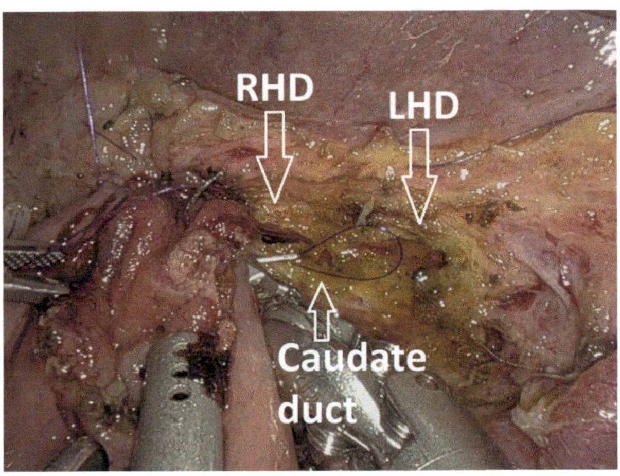

Fig. 24.16 Stitches inserted forming posterior wall of hepaticojejunostomy anastomosis between separate right (RHD), left (LHD), and caudate ducts and roux limb of jejunum

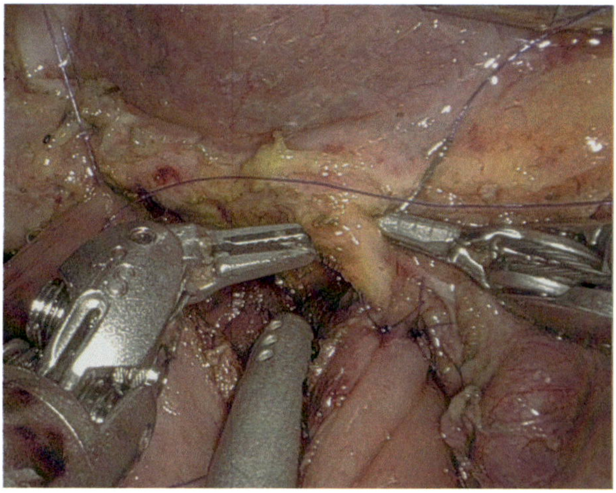

Fig. 24.17 Anterior wall of hepaticojejunostomy sutured with interrupted stitches

suture. If there are two bile duct stumps that are too short to be combined into one, it is often easier to complete the back wall stitches on both ducts before starting on the front walls of the anastomoses (Fig. 24.17).

Conclusion

The robotic platform provides some advantages over conventional laparoscopic technique for complex hepatobiliary surgery. Robotic instrumentation enables meticulous dissection of the liver hilum, enabling isolation of inflow vessels, dissection of the biliary tree, and biliary anastomosis. Adjuncts can be utilized, such as ICG cholangiogram, multi-image display to facilitate identification of biliary anatomy, and intraoperative ultrasound to guide liver resection. We are still in the early stages of adoption of this minimally invasive approach in hepatobiliary surgery, and larger multicenter studies are needed to define standardized techniques and investigate surgical and oncological outcomes.

References

1. Reich H, McGlynn F, DeCaprio J, Budin R. Laparoscopic excision of benign liver lesions. Obstet Gynecol. 1991;78(5 Pt 2):956–8.
2. Scatton O, Brustia R, Belli G, Pekolj J, Wakabayashi G, Gayet B. What kind of energy devices should be used for laparoscopic liver resection? Recommendations from a systematic review. J Hepatobiliary Pancreat Sci. 2015;22:327–34.
3. Giulianotti PC, Coratti A, Angelini M, Sbrana F, Cecconi S, Balestracci T, Caravaglios G. Robotics in general surgery: personal experience in a large community hospital. Arch Surg. 2003;138(7):777–84.
4. Wakabayashi T, Cacciaguerra AB, Abe Y, Bona ED, Nicolini D, Mocchegiani F, Kabeshima Y, Vivarelli M, Wakabayashi G, Kitagawa Y. Indocyanine green fluorescence

navigation in liver surgery: a systematic review on dose and timing of administration. Ann Surg. 2022;275(6):1025–34.
5. Di Benedetto F, Magistri P, Di Sandro S, et al. Safety and efficacy of robotic vs open liver resection for hepatocellular carcinoma. JAMA Surg. 2023;158(1):46–54.
6. Ciria R, Berardi G, Alconchel F, Briceño J, Choi GH, Wu YM, Sugioka A, Troisi RI, Salloum C, Soubrane O, Pratschke J, Martinie J, Tsung A, Araujo R, Sucandy I, Tang CN, Wakabayashi G. The impact of robotics in liver surgery: a worldwide systematic review and short-term outcomes meta-analysis on 2,728 cases. J Hepatobiliary Pancreat Sci. 2022;29(2):181–97.
7. Chen PD, Wu CY, Hu RH, Chou WH, Lai HS, Liang JT, Lee PH, Wu YM. Robotic versus open hepatectomy for hepatocellular carcinoma: a matched comparison. Ann Surg Oncol. 2017;24(4):1021–8.
8. Chen PD, Wu CY, Hu RH, Chen CN, Yuan RH, Liang JT, Lai HS, Wu YM. Robotic major hepatectomy: is there a learning curve? Surgery. 2017;161(3):642–9.
9. Sucandy I, Shapera E, Crespo K, Syblis C, Przetocki V, Ross S, Rosemurgy A. The effect of the robotic platform in hepatectomy after prior liver and non-liver abdominal operations: a comparative study of clinical outcomes. J Robot Surg. 2022;16(5):1067–72.
10. Hackl F, Nazemian R, Saeed A, Cheah YL, Kaufman MD. Anesthesia and enhanced recovery for robotic living donor hepatectomy—a narrative review. J Liver Transplant. 2023;9:100148.
11. Joliat GR, Kobayashi K, Hasegawa K, Thomson JE, Padbury R, Scott M, Brustia R, Scatton O, Tran Cao HS, Vauthey JN, Dincler S, Clavien PA, Wigmore SJ, Demartines N, Melloul E. Guidelines for perioperative care for liver surgery: Enhanced Recovery After Surgery (ERAS) Society Recommendations 2022. World J Surg. 2023 Jan;47(1):11–34.
12. Choi GH, Chong JU, Han DH, Choi JS, Lee WJ. Robotic hepatectomy: the Korean experience and perspective. Hepatobiliary Surg Nutr. 2017;6(4):230–8.
13. Ortiz Galindo SA, Haber PK, Benzing C, Krenzien F, Riddermann A, Frisch O, Schöning W, Schmelzle M, Pratschke J, Feldbrügge L. Safety of intermittent Pringle maneuver during minimally invasive liver resection in patients with hepatocellular carcinoma with and without cirrhosis. Langenbeck's Arch Surg. 2022;407(1):235–44.
14. Huang JW, Su WL, Wang SN. Alternative laparoscopic intracorporeal Pringle maneuver by Huang's loop. World J Surg. 2018;42(10):3312–5.
15. Dahmane R, Morjane A, Starc A. Anatomy and surgical relevance of Rouviere's sulcus. ScientificWorldJournal. 2013;2013:254287.
16. Lee H, Kwon W, Han Y, Kim JR, Kim SW, Jang JY. Comparison of surgical outcomes of intracorporeal hepaticojejunostomy in the excision of choledochal cysts using laparoscopic versus robot techniques. Ann Surg Treat Res. 2018 Apr;94(4):190–5.
17. Cuendis-Velázquez A, Trejo-Ávila M, Bada-Yllán O, Cárdenas-Lailson E, Morales-Chávez C, Fernández-Álvarez L, Romero-Loera S, Rojano-Rodríguez M, Valenzuela-Salazar C, Moreno-Portillo M. A new era of bile duct repair: robotic-assisted versus laparoscopic hepaticojejunostomy. J Gastrointest Surg. 2019;23(3):451–9.

25 Robotic-Assisted Pancreaticoduodenectomy (Whipple)

Ahmad Abou Abbass and Mohamad Othman El Helou

Abbreviations

BD	Bile duct
CHA	Common hepatic artery
ERAS	Early recovery after surgery
GDA	Gastroduodenal artery
IPDA	Inferior pancreaticoduodenal artery
IVC	Inferior vena cava
MIS	Minimally invasive surgery
PV	Portal vein
SMA	Superior mesenteric artery
SMV	Superior mesenteric vein

Robotic Whipple

Over the last decade, there has been a global surge in interest in the robotic approach for hepatobiliary surgery [9]. Notably, there has been a significant rise in the worldwide adoption of the robotic Whipple procedure, with the majority of major medical centers in the United States now offering this robotic approach to patients. Both patients and referring physicians have shown a growing curiosity about the benefits of the robotic [17].

A. Abou Abbass (✉)
Directory of Hepatobiliary Surgery, Mission Hospital, Mission Viejo, CA, USA

M. O. El Helou
Department of Surgery, Yale New Haven Hospital, Yale School of Medicine, New Haven, CT, USA

Department of Surgery, Henry Ford Providence Hospital, Southfield, MI, USA

S. Samreen et al. (eds.), *The SAGES Manual of Robotic Surgery*,
https://doi.org/10.1007/978-3-031-86927-3_25

Minimally invasive surgery (MIS) has demonstrated its equivalency or superiority to open surgery in various cases, characterized by reduced pain, shorter hospital stays, minimized fluid shifts, and improved cosmetic outcomes [17, 19]. In the context of colorectal surgery, MIS has been proven to yield comparable oncologic outcomes in terms of surgical margins, harvested lymph nodes, patient survival, and the occurrence of local or distant colon cancer recurrences [11].

These advantages are not exclusive to colorectal surgery and are also applicable to pancreatic cancer cases. Patients undergoing robotic surgery for pancreatic cancermay experience faster recovery times, enabling them to commence adjuvant therapy sooner. This prompt initiation of treatment could potentially translate into improved long-term survival rates [5, 12].

Since its introduction in 1994, laparoscopic Whipple has been shown to be a safe alternative to open procedures, demonstrating comparable short- and long-term outcomes. Notably, some studies reported fewer complications, shorter hospital stays, and reduced postoperative pain compared to open procedures [7].

Despite these advantages, the adoption of laparoscopic Whipple procedures has been limited within the surgical community due to inherent challenges. The complexity of resection, particularly in terms of reconstruction, places a significant physical burden on surgeons, making the procedure demanding and challenging. Consequently, only a small number of surgeons in the United States regularly perform laparoscopic Whipple procedures [3, 16].

In contrast, the robotic approach offers a more viable solution. With a stable platform, a three-dimensional view, and articulated instruments, it addresses the challenges faced by laparoscopic Whipple procedures, facilitating both dissection and reconstruction [15]. Moreover, the robotic approach enhances surgeon comfort as they can sit throughout the procedure, which can last between 4 and 8 hours (Fig. 25.1) [15]. This combination of technical advantages and increased comfort may contribute to the broader acceptance of robotic approaches within the surgical community.

The stable three-dimensional view and articulated instruments enable surgeons to navigate critical dissection around major vessels with increased precision. Moreover, the robotic platform facilitates the execution of demanding anastomoses, specifically those involving the pancreas and biliary system (Fig. 25.2). This technical prowess not only enhances the overall feasibility of the procedure but also positions the robotic approach as a valuable option for surgeons engaged in intricate surgeries like the Whipple procedure [13].

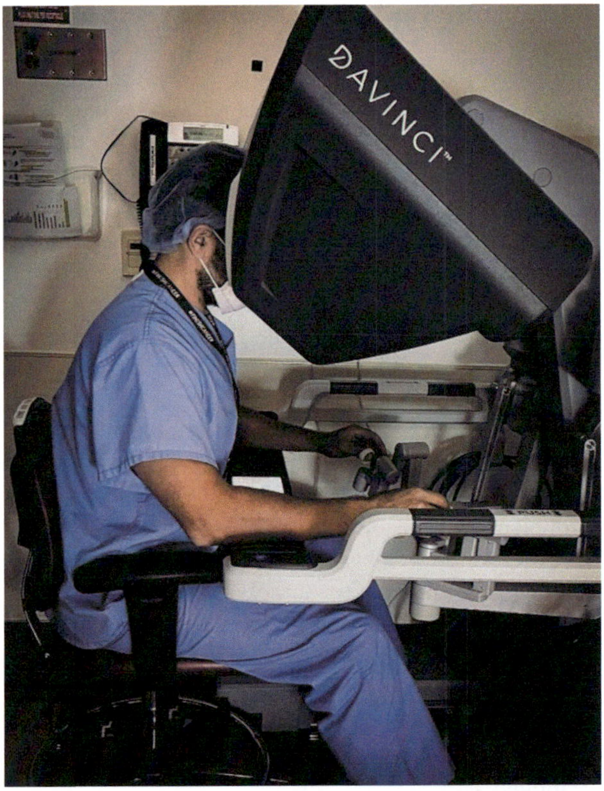

Fig. 25.1 Surgeon working on the robotic console

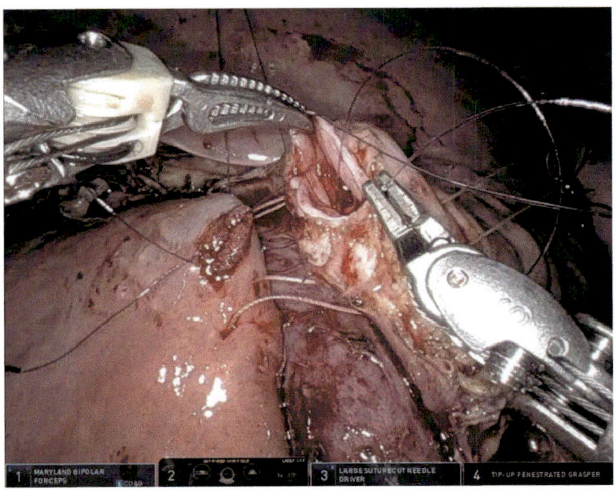

Fig. 25.2 Surgeon performing demanding anastomosis using the robotic system

Pathway to Building a Robotic Whipple Program

Currently, the predominant approach for Whipple procedures among surgeons in the United States is the open method, and training programs predominantly focus on imparting skills related to this traditional approach. However, there is a growing acknowledgment of the feasibility of transitioning to a robotic approach, particularly for practicing surgeons already proficient in open Whipple surgeries [22]. Venturing into robotic Whipple procedures necessitates two key prerequisites: proficiency in both open Whipple techniques and prior experience in robotic surgery.

For a surgeon to successfully adopt the robotic approach, a requisite level of expertise and caseload volume is essential. Rapidly gaining experience and overcoming the learning curve is facilitated by performing multiple robotic cases in a condensed timeframe [22]. It is important to note that a surgeon regularly performing Whipple procedures every few months, albeit safely, might find it more beneficial to adhere to the open approach. Thus, the decision to transition to a robotic approach should be a deliberate and informed one, grounded in the surgeon's dual proficiency and readiness for the complexities of robotic Whipple procedures.

Furthermore, embarking on a robotic Whipple procedure should not mark the initial foray into robotic surgery for a surgeon. Instead, a surgeon contemplating such complex robotic interventions must possess a high level of proficiency with the robotic platform, having gained extensive experience and familiarity with its capabilities and nuances. While the precise number of cases required varies for each surgeon, it is generally recommended that a surgeon accumulates a substantial experience base, potentially in the hundreds of cases, before considering a robotic Whipple.

Establishing a robust robotic practice follows a strategic progression, commencing with smaller, less complex cases and gradually advancing toward more intricate procedures, culminating in the Whipple. This step-up approach is underlined by a synergistic effect, where skills honed in various robotic procedures, such as dissecting the pancreatic neck in a distal pancreatectomy or harvesting the hilar lymph nodes for a radical cholecystectomy, contribute to the proficiency needed for a Whipple.

Crucially, a surgeon's journey to becoming proficient in robotic surgery hinges on adopting an "all in" approach. Embracing this mindset entails prioritizing robotic methods over laparoscopic or open approaches in the majority of cases. This immersive commitment is key to accelerating the learning curve and cultivating the necessary skills for mastering complex robotic surgeries like the Whipple procedure [10].

Initiating a robotic Whipple program demands unwavering commitment from the surgeon, along with support from both the department and hospital administration. A dedicated team is indispensable, encompassing a proficient bedside assistant, skilled scrub tech, and adept circulating nurses [14]. The collaborative efforts of this team are pivotal in executing the intricate surgery.

The primary robotic platform employed in nearly all robotic Whipple procedures is the Da Vinci XI Surgical System by Intuitive. Early collaboration with Intuitive, specifically their local representative, is crucial. They serve as a valuable resource, connecting the surgeon with experienced mentors, facilitating case observations, providing advanced courses on simulated models, and arranging for surgeon support and proctoring during initial cases.

A practical starting point involves leveraging digital resources to observe robotic Whipple procedures. Platforms like "YouTube" offer a wealth of videos from surgeons worldwide, showcasing diverse techniques and tools. However, advancing from virtual observation to in-person experiences is paramount. Being physically present in the operating room enables real-time communication with the surgeon, an understanding of the entire workflow, and the ability to learn troubleshooting should something go wrong. Ideally, the entire team should participate in these observations to enhance collaborative learning.

For hands-on preparation, Intuitive offers two robotic hepatobiliary courses hosted by seasoned surgeons across multiple locations in the United States. Planning a series of cases immediately following the training optimizes the application of newly acquired skills. Collaboration with Intuitive beforehand ensures the availability of a proctoring surgeon on selected dates, offering invaluable support for the initial cases.

Patient Selection

Choosing the right patients is crucial, especially when starting with robotic surgeries. It's recommended to begin with early-stage, clearly resectable cancer cases. Cases involving non-pancreatic cancers like ampullary or duodenal tumors, as well as pancreatic neuroendocrine tumors, are also ideal for the initial robotic approach. These cases are advantageous because they require less extensive dissection around major blood vessels like the superior mesenteric vein (SMV) or artery (SMA). Early on, surgeons may find working closely with these vessels challenging, but as they gain experience, they'll become more comfortable with the intricate dissection. One potential challenge might be a harder pancreatic anastomosis with a soft pancreas and small duct, but the robotic platform makes the process feasible.

While vascular resection and reconstruction have been reported in the literature and are technically achievable, it is recommended to avoid these cases until the surgeon has gained substantial experience in robotic Whipple procedures. Some surgeons may choose to never perform robotic vascular resections, especially if they do not perform them using an open approach and prefer vascular surgeons to handle the actual anastomosis [1]. This cautious approach ensures a gradual and safe progression in adopting complex robotic techniques.

Furthermore, it is advisable to steer clear of cases that pose challenging dissections, such as those involving obese patients, individuals with a history of pancreatitis, or those who have undergone radiation therapy. Patients with a surgical history that includes procedures like surgery for peptic ulcer disease or gastric bypass should also be avoided. However, a previous abdominal cholecystectomy is generally not a concern. For patients with a history of exploratory laparotomy, there may be extensive small bowel adhesions, potentially complicating the mobilization of the jejunum enough to perform anastomoses.

Achieving favorable outcomes in robotic Whipple procedures requires selecting patients who are suitable candidates for major surgery, akin to open procedures. Preoperative optimization is crucial, encompassing cardiovascular, nutritional, and physical aspects. In cases where surgery is delayed, addressing jaundice is essential. Additionally, resolving any existing infections prior to surgery contributes to the overall readiness and well-being of the patient, laying the groundwork for a successful robotic Whipple procedure [8, 20].

Operating Room Setup and Instrumentation

A robotic Whipple procedure is typically conducted in a specialized robotic room designed to accommodate the robot, console, and laparoscopy towers, ensuring ample space for seamless operation. Essential equipment includes an ultrasound machine featuring a dedicated robotic probe, such as the BK5000 (R). The surgical setup involves utilizing laparoscopic and robotic trays, with open trays and an open retractor readily available in case a conversion to an open procedure becomes necessary (Figs. 25.3a, b).

The robotic instruments employed in a Whipple procedure commonly include a hook, monopolar scissors, fenestrated bipolar, tip-up instrument, and an energy device like the vessel sealer or synchro seal. Additionally, a robotic stapler, requiring a 12 mm robotic port, or a laparoscopic stapler used by the assistant can be incorporated. For fine dissection, a Maryland instrument is effective, while a large suture cut is suitable for suturing. Various clip appliers in large, medium, and small sizes are available for vessels like the gastroduodenal artery (GDA).

Sutures utilized during a robotic Whipple are often similar to those used in an open Whipple, but they need to be shorter, typically ranging from 6 to 8 inches. The choice of sutures includes 3–0 silk for the outer layer of the pancreatic anastomosis, 4–0 or 5–0 Monocryl for the duct-to-mucosa anastomosis, 4–0 PDS for the hepaticojejunostomy, 3–0 V-Loc sutures for the gastrojejunostomy, and 4–0 Prolene for controlling bleeding if necessary (Fig. 25.4).

The presence of vascular clamps is critical in an open Whipple procedure, making it essential to ensure availability of clamps that can pass through a 12 mm trocar and be easily applied in both laparoscopic and robotic settings (Fig. 25.5). Many hospitals typically already have these clamps readily accessible, as they are commonly used by urologists during procedures such as partial nephrectomies.

Airseal (R) can be beneficial as it maintains pneumoperitoneum in cases suction is needed for bleeding. That can be used with a dedicated assistant 12 mm trocar.

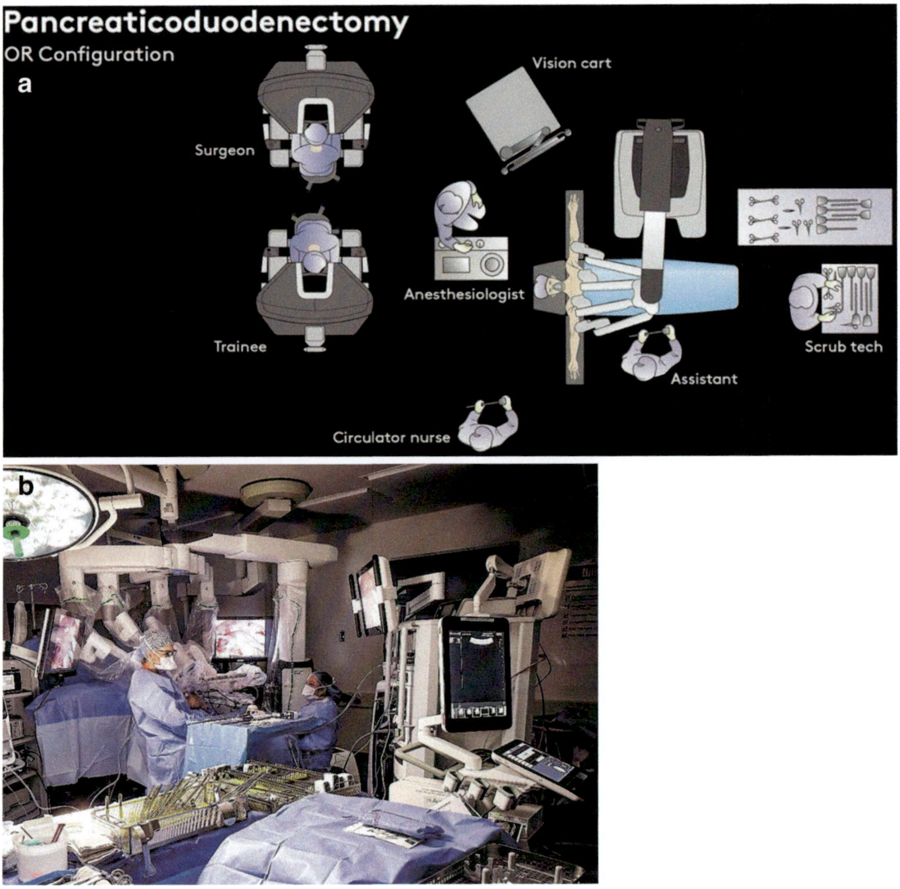

Fig. 25.3 (**a**) Operating room configuration for robotic Whipple. (**b**) Room setup for robotic Whipple. The robot comes from the left side. All needed robotic instruments are on the table, and open trays are readily available. Ultrasound machine is connected to the vision cart for picture-in-picture view when needed

Fig. 25.4 Sutures used in a robotic Whipple

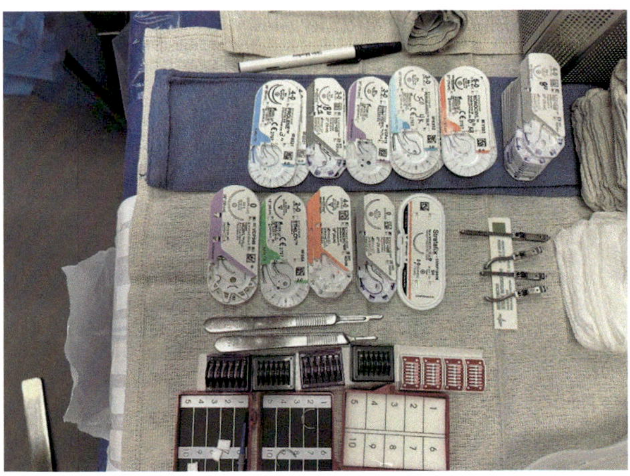

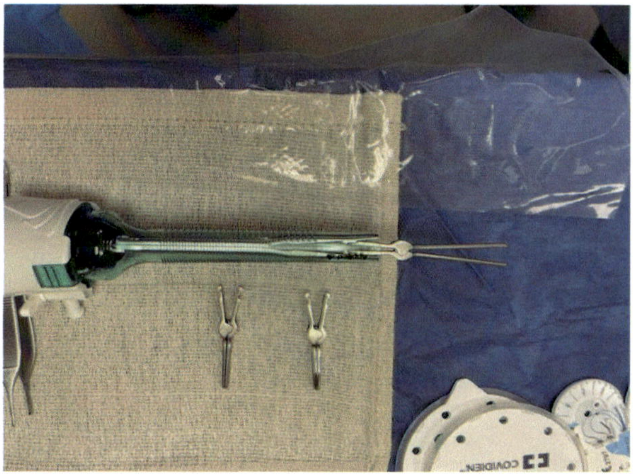

Fig. 25.5 Scanlan (R) vascular clamps

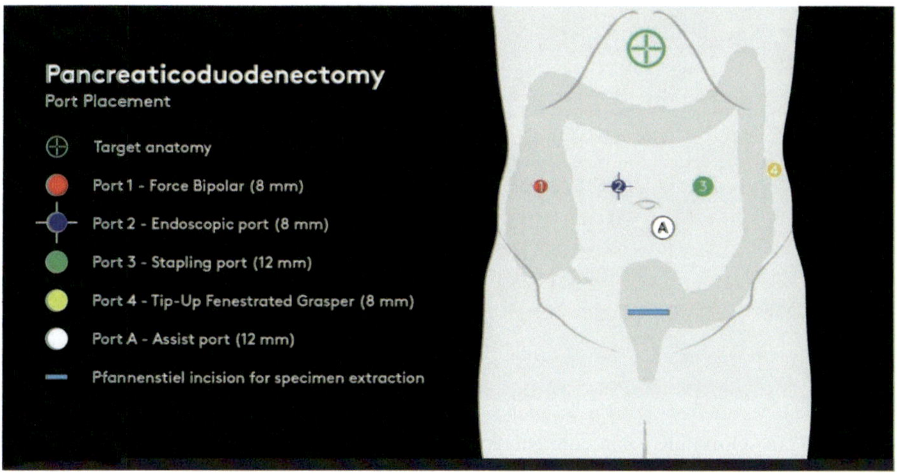

Fig. 25.6 Robotic Whipple port placement

Operative Steps

The patient is placed supine on the operating table with the arms extended. Access to the abdominal cavity is achieved and the abdomen is insufflated. The camera port is placed right to the umbilicus as that provides optimal view for uncinate dissection and for the pancreatic anastomosis. A diagnostic laparoscopy is performed to rule out occult peritoneal or liver metastases. Then an 8 mm port is placed to the right of the camera port and a 12 mm robotic port is placed on the left side. Another 8 mm port is placed on the left side of the 12 mm port. All the ports are placed in a straight line facing the target anatomy, and 8–10 cm apart. An assistant 12 mm port is placed in the left lower quadrant below and between the camera and the 12 mm robotic ports. Another 5 mm port can be placed in the right lower quadrant. (Figs. 25.6 and 25.7).

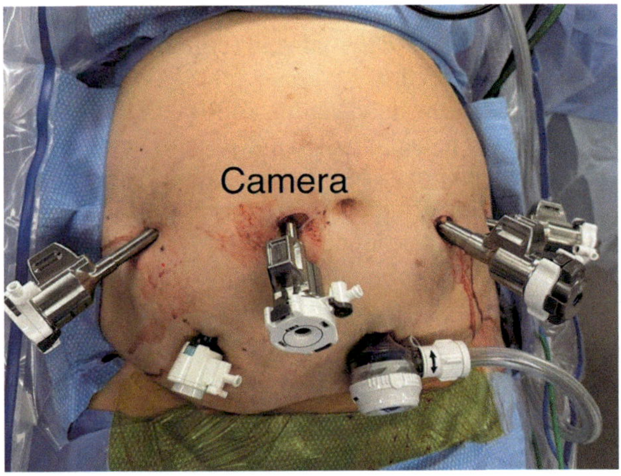

Fig. 25.7 Robotic Whipple port placement

The patient is then placed in 15–18 degrees of reverse Trendelenburg and the robot is docked. The instruments are placed under direct visualization and the surgeon then scrubs out and goes to the console.

The conduct of the operation follows a stepwise approach identical to open approach. The surgeon should follow a basic plan but allow for improvisation based on each individual case. If a step appears difficult, the surgeon can move on and come back to that step later and leave the most challenging step till the end of the dissection. The first few Whipples will take a long time, so it is best if the surgeon is prepared and have no other cases booked for the day. As the experience build up, the efficiency will improve, and the operative times will shorten.

The operation is performed almost entirely by the console surgeon, and the bedside assistant provides retraction and suction as needed as well as instrument exchange. Some centers adopted a hybrid approach where the bedside surgeon does a lot of the energy device division, clipping, and stapling.

Entering the Lesser Sac, Colon Mobilization

The first step after docking the robot is to divide the gastrocolic omentum and expose the pancreas. Dissection is carried toward the right side and the right colon is mobilized all the way to expose the head of the pancreas and duodenum. Gravity will retract the colon downward which helps in subsequent steps.

Kocher Maneuver, Ligament of Treitz Dissection

After the duodenum has been fully exposed, it is mobilized from the retroperitoneum and retracted to the left side by the third robotic arm. This dissection is carried by either hook or vessel sealer. This will expose the inferior vena cava (IVC) and left renal vein. Dissection is carried until the origin of the SMA is exposed as it crossed above the left renal vein (Fig. 25.8). The artery doesn't need to be circumferentially isolated.

Afterward, the duodenum is followed distally toward the ligament of Treitz and the proximal jejunum pulled to the right underneath the mesentery (Fig. 25.9). The proximal jejunum is then divided with robotic white load stapler.

If this step is difficult, then the transverse colon can be elevated and the ligament of Treitz dissection done to the left of the mesentery. Then the jejunum can be divided, and the proximal end is pulled from under the mesentery to the right upper quadrant.

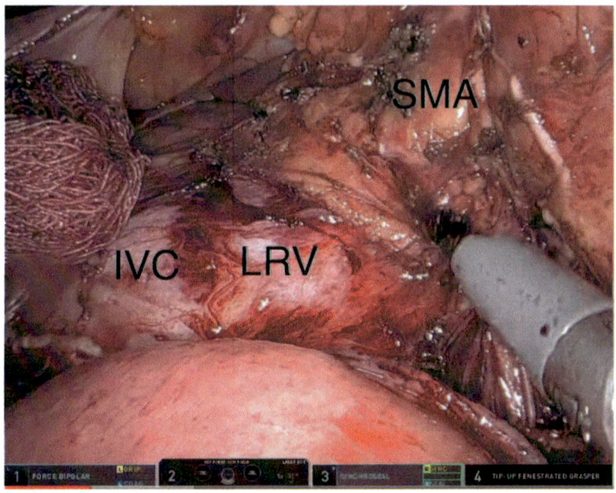

Fig. 25.8 Dissection of SMA over the IVC and left renal vein (LRV)

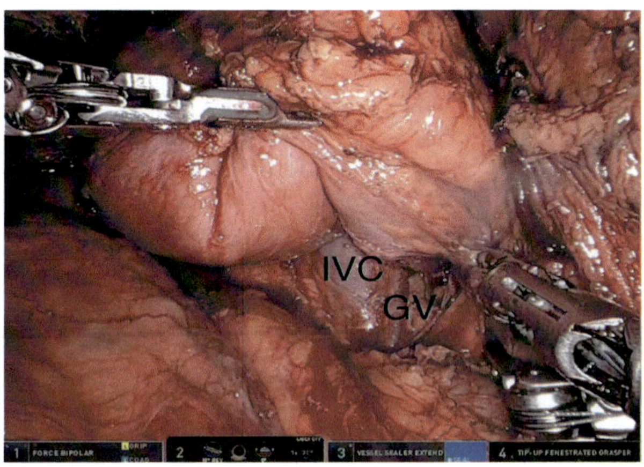

Fig. 25.9 Ligament of Treitz dissection from the right side of the mesentery. IVC inferior vena cava. GV gonadal vein

Infra-pancreatic Neck Dissection, Isolating the SMV

It is important to expose the SMV under the neck of the pancreas and see how easy it separates from the pancreas to assess resectability and possible need for vascular control. The SMV is exposed under the neck of the pancreas with gentle retraction on the pancreas and division of the areolar tissues with fine instruments like the hook until the vein is exposed (Fig. 25.10). It can be helpful to follow the middle colic vein backward toward the SMV. If there's a lot of fatty tissue, intro ultrasound can be very useful in finding the vein and save time trying to locate the vein.

After the vein is located, it is dissected anteriorly and separated from the neck of the pancreas starting the tunnel, which will be completed later.

The SMV is then followed distally separating it from the uncinate process. This is continued until the first jejunal vein is exposed. The right gastroepiploic vein will be encountered and needs to be divided which will further improve the exposure of the SMV (Fig. 25.11).

Once the vein has been dissected and it appears easily separable from the pancreatic headband uncinate process, then resectability is confirmed and the surgeon can proceed with the rest of the procedure.

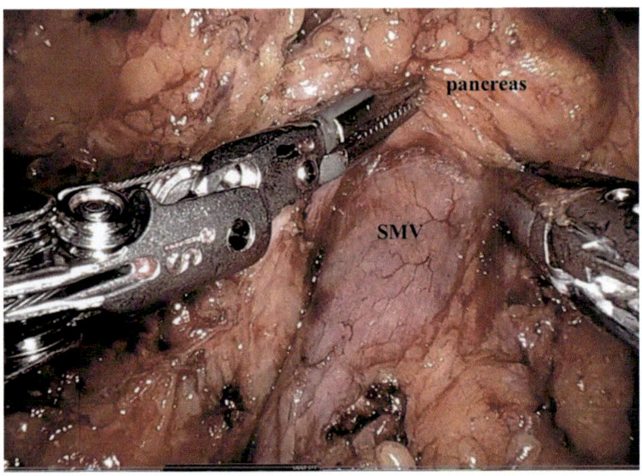

Fig. 25.10 SMV exposed below the pancreatic neck

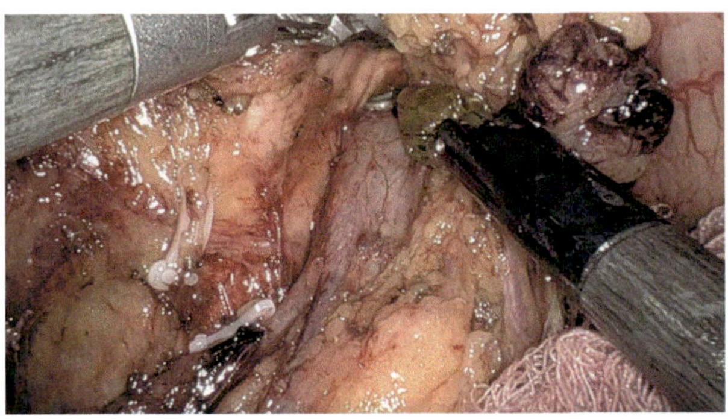

Fig. 25.11 The SMV appears to easily separate from the uncinate process, a good indicator of resectability. The right gastroepiploic vein has been divided between hemolock clips

Supra-pancreatic/Hilar Dissection

This step is started by division of the stomach as that gives better caudal access to the area. The stomach is divided with robotic stapler green or blue loads. If pylorus preservation is being done, the duodenum is divided with stapler distal to the pylorus.

Exposure of the liver hilum requires some sort of liver retraction. Both the falciform ligament and the gallbladder are sutured to the abdominal wall, which provides great exposure without the need for an external retractor (Figs. 25.12 and 25.13).

After the exposure is achieved, the hepatic artery lymph node (8A) is resected, which provides access to the common hepatic artery (CHA) . The artery is dissected distally until the gastroduodenal artery is encountered and isolated. It is then divided between hemlock clips with a tie or with a stapler (Fig. 25.14).

Dividing the GDA provides access to the underlying portal vein (PV), which is then exposed anteriorly and separated from the common bile duct on the right side. Any venous branches can be divided. The bile duct is isolated and either divided now or at the end of the resection to minimize bile spillage. This concludes the hilar dissection (Fig. 25.15). The cholecystectomy is done after the bile duct anastomosis as it is sutured to the abdominal wall to provide exposure.

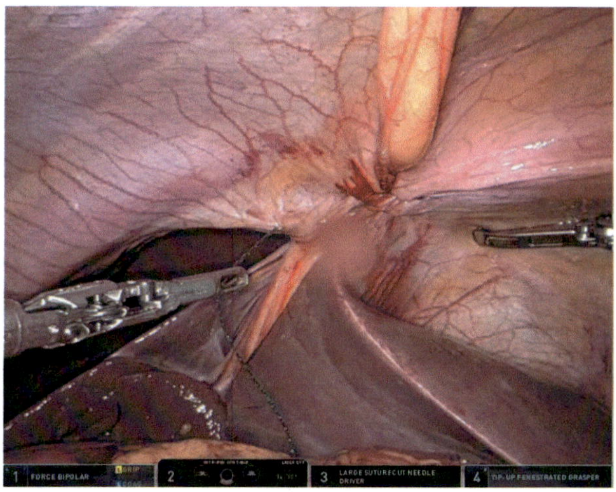

Fig. 25.12 Suturing of the falciform ligament to the abdominal wall

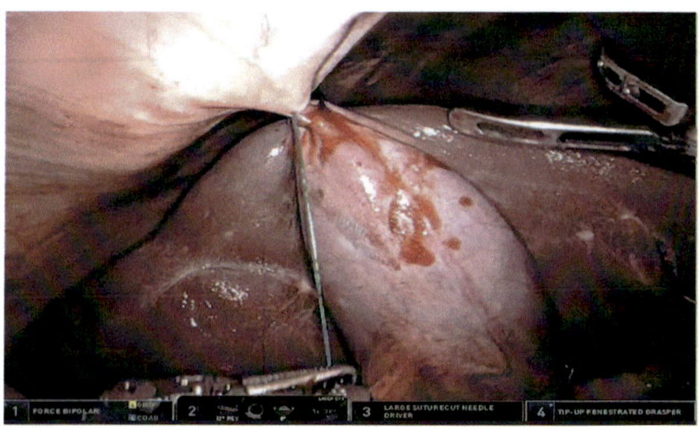

Fig. 25.13 Suturing of the gallbladder to the abdominal wall

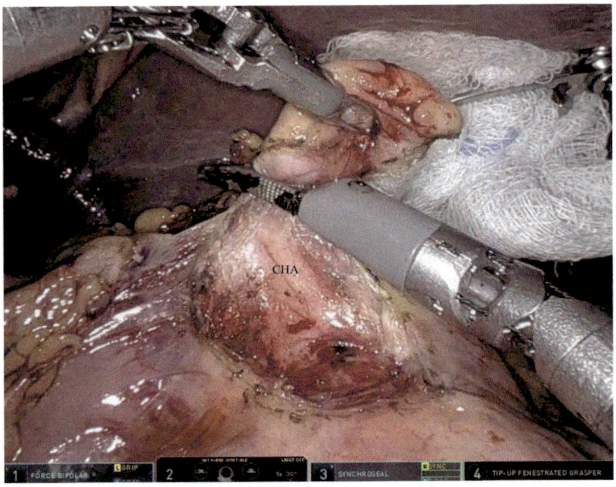

Fig. 25.14 Removal of the hepatic artery lymph nodes exposes the underlying common hepatic artery CHA

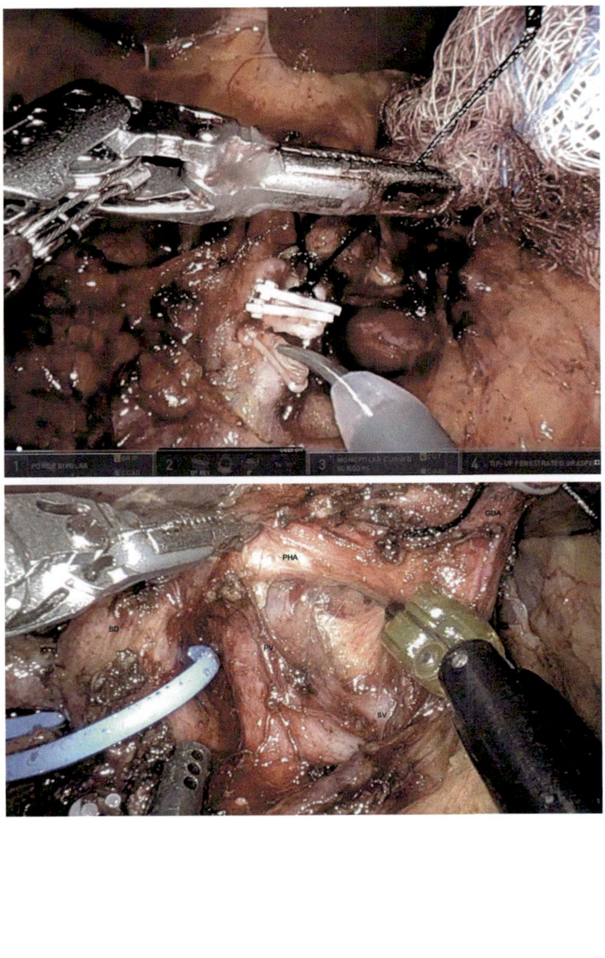

Fig. 25.15 The hilar dissection has been completed. The portal vein (PV) is well exposed. The bile duct (BD) has been encircled with a vessel loop to be divided later. SV (splenic vein)

Creating the Tunnel/Pancreatic Transection

Attention is then turned toward dividing the pancreas. After exposing the PV above and the SMV below the neck of the pancreas, the SMV is gently peeled off the overlying pancreatic neck using a blunt instrument like the Maryland bipolar forceps or synchro seal as there are no venous branches anteriorly. The tip-up forceps are great to complete the tunnel all the way to the other side as it is blunt and long enough (Fig. 25.16).

Sometimes, the pancreas is too stuck to the vein even if there's no tumor involvement particularly in patients with history of pancreatitis or radiation. In these cases, creating the full tunnel might be very difficult or even dangerous. So in these cases, it's best to start dividing the pancreas and dissecting it off the SMV in small steps at the same time until the pancreatic neck is fully divided.

The pancreatic neck is divided with monopolar scissors using energy. There's no need to place any sutures in the pancreas. The bleeders are easily controlled with monopolar energy. Once the pancreatic duct is reached, it is divided sharply with the scissors with a 1–2 mm stump which makes subsequent anastomosis easier (Fig. 25.17).

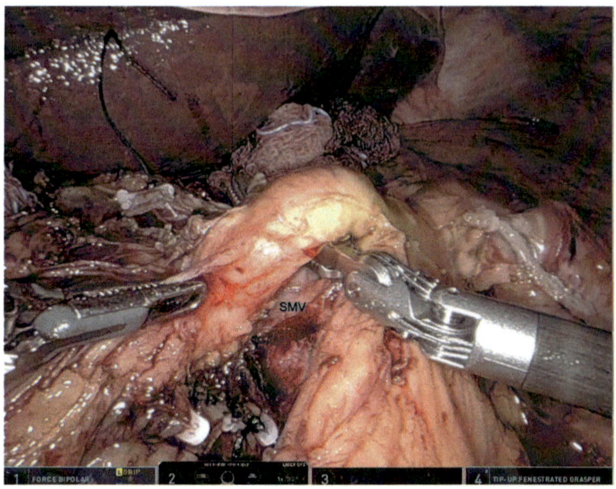

Fig. 25.16 Creating the tunnel for pancreatic transection

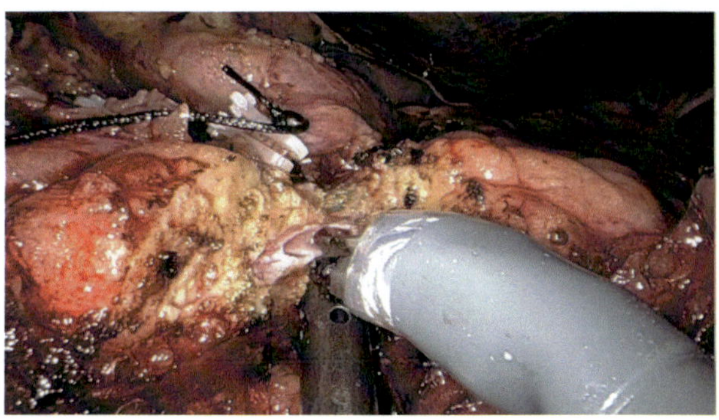

Fig. 25.17 Pancreatic neck division with scissors. The assistant protects the PV by pushing down on it with suction

A piece of pancreas from the specimen side is cut out and sent to pathology for frozen section if indicated.

Uncinate Dissection

This is the challenging part of the dissection as it involves being very close to the SMA and SMV and there's a risk of bleeding that can be difficult to control. The dissection is started in the caudal to cranial direction dissecting the SMV first then exposing and dissecting the SMA. This is started by retracting the specimen to the right by the left hand and exposing the first jejunal vein. There is usually a branch to the uncinate that needs to be divided (Fig. 25.18).

The SMV is then gently separated from the uncinate process with blunt dissection using the robotic hook. Any branches can be controlled with vessel sealing device. After the vein is freed, it is rolled to the left by the third arm exposing the underlying SMA. The SMA is surrounded with thick fibrous and nerve tissue, and it is best to do this dissection to use a fine instrument like the hook cautery. This will gradually expose the SMA for a good oncologic dissection and prevent injury to the artery and its branches. If the artery is difficult to locate, an intraoperative ultrasound is invaluable as one cannot feel for the pulse of the SMA (Fig. 25.19).

Once the artery is identified, it is skeletonized for 180 degrees on the right side with the hook cautery. The inferior pancreaticoduodenal artery (IPDA) is dissected and ligated close to the SMA with hemlock clips. There might be more than one arterial branch so extreme care is taken until the SMA is completely dissected (Fig. 25.20).

The SMA is followed down to its origin from the aorta which was exposed early in the procedure. All the lymph vascular tissues behind the PV including lymph node stations 12 P and B are brought with the specimen. If there's a replaced right hepatic artery off the SMA, extra care is taken to identify and preserve it.

At this point, the specimen is only attached by the bile duct, which is divided with scissors or stapler to minimize bile spillage (Fig. 25.21). The specimen is parked in the right lower quadrant to be removed at the end of the procedure.

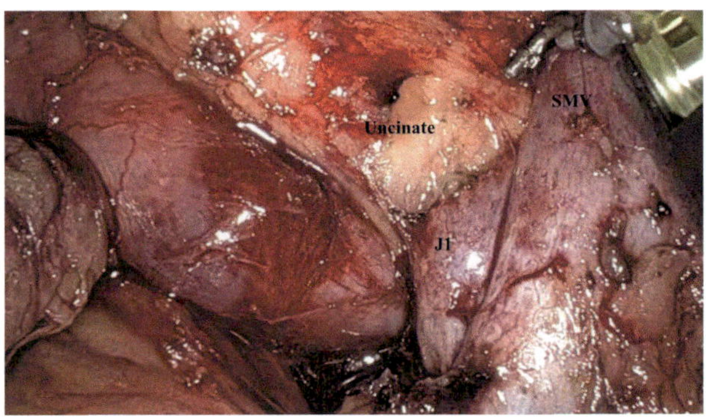

Fig. 25.18 Beginning of uncinate dissection. J1: first jejunal vein

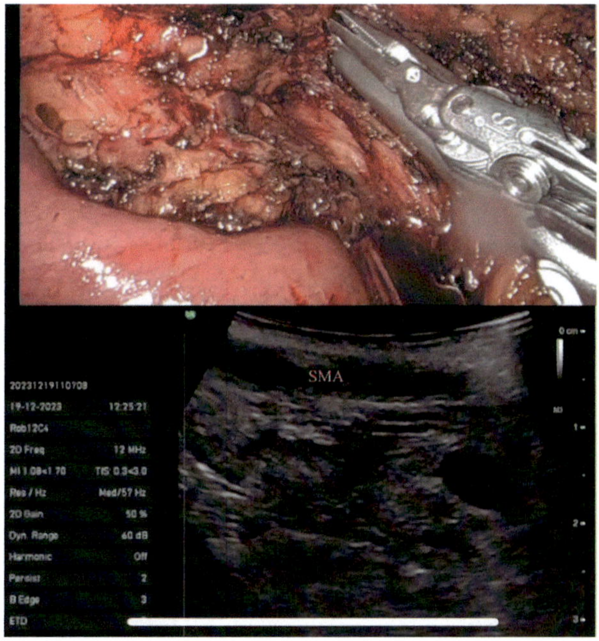

Fig. 25.19 Exposing the SMA and the use of intraoperative ultrasound for detection

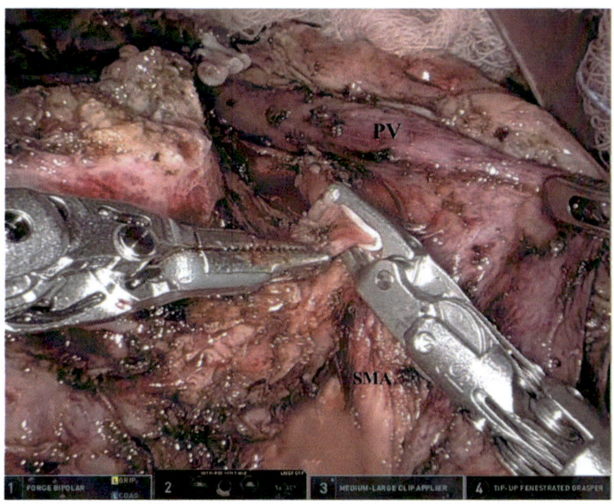

Fig. 25.20 IPDA is divided close to its origin between hemlock clips. The tip-up instrument is used in the third arm, and it gently retracts the SMV to the left to provide full exposure to the SMA. The SMA can even be grabbed with the tip-up

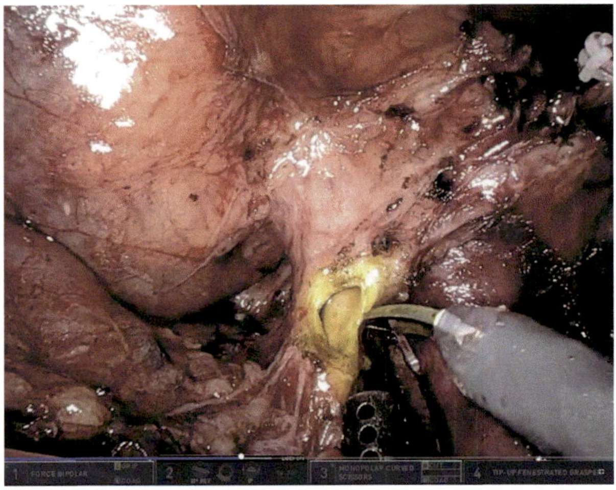

Fig. 25.21 Using the monopolar scissors to divide the specimen from the bile duct

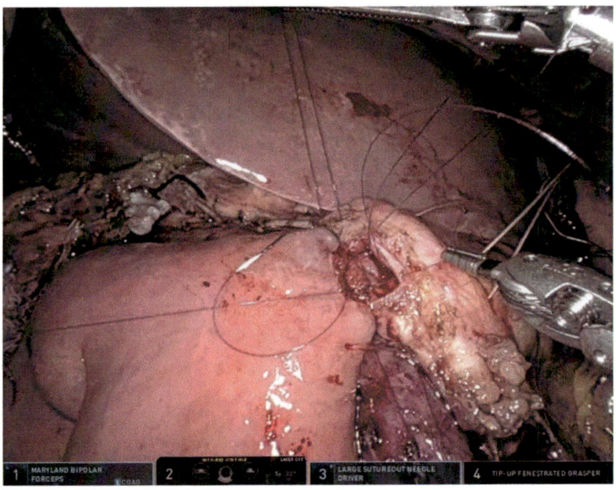

Fig. 25.22 Pancreaticojejunostomy

Reconstruction Phase

This phase is much less risky than the resection phase. However, it is very critical to perform a perfect anastomosis to minimize postoperative complications. The surgeon should take a short break at this time to be prepared for the reconstruction.

Pancreaticojejunostomy (Fig. 25.22)

The jejunum is brought through the natural ligament of Treitz opening or through a defect in the mesocolon, and the pancreatic anastomosis is performed. A modified Blumgart technique is done with outer seromuscular layer through and through pancreas using 3–0 silk sutures using the large suture cut instrument. The duct to mucosa anastomosis is done with interrupted 5–0 Monocryl over a 5- or 7-French stent. The technique is the same as open; only the sutures are much shorter (4–6 inches). The camera placement to the right of the umbilicus provides excellent view for the anastomosis, and the articulated robotic instrument with the magnification makes it easy to take perfect sutures.

Hepaticojejunostomy (Fig. 25.23), Cholecystectomy

Around 15–20 cm distal to the pancreaticojejunostomy, an enterotomy is made in the jejunum and the bile duct anastomosis is made. The bile duct is divided above the level of the cystic duct sharply with scissors. The cystic duct and artery are divided but the gallbladder is left in place as it's sutured to the abdominal wall to provide exposure. A 4–0 PDS is used, running for the posterior and interrupted for the anterior layer. Alternatively, a 3–0 V-Loc suture can be used to run the whole anastomosis. The anastomosis is checked for bile leak.

Then the gallbladder is removed off the liver bed with electrocautery and parked over the liver to be removed later.

Gastrojejunostomy (Fig. 25.24)

The transverse colon is lifted up and the mesenteric defect around the jejunum is closed with sutures. The jejunum is followed distally for around 50 cm and brought over the transverse colon to lie next to the stomach without tension. The GJ is done using robotic stapler and the common enterotomy is closed with 3–0 V-Loc in two layers. If a pylon preserving Whipple is done, the duodenal apple line is removed,

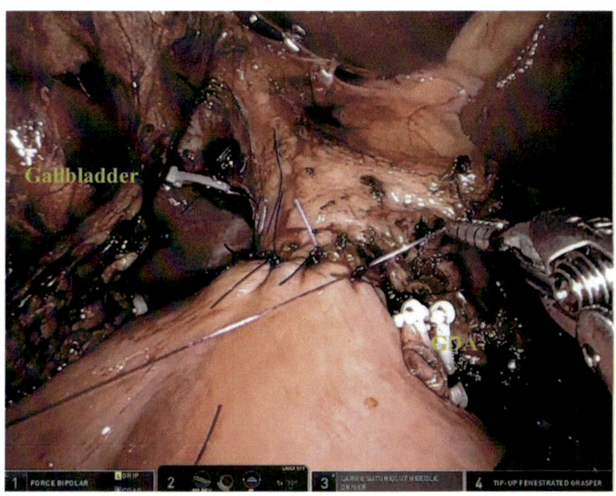

Fig. 25.23 Completed hepaticojejunostomy

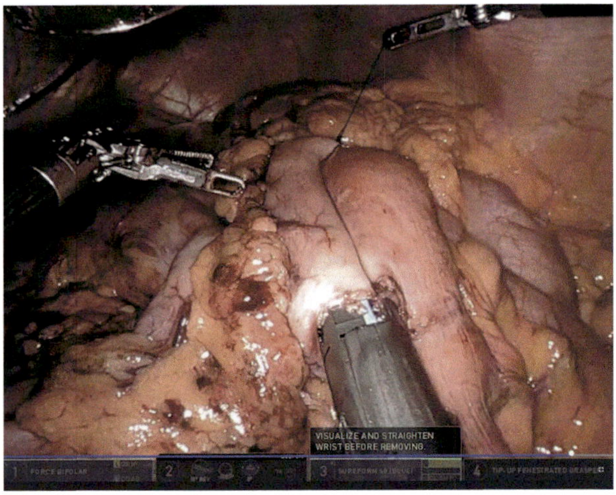

Fig. 25.24 Completed gastrojejunostomy

an enterotomy is made, and a single- or double-layer end to side duodenojejunostomy is performed with 3–0 V-Loc sutures.

Final Steps

The procedure is almost done. A falciform flap can be harvested and placed over the pancreatic anastomosis. The robot is undocked. A Pfannenstiel incision is made, and a wound protector is placed. The two specimens are removed and sent to pathology. The Pfannenstiel incision is closed. The abdomen is insufflated for final look and check for any bleeding or bile leak. A 19-F Blake drain is brought through the right-sided trocar and placed anterior to the pancreatico-jejunal and hepato-jejunal anastomosis. Any 12 mm port sites are closed with 0 Vicryl for fascia. All tracers are then removed, and skin closed.

Vascular Resections

It is important for the surgeon early in the robotic Whipple experience to select clearly resectable cases without any evidence of vascular invasion. If intraoperatively there appears to be any concerns for venous involvement, the safest thing to do is to convert to an open procedure. Venous resections however are doable with the robot. A surgeon can consider attempting a venous resection only after certain mastery with robotic Whipple has been achieved and the surgeon is experienced with venous resection and reconstruction open.

The actual venous reconstruction is easy on the robot as there's a magnified view and articulated instruments that are suitable for fine suturing. The challenge is with the dissection as it is more difficult in these cases. The goal is to obtain

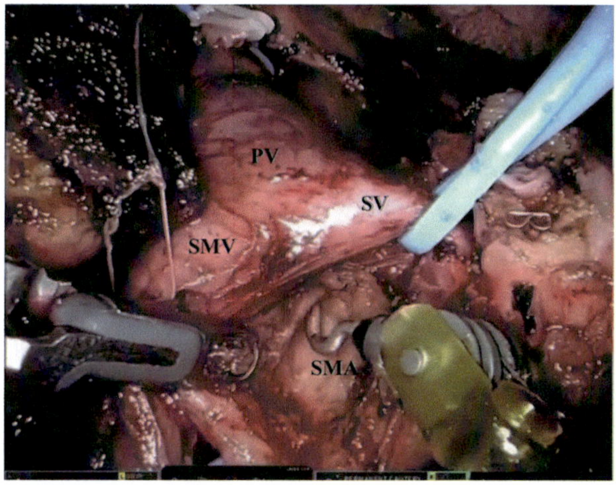

Fig. 25.25 SMA first approach. The SMA is accessed from the left side. This is achieved by retracting the SMV to the right and the splenic vein superiorly by vessel loops. Intraoperative US is very useful in finding the SMA in these cases

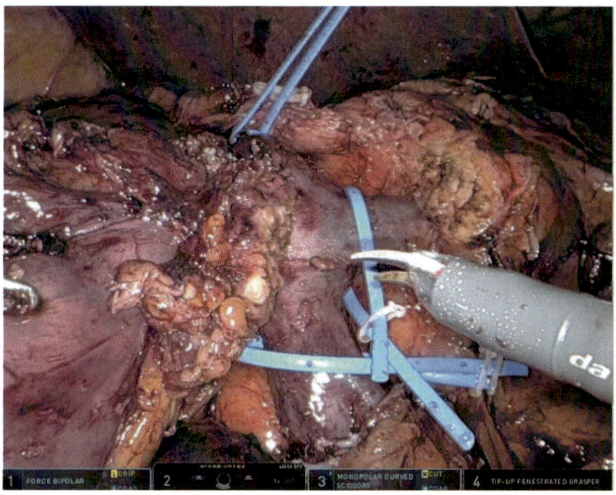

Fig. 25.26 The tumor has been dissected off completely and is only attached to the PV. Vessel loops have been placed on the SMV, PV, and SV

proximal and distal control of the SMV and PV and any side branches like the splenic vein. This is achieved by dissecting the tumor with the involved vein en bloc and then performing the venous resection and reconstruction as the last step. The tumor shouldn't be attached to anything else at this point. In these cases, it might not be feasible to access and dissect the SMA from the right side. In these cases, the SMA is easier accessed and dissected from the left side, what is called SMA first approach (Fig. 25.25).

Once the tumor is dissected completely and is only attached to the vein, vessel loops are placed on the SMV, PV, and splenic vein (Fig. 25.26). Vascular clamps are then placed on each of these vessels, and part of the vein is resected with the tumor (Fig. 25.27).

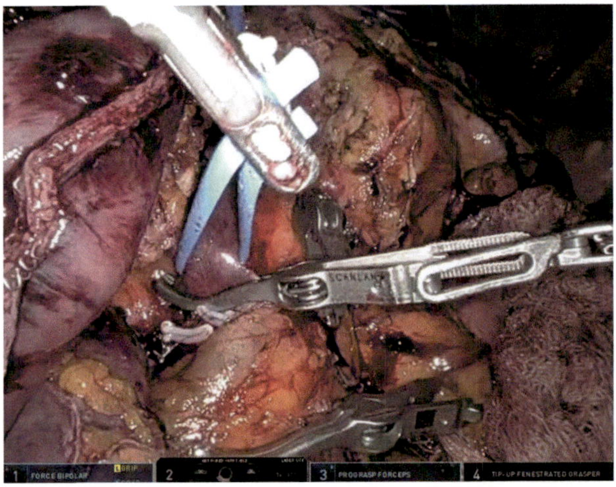

Fig. 25.27 Scanlan bulldogs are easily introduced into the abdominal cavity through 12 mm trocars and placed using ProGrasp forceps

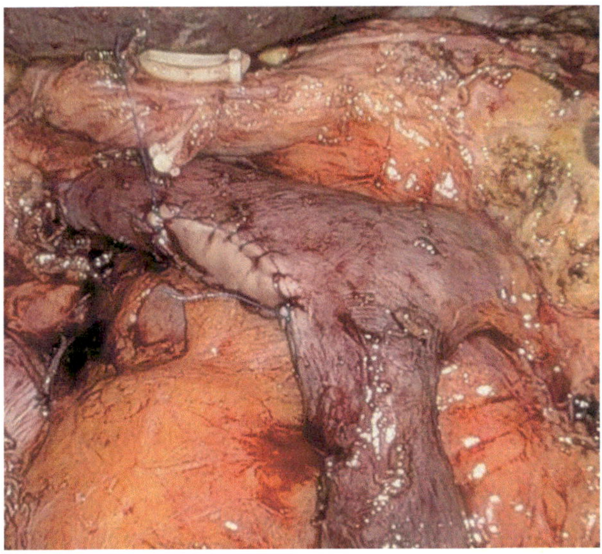

Fig. 25.28 Bovine pericardium patch

Most of the time, the tumor is only attached to the lateral vein wall and all what is needed is a lateral venorrhaphy which can be done with 5–0 or 6–0 Prolene or Gore-Tex sutures. If there's a larger defect, then a simple venorrhaphy would narrow the vein and then a bovine pericardium patch can be used (Fig. 25.28). If a circumferential resection of the vein is needed, then a primary end-to-end anastomosis can be done as long as the distance between the two ends is less than 5 cm. For a longer distance, then an interposition graft might need to be used. It might be better in these situations to open before the portal vein is clamped unless the surgeon is extremely comfortable with both robotic and vascular suturing.

Postoperative Care

The patient is transferred to the surgical floor. An early recovery after anesthesia (ERAS) protocol is implemented with minimization of narcotics. Foley and NGT are removed on postoperative day 1. Patients are typically walking in the hallway the morning after surgery. Patient is started on clear liquid diet and advanced when patient has return of bowel function. Drain amylase is checked on postoperative day 3 and drain is removed if it's < 3x upper normal blood level. Patient is discharged when they meet discharge criteria.

Evidence to Support Robotic Whipple

Robotic Whipple is a relatively new approach, primarily documented by individual centers detailing early experiences, with the University of Pittsburgh presenting the most extensive report, showcasing favorable short-term outcomes [21]. Current literature on robotic Whipple is from centers reporting their early experience which emphasizes outcomes within the learning curve, but as experience grows and larger series are conducted, we anticipate increased support for robotic Whipple. Existing studies on the robotic approach suggest comparable and even superior outcomes compared to the open counterpart, with reports highlighting less gastric emptying, less blood loss, shorter hospital stay, and lower wound infection risk [2, 4, 6]. Oncologic outcomes, including margins and lymph node harvest, appear uncompromised or potentially enhanced with the robotic approach, attributed to magnification benefits for meticulous dissection around critical vessels like the SMA to get the uncinate margin and to perform a complete lymphadenectomy [4, 5]. Moreover, the robotic approach holds promise for improving long-term outcomes by potentially expediting post-surgery recovery, facilitating prompt initiation of adjuvant chemotherapy, a crucial factor for enhanced survival in resectable pancreatic cancer patients [18].

Conclusion

Minimally invasive techniques have been slow to integrate into hepatobiliary surgery, particularly for complex procedures like the Whipple operation. However, the introduction of robotic technology has marked a significant advancement in this field. Robotic surgery is experiencing exponential growth, with an increasing number of surgeons incorporating robotic Whipple procedures into their routine practices. While robotic Whipple surgeries currently exhibit longer operative times and higher costs, these drawbacks are expected to diminish with improved proficiency, potentially offsetting expenses through reduced hospital stays and fewer complications, particularly those requiring reinterventions. Although the robotic approach won't entirely replace open Whipple surgery, it will undoubtedly play a crucial role. Effective case selection will be key in determining which patients stand to benefit most from each approach.

Conflict of Interest Dr. Ahmad Abou Abbass is a proctor and instructor at Intuitive. There are no other conflicts of interest to disclose.

References

1. Allan BJ, Novak SM, Hogg ME, Zeh HJ. Robotic vascular resections during Whipple procedure. J Vis Surg. 2018;4:13. https://doi.org/10.21037/jovs.2017.12.15.
2. Cai J, Ramanathan R, Zenati MS, Al Abbas A, Hogg ME, Zeh HJ, Zureikat AH. Robotic pancreaticoduodenectomy is associated with decreased clinically relevant pancreatic fistulas: a propensity-matched analysis. J Gastrointest Surg. 2020;24(5):1111–8. https://doi.org/10.1007/s11605-019-04274-1.
3. Coppola A, Stauffer JA, Asbun HJ. Laparoscopic pancreatoduodenectomy: current status and future directions. Updat Surg. 2016;68(3):217–24. https://doi.org/10.1007/s13304-016-0402-z.
4. Cunningham KE, Zenati MS, Petrie JR, Steve JL, Hogg ME, Zeh HJ 3rd, Zureikat AH. A policy of omitting an intensive care unit stay after robotic pancreaticoduodenectomy is safe and cost-effective. J Surg Res. 2016;204(1):8–14. https://doi.org/10.1016/j.jss.2016.04.023.
5. Da Dong X, Felsenreich DM, Gogna S, Rojas A, Zhang E, Dong M, Azim A, Gachabayov M. Robotic pancreaticoduodenectomy provides better histopathological outcomes as compared to its open counterpart: a meta-analysis. Sci Rep. 2021;11(1):3774. https://doi.org/10.1038/s41598-021-83391-x.
6. Fong ZV, Lwin TM, Aliaj A, Wang J, Clancy TE. Four-day robotic whipple: early discharge after robotic pancreatoduodenectomy. J Am Coll Surg. 2023;236(6):1172–9. https://doi.org/10.1097/xcs.0000000000000560.
7. Gagner M, Palermo M. Laparoscopic Whipple procedure: review of the literature. J Hepato-Biliary-Pancreat Surg. 2009;16(6):726–30. https://doi.org/10.1007/s00534-009-0142-2.
8. Garcia-Ochoa C, McArthur E, Skaro A, Leslie K, Hawel J. Pre-operative stenting and complications following pancreatoduodenectomy for pancreatic cancer: an analysis of the ACS-NSQIP registry. Surg Endosc. 2021;35(12):6604–11. https://doi.org/10.1007/s00464-020-08160-9.
9. Gonzalez-Ciccarelli LF, Quadri P, Daskalaki D, Milone L, Gangemi A, Giulianotti PC. Robotic approach to hepatobiliary surgery. Chirurg. 2017;88(Suppl 1):19–28. https://doi.org/10.1007/s00104-016-0223-0. (Roboterassistierte hepatobiliäre Chirurgie.)
10. Jones LR, Zwart MJW, Molenaar IQ, Koerkamp BG, Hogg ME, Hilal MA, Besselink MG. Robotic pancreatoduodenectomy: patient selection, volume criteria, and training programs. Scand J Surg. 2020;109(1):29–33. https://doi.org/10.1177/1457496920911815.
11. Lin KM, Ota DM. Laparoscopic colectomy for cancer: an oncologic feasible option. Surg Oncol. 2000;9(3):127–34. https://doi.org/10.1016/s0960-7404(01)00002-0.
12. Ma SJ, Oladeru OT, Miccio JA, Iovoli AJ, Hermann GM, Singh AK. Association of timing of adjuvant therapy with survival in patients with resected stage I to II pancreatic cancer. JAMA Netw Open. 2019;2(8):e199126. https://doi.org/10.1001/jamanetworkopen.2019.9126.
13. Mantzavinou A, Uppara M, Chan J, Patel B. Robotic versus open pancreaticoduodenectomy, comparing therapeutic indexes; a systematic review. Int J Surg. 2022;101:106633. https://doi.org/10.1016/j.ijsu.2022.106633.
14. Nota CL, Zwart MJ, Fong Y, Hagendoorn J, Hogg ME, Koerkamp BG, Besselink MG, Molenaar IQ. Developing a robotic pancreas program: the Dutch experience. J Vis Surg. 2017;3:106. https://doi.org/10.21037/jovs.2017.07.02.
15. Palep JH. Robotic assisted minimally invasive surgery. J Minim Access Surg. 2009;5(1):1–7. https://doi.org/10.4103/0972-9941.51313.
16. Qin R, Kendrick ML, Wolfgang CL, Edil BH, Palanivelu C, Parks RW, Yang Y, He J, Zhang T, Mou Y, Yu X, Peng B, Senthilnathan P, Han HS, Lee JH, Unno M, Damink S, Bansal VK, Chow P, et al. International expert consensus on laparoscopic pancreaticoduodenectomy. Hepatobil Surg Nutr. 2020;9(4):464–83. https://doi.org/10.21037/hbsn-20-446.

17. Rashid OM, Mullinax JE, Pimiento JM, Meredith KL, Malafa MP. Robotic whipple procedure for pancreatic cancer: The moffitt cancer center pathway. Cancer Control. 2015;22(3):340–51. https://doi.org/10.1177/107327481502200313.
18. Shyr YM, Wang SE, Chen SC, Shyr BU. Robotic pancreaticoduodenectomy in the era of minimally invasive surgery. J Chin Med Assoc. 2020;83(7):639–43. https://doi.org/10.1097/jcma.0000000000000333.
19. Veenhof AA, Vlug MS, van der Pas MH, Sietses C, van der Peet DL, de Lange-de Klerk ES, Bonjer HJ, Bemelman WA, Cuesta MA. Surgical stress response and postoperative immune function after laparoscopy or open surgery with fast track or standard perioperative care: a randomized trial. Ann Surg. 2012;255(2):216–21. https://doi.org/10.1097/SLA.0b013e31824336e2.
20. Ward-Boahen D, Wallace-Kazer M. Improving surgical outcomes in pancreatic surgery with preoperative nutrition. J Adv Pract Oncol. 2014;5(2):100–6. https://doi.org/10.6004/jadpro.2014.5.2.4.
21. Zureikat AH, Beane JD, Zenati MS, Al Abbas AI, Boone BA, Moser AJ, Bartlett DL, Hogg ME, Zeh HJ 3rd. 500 minimally invasive robotic pancreatoduodenectomies: One decade of optimizing performance. Ann Surg. 2021;273(5):966–72. https://doi.org/10.1097/sla.0000000000003550.
22. Zwart MJW, van den Broek B, de Graaf N, Suurmeijer JA, Augustinus S, Te Riele WW, van Santvoort HC, Hagendoorn J, Borel Rinkes IHM, van Dam JL, Takagi K, Tran KTC, Schreinemakers J, van der Schelling G, Wijsman JH, de Wilde RF, Festen S, Daams F, Luyer MD, et al. The feasibility, proficiency, and mastery learning curves in 635 robotic pancreatoduodenectomies following a multicenter training program:"standing on the shoulders of giants". Ann Surg. 2023;278(6):e1232–41. https://doi.org/10.1097/sla.0000000000005928.

26 Right Hemicolectomy

Ibrahim H. Ozata and Emre Balık

Introduction

Complete mesocolic excision has recently been the gold standard for the treatment of nonmetastatic colon cancer demonstrating improved oncological outcomes and lowered recurrence risk [1–5]. Similarly in the last years, minimally invasive colon surgery has become increasingly popular meeting the standards established by open surgery. This includes ligation of the vascular pedicles at their origin, oncologic lymphadenectomy, and distal and radial clearance of the tumor from the resection margins. The newest of these techniques is robotic surgery.

Robotic surgery offers great promise due to the fact that it involves smaller incisions, specialized instruments, and enhanced precision. It enables surgeons to operate with enhanced dexterity, as the instruments can mimic human hand movements. This results in improved surgical outcomes allowing for less tissue damage, reduced blood loss, a lower risk of infection, and shorter patient recovery time compared to open surgery [6].

Indications

Right colectomy is indicated for invasive cancers or noninvasive neoplastic lesions located in in the right colon that cannot be endoscopically removed. In addition, it is also performed for appendiceal neoplasm with certain conditions and neoplastic

Supplementary Information The online version contains supplementary material available at https://doi.org/10.1007/978-3-031-86927-3_26.

I. H. Ozata
Department of General Surgery, Koç University School of Medicine, Istanbul, Turkey

E. Balık (✉)
Maltepe Mahallesi, Zeytinburnu, Istanbul, Turkey
e-mail: ebalik@ku.edu.tr

S. Samreen et al. (eds.), *The SAGES Manual of Robotic Surgery*,
https://doi.org/10.1007/978-3-031-86927-3_26

polyps where resection margins are incomplete or there is a high risk of nodal metastasis.

Factors that influence the decision to perform a right hemicolectomy for appendiceal neoplasms include tumor size, extent of invasion, malignant potential, lymph node involvement, specific histopathological features, and the presence of certain types of neoplasms.

An extended right hemicolectomy, characterized by ligation of middle colic pedicle in addition to standard right hemicolectomy, is recommended for lesions that are located in hepatic flexure to mid-transverse colon. This modification is necessary because of the potential for regional lymph nodes metastases around the arterial blood supply.

The surgical approach to colon cancer has been significantly influenced by Hohenberger's concept of complete mesocolic excision (CME). CME entails meticulous dissection along the avascular embryonic plane separating the parietal retroperitoneum and visceral peritoneum of the mesocolon. This procedure ensures an adequate longitudinal resection of the bowel and involves ligating the central blood vessels at the origins of the supplying arteries and draining veins. This precise technique aims to completely remove the mesocolon while preserving its integrity, adhering to anatomical and embryological principles in order to achieve the best possible outcomes in terms of cancer treatment. The underlying philosophy of CME is to apply the principles of total mesorectal excision to surgery involving the colon. Through the process of dissecting along the embryological planes and ensuring the complete removal of the mesocolon, CME offers a more thorough and standardized surgical approach for treating colon cancer.

While there are no absolute contraindications for robotic surgery, conditions such as severe cardiovascular disease, pulmonary disease, large bulky tumors, intestinal obstruction, and extensive adhesions resulting from previous surgeries are considered relative contraindications in robotic surgery, similar to laparoscopic surgery. On the other hand, the surgeon's history and experience with robotic surgery will also be determinative in both the indication and the decision regarding the surgical technique.

In light of all these considerations, the surgical technique should be chosen in a way that maximizes benefit to the patient.

Preparation

Obtaining informed consent from patients before surgery is a crucial component of ethical and legal standards in healthcare. It is essential to prepare the patient psychologically and emotionally for the surgical treatment by informing them of what to expect, the potential risks and advantages, and any accessible alternatives [7]. Before surgery, patients undergo a thorough evaluation process to achieve the best possible results. This assessment usually includes a comprehensive review of the patient's medical history and an in-depth physical examination. A comprehensive family history is gathered to uncover any possible hereditary illnesses. Regular laboratory tests are performed, which involves measuring carcinoembryonic antigen levels to establish a reference point and employ it for the purpose of monitoring. Radiographic staging is an essential part of the preoperative assessment, which includes a CT scan of the chest, abdomen, and pelvis using both oral and intravenous contrast to precisely determine the disease's severity. If abnormalities are found on the CT scan that need more explanation for surgical planning, MRI and PET scans may be used as needed. Additionally, it is crucial to conduct a comprehensive examination of the colon, including histologic study of any detected lesions, before starting treatment. Preoperative medical consultation is requested to assess the patient's risk level according to their medical history. This thorough preoperative assessment guarantees that patients are well prepared for surgery and that necessary steps are implemented to enhance their surgical results.

Patients are initiated on a clear diet the day before surgery, along with bowel preparation and oral antibiotics. Castagneto-Gissey et al. [8] conducted a study that examines the relationship between mechanical bowel preparation with oral antibiotics before to elective colorectal surgery and its effects on surgical site infections and anastomotic leaks [8]. The meta-analysis examined 13 randomized clinical studies with 4334 participants and concluded that combining mechanical bowel preparation with oral antibiotics was associated with reduced rates of anastomotic leakage and surgical site infections. Using bowel preparation along with oral antibiotics is offered to avoid postoperative complications. A technical concern regarding this topic is that bowel preparation decreases feces bulk, which consequently results in diminished contamination when utilizing stapler devices during anastomosis. Additionally, manipulating the colon during dissection and anastomosis will be facilitated with more space in the abdomen.

At our institution, we do not administer oral bowel cleansing. Despite the existence of studies recommending it, we prefer for cleansing using enemas.

Low molecular weight heparin is recommended for prophylaxis before and after surgery. Additionally, to reduce the risk of thromboembolism, it is advised to use intraoperative sequential compression devices and encourage early ambulation [9].

Patient Positioning

The patient is placed on an anti-slip surface in a supine position. During general anesthesia, care should be taken not to give excessive air to the stomach and the small bowel. Additionally, an orogastric catheter should be inserted to deflate the stomach and to prevent loss of space. A urinary catheter is inserted to monitor, prophylactic antibiotics are administered on induction, and sequential compression devices are used for deep vein thrombosis prophylaxis. The patient is sterilized and draped. The robot is positioned on the right side of the patient (Fig. 26.1). When docking and positioning the robot, careful attention must be paid to the maintenance of each body part. Over the years, the table motion technology of the Da Vinci robotic surgery platform has made significant breakthroughs. The da Vinci Xi Surgical System is equipped with Integrated Table Motion, which allows for the connection between the system and the operating table. This enables the surgeon to dynamically position the patient while doing the operation.

Surgical Technique Using the Da Vinci Platform

The Veress technique serves as a standard method for establishing pneumoperitoneum in minimally invasive surgical procedures. In robotic surgery (Video 26.1 for robotic right hemicolectomy), a configuration involving four robotic trocars and one assistant trocar is commonly employed to facilitate the robotic approach. The strategic placement of ports to the left of the midline is typically preferred to optimize

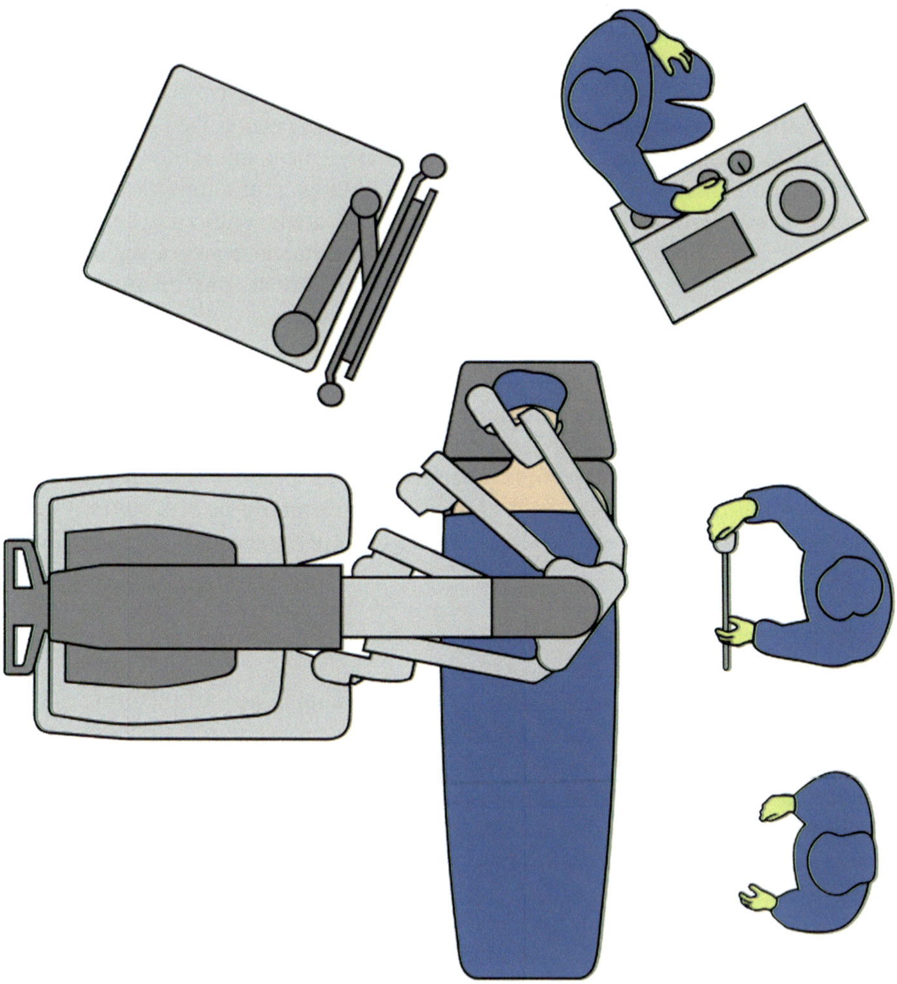

Fig. 26.1 Operation room configuration

the surgical workspace and provide maximal access for the robotic instruments during the procedure (Fig. 26.2). This port arrangement allows for enhanced maneuverability and precision in performing right hemicolectomy using the da Vinci Xi robotic platform, ensuring efficient and effective completion of the surgical intervention.

The AirSeal® system is a trocar without valves that enables a stable pneumoperitoneum and ongoing removal of smoke during surgical procedures. This technology has been associated with enhanced visualization, decreased abdominal pressures, and subsequently, a decrease in cardiopulmonary complications, ileus, and postoperative pain [10].

On the other hand, table motion technology in robotic surgery improves surgical precision and efficiency by enabling better maneuverability and positioning during procedures. This integration allows surgeons to easily modify the orientation and alignment of the robotic arms and instruments, thereby improving overall dexterity and range of motion during surgery.

The abdominal cavity is systematically examined upon entry, dividing the assessment into four quadrants for a thorough evaluation. Simultaneously, a comprehensive assessment is conducted on the liver surface and peritoneum to detect any abnormalities (Fig. 26.3). The colon and omentum are repositioned over the falciform ligament to improve exposure and access. This maneuver improves the clarity and ease of access to the right colon. The small bowel is then moved to the left lower quadrant. This repositioning enables the accurate identification of the ileocolic pedicle, a crucial step in robotic right hemicolectomy.

The robotic cart is positioned to approach the patient from the right side in an orientation. The system utilizes automatic targeting to align the robotic arms optimally, enhancing their range of motion and reducing the chance of collisions. This feature directs the camera toward the patient's anatomy. The 30° robotic endoscope is inserted through Port 2, situated above the umbilicus (Fig. 26.4). The initial robotic arm is outfitted with either monopolar curved scissors or a robotic vessel

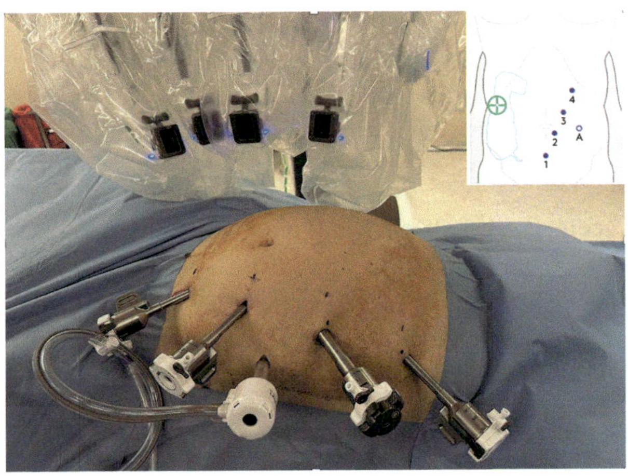

Fig. 26.2 Placement of the ports

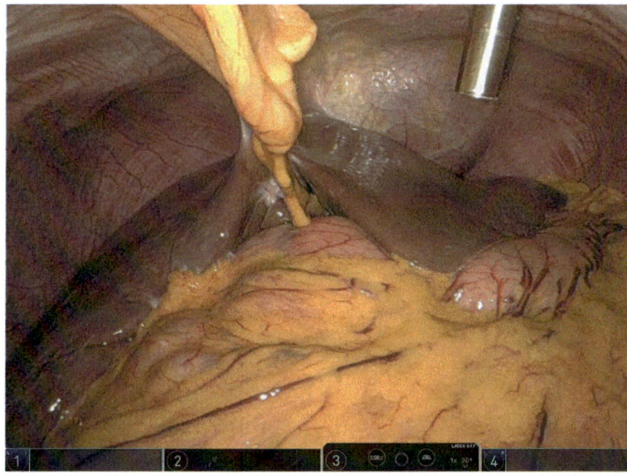

Fig. 26.3 Liver surface and peritoneum

sealing device. The third robotic arm uses a fenestrated bipolar instrument, and the fourth arm employs a Cadiere grasper for tissue manipulation. An 8–10 mm assistant port is used to hold gauze or instruments such as the suction irrigator or a laparoscopic bowel grasper. To enhance visibility in challenging situations, consider adding a 5-mm assistant port to the surgical field.

In a medial-to-lateral technique, arm 4 is used to retract the terminal ileum/cecum to elevate and apply tension to the ileocolic pedicle. The peritoneum below the ileocolic pedicle is incised using a fenestrated monopolar grasper in arm 1 and a bipolar scissor in arm 3 while holding the fatty tissue containing the vessels (Fig. 26.5). This maneuver exposes the vascular pedicle for dissection, followed by the dissection, ligation, and division of the vessels (Fig. 26.6). Following the dissection, the superior mesenteric vein is observed with the presence of clips, as well as the middle colic vein with attached clips (Fig. 26.7). The submesenteric dissection begins directly beneath the mesenteric opening. The dissection process is ongoing following the embryologic planes, revealing the retroperitoneal structures such as the duodenum, head of the pancreas, gonadal vessels, and right ureter (Fig. 26.8). The dissection extends sideways to the abdominal wall, downward to the sacral promontory, and upward revealing the duodenum and head of the pancreas (Fredet fascia-anterior duodenopancreatic fascia). The identification of the pancreatic and colic branches of the gastrocolic trunk of Henle is confirmed (Fig. 26.9).

The dissection will proceed along the superior mesenteric vein until reaching the middle colic vein. In a standard right colectomy, the right branch of the middle colic pedicle is tied off and cut. If present, the right colic artery is tied off. Ligation of any additional vessel structures, such as the right colic vein in the mesentery of the right colon, is performed. The mesentery is separated into the transverse colon (Fig. 26.10). A gauze is positioned as a marker to be located horizontally. The omentum is separated from the distal transverse colon, allowing access to the lesser sac, and then included in the specimen side. Omentectomy, the partial or complete removal of the omentum, is a surgical option that may be considered during right

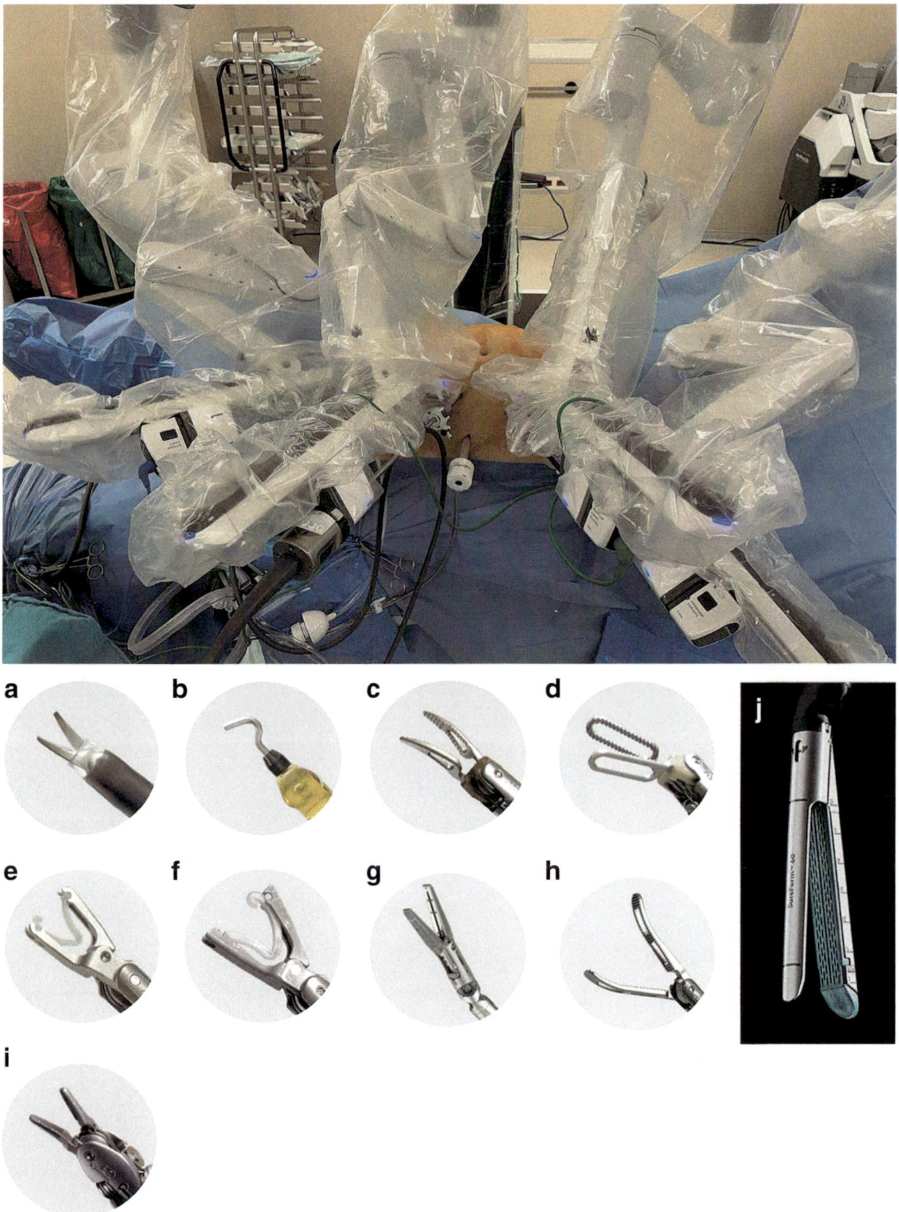

Fig. 26.4 Robotic arms and instruments. (**a**) Monopolar curved scissors (**b**) Monopolar hook (**c**) Maryland bipolar forceps. (**d**) Fenestrated bipolar forceps. (**e**) Medium-large clip applier. (**f**) Large clip applier (**g**) Vessel sealer (**h**) Tip-up fenestrated grasper. (**i**) Large needle driver. (**j**) SureForm® stapler

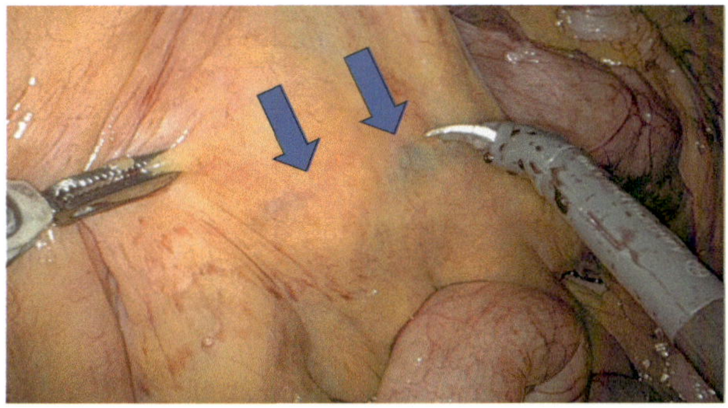

Fig. 26.5 Ileocolic pedicle in mesenterium

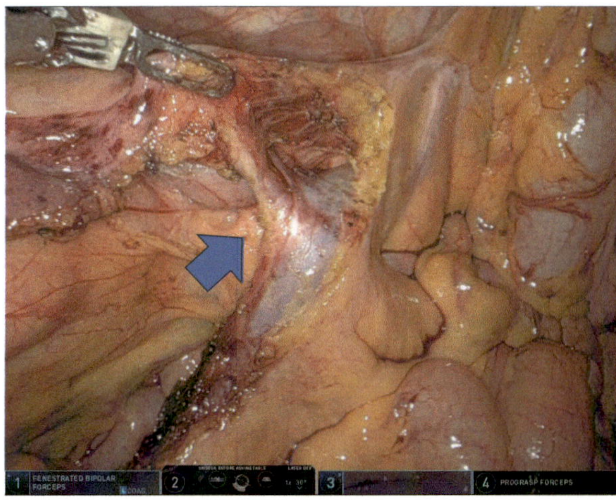

Fig. 26.6 Ileocolic pedicle originating from the superior mesenteric vein

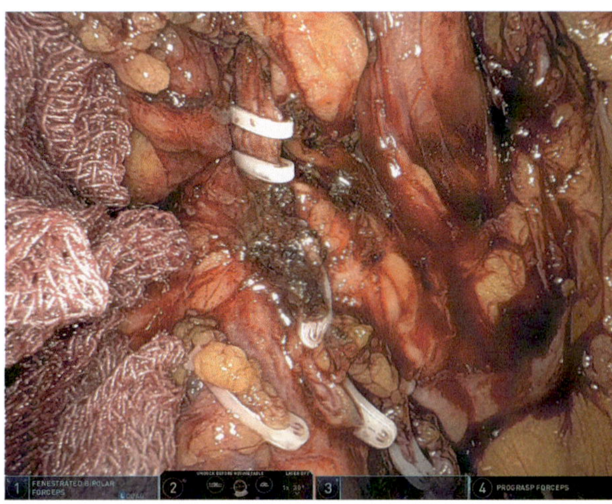

Fig. 26.7 Superior mesenteric vein with clips and middle colic vein with attached clips

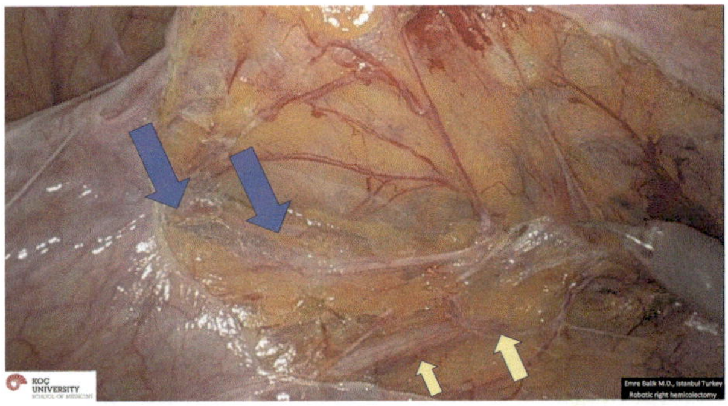

Fig. 26.8 Right ureter and right gonadal vein

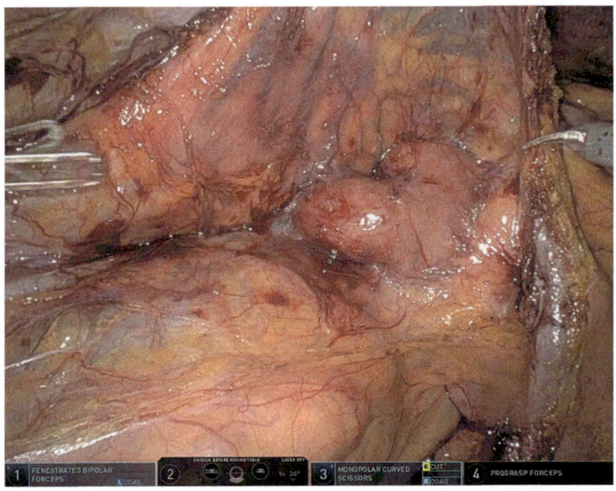

Fig. 26.9 Duodenum and gastrocolic trunk

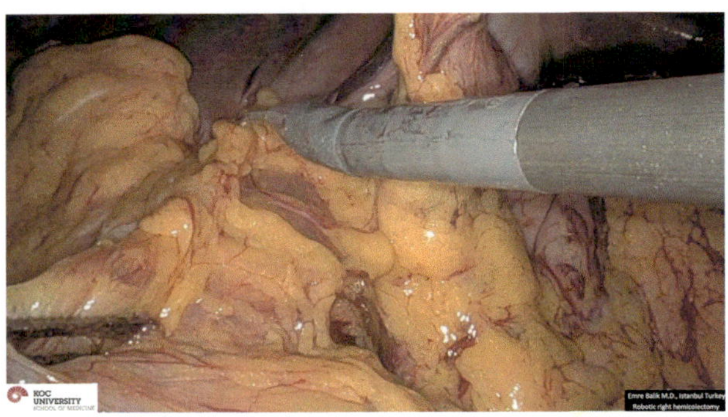

Fig. 26.10 Separation of mesentery

hemicolectomy for colon tumors, depending on factors such as the location of the tumor, the extent of the disease, and preoperative radiologic findings. The transverse colon is repositioned to the cephalic side, and the remaining omental and colonic attachments are cut. This dissection is made easier by the prior submesenteric dissection, which involves detecting the landmark gauze.

The cecum, appendix, and terminal ileum are freed by cutting the peritoneal attachments in the right lower quadrant. The mesentery of the terminal ileum is cut about 10 cm prior to ileocecal valve reaching the small intestine wall. Robotic stapler is used to divide the terminal ileum and the transverse colon. Arterial blood supply is controlled by administering indocyanine green intravenously and examining the terminal ileum and transverse colon using Firefly® mode (Fig. 26.11).

The Firefly® system, which is incorporated into the da Vinci surgical platform, employs near-infrared light to observe the absorption of indocyanine green (ICG) by tissues. This technology enables the immediate and accurate identification of important landmarks during surgical procedures, using image guidance enhancing the precision and accuracy [11]. The Firefly® technology utilizes ICG fluorescence imaging to enhance the visualization of crucial anatomical structures. This aids surgeons in detecting minute and imperceptible lesions, as well as guiding procedures like central lymph node mapping and identifying regions with inadequate blood circulation during surgical operations.

A side-to-side anastomosis is created using isoperistaltic technique. An enterotomy incision is made in the terminal ileum and the transverse colon, and robotic stapler, SureForm®, is then inserted which uses SmartFire technology to monitor tissue compression before and during firing. Typically, the wider jaw of the stapler is inserted into the colon, followed by bringing the ileum over and inserting the narrower stapler jaw (Fig. 26.12). SureForm® is fired to create the

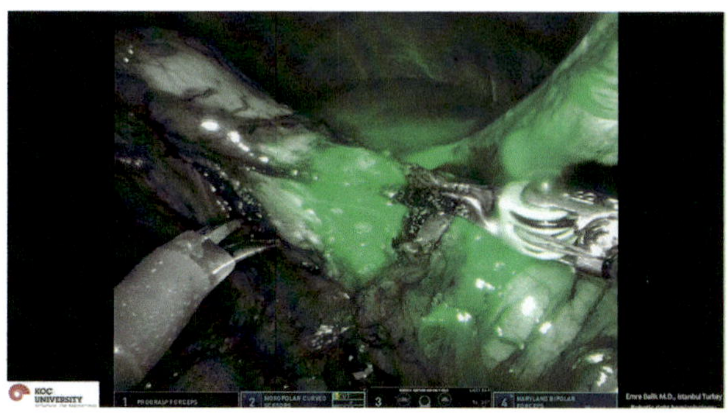

Fig. 26.11 Firefly® mode with indocyanine green

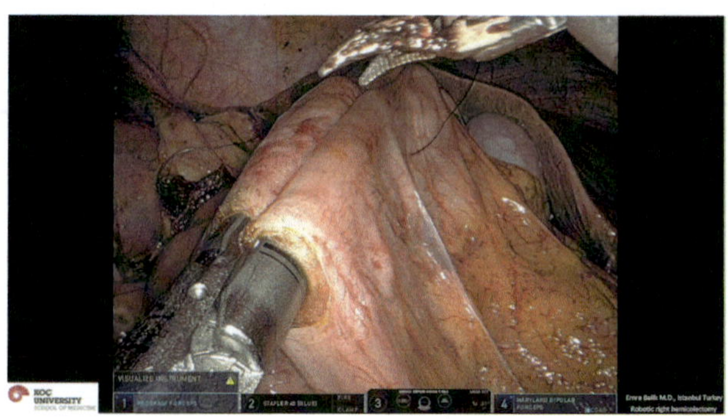

Fig. 26.12 Colon and ileum with SureForm® stapler

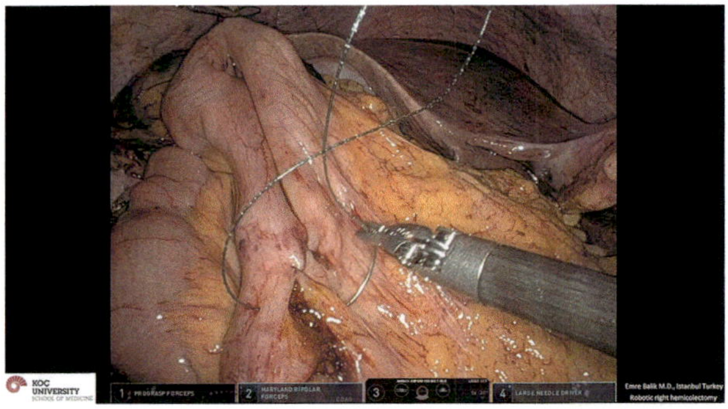

Fig. 26.13 Suturing intestinal opening

anastomosis, and the intestinal opening is then closed with a continuous suture (Fig. 26.13). Pfannenstiel incision is made and the specimen is removed using a wound protector. Next, the wound protector is sealed, the process of introducing gas into the abdomen is resumed, a thorough examination of the abdomen is conducted to ensure there is no bleeding, and the ports are taken out while being directly observed in low pressure. The decision to utilize drains in surgical procedures, lacking substantial evidence, typically relies on the surgeon's expertise and approach.

Recovery After the Surgery

Postoperative discharge following colorectal surgery is a critical component of patient care that requires careful consideration to ensure patient safety and promote the best possible recovery. Criteria for discharge commonly include factors like tolerance of oral nutrition, effective pain management, bowel recovery, and autonomy in daily living activities as stated by Biondi et al. [12]. Biomarkers such as C-reactive protein and procalcitonin have been suggested as early indicators of septic complications and dehiscence, aiding in a safe hospital discharge [13, 14]. Early discharge has been associated with positive patient experiences and enhanced recovery. However, it is crucial to weigh the benefits of early discharge against the risks of readmission and postoperative complications [15, 16]. Therefore, a comprehensive assessment of patient recovery, compliance with enhanced recovery protocols, and individual risk factors is essential in determining the appropriate timing for discharge after surgery.

After colorectal surgery, patients undergo a period of recovery and adaptation to resume their usual daily routines and quality of life. Research has emphasized the influence of colorectal surgery on patients' well-being, underscoring the significance of monitoring postoperative complications and quality of life results. Understanding the physical, emotional, and social components of life following colorectal surgery is essential for healthcare professionals to assist patients in their recovery process and improve their postoperative health.

Conclusion

Robotic right hemicolectomy represents the highest achievement in minimally invasive surgical methods for treating colon cancer. It provides improved accuracy, less damage to the body, and faster recovery, all while following oncologic principles. This approach not only adheres to the highest standard of complete mesocolic excision but also offers benefits such as reduced risk of infection and enhanced surgical outcomes. The success of this procedure relies heavily on the preparation, positioning of the patient, and recovery phases. This emphasizes the significance of conducting a thorough preoperative assessment and providing comprehensive postoperative care. With advancements in technology and increasing surgeon expertise, robotic surgery offers the potential to enhance the treatment of colon cancer by maximizing patient advantages and advancing surgical techniques.

References

1. Wang C, Gao Z, Shen K, Shen Z, Jiang K, Liang B, et al. Safety, quality and effect of complete mesocolic excision vs non-complete mesocolic excision in patients with colon cancer: a systemic review and meta-analysis. Color Dis. 2017;19(11):962–72. https://doi.org/10.1111/codi.13900.
2. Bertelsen C, Gundestrup A, Olsen A, Bols B, Ingeholm P, Kleif J. Association between plane of mesocolic dissection and recurrence after complete mesocolic excision for right-sided colon cancer: a cohort study. Color Dis. 2023;25(7):1392–402. https://doi.org/10.1111/codi.16551.
3. Trilling B, Delattre F, Faucheron J. Comment on "efficacy and safety of complete mesocolic excision in patients with colon cancer: three-year results from a prospective, nonrandomized, double-blind, controlled trial". Ann Surg. 2020;274(6):e788–9. https://doi.org/10.1097/sla.0000000000004403.
4. Aziz M, El-Deen A, Hasanien A, Attia A, Hafez A. Laparoscopic complete mesocolic excision with central vascular ligation for right colonic cancer (feasibility & safety). Minia J Med Res. 2020;31(1):262–7. https://doi.org/10.21608/mjmr.2022.221517.
5. Tribuzi A, Marzano M, Paolini C, Bencini L, Marino M, Coratti A. Robotic extended right colectomy with complete mesocolic excision. Color Dis. 2020;22(11):1807. https://doi.org/10.1111/codi.15246.
6. Ng KT, Tsia AKV, Chong VYL. Robotic versus conventional laparoscopic surgery for colorectal cancer: a systematic review and meta-analysis with trial sequential analysis. World J Surg. 2019;43(4):1146–61. https://doi.org/10.1007/s00268-018-04896-7.
7. Childers R, Lipsett PA, Pawlik TM. Informed consent and the surgeon. J Am Coll Surg. 2009;208(4):627–34. https://doi.org/10.1016/j.jamcollsurg.2008.12.012.
8. Castagneto-Gissey L, Russo MF, Casella-Mariolo J, Serao A, Marcellinaro R, D'Andrea V, Carlini M, Casella G. The role of antibiotic prophylaxis in anastomotic leak prevention during elective colorectal surgery: systematic review and meta-analysis of randomized controlled trials. Antibiotics (Basel, Switzerland). 2023;12(2):397. https://doi.org/10.3390/antibiotics12020397.
9. Anderson DR, Morgano GP, Bennett C, Dentali F, Francis CW, García D, et al. American society of hematology 2019 guidelines for management of venous thromboembolism: prevention of venous thromboembolism in surgical hospitalized patients. Blood Adv. 2019;3(23):3898–944. https://doi.org/10.1182/bloodadvances.2019000975.

10. Razdan S, Üçpınar B, Okhawere K, Badani KK. The role of airseal in robotic urologic surgery: a systematic review. J Laparoendosc Adv Surg Tech. 2023;33(1):21–31. https://doi.org/10.1089/lap.2022.0153.
11. Koerner C, Rosen S. How robotics is changing and will change the field of colorectal surgery. World J Gastrointest Surg. 2019;11(10):381–7. https://doi.org/10.4240/wjgs.v11.i10.381.
12. Biondi A, Mele MC, Agnes A, Lorenzon L, Cintoni M, Rinninella E, et al. Feasibility of discharge within 72 hours of major colorectal surgery: lessons learned after 5 years of institutional experience with the eras protocol. BJS Open. 2022;6(1) https://doi.org/10.1093/bjsopen/zrac002.
13. Ortega-Deballon P, Radais F, Facy O, d'Athis P, Masson D, Charles P, et al. C-reactive protein is an early predictor of septic complications after elective colorectal surgery. World J Surg. 2010;34(4):808–14. https://doi.org/10.1007/s00268-009-0367-x.
14. Giaccaglia V, Salvi PF, Antonelli M, Nigri G, Pirozzi F, Casagranda B, et al. Procalcitonin reveals early dehiscence in colorectal surgery. Ann Surg. 2016;263(5):967–72. https://doi.org/10.1097/sla.0000000000001365.
15. Jakobsson J, Idvall E, Wann-Hansson C. Patient-reported recovery after enhanced colorectal cancer surgery: a longitudinal six-month follow-up study. Int J Color Dis. 2014;29(8):989–98. https://doi.org/10.1007/s00384-014-1939-2.
16. Azevedo J, Mendes CRS, Lima MLD, Pessoa JCSDP, Julião GPS, Perez RO, et al. Laparoscopic colorectal surgery and discharge within 24 h—who is at risk for readmission? Color Dis. 2021;23(10):2714–22. https://doi.org/10.1111/codi.15791.

27 Left Hemicolectomy and Total Colectomy

Kamil Erozkan and Emre Gorgun

Background

With the advent of minimally invasive surgical strategies, the landscape of surgical practice has undergone a paradigm shift. Laparoscopic colectomy, which is now widely performed for benign and malignant conditions, has demonstrated advantages, such as reduced pain, lower incidence of ileus, and shorter hospital stays. These outcomes have propelled surgeons to explore newer, minimally invasive approaches to diminish the operative trauma, shorten hospital stays, and enhance operative visualization and dexterity. Surgeons, drawn to less-invasive techniques with comparable efficacy, are now immersed in the discourse surrounding robotic surgery [1, 2].

The inherent technical challenges of laparoscopic colon surgery, characterized by anatomical complexities and a demanding learning curve, have led to increased adoption of robotic systems. Particularly advantageous in challenging anatomical regions such as the pelvis, these systems provide high-definition three-dimensional vision, surgeon motion filtration, articulating instrument movements, stable camera control, retraction, and improved ergonomics [3]. The fatigue associated with unnatural positions during laparoscopy can be mitigated using robotic technology [4]. These advantages address the limitations of laparoscopic surgery and potentially reduce the learning curve of minimally invasive colorectal surgery [5].

Supplementary Information The online version contains supplementary material available at https://doi.org/10.1007/978-3-031-86927-3_27.

K. Erozkan · E. Gorgun (✉)
Department of Colorectal Surgery, Digestive Disease and Surgery Institute, Cleveland Clinic, Cleveland, OH, USA
e-mail: erozkak@ccf.org; gorgune@ccf.org

S. Samreen et al. (eds.), *The SAGES Manual of Robotic Surgery*,
https://doi.org/10.1007/978-3-031-86927-3_27

The da Vinci® robotic surgical system (Intuitive Surgical, Inc., Sunnyvale, CA, USA) has further catalyzed this evolution, particularly in colon and rectal surgeries. Since its first reported application in 2002, robotic colorectal surgery has gained momentum for both benign and malignant resections. Insights from a population-based study involving patients undergoing colectomy have revealed a noteworthy surge in the use of robotic colectomy. Robotic colorectal surgery increased from 0.7% in 2006 to 10.9% in 2010 within all colorectal procedures across all hospitals. Furthermore, in hospitals with the highest adoption rate of robotic colectomy, the utilization of robotic colectomy escalated even more significantly, moving from 0.8 to an impressive 32.8% among all colectomies [6]. Another study from 2012 to 2018 echoed this trend, reporting a substantial rise in the prevalence of robotic colectomy from 2.5% to 16.3% [1].

Despite its advantages, robotic surgery has several limitations. A notable data gap exists concerning the long-term oncological outcomes of robotic colon cancer surgery, and the escalated cost associated with robotic techniques is a considerable hurdle to its widespread adoption. In addition, maintenance requirements and extra training are additional limitations. While the predominant focus on the application of robotics in colorectal surgery has been directed toward rectal cancer and dissection within the narrow pelvis, it is imperative to underscore its pivotal role in other procedures, particularly left hemicolectomy and total colectomy. This chapter delves into the evolving landscape of robotic left hemicolectomy and total colectomy, emphasizing the indications, operative steps, and future directions. By meticulously exploring these procedures, we aimed to contribute to a broader understanding of robotic colectomies, their challenges, and potential avenues for improvement, thereby facilitating the continued evolution of minimally invasive colorectal surgery.

Indications

Left hemicolectomy and total colectomy represent crucial surgical interventions employed for various indications, and the decision to perform robotic colectomy is typically based on the patients' specific condition and surgeons' proficiency. The indications for robotic surgery are similar to those for laparoscopic surgery. Precancerous polyps, endometriosis involving the colon, diverticular disease, left hemicolectomy, or sigmoid resection are the preferred surgical interventions for left-sided colon cancer. The preferred surgical intervention for tumors situated in the segment of the colon between the left colic vessels and the initial sigmoidal branches is a "true" left hemicolectomy [7]. This procedure entails complete removal of the left colon, including the origin of the inferior mesenteric artery (IMA) and its associated lymphatic territory. Alternatively, tumors in this location may undergo segmental resection. This less invasive approach involves only the division of the left branch of the middle colic and left colic vessels while preserving the root of the IMA and main sigmoidal vessels. Importantly, this method does not compromise oncological outcomes [8].

However, it is crucial to note that indications for total colectomy are limited. Despite the restricted scope, we believe that a comprehensive discussion on these indications is valuable. Depending on the tumor location, synchronous cancer may require total colectomy [9, 10]. Conditions such as familial adenomatous polyposis, juvenile polyposis, MUTYH-associated polyposis, and Peutz-Jeghers syndrome, characterized by diffuse adenomatosis of the colon, are additional indications for total colectomy to reduce the risk of colorectal cancer development [10, 11]. Total colectomy is recommended for patients with hereditary nonpolyposis colorectal cancer (HNPCC) syndrome because of the elevated risk of synchronous or metachronous colorectal cancers [12]. Inflammatory bowel diseases, including ulcerative colitis and Crohn's disease, may prompt total colectomy when medical management fails or in the presence of complications such as refractory disease, dysplasia, or severe inflammation [13–15]. Surgical management is indicated for patients with Clostridium difficile infections who do not respond to medical treatment [16]. When conservative measures are ineffective, conditions marked by impaired colonic motility, such as slow-transit constipation or colonic inertia, can be addressed with total robotic colectomy [17, 18]. Total robotic colectomy may be considered in cases of endometriosis or diverticular disease involving the different sides of the colon.

However, surgical emergencies, previous abdominal surgery with extensive adhesions, cardiovascular or respiratory disease preventing safe pneumoperitoneum, or highly complex diseases may pose contraindications to most minimally invasive approaches including robotics. Notably, obesity does not serve as a contraindication to robotic surgery, as evidenced by the comparable short-term outcomes between the robotic and laparoscopic approaches in obese patients. Moreover, the robotic approach has shown accelerated postoperative recovery compared with its laparoscopic counterpart [19]. It is paramount to emphasize that the decision to perform robotic left hemicolectomy and total colectomy is personalized, considering many factors encompassing the patients' overall health and surgeons' expertise. This individualized approach ensures optimal patient outcomes and aligns with the evolving landscape of colorectal surgery.

Preoperative Planning and Room Setup

Proper patient selection is paramount in preoperative planning and candidates should be medically fit and capable of tolerating laparoscopy. A comprehensive evaluation, including a detailed history and physical examination, is essential for all patients undergoing colon surgery.

Preoperative colonoscopy and flexible sigmoidoscopy are recommended in patients with left-sided colonic or rectal lesions. Flexible sigmoidoscopy provides valuable information regarding the distance from the anal verge to the lower edge of the tumor, aiding operative planning. It is imperative to underscore the role of total colonoscopy in eligible patients to rule out the potential presence of synchronous tumors effectively. Patients are given mechanical bowel preparation with oral

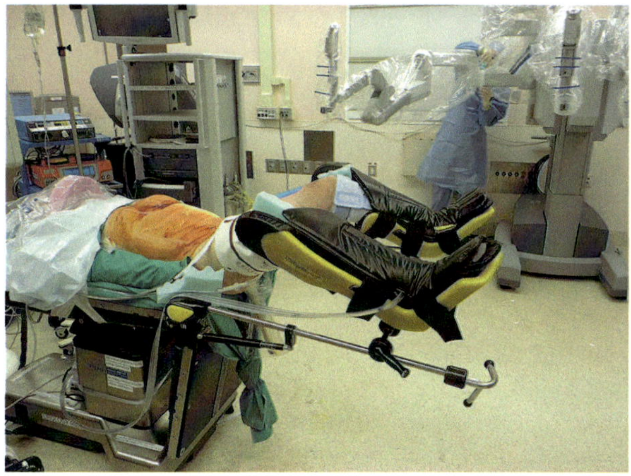

Fig. 27.1 Modified lithotomy position in robotic surgery

antibiotics as part of the preoperative preparation. This protocol is rigorously enforced in our practice to maintain a low incidence of postoperative site infections. Preoperative intravenous antibiotics are administered within 30–60 min of incision, ensuring adequate concentration at the outset [20]. Deep venous prophylaxis includes the use of sequential compression devices coupled with chemical prophylaxis, in the form of preoperative heparin.

After informed consent is obtained, intravenous induction is performed, followed by endotracheal intubation. A urinary catheter and orogastric tube are placed in all cases. During the surgical procedure, patients are positioned in a modified lithotomy position, with Allen® Yellofin® or Yellofin Elite™ Stirrups (Allen Medical, Acton, MA, USA) utilized to prevent peroneal nerve injury (Fig. 27.1). This positioning offers the advantage of creating additional space for an assistant, easy access to the anus for intraoperative colonoscopy if needed, and transanal stapler use and facilitates anastomosis formation. Both arms are tucked at the sides. Gel pads are used for decubitus support and additional stability. The operating table is adjusted in slightly Trendelenburg position during the procedure. To prevent injuries and ensure patient safety, we prefer to secure the patient further with a strong tape around the chest area, mitigating the potential risk for patient sliding. The entire abdomen is prepared using standard sterile surgical draping. Two monitors on both sides of the table should be routine in laparoscopic surgery, and a robotic view should be added to these monitors via a wire connection for the bedside assistant. This setup is also helpful in hybrid procedures in which part of the operation is performed using a laparoscopic approach.

This meticulous approach to patient selection and preoperative planning aims to optimize outcomes, minimize complications, and create a conducive environment for successful execution of colon and rectal surgical procedures.

Operation Steps

Left Hemicolectomy

The patient's cart is positioned to the left of the patient (Fig. 27.2), legs kept slightly separated, and positioned in Trendelenburg position, typically angled at 10–15°, with a lateral tilt to the right, also approximately 10–15° head down. This specific positioning aids in moving the omentum and intestines cephalad, thereby facilitating a clear view of the sigmoid/left colon during the procedure. In cases where the small intestine obstructs the view and dissection planes, RAY-TEC X-Rayable Sponge (Johnson & Johnson Medical, Inc., Arlington, TX, USA) can be introduced through the 8 mm assistant trocar, allowing the assistant to gently push it on, moving the small bowel as a single unit out of the surgical field. Alternatively, enveloping the small intestine like a cocoon using a RAY-TEC X-Rayable Sponge inserted through the Pfannenstiel incision can be another solution after the Pfannenstiel incision. However, this is not our choice of approach as it requires an additional incision side. Before docking the robotic system, adjustments to the patient's position are crucial to ensure optimal exposure of the surgical field. It is important to note that the robotic system is docked and the operating table cannot be moved unless it is equipped with a motion-activating table such as TruSystem® 7000dV (Trumpf Medizin Systeme GmbH & Co. KG software, Saalfeld, Germany). TruSystem® 7000dV is an advanced motion-activating table that enables precise surgical table movement across multiple quadrants [21].

To perform robotic left colectomy or sigmoid resection, five ports, including the camera and assistant ports, are required [22]. The choice of port placement technique depends on the location of the pathology and surgeon's preference. For sigmoid and distal descending colon resections, a line is drawn from the right lower quadrant to the left midclavicular line intersecting the left subcostal border. Port 2 is initially placed at the junction of this line with the midline. After camera insertion, the procedure begins with an examination of the abdominal cavity to rule out metastatic disease. Subsequent trocars are positioned at least 8 cm apart following the pneumoperitoneum under direct visualization (Fig. 27.3). Different port placement techniques can be used in some centers (Fig. 27.4). In cases involving the proximal descending colon and splenic flexure lesions, ports are inserted, as shown in Fig. 27.5. This alternative port placement technique facilitates a single-docking surgical procedure during splenic flexure mobilization. As in the authors of this chapter, we generally use the alternative port placement technique in all left-sided colectomies. The assistant port is strategically placed as far as possible from the da Vinci® ports and lateral to the right of the midclavicular line. These assistant ports play a crucial role in small bowel and colon retraction, and suction irrigation. Subsequently, the greater omentum is retracted cephalad and extended over the

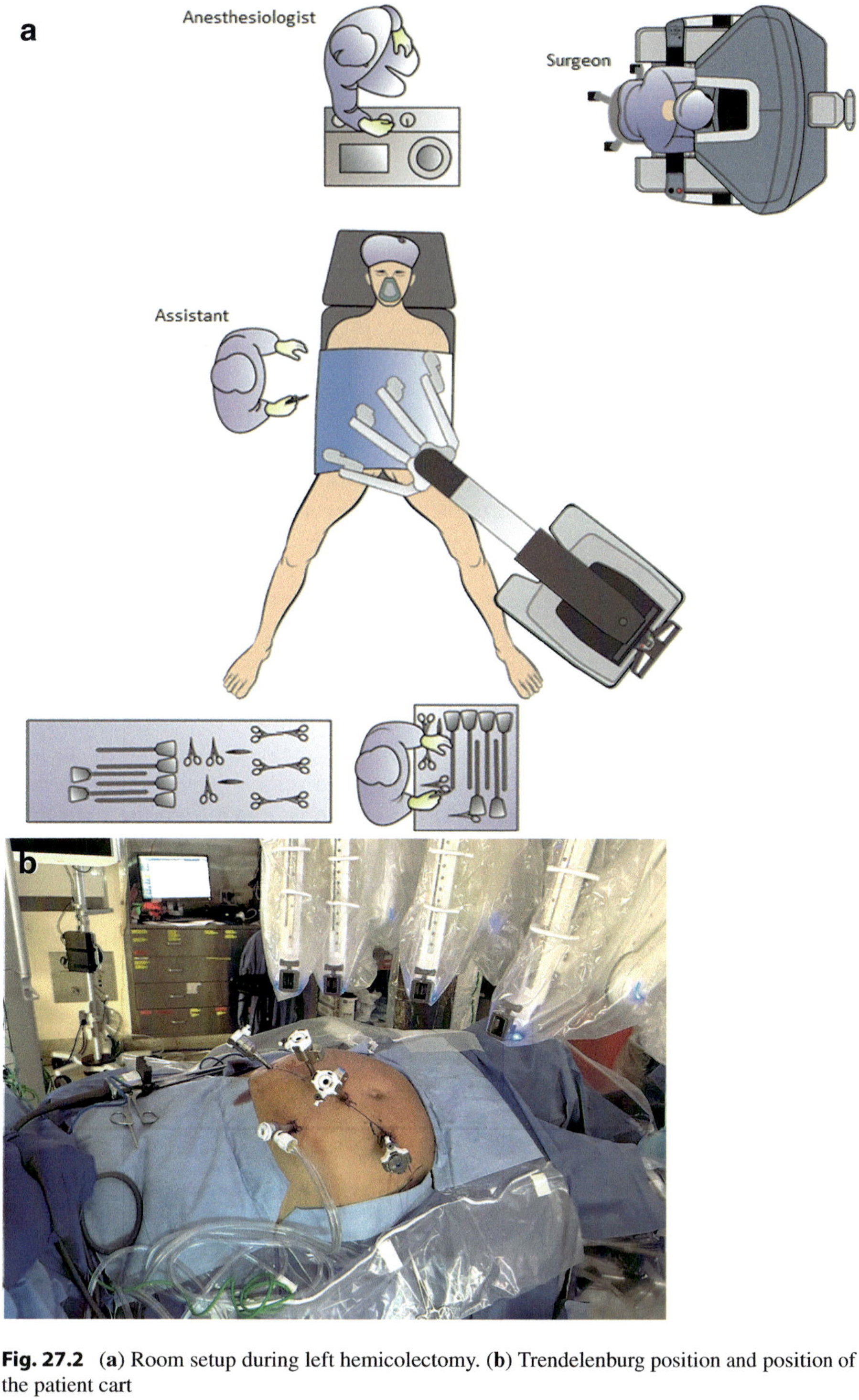

Fig. 27.2 (**a**) Room setup during left hemicolectomy. (**b**) Trendelenburg position and position of the patient cart

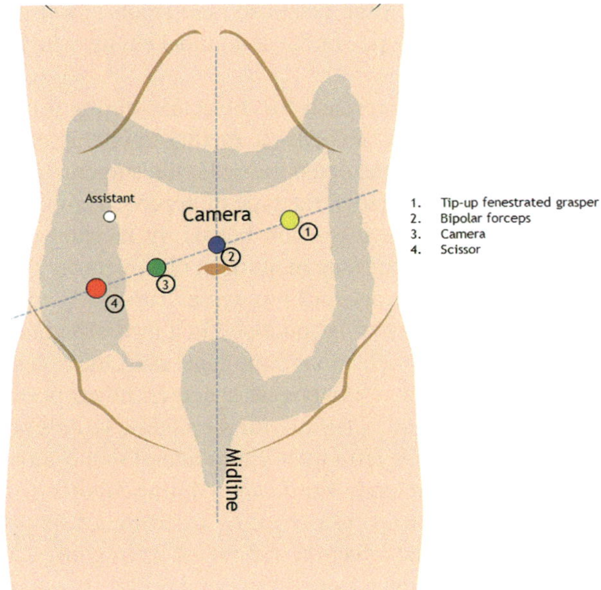

Fig. 27.3 Port placement during left hemicolectomy (double docking)

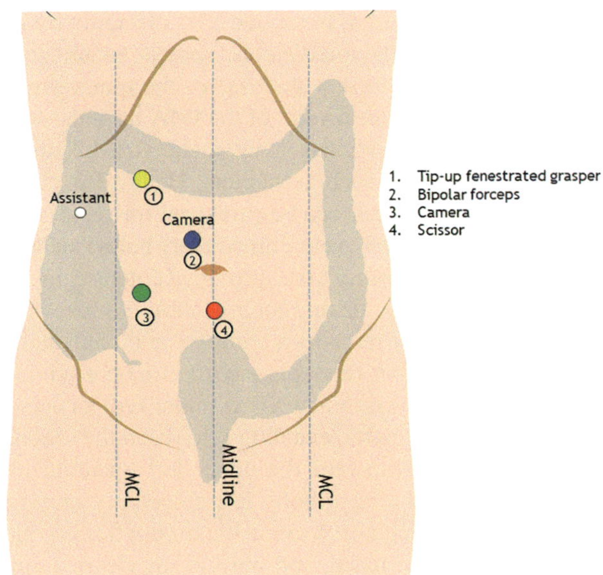

Fig. 27.4 Alternative port placement for proximal descending colon and splenic flexure lesions

transverse colon. Simultaneously, the small bowel is retracted medially and positioned on the right side of the abdominal cavity, which revealed the mesentery of the left colon.

The preferred approach for dissection during robotic left colectomy or sigmoid resection generally involves a medial-to-lateral orientation, although the lateral approach can be considered based on the surgeon's comfort level. Comparable outcomes were identified in the type of approach employed in colorectal cancer operations [23, 24]. The dissection begins by incising the right lateral superior pelvic peritoneal reflection using monopolar electrocautery. This incision starts inferiorly to the sacral promontory and progresses superiorly to the inferior mesenteric artery (IMA). The dissection is continued in a medial-to-lateral direction, reaching the left lateral peritoneal reflection. Simultaneously, the superior rectal artery is swept anteriorly, and the superior hypogastric nerves moved posteriorly. Identification and ligation of the superior rectal/inferior mesenteric vessels occur after the visualization and preservation of the left ureter. Intraureteral indocyanine green (ICG) can be used as an adjunct for ureteral identification during robot-assisted surgeries. This can be performed using a rigid cystoscope by inserting a 5 Fr open-ended ureteral catheter up to 20 cm. A gentle injection of 5 mL of 2.5 mg/mL ICG is performed as the ureteral catheter is withdrawn from the ureteral orifice. No stent is left in place, and the intraureteral ICG is detected using robotic near-infrared laser fluorescence technology. Depending on the surgical indication, high ligation of the IMA or its branches may or may not be required. In robotic left colectomy for cancer, it is preferable to ligate the left branch of the middle colic vessels, identified at the root of the small bowel mesentery, and divided at the base of the transverse mesocolon. If high ligation is deemed necessary, the takeoff of the IMA from the aorta is meticulously dissected to avoid injury to the lumbar sympathetic (L1–L3) and superior hypogastric nerves. Various modalities, such as staplers, Hem-o-lok clips, sutures, and robotic vessel-sealing energy devices, can be employed for vessel ligation. Additionally, ligation of the inferior mesenteric vein immediately below the level of the pancreatic body provides increased mobility to the proximal colon segment and entering to the lesser sac.

Although splenic flexure mobilization is somewhat easier with the da Vinci Xi® system [25, 26], it remains a complex and challenging step. Some centers opt for double docking, but this approach is time-consuming. After working on the first target anatomy, the da Vinci Xi® is undocked, its boom is rotated 180°, and it docks again to the same ports, enabling it to reach the second target anatomy. The robotic arms are oriented toward the upper left quadrant of the patient to mobilize the splenic flexure during robotic left colectomy or sigmoid resection. This process begins by adjusting arm 1 to the maximum flexion, aiming to create space between the arms, enhance reach, and prevent interference. In our practice, we deviate the standard port placement line 15–20° counterclockwise and favor a single-docking cross-armed approach (Fig. 27.5).

In our practice, we prefer single-docking crossed-arm technique. Using a tip-up fenestrated grasper through port number one, we retract the descending colon medially and inferiorly toward the cecum (Fig. 27.6a). Subsequently, we cross the arms

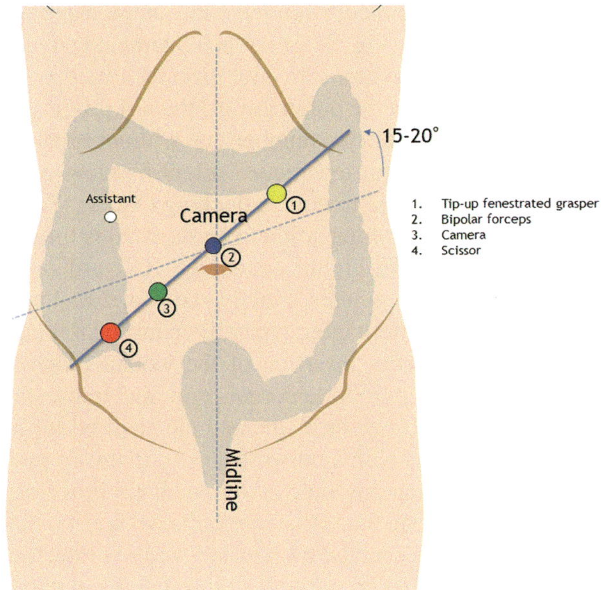

Fig. 27.5 Alternative port placement for single-docking cross-armed technique

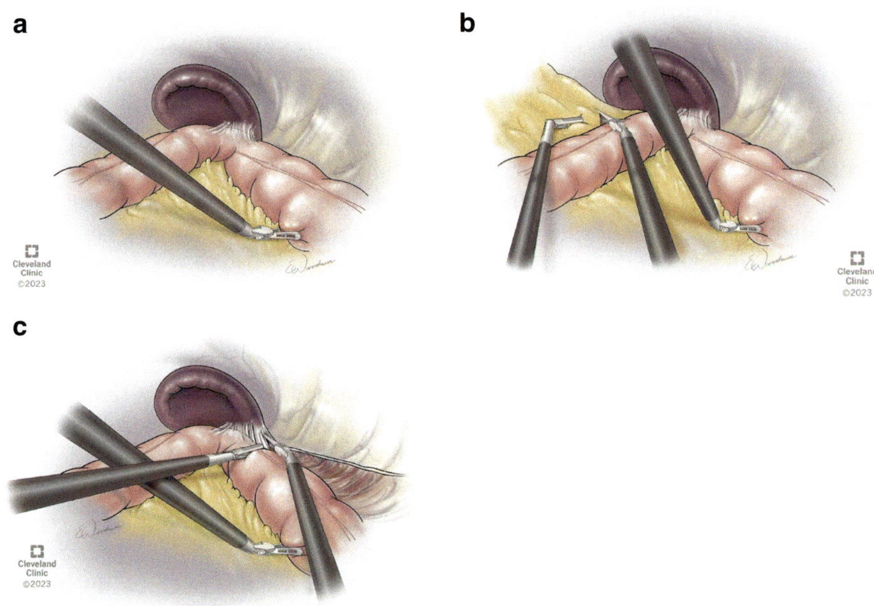

Fig. 27.6 (**a**) Traction of descending colon. (**b**) Lateral aspect of arm one. (**c**) Medial aspect of arm one

without robotic arm collision from the lateral aspect of arm one, facilitating splenic flexure takedown (Fig. 27.6b). Once lateral side dissection is completed, we adjust the instrument positions to mobilize the transverse colon. The tip-up grasping instrument retracts the colon toward the left lower quadrant, allowing us to work in the medial aspect of port number one without restriction (Fig. 27.6c). This "single-docking crossed-arm technique" offers freedom of movement and efficiency and saves time compared to double docking (Video 27.1) [27].

The mesentery of the colon to be resected is fully divided intracorporeally using a vessel sealer. We highly encourage ICG utilization to assess perfusion in the remaining colon segments. Finally, the bowel wall is transected proximally and distally using a robotic stapler, typically requiring a single firing depending on the level of transection. After insertion of the wound protector, the specimen is extracted through the 12 mm robotic port#4. Proximal transection can be performed extracorporeally using scissor or blade, and the anvil head placed into the proximal bowel. The anvil is fixed with a purse string. To maintain pneumoperitoneum, we prefer to use the Alexis® laparoscopic system with Kii Fios First Entry wound protectors with a cap (Applied Medical, Rancho Santa Margarita, CA, USA) or simply by using a Penrose drain around the trocars and wound protector. The anastomosis is achieved with a circular stapler, introduced through the rectum.

Alternatively, side-to-side isoperistaltic intracorporeal anastomosis can be created by anastomosing the small enterotomies on the proximal and distal portions of the colon. The lumen of the anastomosis is formed using one or two firings of the blue-loaded robotic stapler. Enterotomy defects can be closed using barbed sutures [7]. For intracorporeal anastomosis with a circular stapler, the anvil can be passed intra-abdominally through the Pfannenstiel incision wound protector. Approximately 2 cm proximal to the proximal transection point, a small pinpoint colotomy is performed at the anvil post-exit point. After introducing and positioning the anvil, the distal colotomy is closed using running barbed sutures [28]. Some surgeons prefer those alternative techniques. However, we don't believe these approaches provide additional benefits on minimizing extraction site incision size or recovery benefits.

Once the anastomosis completed and hemostasis confirmed especially at the vascular pedicle sites, ports are then removed under direct vision (Video 27.2).

Although the long-term oncological advantages of robotic surgery for rectal and colon cancers have not been conclusively demonstrated, notable short-term benefits are associated with robotic surgery. Alharthi et al. found that robotic left hemicolectomy is associated with a shorter length of hospital stay and higher total hospital costs than laparoscopic left hemicolectomy while maintaining comparable postoperative complication rates [29]. Additionally, Bastawrous et al. reported a lower rate of conversion to open surgery in robotic left hemicolectomy than in laparoscopic left hemicolectomy [30]. Studies addressing benign lesions, such as diverticula, have also suggested the feasibility of robotic left hemicolectomy for both simple and complicated diverticular diseases of the sigmoid colon [31]. The robotic system has demonstrated effective performance in mobilizing the colonic splenic flexure [32]. Furthermore, increasing evidence supports the safety and effectiveness of robotic intracorporeal anastomosis in left-sided colon resection. This technique has been associated with faster gastrointestinal recovery, shorter hospital stays, and lower postoperative hernia rates [33]. Although the long-term oncological benefits remain a subject of ongoing research, these short-term advantages highlight the potential of robotic left hemicolectomy.

Total Colectomy

The technique for total abdominal colectomy incorporates the combination of right hemicolectomy into the previously described left hemicolectomy procedure. The process involves sequential division of branches originating from the superior mesenteric artery, commencing with the ileocecal and right colic vessels, followed by the middle colic vessels. The IMA can be divided at its origin, or the superior rectal artery can be preserved depending on the nature of the operative indication.

Multiple quadrant access is usually necessary for this intricate procedure. For this purpose, the most commonly preferred approach for the patient cart is from the right or left side of the operating table. Rotation of the boom from right to left enables precise maneuvering of both sides of the abdomen (Fig. 27.7a). The surgeon initially gains access to the right side, followed by access to the left side, which is achieved by turning the boom where the arms are anchored. Alternatively, the patient's cart can be placed between the patient's legs (Fig. 27.7b), associated with a similar operative time [10]. A meticulous approach to docking is imperative, necessitating the accurate alignment of the patient cart and robotic arms. In total colectomy, the surgeon initiates the procedure by accessing the abdominal cavity using established techniques such as the Hasson technique, VisiPort™ Trocars (Medtronic, Minneapolis, MN, USA), or a Veress needle. This entry point allows a comprehensive examination of the abdominal anatomy, focusing on critical structures such as the ileocolic artery and duodenum. Pre-docking intra-abdominal inspection is recommended to reveal anatomical details and avoid platform-positioning complications. Port placement, a critical consideration, involves strategic positioning of trocars to ensure effective access to all four quadrants of the abdomen. The typical configuration includes a 12 mm robotic port in the right iliac fossa; 8 mm robotic ports in the umbilical region, left iliac fossa, and right and left upper quadrants; and 5 mm assistant ports in the right and left flanks (Fig. 27.8). Alternative port placements and patient cart positions can be considered based on the procedure and the surgeon's preferences. As the authors of this chapter, we do not prefer a robotic approach for total colectomy. Consequently, we do not advocate a specific preferred patient cart position or port placement technique.

After port placement and docking, the operation starts with isolation and division of the ileocolic artery, with careful dissection to prevent harm to the duodenum and the right ureter. Mobilization of the right colon and hepatic flexure ensues with medial-to-lateral and lateral-to-medial dissections performed sequentially to facilitate smooth and safe mobilization. Next, the middle colic pedicle is tackled, skeletonized, and ligated. Subsequently, the robotic system is docked using a multidocking approach to focus on the distal transverse colon and splenic flexure. Final docking

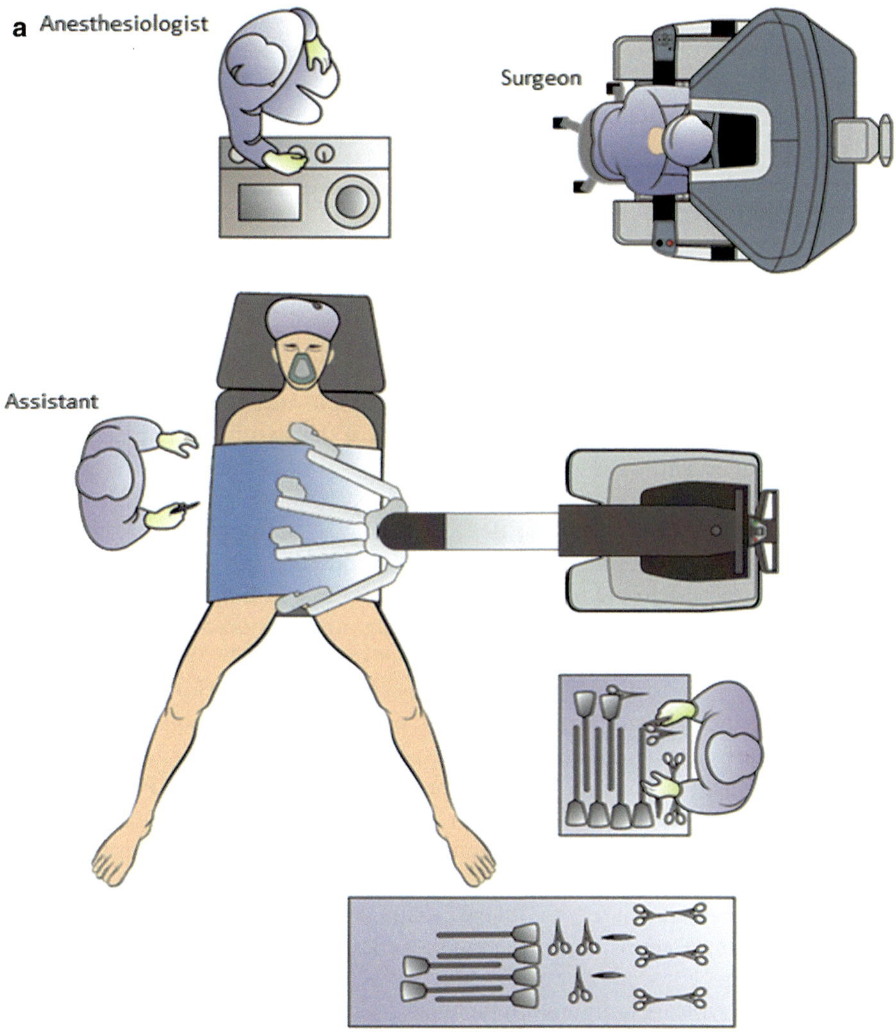

Fig. 27.7 Room setup during total colectomy. (**a**) Lateral patient cart docking. (**b**) Docking between the legs

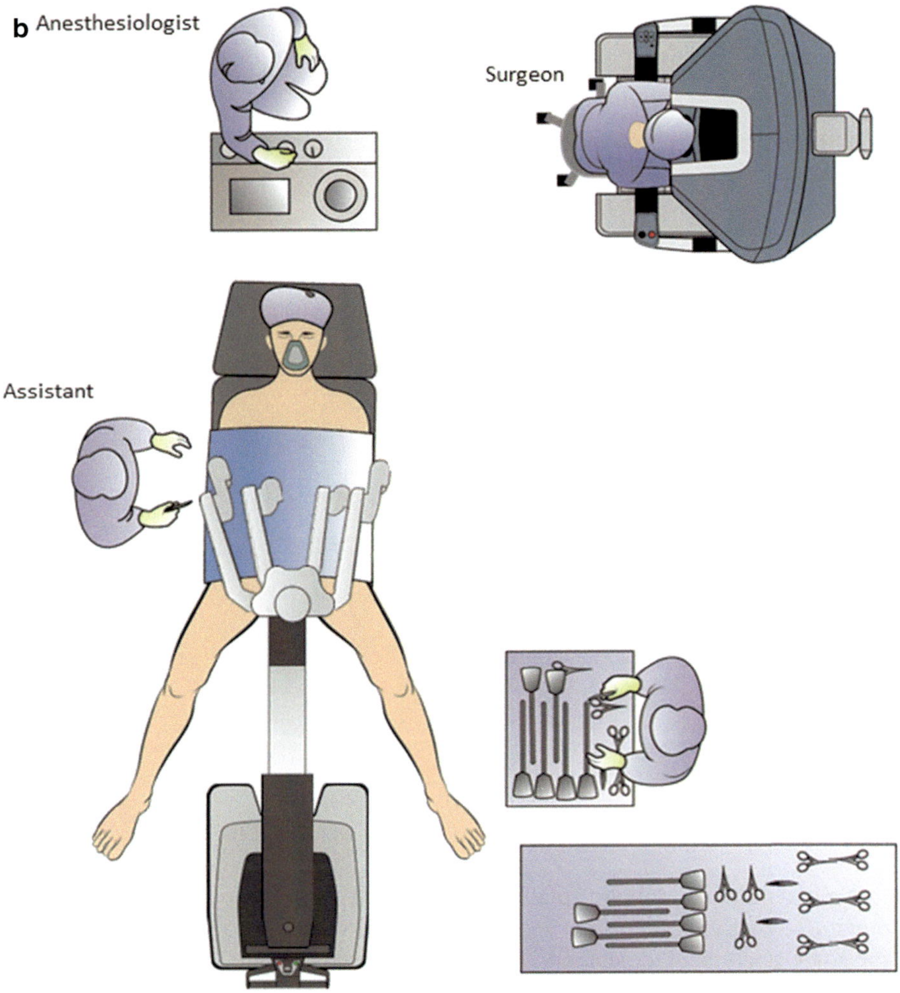

Fig. 27.7 (continued)

enables the dissection of the descending and rectosigmoid colon. The rectosigmoid junction is divided by using a robotic stapler mounted on arm #1 and docked in the right lower quadrant. The specimen is extracted through a Pfannenstiel incision, and the small bowel is transected. An anvil is placed at the proximal transection point. Ileorectal anastomosis is performed under direct visualization, using a circular stapler inserted through the anus. Flexible sigmoidoscopy is used to assess the integrity and level of anastomosis.

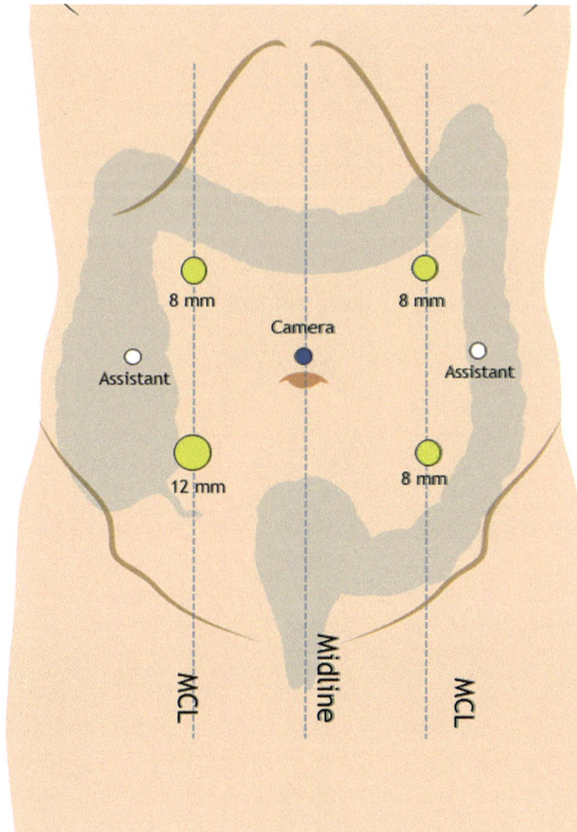

Fig. 27.8 Port placement for total colectomy

New-generation robotic platforms represent a notable advancement over previous-generation platforms and are associated with comparable operative times for total abdominal colectomy [10]. Utilizing the boom system and motion-activating table with newer-generation robotic platforms has proven advantageous in seamlessly performing anatomical dissection during total colectomy [32]. Additionally, robotic total colectomy offers a lower conversion rate and more number of harvested lymph nodes than laparoscopic methods [32, 34]. It is worth noting that despite its advantages in terms of dissection, there are financial considerations associated with robotic surgery. The total hospital charges are significantly higher in robotic surgery than the laparoscopic approach [35].

Postoperative Care and Complication Management

Patients undergoing robotic colectomy typically recover seamlessly especially with the addition of enhanced recovery pathways [36]. Early ambulation is encouraged on the day of the surgery or next morning after surgery [7]. Minimizing postoperative intravenous fluids and advocating limited use of narcotics are highly recommended to reduce postoperative ileus [37]. Starting from the day of the surgery, all patients are placed on a liquid diet, progressing to regular diet as tolerated. Administration of IV antibiotics is limited only for perioperative use, and urinary catheter removal occurs on postoperative day number one to mitigate potential urinary tract infections and promote early mobilization [38]. Stoma care and education are prerequisites for patients undergoing ileostomy before discharge to their homes. Patients undergoing colorectal surgery benefit from an enhanced recovery pathway, demonstrating a decreased length of hospital stay and cost without increased complications [39].

A systematic review comparing laparoscopic and robot-assisted colectomies includes randomized and nonrandomized studies, indicating a lower morbidity in robotic surgery. However, it is noteworthy that extended operative times and increased costs may counterbalance this advantage compared to laparoscopic approach [40]. It is crucial to emphasize that these findings are not reproduced in randomized controlled trials, as there are limited randomized controlled studies evaluating robotic colectomies. According to the ROLLAR Study, robotic-assisted laparoscopic surgery did not significantly reduce the risk of conversion to open laparotomy compared to conventional laparoscopic surgery [41]. It's important to note that our chapter differs from the ROLLAR Study, which focuses on rectal cancer patients.

Postoperative symptomatic impediments following total abdominal colectomy often manifest as chronic diarrhea, fecal urgency, and accidental bowel leakage [42]. The use of bulking agents, such as fiber supplements, and antidiarrheal agents, such as loperamide and diphenoxylate/atropine, is beneficial after excluding infectious, inflammatory, and dietary causes [42]. Cholestyramine is particularly effective for patients with a history of cholecystectomy. Endoscopic assessment of the rectum is imperative after total colectomy for inflammatory bowel disease and polyposis syndromes, which dictates the necessity for completion proctectomy, either with end ileostomy or ileal pouch anastomosis [42]. The risk of rectal neoplasia in patients with polyposis syndrome after ileorectal anastomosis is a significant concern, necessitating frequent endoscopic surveillance with biopsies and a multidisciplinary discussion and approach.

Learning Curve

Publications on the learning curve usually concentrate on robotic proctectomy rather than on robotic colonic resection procedures. However, several comprehensive robotic colorectal learning curve studies have included both left hemicolectomy and total colectomy. The robotic colorectal surgery learning curve has three stages [43, 44]. Various studies have reported different numbers of cases in the initial phase of the learning curve. Typically, this phase spans between 27 and 45 cases, with certain studies assuming that practitioners have prior experience in laparoscopic colorectal surgery [45–48]. The learning curve has the potential to be expedited through the use of simulators and video-based education [49, 50]. The rapid adoption of robotic colorectal resections has led to a significant proportion of procedures being performed by surgeons in their initial phases. However, during this phase, they exhibit a higher incidence of iatrogenic complications [51]. Upon completing the initial phase, surgeons proceed to the competent and challenging phase, performing more intricate and demanding procedures [43]. After completing the learning, robot-assisted surgery can be effectively performed within diverse colorectal practices, demonstrating minimal conversion rates and postoperative complications [47].

Whether robotic surgery has shorter learning curve than laparoscopic colorectal surgery remains controversial. Various reports suggest that robotic technology shortens the learning curve for complex tasks compared to conventional laparoscopy [52]. Conversely, another study contended that the learning curves for both robotic and laparoscopic approaches were similar [44]. Nevertheless, additional research is required to further shed light to this topic and clarify the debated points regarding differences between robotic and laparoscopic colon resection.

Future Directions

Suprapubic Approach

The suprapubic surgical approach involves colonic resection with horizontally and linearly placed ports in the suprapubic region and is primarily utilized for robotic right hemicolectomy procedures. The trocars are placed horizontally below the line between the anterior superior iliac spines, with a 12 mm trocar on the left and three trocars of 8 mm spaced 4 cm apart (Fig. 27.9). Investigation of the optimization of the suprapubic method is clinically significant. Suprapubic incision is known to

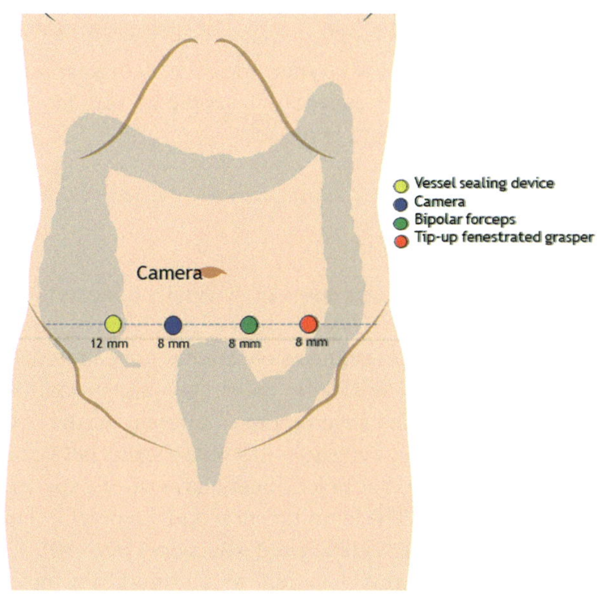

Fig. 27.9 Suprapubic approach port placement

provide better cosmesis, less pain, and a lower risk of incisional hernia than midline incision. A streamlined surgical approach can enhance the operational efficiency and minimize collisions across the robotic arms.

A few studies have described a suprapubic approach for robotic total colectomy [53]. The patient cart is strategically positioned between the patient's legs, initially targeting the mesentery and the upper abdominal region. Subsequently, the instruments and camera are reoriented to focus on the pelvic region. The surgical procedure commences in the upper rectal region by dissecting the rectosigmoid mesocolon. The sigmoid and left colon are mobilized, and the dissection is advanced toward the splenic flexure. However, due to the substantial distance of the splenic flexure from the suprapubic access point, first mobilization of the transverse colon is performed to facilitate takedown of the flexure. Subsequently, splenic flexure mobilization is performed. Ultimately, the final stages of dissection involve mobilization of the right colon in order to achieve tension-free anastomosis using the ileum. It is noteworthy that the procedure can hypothetically be performed also for the left colon resection up to the transverse colon; however, there are limited studies addressing this aspect in the existing literature. Yeo et al. tested the feasibility of a suprapubic approach for robotic left hemicolectomy in cadaveric models and adapted it for the first clinical case [54].

A comparison between the suprapubic approach and traditional port placement revealed the advantages of the suprapubic approach, including reduced operation time, lower conversion rates, decreased complications, and shorter hospital stay [55, 56]. Other studies have proposed a suprapubic approach for robotic colectomy, integrating complete mesocolic excision and D3 lymphadenectomy, demonstrating potential feasibility [57, 58]. Some case reports have demonstrated the feasibility and efficiency of the suprapubic approach using the da Vinci Single-Port (SP®) system (Intuitive Surgical, Inc., Sunnyvale, CA, USA) [59].

The collective findings suggest optimism for the future application of the suprapubic surgical approach, pending further clarification of the application conditions and long-term efficacy.

Single-Site Robotic Surgery

As engineering and technology continue to advance, enhancements in surgical robots are aimed at overcoming the challenges encountered in traditional approaches. Single-incision laparoscopic surgery (SILS) was introduced to mitigate port-related trauma and complications. However, technical challenges, particularly in complex operations requiring delicate tissue manipulation, have impeded the progress of SILS. Robotic surgery, characterized by increased articulation and reduced risk of instrument collision, presents a solution to these limitations [60]. Surgeons strive to minimize the number of robotic ports used in colonic resections to enhance cosmetic outcomes and expedite recovery. The integration of both surgical concepts holds the potential to achieve a relatively "scarless" operation with improved surgical dynamics.

Single-site robotic surgery for total colectomy has been introduced in case reports, demonstrating its feasibility with comparable operative times [61]. The procedure is also safe and feasible for left-sided colectomies and exhibits surgical and pathological outcomes similar to those of the laparoscopy [62]. Bae et al. introduced 23 cases of single-site robotic left colectomy with an additional assistant port, confirming the feasibility and safety of this method [63]. A systematic review indicated that current studies support the safety and feasibility of single-port robotic colectomy, although the evidence is limited [64]. Concerns persist regarding whether surgeons can achieve surgical and oncological outcomes comparable to those of conventional multiport laparoscopic and robotic colonic resection. Challenges include limited mobilization and countertraction due to the single-site entrance, as well as the constrained range of motion of the robotic arms hindering multiquadrant abdominal surgery. Issues such as docking and repositioning of the robot, particularly in extended colectomies, limit the utility of robotic surgery. Despite advancements in single-access ports, robotic arm configurations, and surgical platforms for single-port robotic surgery in the colorectal field, significant improvements are still required such as the need for vessel sealing robotic tools and stapling [63, 64]. The development of novel robotic platforms specifically designed for single-site surgery is essential to overcome the current limitations, and these efforts signify the potential of robotic surgery to overcome the limitations of conventional approaches.

da Vinci SP® Surgical System

The da Vinci SP® surgical system (Intuitive Surgical, Sunnyvale, CA, USA) is specifically designed for single-port surgery. It features a singular arm comprising a shaft with three multijointed, fully articulated instruments and a jointed high-resolution camera. The system is specifically designed to operate in narrow, hard-to-reach areas, such as anorectal surgery, prostatectomy, and tonsillectomy, and is characterized by a 360-degree boom movement that facilitates full multiquadrant operations in colorectal surgery [27]. The shaft design, which consists of all the instruments, prevents robotic arm collisions during surgery. However, limitations include the inability to use surgical energy devices and robotic staplers as well as the absence of suction irrigation. Furthermore, the grasping and traction forces are comparatively weaker than those in previous models, constraining their use in major surgeries [65].

Pioneering studies have confirmed the feasibility and efficiency of da Vinci SP® (dVSP) in colorectal surgery [66, 67]. Another study, comprising 43 robotic dVSP cases, incorporated six left hemicolectomies, demonstrating comparable short-term outcomes to conventional multiport laparoscopic surgery [68]. The overall efficiency and functionality of the dVSP for robotic colorectal procedures suggests a promising future for the widespread adoption of this technique. The growing interest in dVSP in colorectal surgery underscores its potential use in abdominal procedures and possibly other endoluminal approaches. However, a comprehensive analysis of procedural outcomes and further technological improvements is imperative to properly advance the field.

Conclusion

A meticulous decision-making process based on the surgeon's experience considering patient-specific conditions is paramount, achieving optimal outcomes in colonic interventions.

Advances in preoperative planning and meticulous room setup have enhanced the success of these procedures. A comprehensive examination of the operative steps is essential for successful execution of robotic surgery. The efficacy of robotic platforms, particularly for left hemicolectomy, is underscored by their potential short-term advantages. Technological advancements are poised to augment the significance of robotic surgery in colonic intervention.

References

1. Sheetz KH, Claflin J, Dimick JB. Trends in the adoption of robotic surgery for common surgical procedures. JAMA Netw Open. 2020;3(1):e1918911.
2. Benlice C, Aytac E, Costedio M, Kessler H, Abbas MA, Remzi FH, et al. Robotic, laparoscopic, and open colectomy: a case-matched comparison from the ACS-NSQIP. Int J Med Robot. 2017;13(3) https://doi.org/10.1002/rcs.1783.
3. Lanfranco AR, Castellanos AE, Desai JP, Meyers WC. Robotic surgery: a current perspective. Ann Surg. 2004;239(1):14–21.
4. Uhrich ML, Underwood RA, Standeven JW, Soper NJ, Engsberg JR. Assessment of fatigue, monitor placement, and surgical experience during simulated laparoscopic surgery. Surg Endosc. 2002;16(4):635–9.
5. Maeso S, Reza M, Mayol JA, Blasco JA, Guerra M, Andradas E, et al. Efficacy of the Da Vinci surgical system in abdominal surgery compared with that of laparoscopy: a systematic review and meta-analysis. Ann Surg. 2010;252(2):254–62.
6. Sheetz KH, Norton EC, Dimick JB, Regenbogen SE. Perioperative outcomes and trends in the use of robotic colectomy for medicare beneficiaries from 2010 through 2016. JAMA Surg. 2020;155(1):41–9.
7. Quezada-Diaz F, Pappou EP. Robotic left colectomy. In: Kim J, Garcia-Aguilar J, editors. Minimally invasive surgical techniques for cancers of the gastrointestinal tract: a step-by-step approach. Cham: Springer International Publishing; 2020. p. 193–200.
8. Rouffet F, Hay JM, Vacher B, Fingerhut A, Elhadad A, Flamant Y, et al. Curative resection for left colonic carcinoma: hemicolectomy vs. segmental colectomy. A prospective, controlled, multicenter trial. French Association for Surgical Research. Dis Colon Rectum. 1994;37(7):651–9.
9. Lee BC, Yu CS, Kim J, Lee JL, Kim CW, Yoon YS, et al. Clinicopathological features and surgical options for synchronous colorectal cancer. Medicine (Baltimore). 2017;96(9):e6224.
10. Jimenez-Rodriguez RM, Quezada-Diaz F, Tchack M, Pappou E, Wei IH, Smith JJ, et al. Use of the Xi robotic platform for total abdominal colectomy: a step forward in minimally invasive colorectal surgery. Surg Endosc. 2019;33(3):966–71.
11. Shussman N, Wexner SD. Colorectal polyps and polyposis syndromes. Gastroenterol Rep (Oxford). 2014;2(1):1–15.
12. Schlussel AT, Gagliano RA Jr, Seto-Donlon S, Eggerding F, Donlon T, Berenberg J, et al. The evolution of colorectal cancer genetics-Part 2: clinical implications and applications. J Gastrointest Oncol. 2014;5(5):336–44.
13. Zimmern A, Prasad L, Desouza A, Marecik S, Park J, Abcarian H. Robotic colon and rectal surgery: a series of 131 cases. World J Surg. 2010;34(8):1954–8.

14. Delaney CP, Lynch AC, Senagore AJ, Fazio VW. Comparison of robotically performed and traditional laparoscopic colorectal surgery. Dis Colon Rectum. 2003;46(12):1633–9.
15. Kilcoyne A, Kaplan JL, Gee MS. Inflammatory bowel disease imaging: current practice and future directions. World J Gastroenterol. 2016;22(3):917–32.
16. Al-Jashaami LS, DuPont HL. Management of clostridium difficile infection. Gastroenterol Hepatol (N Y). 2016;12(10):609–16.
17. Bokhari MB, Patel CB, Ramos-Valadez DI, Ragupathi M, Haas EM. Learning curve for robotic-assisted laparoscopic colorectal surgery. Surg Endosc. 2011;25(3):855–60.
18. Beck DE. Evaluation and management of constipation. Ochsner J. 2008;8(1):25–31.
19. Gorgun E, Ozben V, Costedio M, Stocchi L, Kalady M, Remzi F. Robotic versus conventional laparoscopic rectal cancer surgery in obese patients. Color Dis. 2016;18(11):1063–71.
20. Gorgun E, Rencuzogullari A, Ozben V, Stocchi L, Fraser T, Benlice C, et al. An effective bundled approach reduces surgical site infections in a high-outlier colorectal unit. Dis Colon Rectum. 2018;61(1):89–98.
21. Palmeri M, Gianardi D, Guadagni S, Di Franco G, Bastiani L, Furbetta N, et al. Robotic colorectal resection with and without the use of the new Da Vinci table motion: a case-matched study. Surg Innov. 2018;25(3):251–7.
22. Parra-Davila E, Diaz-Hernandez JJ. Totally robotic left colectomy. J Robot Surg. 2011;5(1):57–64.
23. ErÖZkan K, Vatansever S, Tamam S, Benk MŞ, Azili C, Bayar S, et al. Laparoscopic right hemicolectomy: comparison of medial and lateral approach. Ege Tıp Dergisi. 2023;62(3):339–45.
24. Hajibandeh S, Hajibandeh S, Navid A, Sarma DR, Eltair M, Mankotia R, et al. Meta-analysis of medial-to-lateral versus lateral-to-medial colorectal mobilisation during laparoscopic colorectal surgery. Int J Color Dis. 2019;34(5):787–99.
25. Ozben V, Cengiz TB, Atasoy D, Bayraktar O, Aghayeva A, Erguner I, et al. Is da Vinci Xi Better than da Vinci Si in robotic rectal cancer surgery? Comparison of the 2 generations of da Vinci systems. Surg Laparosc Endosc Percutan Tech. 2016;26(5):417–23.
26. Protyniak B, Jorden J, Farmer R. Multiquadrant robotic colorectal surgery: the da Vinci Xi vs Si comparison. J Robot Surg. 2018;12(1):67–74.
27. Erozkan K, Gorgun E. Robotic colorectal surgery and future directions. Am J Surg. 2023;230:91.
28. Achilli P, Perry W, Grass F, Abd El Aziz MA, Kelley SR, Larson DW, et al. Completely intracorporeal anastomosis in robotic left colonic and rectal surgery: technique and 30-day outcomes. Updat Surg. 2021;73(6):2137–43.
29. Alharthi S, Reilly M, Arishi A, Ahmed AM, Chulkov M, Qu W, et al. Robotic versus laparoscopic sigmoid colectomy: Analysis of healthcare cost and utilization project database. Am Surg. 2020;86(3):256–60.
30. Bastawrous AL, Landmann RG, Liu Y, Liu E, Cleary RK. Incidence, associated risk factors, and impact of conversion to laparotomy in elective minimally invasive sigmoidectomy for diverticular disease. Surg Endosc. 2020;34(2):598–609.
31. Grass F, Crippa J, Mathis KL, Kelley SR, Larson DW. Feasibility and safety of robotic resection of complicated diverticular disease. Surg Endosc. 2019;33(12):4171–6.
32. Kim JC, Lee JL, Yoon YS, Kim CW, Park IJ, Lim SB. Robotic left colectomy with complete mesocolectomy for splenic flexure and descending colon cancer, compared with a laparoscopic procedure. Int J Med Robot. 2018;14(5):e1918.
33. Al Natour RH, Obias V, Albright J, Wu J, Ferraro J, Akram WM, et al. A propensity score matched comparison of intracorporeal and extracorporeal techniques for robotic-assisted sigmoidectomy in an enhanced recovery pathway. J Robot Surg. 2019;13(5):649–56.
34. Ozben V, de Muijnck C, Karabork M, Ozoran E, Zenger S, Bilgin IA, et al. The da Vinci Xi system for robotic total/subtotal colectomy vs. conventional laparoscopy: short-term outcomes. Tech Coloproctol. 2019;23(9):861–8.
35. Moghadamyeghaneh Z, Hanna MH, Carmichael JC, Pigazzi A, Stamos MJ, Mills S. Comparison of open, laparoscopic, and robotic approaches for total abdominal colectomy. Surg Endosc. 2016;30(7):2792–8.

36. Carmichael JC, Keller DS, Baldini G, Bordeianou L, Weiss E, Lee L, et al. Clinical practice guidelines for enhanced recovery after colon and rectal surgery from the American Society of Colon and Rectal Surgeons and Society of American Gastrointestinal and Endoscopic Surgeons. Dis Colon Rectum. 2017;60(8):761–84.
37. Lee L, Liberman S, Charlebois P, Stein B, Kaneva P, Carli F, et al. The impact of complications after elective colorectal resection within an enhanced recovery pathway. Tech Coloproctol. 2018;22(3):191–9.
38. Hung LY, Benlice C, Jia X, Steele SR, Valente MA, Holubar SD, et al. Outcomes after early versus delayed urinary bladder catheter removal after proctectomy for benign and malignant disease in 2,429 patients: An Observational Cohort Study. Surg Infect. 2021;22(3):310–7.
39. Liska D, Novello M, Cengiz BT, Holubar SD, Aiello A, Gorgun E, et al. Enhanced recovery pathway benefits patients undergoing nonelective colorectal surgery. Ann Surg. 2021;273(4):772–7.
40. Lorenzon L, Bini F, Balducci G, Ferri M, Salvi PF, Marinozzi F. Laparoscopic versus robotic-assisted colectomy and rectal resection: a systematic review and meta-analysis. Int J Color Dis. 2016;31(2):161–73.
41. Jayne D, Pigazzi A, Marshall H, Croft J, Corrigan N, Copeland J, et al. Effect of robotic-assisted vs conventional laparoscopic surgery on risk of conversion to open laparotomy among patients undergoing resection for rectal cancer: The ROLARR Randomized Clinical Trial. JAMA. 2017;318(16):1569–80.
42. Jimenez-Rodriguez R, Quezada-Diaz F, Garcia-Aguilar J. Robotic total abdominal colectomy: A step-by-step approach. In: Kim J, Garcia-Aguilar J, editors. Minimally invasive surgical techniques for cancers of the gastrointestinal tract: A step-by-step approach. Cham: Springer International Publishing; 2020. p. 227–32.
43. Park EJ, Baik SH. Robotic surgery for colon and rectal cancer. Curr Oncol Rep. 2016;18(1):5.
44. Park EJ, Kim CW, Cho MS, Kim DW, Min BS, Baik SH, et al. Is the learning curve of robotic low anterior resection shorter than laparoscopic low anterior resection for rectal cancer?: a comparative analysis of clinicopathologic outcomes between robotic and laparoscopic surgeries. Medicine (Baltimore). 2014;93(25):e109.
45. Lin CY, Liu YC, Chen MC, Chiang FF. Learning curve and surgical outcome of robotic assisted colorectal surgery with ERAS program. Sci Rep. 2022;12(1):20566.
46. Hirschburger M, Schneider R, Kraenzlein S, Padberg W, Hecker A, Reichert M. Right colectomy from open to robotic – a single-center experience with functional outcomes in a learning-curve setting. Langenbeck's Arch Surg. 2022;407(7):2915–27.
47. Parascandola SA, Horsey ML, Hota S, Paull JO, Graham A, Pudalov N, et al. The robotic colorectal experience: an outcomes and learning curve analysis of 502 patients. Color Dis. 2021;23(1):226–36.
48. Park EJ, Kim CW, Cho MS, Baik SH, Kim DW, Min BS, et al. Multidimensional analyses of the learning curve of robotic low anterior resection for rectal cancer: 3-phase learning process comparison. Surg Endosc. 2014;28(10):2821–31.
49. Kılınçarslan Ö, Türk Y, Vargör A, Özdemir M, Hassoy H, Makay Ö. Video gaming improves robotic surgery simulator success: a multi-clinic study on robotic skills. J Robot Surg. 2023;17(4):1435–42.
50. Erözkan K, Culcu S, Tamam S, Unal AE. The contribution of laparoscopic distal pancreatectomy videos on YouTube to the learning curve in the COVID-19 pandemic. Medicine (Baltimore). 2022;101(47):e31537.
51. Symer MM, Sedrakyan A, Yeo HL. Case sequence analysis of the robotic colorectal resection learning curve. Dis Colon Rectum. 2019;62(9):1071–8.
52. Park JS, Choi GS, Lim KH, Jang YS, Jun SH. Robotic-assisted versus laparoscopic surgery for low rectal cancer: case-matched analysis of short-term outcomes. Ann Surg Oncol. 2010;17(12):3195–202.
53. Pasquer A. Full robotic total colectomy with a suprapubic approach: technical points. Tech Coloproctol. 2023;27(5):421–2.

54. Yeo SA, Noh GT, Han JH, Cheong C, Stein H, Kerdok A, et al. Universal suprapubic approach for complete mesocolic excision and central vascular ligation using the da Vinci Xi(®) system: from cadaveric models to clinical cases. J Robot Surg. 2017;11(4):399–407.
55. Hamilton AER, Chatfield MD, Johnson CS, Stevenson ARL. Totally robotic right hemicolectomy: a multicentre case-matched technical and peri-operative comparison of port placements and da Vinci models. J Robot Surg. 2020;14(3):479–91.
56. Bianchi PP, Giuliani G, Salaj A, Ferraro L, Opocher E, Toti F, et al. Bottom-up suprapubic approach for robotic right colectomy: technical aspects and preliminary outcomes. Minerva Surg. 2021;76(2):129–37.
57. Schulte Am Esch J, Iosivan SI, Steinfurth F, Mahdi A, Förster C, Wilkens L, et al. A standardized suprapubic bottom-to-up approach in robotic right colectomy: technical and oncological advances for complete mesocolic excision (CME). BMC Surg. 2019;19(1):72.
58. Lee HJ, Choi GS, Park JS, Park SY, Kim HJ, Woo IT, et al. A novel robotic right colectomy for colon cancer via the suprapubic approach using the da Vinci Xi system: initial clinical experience. Ann Surg Treat Res. 2018;94(2):83–7.
59. Choo JM, Kim JS, Cheong JY, Rusli SM, Park H, Kim SH. Application of a single-port robotic system for right colectomy: a novel suprapubic approach. Dis Colon Rectum. 2022;65(11):e1029.
60. Kim SJ, Choi BJ, Lee SC. Overview of single-port laparoscopic surgery for colorectal cancers: past, present, and the future. World J Gastroenterol. 2014;20(4):997–1004.
61. Juo YY, Obias V. Robot-assisted single-incision total colectomy: a case report. Int J Med Robot. 2015;11(1):104–8.
62. Chang TC, Lin EK, Lu YJ, Huang MT, Chen CH. Single-incision robotic colectomy versus single-incision laparoscopic colectomy: a matched case control study. Asian J Surg. 2021;44(5):749–54.
63. Bae SU, Jeong WK, Baek SK. Robot-assisted colectomy for left-sided colon cancer: comparison of reduced-port and conventional multi-port robotic surgery. J Laparoendosc Adv Surg Tech A. 2017;27(4):398–403.
64. Voskens FJ, van Hillegersberg R, Broeders IAMJ, Ruurda J. Single-site systems in general surgery. In: Gharagozloo F, Patel VR, Giulianotti PC, Poston R, Gruessner R, Meyer M, editors. Robotic surgery. Cham: Springer International Publishing; 2021. p. 821–8.
65. Baek SJ, Piozzi GN, Kim SH. Optimizing outcomes of colorectal cancer surgery with robotic platforms. Surg Oncol. 2021;37:101559.
66. Piozzi GN, Kim JS, Choo JM, Shin SH, Kim JS, Lee TH, et al. Da Vinci SP robotic approach to colorectal surgery: two specific indications and short-term results. Tech Coloproctol. 2022;26(6):461–70.
67. Kim HJ, Choi GS, Song SH, Park JS, Park SY, Lee SM, et al. An initial experience with a novel technique of single-port robotic resection for rectal cancer. Tech Coloproctol. 2021;25(7):857–64.
68. Kim HS, Oh BY, Chung SS, Lee RA, Noh GT. Short-term outcomes of single-incision robotic colectomy versus conventional multiport laparoscopic colectomy for colon cancer. J Robot Surg. 2023;17(5):2351–9.

28 Low Anterior Resection

Cigdem Benlice and Bilgi Baca

Background

The practice of colorectal surgery has undergone significant transformation in the past three decades, primarily due to the increasing adoption of minimally invasive techniques following the introduction of laparoscopic colectomy by Jacobs [1]. These minimally invasive approaches have demonstrated enhancements in postoperative recovery, along with reductions in morbidity and length of hospital stay as compared to traditional open surgery for colorectal procedures [2].

In the management of rectal cancer, surgical resection remains the foremost treatment approach for achieving curative resection, accurate staging, determining prognosis, and guiding subsequent therapeutic decisions [3, 4]. However, rectal cancer surgery poses considerable technical challenges due to the confined anatomical boundaries and the intricate nature of the pelvis, where the presacral veins, autonomic and sexual nerves, and organs are in close proximity. The complexities inherent in rectal surgery are further compounded when employing laparoscopic techniques, primarily due to ergonomic limitations in instrument design [5]. Laparoscopic surgeons are tasked with performing multi-quadrant operations similar to open surgery, yet they encounter challenges such as limited tactile feedback and poorly designed instruments. The two-dimensional (2D) visualization adds another layer of difficulty, diminishing in-depth perception and hand-eye coordination.

Undoubtedly, the robotic approach is gaining prominence in the field of colorectal surgery. Three-dimensional visualization, the use of endo-wristed instruments, tremor reduction, and the provision of ergonomic and physical comfort for the surgeon represent several advantages that robotic surgery holds over laparoscopy [6].

C. Benlice · B. Baca (✉)
Department of General Surgery, Acibadem Mehmet Ali Aydinlar University School of Medicine, Istanbul, Turkey

S. Samreen et al. (eds.), *The SAGES Manual of Robotic Surgery*,
https://doi.org/10.1007/978-3-031-86927-3_28

Despite these advantages, there remains a debate about whether this technology will translate into clinical efficiency and contribute to the overall value of care. This chapter aims to assess the impact of the robotic approach on low anterior resection, with a specific focus on rectal cancer surgery.

Rationality and Adaption of Robotic Surgery

The application of robotic surgery has witnessed a remarkable expansion across various surgical disciplines, with a particular focus on colorectal procedures. This surge in adoption can be traced back to the early twenty-first century when initial reports surfaced regarding the successful implementation of robotic technology in colonic and rectal resections [4, 7]. In a recent extensive analysis encompassing a 16-year period and involving a substantial cohort of 318,548 patients with rectal adenocarcinoma in the United States, notable shifts in treatment modalities and outcomes were identified. The study brought to light a substantial decline in the utilization of open surgery, showing a significant 50% reduction from 60.1% during period 2 to 30.1% in period 4. In tandem with this decline in open surgery, there was a noteworthy surge in the adoption of minimally invasive surgery, with robotic surgery leading the way with a remarkable more than five-fold increase [4]. This paradigm shift in surgical approaches can be attributed, in large part, to the perceived advantages associated with robotic surgery. The heightened precision, improved visualization provided by a three-dimensional view, stable camera function, and articulated instruments are factors that have contributed to the growing appeal of robotic-assisted procedures. Among the minimally invasive options, robotic surgery has particularly stood out as a favored choice. The pivotal year 2015 emerges as a key turning point in this trend. This coincides with a notable uptick in the adoption of robotic surgery. Intriguingly, this timeframe aligns with the publication of the ALaCaRT trial in the same year [8]. The ALaCaRT trial findings were instrumental, revealing that laparoscopic surgery did not establish non-inferiority compared to open surgery for patients with T1 to T3 rectal cancers. The uncertainties arising from this trial seemingly influenced the medical community's approach to rectal cancer treatment, prompting a shift toward alternative methods, with robotic surgery emerging as a compelling choice. In summary, the findings from this comprehensive study underscore a substantial evolution in the landscape of rectal adenocarcinoma treatment in the United States. The significant decline in open surgery, coupled with the remarkable increase in minimally invasive approaches, particularly robotic surgery, reflects a dynamic response to emerging clinical evidence and a pursuit of more advanced and effective treatment strategies in the ever-evolving field of oncology.

The purported advantages of utilizing the robotic platform are not only underscored in observational studies [9, 10] but are also synthesized from comprehensive literature reviews [11, 12]. However, despite the promising outlook, findings from randomized control trials (RCTs) and a meta-analysis incorporating RCT data have, up until now, indicated a state of non-inferiority [13, 14]. A pivotal contribution to this discourse comes from the ROLARR RCT, which examined 471 cases across 10 different countries involving 40 surgeons, comparing the outcomes of laparoscopic and robotic rectal surgery. Notably, while there was no discernible decrease in conversion rates with robotic surgery within the primary patient cohort, a reduction in conversion rates was identified in male robotic cases as opposed to laparoscopic cases [13].

In parallel, a spectrum of other studies has brought to light compelling benefits associated with robotic colorectal surgery. These encompass significantly reduced conversion rates [15, 16], enhanced oncological outcomes [17, 18], and improved autonomic nerve preservation in cases where the robotic platform was employed. Despite these positive indicators, concerns have been raised regarding operating time and cost as potential drawbacks of robotic colorectal surgery. Nevertheless, it is worth noting that as surgeon experience with robotic technology deepens and the availability of robotic platforms becomes more widespread, the trajectory points toward reduced operating times and costs [19]. This hints at a potential paradigm shift in the perception of drawbacks, making robotic colorectal surgery an increasingly viable and advantageous option in the evolving landscape of surgical techniques.

Comparison of Different Surgical Approaches

The advancement of total mesorectal excision (TME) has established a standard for improving local recurrence and survival in rectal cancer surgery. However, the ongoing debate centers on whether a laparoscopic approach can achieve comparable oncological outcomes to open surgery [8]. Although open TME is linked to favorable pathologic and oncologic results, it deprives patients of the well-established advantages associated with minimally invasive surgery [20]. These benefits include a shorter length of stay, reduced analgesic requirements, and an earlier return of bowel function [21]. Despite decades of experience with laparoscopy in colon cancer treatment, its widespread acceptance for rectal cancer surgery has been hindered by technical challenges, specifically related to using in-line, non-articulating instruments in a confined pelvis [4]. The limitations linked to an assistant-dependent laparoscopic (two-dimensional, 2D) view, constrained dexterity, and straight instruments have prolonged the learning curve for laparoscopic rectal resections, impeding widespread adoption and potentially influencing oncological outcomes. However, it's crucial to recognize and consider drawbacks, such as the absence of haptic feedback, when planning and executing robotic procedures.

The increasing popularity of robotic surgery may suggest perceived or actual advantages over traditional laparoscopy. These advantages often include a three-dimensional (3D) view for the operating surgeon, a stable camera, and articulated instruments. In colorectal practice, these benefits become particularly relevant in restorative resections of mid- and low-rectal cancers [21].

Cohort studies and meta-analyses indicate that robotic surgery for rectal cancer is associated with a significantly lower positive circumferential resection margin (CRM) rate compared to laparoscopic surgery [2, 19, 22, 23]. Additionally, robotic surgery exhibits lower open conversion rates, reduced postoperative complications, and shorter hospital stays [24]. Moreover, there is evidence suggesting better recovery of urinary and sexual function. This suggests that, despite acknowledged disadvantages, the robotic approach demonstrates promising oncological outcomes and may serve as a valuable alternative in rectal cancer surgery [25]. It's important to note that the current evidence is of low quality [26]. A Korean study conducted a comparative analysis of robotic, open, and laparoscopic TME, revealing comparable and excellent oncological outcomes [27]. These included 3-year local recurrence rates ranging from 2.5% to 3.4% and low rates of CRM positivity, specifically less than 2.5%. As anticipated, both robotic and laparoscopic minimally invasive proctectomy demonstrated advantages such as a shorter length of stay, reduced pain, and fewer surgical site infections. Additionally, the robotic approach exhibited a significant association with sphincter preservation and a lower conversion rate when compared to laparoscopic TME as reported in published studies [28].

Learning Curve

The advantage of robotic surgery in low anterior resection lies in its freedom of movements and precision during pelvic dissection. However, the duration of the learning curve is a subject of debate. Significantly, emerging evidence suggests that the learning curve associated with robotic surgery in procedures such as rectal cancer surgery is notably shorter compared to that required for laparoscopic surgery, as illuminated by several studies. Several studies have explored the learning curve for robot-assisted rectal cancer surgery, with reported values ranging from 20 to 50 cases [29–31]. This sharply contrasts with the frequently mentioned 30 to 70 surgeries associated with the laparoscopic approach [32]. However, it's essential to note that some authors have raised concerns about potential bias due to the relatively small number of cases included in these series (less than 50 each) [33]. These considerations underscore the evolving understanding of the learning curve in robot-assisted rectal cancer surgery and the importance of methodological rigor in assessing this crucial aspect of surgical adoption. Despite the existence of recently published studies [34], it's crucial to acknowledge that the experience of laparoscopic surgeons should be recognized as a significant influencing factor in the learning of robot-assisted techniques. Surgeons with prior experience in laparoscopic procedures may benefit from their familiarity with tactless surgery and prior optical handling, potentially leading to a decreased learning curve and a more efficient acquisition of expertise in robot-assisted techniques. This interplay between prior surgical skills and the adoption of innovative technologies highlights the importance of leveraging existing expertise to facilitate the integration of newer surgical approaches.

Training Program

The inherent advantages offered by robotic technology play a pivotal role in potentially streamlining the learning process, potentially reducing the number of cases necessary to attain optimal surgical proficiency. The intricacies of rectal cancer surgery, a procedure known for its complexity, may benefit substantially from the precision and enhanced capabilities of robotic systems, thereby accelerating the surgeon's journey toward mastery. Without mentoring, it has been observed to take over 50 procedures to achieve proficiency in robotic proctectomy. A dedicated training process holds the potential to reduce the duration of this learning curve and contribute to identifying new parameters for defining surgeons' expertise in robotic procedures. It's noteworthy that in expert centers, robotic surgery may not always exhibit longer durations than laparoscopy, emphasizing the importance of specialized training and expertise in optimizing the benefits of robotic techniques [35, 36].

The establishment and implementation of a rigorous training program for robotic rectal surgery are critical components in shaping a proficient surgical workforce. Standardization and structured training play pivotal roles in ensuring a consistent and high-quality educational experience for surgeons venturing into this complex field. A standardized curriculum serves as a foundational guide, covering essential aspects ranging from mastering robotic console control to intricate pelvic dissection techniques [37]. For instance, initiatives like the Robotic-Assisted Colorectal Training (RACT) program have demonstrated the efficacy of structured training in enhancing surgeon proficiency [38]. This comprehensive program encompasses didactic modules, virtual reality simulation, and hands-on training, contributing to a well-rounded educational experience. Moreover, standardized training ensures consistency in skill acquisition across diverse surgical environments. Studies emphasize the importance of standardized training in minimizing variations in surgical performance and promoting uniformity in the adoption of robotic techniques [39]. Structured training programs not only facilitate a more streamlined learning curve but also aid in the objective assessment of surgeons' competencies. Given this information, the implementation of a standardized and structured training program for robotic rectal surgery is instrumental in shaping a skilled and confident surgical workforce. By drawing insights from various studies and initiatives, we can appreciate the multifaceted benefits of such programs in optimizing surgical outcomes and advancing the field of robotic rectal surgery.

Genitourinary Function

Robotic rectal surgery distinguishes itself with its advanced capabilities, providing unparalleled optics and heightened visualization of the intricate autonomic nervous plexus within the pelvis. This elevated visual acuity serves as a powerful tool for precision, empowering surgeons to engage in meticulous preservation of nerves. Advocates of the total robotic technique posit that this meticulous preservation, especially concerning both pelvic and periaortic nerves, holds the promise of a substantial reduction in postoperative complications. Specifically, there is an anticipation of minimizing the risk of complications such as sexual and bladder dysfunction. The integration of superior optics into robotic rectal surgery not only underscores the technological advancements in the field but also underscores the potential for improved patient outcomes and enhanced quality of life following such intricate surgical procedures [40–42]. This perspective accentuates the multifaceted advantages that robotic rectal surgery can bring to the forefront, promising not only heightened surgical precision but also a potential positive impact on patients' genitourinary function during the critical postoperative phase. The integration of robotic technology not only elevates the technical aspects of the surgical procedure but also holds the potential to contribute significantly to the overall well-being of patients by addressing genitourinary concerns. This holistic approach aligns with the evolving landscape of surgical advancements, where innovations extend beyond procedural efficacy to encompass broader considerations for patient outcomes and postoperative quality of life. Recent two randomized controlled trials, which assessed minimally invasive techniques, incorporated sexual and urinary function metrics as outcome measures [13, 14]. The initial trial revealed no statistically significant difference between the two groups concerning urinary and sexual function for both males and females at the 6-month mark. In contrast, the second study reported that sexual function 1-year post-surgery was notably superior in the robotic-assisted group when compared to the laparoscopic group. A robotic platform serves as a tool that enhances visibility in the operating field and offers increased precision. Nevertheless, it merely mimics the movements of the surgeon's hands. Therefore, a thorough understanding of pelvic neuroanatomy and the principles of nerve-sparing total mesorectal excision is essential to minimize the potential for iatrogenic injury to the hypogastric plexus [43].

Preoperative Planning

The meticulous selection of patients is paramount for effective preoperative planning, necessitating individuals who are not only medically fit but also capable of tolerating minimally invasive surgery. A comprehensive evaluation, including a detailed history and physical examination, is essential for all patients. For those with rectal lesions, a preoperative full colonoscopy is strongly recommended, particularly for identifying tumor location and potential synchronous colorectal lesions.

As part of the preoperative preparation for rectal surgery, patients undergo mechanical bowel preparation along with oral antibiotics. Preoperative broad-spectrum intravenous antibiotics are administered within 30–60 min of the incision time to ensure optimal concentration from the outset. Deep venous prophylaxis involves the use of sequential compression devices and chemical prophylaxis (preoperative heparin). A Foley catheter and intraoperative orogastric tube are routinely placed in all cases. Additionally, patients receive counseling from the colorectal nurse, who marks the site of the ileostomy.

Operative Procedure

Room Setup

When performing robotic low anterior resection with da Vinci® Xi Surgical Systems, the patient is positioned in a modified lithotomy stance utilizing adjustable lithotomy stirrups. The assistant surgeon maintains a position on the right side of the patient, providing support to the console surgeon through one assistant port. Robot was docked from the left side of the patient (edited and narrated video clip showing surgical steps for robotic low anterior resection).

Patient Positioning

The lithotomy position proves advantageous for the surgical team, particularly when operating in the upper quadrants of the abdomen, as it allows them to stand between the patient's legs. Padded stirrups or yellow fins are utilized, and meticulous attention is given to preventing perineal nerve injury. Both arms are tucked at the patient's sides. A gel pad on the operating table can offer additional decubitus support and stability against extreme table tilting. To mitigate the risk of nerve injury, caution is exercised during changes in the operation table position, as subsequent patient sliding may lead to pressure from the stirrup on the posterior aspect of the lower extremity. To prevent such occurrences, we opt to secure patients on the operating table using strong tape anteriorly, encircling the chest, thus minimizing the potential for sliding during maneuvers.

Port Placement and Docking

To facilitate robotic low anterior resection, a total of five ports are necessary, including camera and assistant ports. Figure 28.1 illustrates the placement of ports for three robotic arms, camera, and assistant ports. The port placement strategy involves an 8 mm port in the supraumbilical area using a Veress needle technique. An 8 mm port is situated in the left upper quadrant lateral to the umbilicus, 10 cm apart; two additional 8 mm ports are placed on the right lower quadrant. An assistant port is inserted on the right lateral side of the robotic ports, equidistant from the right upper or lower quadrant (Fig. 28.1).

After docking the da Vinci patient cart as described, the arms are arranged according to figure. A monopolar curved scissor (da Vinci® Surgical System, Intuitive Surgical, Sunnyvale, CA) is inserted through the port just right side of the camera port. A bipolar grasper (double fenestrated) (da Vinci® Surgical System, Intuitive Surgical, Sunnyvale, CA) is inserted through the port just left side of the camera port. A double fenestrated tip-up grasper (da Vinci® Surgical System, Intuitive Surgical, Sunnyvale, CA) is placed at the leftmost port. Typically, the

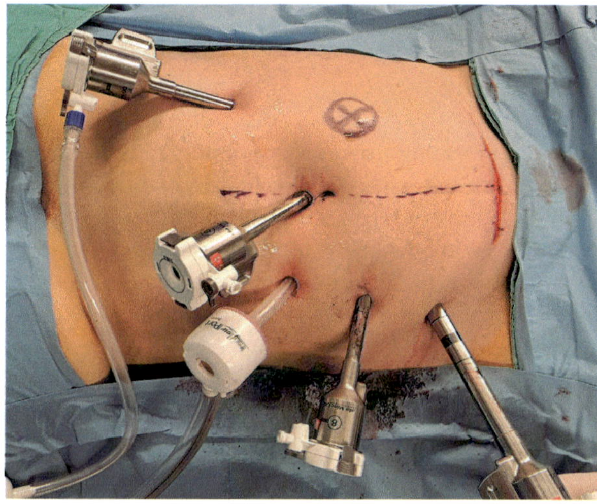

Fig. 28.1 Robotic low anterior resection port placement

assistant instrument consists of a laparoscopic bowel grasper or suction device. During the surgery, the port used for monopolar scissors is changed to 12 mm robotic trocar to insert robotic stapler for the transection of the bowel.

Technique

After establishing pneumoperitoneum, the camera is introduced, and additional trocars are placed under direct vision. The patient is repositioned in a right-side-down and slight Trendelenburg position to aid in displacing the small bowel and the cecum out of the pelvis. Subsequently, the robot is then docked. Initially, utilizing the robot, a medial-to-lateral mobilization of the left colon is carried out, representing our preferred approach. However, depending on the surgeon's comfort level, a lateral approach can also be employed. This flexibility allows for adaptation to individual surgeon preferences and patient-specific considerations during the procedure.

After the initial exposure, the peritoneum was incised at the sacral promontory level, and the aorta-mesenteric window was opened using monopolar scissors and bipolar forceps (Fig. 28.2). The inferior mesenteric artery (IMA) was then exposed and cleared at its origin from the aorta, ensuring preservation of the inferior mesenteric plexus (Fig. 28.3). Subsequently, the IMA was ligated with Hem-o-Lok clips and transected 1 cm away from the aorta (Fig. 28.4). Following the ligation of the IMA, autonomic nerves innervating the descending and sigmoid colon were meticulously dissected and cut separately using monopolar scissors set to level 2. This approach is adopted to prevent lateral thermal injury to the autonomic nerves that innervate pelvic organs.

In a medial-to-lateral fashion, the dissection was systematically extended to identify the inferior mesenteric vein (IMV). The IMV was isolated at the inferior border of the pancreas, ligated with Hem-o-Lok clips, and subsequently divided

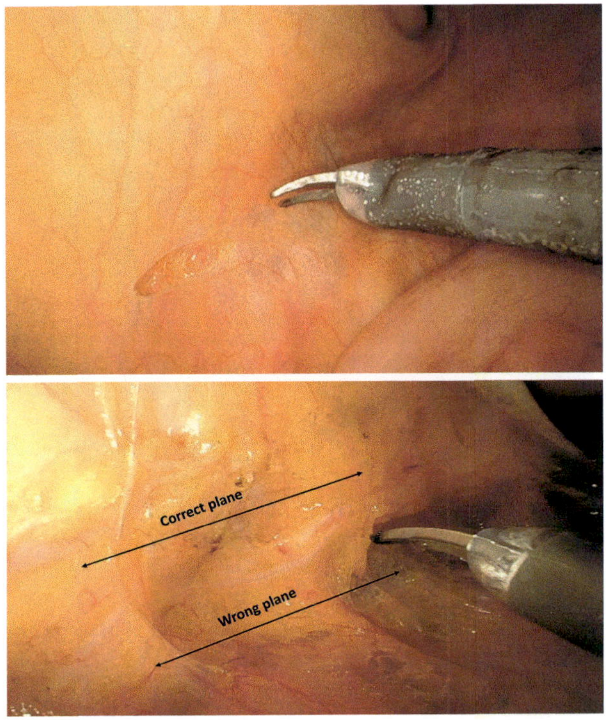

Fig. 28.2 Initial peritoneal incision and dissection of the aorta-mesenteric window

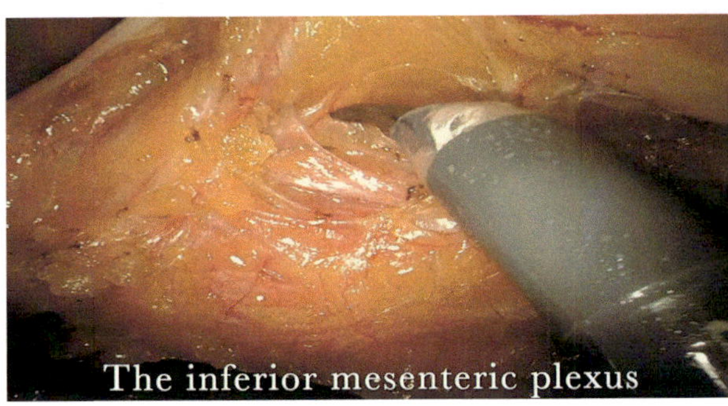

Fig. 28.3 Demonstration of the inferior mesenteric plexus

(Fig. 28.5). The dissection process continued along the embryological planes over Gerota's and Toldt's fasciae (Fig. 28.6), with careful preservation of the left ureter, gonadal vessels, and autonomic nerves (Fig. 28.7). During the medial dissection, the superior hypogastric plexus, left ureter, and gonadal vessels were exposed and deliberately preserved (Fig. 28.8). This approach ensures meticulous dissection while safeguarding critical anatomical structures, contributing to the overall success and safety of the procedure.

After completing the abdominal portion, attention was directed to the pelvis. Initially, the peritoneal reflection just below the sacral promontory was incised, and the rectum was mobilized posteriorly through sharp dissection in the "holy plane"

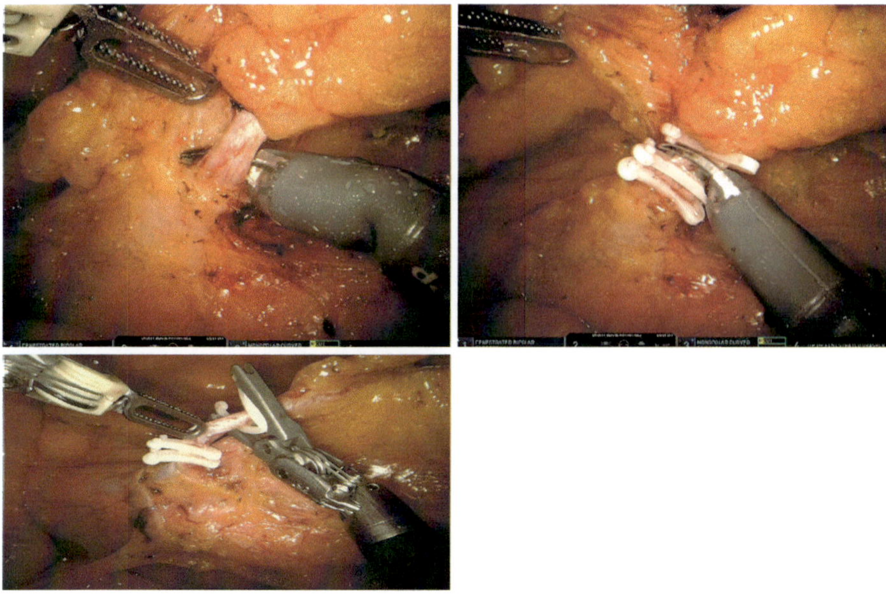

Fig. 28.4 Dissection and ligation of the inferior mesenteric artery

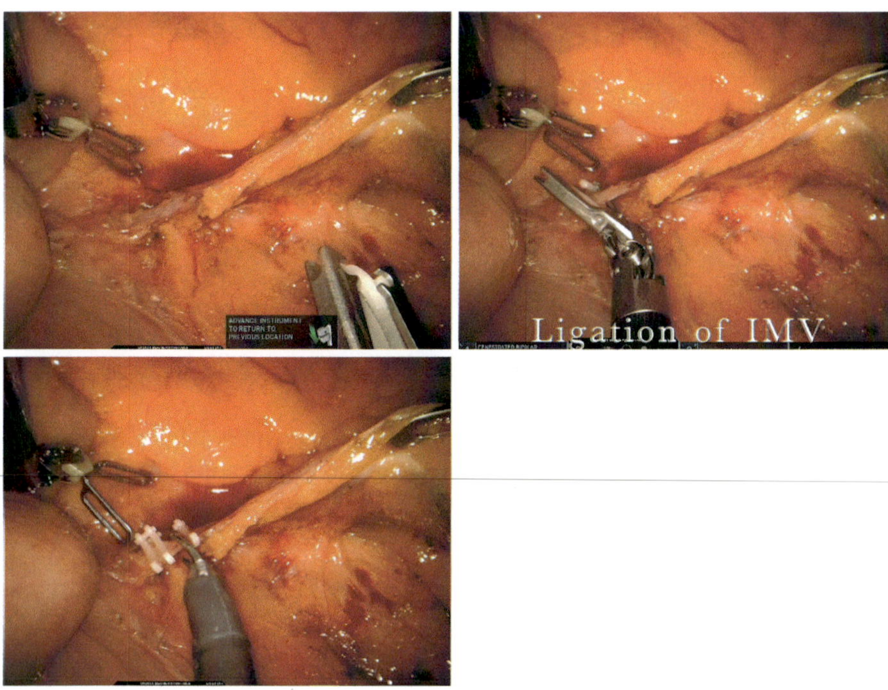

Fig. 28.5 Dissection and ligation of the inferior mesenteric vein

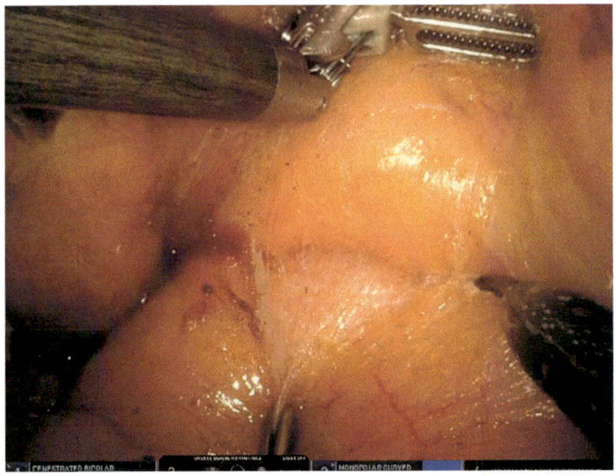

Fig. 28.6 Demonstration of the Toldt's line during medial to lateral dissection

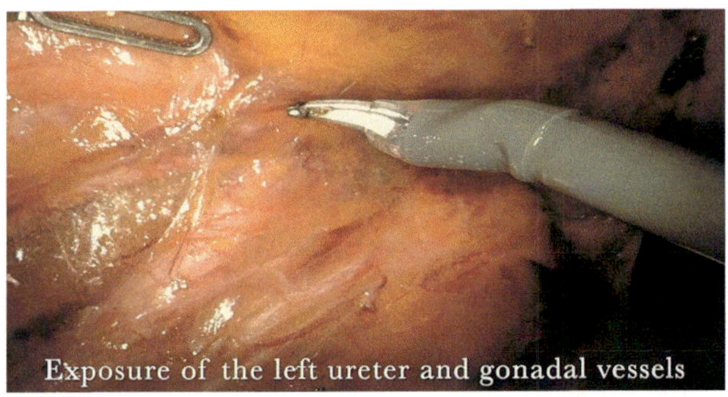

Fig. 28.7 Demonstration of the left ureter and gonadal vessels during medial to lateral dissection

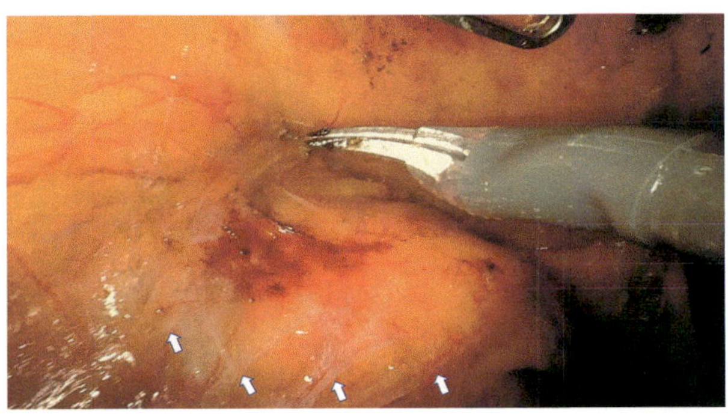

Fig. 28.8 Demonstration of the superior hypogastric plexus at the level of sacral promontorium

(Fig. 28.9). In a medial-to-lateral dissection, the right and left hypogastric nerves were sequentially identified at the level of the pelvic brim (Fig. 28.10). During the initial medial dissection at the sacral promontory level, there exists a risk of injuring the hypogastric nerves if working in the incorrect anatomical plane. The robot's magnification, stable traction, and vaporization from the monopolar scissors play

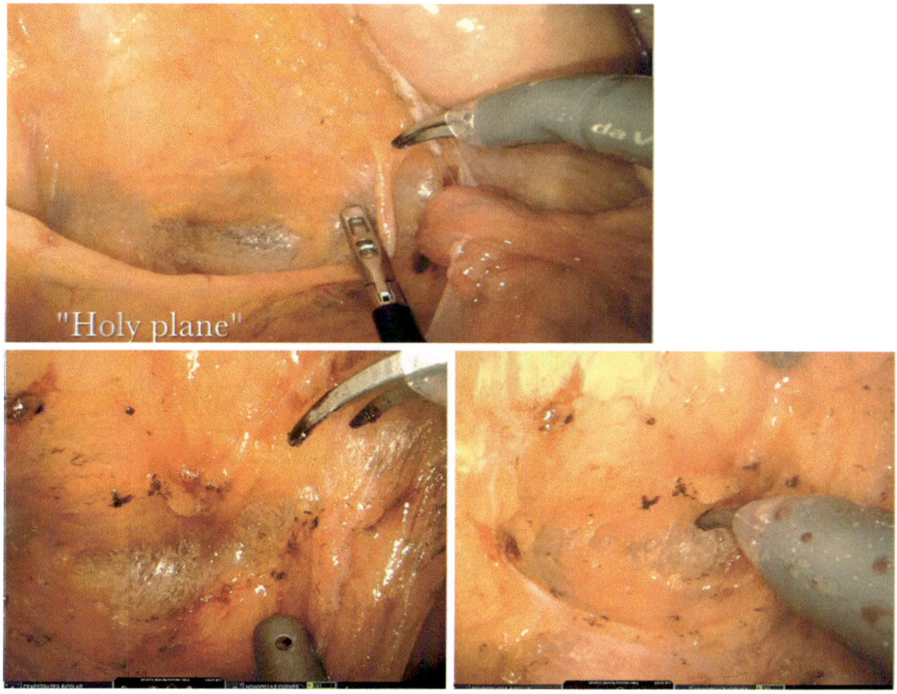

Fig. 28.9 Demonstration of the holy plane and posterior wall dissection

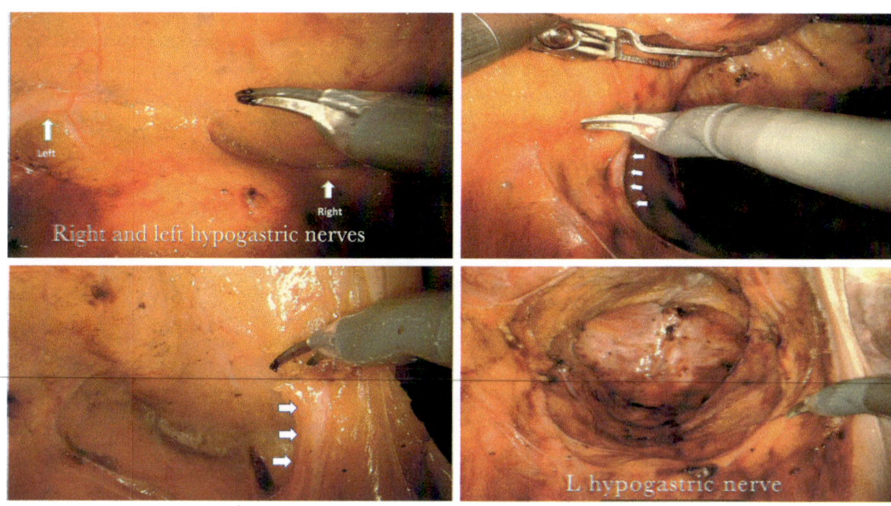

Fig. 28.10 Demonstration of the right and left hypogastric nerve

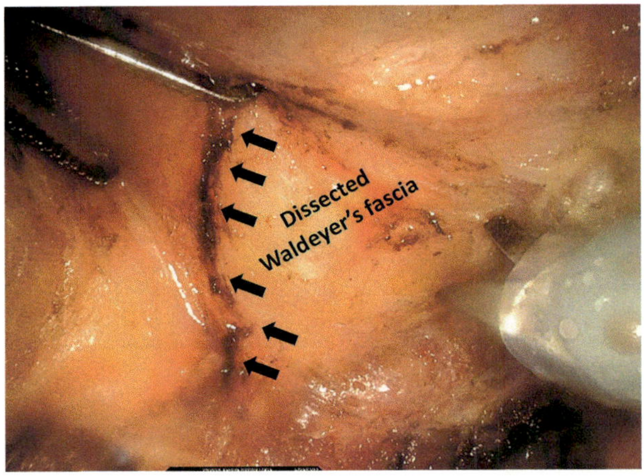

Fig. 28.11 Demonstration of the Waldeyer's fascia

crucial roles in identifying the correct plane and minimizing such risks. Posterior pelvic dissection is then performed along the fascia propria recti, exposing the holy plane at the level of the sacral promontory, which encompasses the loose areolar connective tissue between the rectal proper fascia and the prehypogastric nerve fascia (Fig. 28.11).

Dissecting the posterior mesorectum first provides the surgeon with better control over the mesorectum, facilitating subsequent lateral dissection. The right lateral side of the mesorectum was then mobilized, followed by the mobilization of the left side. Conducting posterior dissection all the way down to the pelvic floor and levator ani muscles is crucial for preventing injury to the inferior hypogastric plexus during lateral dissection (Fig. 28.11). Once adequate mobilization is achieved bilaterally, attention shifts to the anterior mesorectum. Anterior dissection commences by incising the anterior peritoneal reflection. The anterior dissection plane is exposed, and the dissection proceeds posteriorly to the seminal vesicle or the vagina. Stable traction with the third robotic arm facilitates more convenient and easier anterior dissection. The magnified robotic view enhances the surgeon's ability to determine the correct surgical plane. This systematic approach ensures precise dissection and minimizes the risk of complications during the procedure. If the tumor is located anteriorly, the dissection proceeds in front of Denonvilliers' fascia. Nerve fibers from the pelvic plexus traverse underneath the seminal vesicles to reach the bladder. In men, Denonvilliers' fascia is identified at the level of the seminal vesicle, located behind the seminal vesicles and in front of the rectum. Dissecting anterior to Denonvilliers' fascia poses a significant risk of nerve injury (Fig. 28.12). Conversely, if the tumor is posterior, the optimal dissection plane is posterior to Denonvilliers' fascia, ensuring a safe plane for nerve preservation. For continued dissection, an avascular plane can be created between the mesorectum and the neurovascular bundles to prevent injury. Excessive traction of the seminal vesicle to

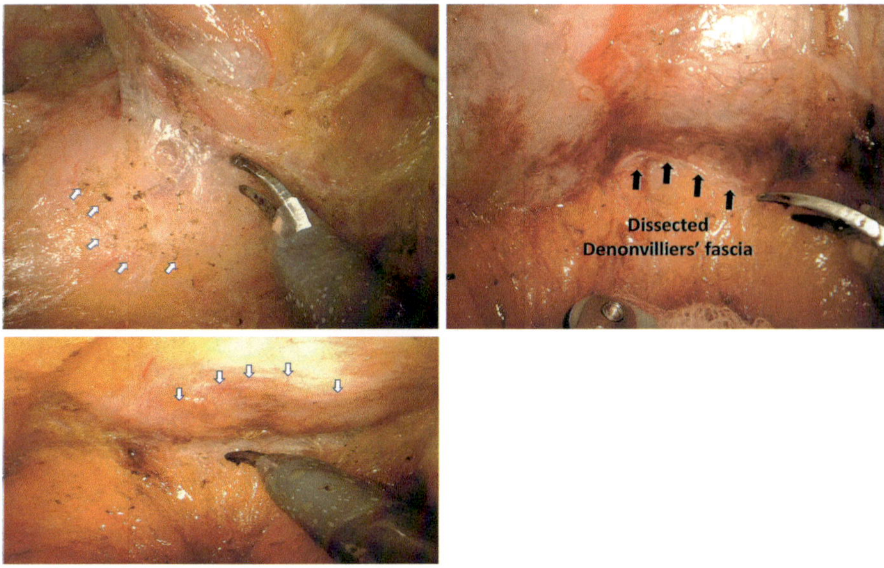

Fig. 28.12 Demonstration of the Denonvilliers' fascia

Fig. 28.13 Demonstration of the neurovascular bundle of the Walsh

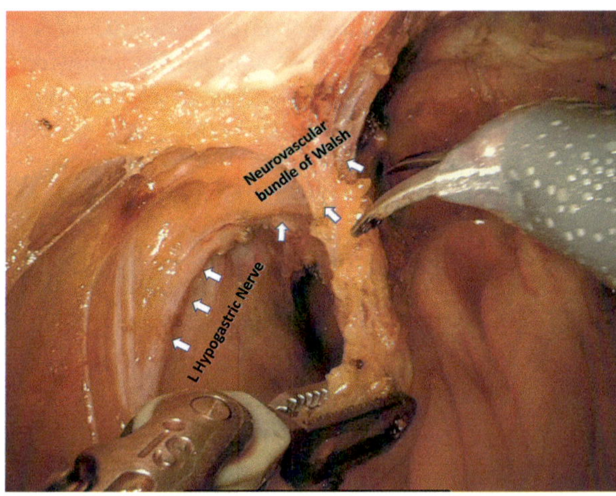

establish the operative field may result in nerve injury. Stable traction and the use of multi-angled instruments contribute to effective and safer dissection. The neurovascular bundles travel through the 2 o'clock and 10 o'clock directions, extending toward the genitalia (Fig. 28.13). A U-shaped incision in the anterior rectum may be employed to prevent nerve damage. The magnified robotic view enhances the clear identification and tracking of neurovascular bundles compared to laparoscopy or naked vision. Additionally, stable traction and countertraction help prevent excessive traction or avulsion damage to the nerves.

During posterior and lateral dissection, meticulous care is essential to preserve both the right and left hypogastric nerves and the inferior hypogastric plexus, respectively. The inferior hypogastric plexus is particularly susceptible to injury during posterolateral and anterolateral mesorectal dissection. The mesorectal dissection is then continued down to the pelvic floor. Upon completing the full mobilization of the mesorectum, a digital rectal examination is performed by the assistant surgeon to determine the appropriate level of rectal transection. A useful estimate of the transection level is achieved by placing the tip of a finger in the anus with the proximal interphalangeal joint at the level of the anal verge. The rectum is divided using a robotic stapler(s) with a green cartridge introduced through the 12 mm trocar. Once adequate mobilization is achieved, the rectum is transected with the robotic stapler. Subsequently, end-to-end colorectal anastomosis is accomplished, and a negative air leak test is conducted to ensure the integrity of the anastomosis.

Conclusion

The adoption of a fully robotic approach in pelvic rectal surgery aims to address technical challenges, offering improved ergonomics and facilitating the intricate task of preserving autonomic nerves within the confined space of the pelvis. By eliminating technical difficulties, which are a distinctive feature of the fully robotic approach, not only does it streamline the surgical process, but it also enhances the surgeon's ability to navigate the complexities of pelvic anatomy with precision. The superior ergonomics provided by robotic systems contribute to reducing physical strain on the surgeon, enabling sustained focus and dexterity throughout the procedure. Additionally, the advanced capabilities of robotic technology empower surgeons to navigate and preserve autonomic nerves in the inherently narrow confines of the pelvis, representing a significant advancement in optimizing outcomes and preserving functional aspects crucial for patient well-being. As surgical innovation continues to advance, ongoing scientific exploration is anticipated to yield further insights into the benefits of such progress. Despite inherent limitations related to cost and potential operative time, there is promise in robotic rectal surgery. There is optimism that ongoing learning and refinement in the field will effectively address these challenges.

State None.

Conflicts of Interest and Source of Funding The authors have no conflicts of interest including relevant financial interests, activities, relationships, and affiliations.

References

1. Jacobs M, Verdeja JC, Goldstein HS. Minimally invasive colon resection (laparoscopic colectomy). Surg Laparosc Endosc. 1991;1:144.
2. De Jesus JP, Valadão M, de Castro Araujo RO, Cesar D, Linhares E, Iglesias AC. The circumferential resection margins status: a comparison of robotic, laparoscopic and open total mesorectal excision for mid and low rectal cancer. Eur J Surg Oncol (EJSO). 2016;42(6):808–12.
3. Carlsen E, Schlichting E, Guldvog I, Johnson E, Heald RJ. Effect of the introduction of total mesorectal excision for the treatment of rectal cancer. Br J Surg. 1998; https://doi.org/10.1046/j.1365-2168.1998.00601.x.
4. Emile SH, Horesh N, Freund MR, Garoufalia Z, Gefen R, Silva-Alvarenga E, et al. Trends in the characteristics, treatment, and outcomes of rectal adenocarcinoma in the US from 2004 to 2019: a national cancer database analysis. JAMA Oncol. 2023;9(3):355–64.
5. Bosio RM, Pigazzi A. Emerging and evolving technology in Colon and Rectal Surgery. Clin Colon Rectal Surg. 2015;28(3):152–7.
6. Nezhat C, Vu M, Vang N, Chavali KS, Nezhat A. The journey from video laparoscopy to robotic and digital surgery. In: Robotic surgery; 2021. p. 3–10.
7. Giulianotti PC, Coratti A, Angelini M, Sbrana F, Cecconi S, Balestracci T, et al. Robotics in general surgery: personal experience in a large community hospital. Arch Surg. 2003;138(7):777–84.
8. Stevenson ARL, Solomon MJ, Lumley JW, Hewett P, Clouston AD, Gebski VJ, et al. Effect of laparoscopic-assisted resection vs open resection on pathological outcomes in rectal cancer: the ALaCaRT randomized clinical trial. JAMA. 2015;314(13):1356–63.
9. Bilgin IA, Bas M, Aytac E, Benlice C, Esen E, Kirbiyik E, et al. Operative and long-term oncological outcomes in patients undergoing robotic versus laparoscopic surgery for rectal cancer. Int J Med Robot Comput Assisted Surg. 2020;16(6):1–10.
10. Baek SJ, Kim SH, Cho JS, Shin JW, Kim J. Robotic versus conventional laparoscopic surgery for rectal cancer: a cost analysis from a single institute in Korea. World J Surg. 2012;36:2722–9.
11. Katsuno H, Hanai T, Masumori K, Koide Y, Ashida K, Matsuoka H, et al. Robotic surgery for rectal cancer: operative technique and review of the literature. J Anus Rectum Colon. 2020;4(1):14–24.
12. Huang YJ, Kang YN, Huang YM, Wu ATH, Wang W, Wei PL. Effects of laparoscopic vs robotic-assisted mesorectal excision for rectal cancer: an update systematic review and meta-analysis of randomized controlled trials. Asian J Surg. 2019;42(6):657–66.
13. Jayne D, Pigazzi A, Marshall H, Croft J, Corrigan N, Copeland J, et al. Effect of robotic-assisted vs conventional laparoscopic surgery on risk of conversion to open laparotomy among patients undergoing resection for rectal cancer: the ROLARR randomized clinical trial. JAMA. 2017;318(16):1569–80.
14. Kim MJ, Park SC, Park JW, Chang HJ, Kim DY, Nam BH, et al. Robot-assisted versus laparoscopic surgery for rectal cancer. Ann Surg. 2018;267(2):243–51.
15. Ackerman SJ, Daniel S, Baik R, Liu E, Mehendale S, Tackett S, et al. Comparison of complication and conversion rates between robotic-assisted and laparoscopic rectal resection for rectal cancer: which patients and providers could benefit most from robotic-assisted surgery? J Med Econ. 2018;21(3):254–61.
16. Zhang X, Wei Z, Bie M, Peng X, Chen C. Robot-assisted versus laparoscopic-assisted surgery for colorectal cancer: a meta-analysis. Surg Endosc. 2016;30:5601–14.
17. D'Annibale A, Pernazza G, Monsellato I, Pende V, Lucandri G, Mazzocchi P, et al. Total mesorectal excision: a comparison of oncological and functional outcomes between robotic and laparoscopic surgery for rectal cancer. Surg Endosc. 2013;27:1887–95.
18. Baek JH, McKenzie S, Garcia-Aguilar J, Pigazzi A. Oncologic outcomes of robotic-assisted total mesorectal excision for the treatment of rectal cancer. Ann Surg. 2010;251(5):882–6.
19. Sun Y, Xu H, Li Z, Han J, Song W, Wang J, et al. Robotic versus laparoscopic low anterior resection for rectal cancer: a meta-analysis. World J Surg Oncol. 2016;14:1–8.

20. Jimenez-Rodriguez RM, Flynn J, Patil S, Widmar M, Quezada-Diaz F, Lynn P, et al. Comparing outcomes of robotic versus open mesorectal excision for rectal cancer. BJS Open. 2021;5(6):zrab135.
21. Lim S, Nagai Y, Nozawa H, Kawai K, Sasaki K, Murono K, et al. Surgical outcomes of robotic, laparoscopic, and open low anterior resection after preoperative chemoradiotherapy for patients with advanced lower rectal cancer. Surg Today. 2023;53(1):109–15.
22. Yao Q, Sun QN, Ren J, Wang LH, Wang DR. Comparison of robotic-assisted versus conventional laparoscopic surgery for mid–low rectal cancer: a systematic review and meta-analysis. J Cancer Res Clin Oncol. 2023;149(16):15207–17.
23. Wee IJY, Kuo L, Ngu JC. Urological and sexual function after robotic and laparoscopic surgery for rectal cancer: a systematic review, meta-analysis and meta-regression. Int J Med Robot Comput Assisted Surg. 2021;17(1):1–8.
24. Gavriilidis P, Wheeler J, Spinelli A, de Angelis N, Simopoulos C, Di Saverio S. Robotic vs laparoscopic total mesorectal excision for rectal cancers: has a paradigm change occurred? A systematic review by updated meta-analysis. Color Dis. 2020;22(11):1506–17.
25. Feng Q, Yuan W, Li T, Tang B, Jia B, Zhou Y, et al. Robotic versus laparoscopic surgery for middle and low rectal cancer (REAL): short-term outcomes of a multicentre randomised controlled trial. Lancet Gastroenterol Hepatol. 2022;7(11):991–1004.
26. Hoshino N, Sakamoto T, Hida K, Sakai Y. Robotic versus laparoscopic surgery for rectal cancer: an overview of systematic reviews with quality assessment of current evidence. Surg Today. 2019;49:556–70.
27. Kim JC, Yu CS, Lim SB, Park IJ, Kim CW, Yoon YS. Comparative analysis focusing on surgical and early oncological outcomes of open, laparoscopy-assisted, and robot-assisted approaches in rectal cancer patients. Int J Color Dis. 2016;31:1179–87.
28. Fleshman J, Branda M, Sargent DJ, Boller AM, George V, Abbas M, et al. Effect of laparoscopic-assisted resection vs open resection of stage II or III rectal cancer on pathologic outcomes: the ACOSOG Z6051 randomized clinical trial. JAMA. 2015;314(13):1346–55.
29. Oshio H, Konta T, Oshima Y, Yunome G, Okazaki S, Kawamura I, et al. Learning curve of robotic rectal surgery using risk-adjusted cumulative summation: a 5-year institutional experience. Langenbeck's Arch Surg. 2023;408(1):89.
30. Jiménez-Rodríguez RM, Rubio-Dorado-Manzanares M, Díaz-Pavón JM, Reyes-Díaz ML, Vazquez-Monchul JM, Garcia-Cabrera AM, et al. Learning curve in robotic rectal cancer surgery: current state of affairs. Int J Color Dis. 2016;31:1807–15.
31. Aghayeva A, Baca B. Robotic sphincter saving rectal cancer surgery: a learning curve analysis. Int J Med Robot Comput Assisted Surg. 2020;16(4):e2112.
32. Burghgraef TA, Sikkenk DJ, Verheijen PM, El Moumni M, Hompes R, Consten ECJ. The learning curve of laparoscopic, robot-assisted and transanal total mesorectal excisions: a systematic review. Surg Endosc. 2022;36(9):6337–60.
33. Park EJ, Kim CW, Cho MS, Kim DW, Min BS, Baik SH, et al. Is the learning curve of robotic low anterior resection shorter than laparoscopic low anterior resection for rectal cancer?: a comparative analysis of clinicopathologic outcomes between robotic and laparoscopic surgeries. Medicine. 2014;93(25):e109.
34. Foo CC, Law WL. The learning curve of robotic-assisted low rectal resection of a novice rectal surgeon. World J Surg. 2016;40:456–62.
35. Kolehmainen CSJ, Ukkonen MT, Tomminen T, Helavirta IM, Laukkarinen JM, Hyöty M, et al. Short learning curve in transition from laparoscopic to robotic-assisted rectal cancer surgery: a prospective study from a Finnish Tertiary Referral Centre. J Robot Surg. 2023;17(5):2361–7.
36. Zaepfel S, Marcovei R, Fernandez-de-Sevilla E, Sourrouille I, Honore C, Gelli M, et al. Robotic-assisted surgery for mid and low rectal cancer: a long but safe learning curve. J Robot Surg. 2023;17:1–10.
37. Panteleimonitis S, Popeskou S, Aradaib M, Harper M, Ahmed J, Ahmad M, et al. Implementation of robotic rectal surgery training programme: importance of standardisation and structured training. Langenbeck's Arch Surg. 2018;403:749–60.

38. Younes MM, Larkins K, To G, Burke G, Heriot A, Warrier S, et al. What are clinically relevant performance metrics in robotic surgery? A systematic review of the literature. J Robot Surg. 2023;17(2):335–50.
39. Shu D, Cai Z, Yin X, Zheng M, Li J, Yang X, et al. Structured training curricula for robotic colorectal surgery in China: does laparoscopic experience affect training effects? J Gastrointest Oncol. 2023;14(1):198.
40. Luca F, Valvo M, Ghezzi TL, Zuccaro M, Cenciarelli S, Trovato C, et al. Impact of robotic surgery on sexual and urinary functions after fully robotic nerve-sparing total mesorectal excision for rectal cancer. Ann Surg. 2013;257(4):672–8.
41. Liu Y, Liu M, Lei Y, Zhang H, Xie J, Zhu S, et al. Evaluation of effect of robotic versus laparoscopic surgical technology on genitourinary function after total mesorectal excision for rectal cancer. Int J Surg. 2022;104:106800.
42. Panteleimonitis S, Ahmed J, Harper M, Parvaiz A. Critical analysis of the literature investigating urogenital function preservation following robotic rectal cancer surgery. World J Gastrointest Surg. 2016;8(11):744.
43. Luca F, Craigg DK, Senthil M, Selleck MJ, Babcock BD, Reeves ME, et al. Sexual and urinary outcomes in robotic rectal surgery: review of the literature and technical considerations. Updat Surg. 2018;70:415–21.

Part IV
Miscellaneous

29 Robotic Lateral Transabdominal Adrenalectomy

Felipe B. Maegawa, Justin Malek, and Snehal G. Patel

Introduction

Overall adrenalectomy is indicated for functional adrenal tumors, for proven or suspected malignancy of the adrenal gland, or for tumors larger than 4 cm [1]. As discussing the indications for adrenalectomy is beyond the scope of this chapter, please refer to the guidelines for adrenalectomy recently published by the American Association of Endocrine Surgeons for further details [1]. Although open adrenalectomy remains the standard surgical treatment for adrenocortical carcinoma, minimally invasive approaches are the mainstay therapy for most adrenal tumors [2, 3]. Laparoscopic adrenalectomy was first introduced in the early 1990s and it has been widely adopted, given its association with decreased postoperative pain, intraoperative blood loss, length of stay, and postoperative complications [3]. The robotic platform further elevates the benefits of laparoscopy by enhancing the surgeons' ergonomics, improved 3D visualization, and endowrist articulation. These enhanced features translate into decreased operative time, blood loss, conversion to open, and length of stay for robotic adrenalectomy when compared to laparoscopy [4, 5]. Therefore, we have switched to a robotic approach in our practice. Herein, we describe our routine technique for robotic lateral transabdominal adrenalectomy.

Supplementary Information The online version contains supplementary material available at https://doi.org/10.1007/978-3-031-86927-3_29.

F. B. Maegawa (✉) · J. Malek · S. G. Patel
Department of Surgery, Emory University School of Medicine, Atlanta, GA, USA
e-mail: felipe.antonio.boff.maegawa@emory.edu

S. Samreen et al. (eds.), *The SAGES Manual of Robotic Surgery*,
https://doi.org/10.1007/978-3-031-86927-3_29

Pertinent Anatomy

The adrenal glands are located in the retroperitoneum, and each gland weighs approximately 4 g. The glands have their own capsule; they are surrounded by perirenal fat and enclosed in the Gerota's fascia [6]. The right adrenal gland is in contact with the posterolateral aspect of the retro-hepatic vena cava, and it is surrounded by the right kidney inferolaterally, the bare area of the liver anterosuperiorly, and the diaphragm posteriorly. The left adrenal gland is located between the left kidney and the aorta and it is surrounded by the spleen and the tail of the pancreas anteriorly and the diaphragm posteriorly [6]. The adrenal gland arterial supply is similar and consistent for both sides. It arises from 3 main sources: The inferior phrenic artery gives rise to the superior adrenal artery, the middle adrenal artery branches off the aorta, and the inferior adrenal artery arises from the renal artery. The typical venous drainage of the adrenal glands is through a single vein. The right adrenal vein is quite short and drains directly into the inferior vena cava (IVC) posterolaterally. The left adrenal vein runs inferomedially to empty in the left renal vein after joining the inferior phrenic vein [7]. A large retrospective study of over 500 adrenalectomies revealed the intraoperative variations to the standard anatomy to be as high as 13% [8]. The variations included no main adrenal vein identifiable, additional small veins, two adrenal veins, more than two adrenal veins, and variant drainage to the IVC or to the right hepatic vein or to the inferior phrenic vein. Solid understanding of these anatomical landmarks and possible anatomical variations helps with the surgical dissection along the avascular planes around the adrenal gland, avoiding inadvertent injuries or intraoperative bleeding.

Patient Positioning

For both right and left robotic adrenalectomies, the patient is placed in a full lateral decubitus position with the lower ribs over the break of the bed. With the full lateral decubitus, gravity works as a passive retractor exposing the planes of dissection. The contralateral arm to the decubitus position is supported and secured on an arm board. An axillary roll and appropriate padding are placed. Attention is made to points of potential nerve compression injury and bone prominences. The bed is then flexed opening the space between the costal margin and the iliac crest. After that, the beanbag is connected to suction. Padding is revised and the patient is further secured with safety straps (Fig. 29.1).

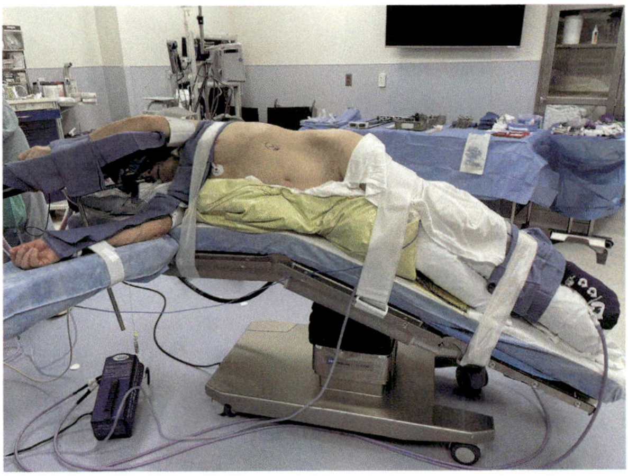

Fig. 29.1 Patient positioning in a 90° lateral decubitus on a beanbag. Adequate padding and safety straps are demonstrated

Robotic Docking and Instrumentation

Regardless of the side, we dock the robot at the patient's right side and deployment set up for the upper abdomen (Fig. 29.2). Once the robot is docked, the targeting feature is used aiming toward the adrenal gland. The instruments are placed under direct visualization. We routinely used the 30° scope, robotic scissors, the forced bipolar, medium-large Hem-O-Lok, vessel sealer, and tip-up grasper.

a

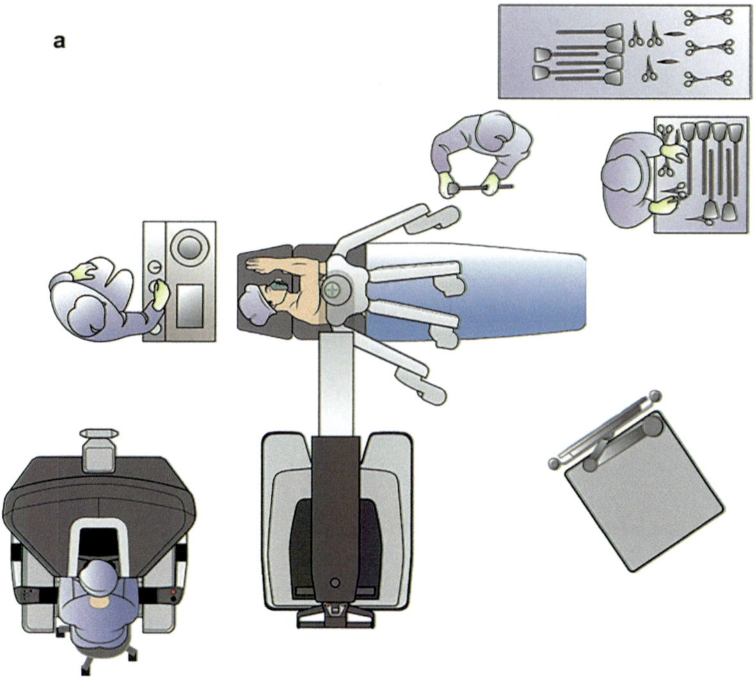

b

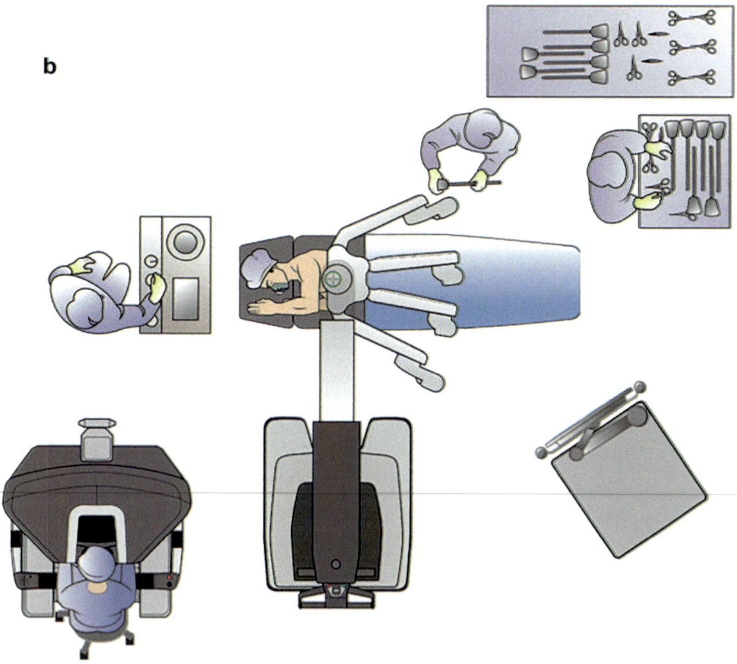

Fig. 29.2 Operating room layout depicting the robot docking and deployment for the right (**a**) and left (**b**) lateral transabdominal adrenalectomy

Right Adrenalectomy

Port Placement

Along with the patient's positioning, the port placement is one of the most critical portion of the operation. The peritoneal cavity is entered using a 5 mm optic view trocar on the right midclavicular line in the lower quadrant (Fig. 29.3a). This 5 mm trocar is left as an assistant port for suction or to be quickly upsized to a 12 mm trocar for placement of baby lap pads and compression, in case of a significant IVC bleeding requiring conversion to open. Once pneumoperitoneum of 15 mmHg is established, the most lateral 8 mm robotic trocar is introduced under direct visualization between the right posterior and midaxillary lines, approximately 1–2 cm from the costal ridge. After that, three other 8 mm robotic trocars are placed from lateral to medial, with at least 6 cm distance between each other, along the costal ridge toward the xyphoid process (Fig. 29.3a). The robotic instrument configuration from lateral to medial is as follows: forced bipolar, camera, scissors, and tip-up grasper (by the xyphoid process for liver retraction).

Technique

We follow the open book technique, which was previously described for laparoscopic adrenalectomy [6]. The first step is to divide the coronal ligament of the right lobe of the liver, allowing the mobilization of the liver anteromedially. This maneuver opens the book that is comprised of the bare surface of the liver on the right-hand page and the kidney and adrenal gland/tumor on the left-hand page. The tip-up grasper is utilized to retract the right lobe of the liver, exposing the IVC. Given how cephalad the right adrenal gland is located, rarely mobilization of the hepatic flexure of the colon or duodenum is required. Different than the laparoscopic technique, we develop the space between the IVC and adrenal gland from inferior to superior (Video 29.1). We perform this dissection layer by layer along the posterolateral

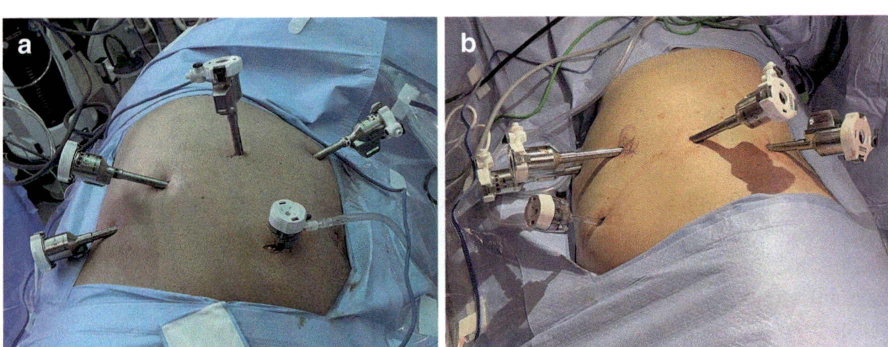

Fig. 29.3 Trocar placements for the robotic right (**a**) and left (**b**) adrenalectomies

aspect of the IVC. We found this technique to be safe, providing us a consistent identification and control of the right adrenal vein and its potential anatomical variations. Once the right adrenal vein is identified and isolated, it is controlled with a medium-large Hem-O-Lok toward the IVC and divided with the vessel sealer device (Video 29.1). After that, the inferolateral aspect of the adrenal gland is dissected and mobilized. The dissection is completed in a circumferential fashion. The arterial branches and retroperitoneal attachments are controlled with the vessel sealer device. Once the gland and tumor are completely free, they are removed from the peritoneal cavity with an extraction bag.

Left Adrenalectomy

Port Placement

The port placement mirrors the steps described for the right adrenalectomy. We enter the peritoneal cavity using a 5 mm optic view trocar on the left midclavicular line in the lower quadrant. Once the pneumoperitoneum is established, the most lateral 8 mm robotic trocar is introduced under direct visualization between the left posterior and midaxillary lines, followed by the remaining three other 8 mm robotic trocars from lateral to medial (Fig. 29.3b). We used the same robotic instruments as described for the right adrenalectomy. The robotic instrument configuration from lateral to medial is as follows: scissors, camera, forced bipolar, and tip-up grasper (by the xyphoid process for retraction of the spleen/pancreas).

Technique

Following the open book technique, the splenophrenic and splenorenal ligaments are divided, allowing the spleen to be mobilized anteromedially. Attention is made to avoid causing injury to the splenic capsule. As the spleen is mobilized medially, the gastric fundus and tail of the pancreas come into view. Careful dissection along the correct avascular plane is critical to avoid injury to the pancreas or splenic vessels. Once this dissection is complete, the right-hand page of the book is comprised by the adrenal gland and kidney, and the left-hand page by the spleen, tail of the pancreas, and gastric fundus (Video 29.2). Depending on the amount of peritoneal adipose tissue and size of the adrenal tumor, mobilization of the splenic flexure of the colon may be necessary, particularly if the inferior limb of the left adrenal gland extends to the renal hilum. The cleft of the book is developed from superior to inferior, toward the inferomedial aspect of the adrenal gland, where usually the adrenal vein is located. If the left phrenic vein is encountered at the medial aspect of the adrenal gland, it can help to identify the adrenal vein, as they join before entering the left renal vein. Once the left adrenal vein is identified, it is encircled and controlled with a medium-large Hem-O-Lok toward the renal vein and divided with the vessel sealer device (Video 29.2). Given the length of the left adrenal vein, usually the dissection and exposure of the renal vein is not necessary. The dissection is continued separating the adrenal gland from the superomedial aspect of the left kidney. Attention is made to avoid injury to a potential polar renal artery. The dissection is completed circumferentially dividing the retroperitoneal attachments and the adrenal arterial branches with vessel sealer device.

Postoperative Care

Patients are admitted for overnight observation with anticipated discharge home postoperative day 1. Diet is resumed the same day of the operation and early mobilization is resumed as for other minimally invasive operations. For pheochromocytoma patients, decision regarding admission to the intensive care unit is determined at the end of the case depending on the need of vasopressor support. Hemodynamically stable patients are admitted to the regular ward. Cushing's syndrome/disease patients receive perioperative steroids and steroid tapering the weeks following their surgery. For patients with preoperative diagnosis of hyperaldosteronism, the potassium supplement is stopped after surgery and serum potassium levels are checked on postoperative day 1 and a week after surgery. Antihypertensive medications are stopped or have their dose reduced depending on their blood pressure after the adrenalectomy.

Limitations

The main criticism to robotic adrenalectomy is the cost when compared to the laparoscopic approach. However, recent data from a large metanalysis and a randomized clinical trial revealed that robotic adrenalectomy is associated with a shorter operative time, reduced intraoperative blood loss, decreased conversion to open, and lower length of stay when compared to laparoscopy [4, 5]. These improved postoperative outcomes might offset some of the associated costs of the robotic approach. Therefore, high-quality cost-effectiveness studies in this subject are needed.

Competing Interests The authors have no competing financial or nonfinancial interests concerning the context of this book chapter.

Ethics Approval The authors followed the ethical standards for human participants as per the Declaration of Helsinki. Informed consents for the use of identifiable images were obtained.

References

1. Yip L, Duh QY, Wachtel H, et al. American Association of Endocrine Surgeons Guidelines for adrenalectomy: executive summary. JAMA Surg. 2022;157:870–7.
2. Giordano A, Feroci F, Podda M, et al. Minimally invasive versus open adrenalectomy for adrenocortical carcinoma: the keys surgical factors influencing the outcomes-a collective overview. Langenbeck's Arch Surg. 2023;408:256.

3. Madani A, Lee JA. Surgical approaches to the adrenal gland. Surg Clin North Am. 2019;99:773–91.
4. Gan L, Peng L, Li J, et al. Comparison of the effectiveness and safety of robotic-assisted and laparoscopic in adrenalectomy: a systematic review and meta-analysis. Int J Surg. 2022;105:106853.
5. Ma W, Mao Y, Zhuo R, et al. Surgical outcomes of a randomized controlled trial compared robotic versus laparoscopic adrenalectomy for pheochromocytoma. Eur J Surg Oncol. 2020;46:1843–7.
6. Yeh MW, Livhits M, Duh QY. Chapter 40: The adrenal glands. In: Sabiston textbook of surgery: the biological basis of modern surgical practice. St. Louis: Elsevier; 2021. p. 964–97.
7. Standring S. Gray's anatomy – the anatomical basis of clinical practice. 42th ed. Elsevier; 2021.
8. Scholten A, Cisco RM, Vriens MR, et al. Variant adrenal venous anatomy in 546 laparoscopic adrenalectomies. JAMA Surg. 2013;148:378–83.

30 Thyroid and Parathyroid Surgery

Micaela Piccoli, Alice Francescato, and Barbara Mullineris

Introduction

In recent years, multiple minimally invasive and remote access techniques for thyroid and parathyroid surgery have been developed to avoid anterior neck scars with good cosmetic results, without compromising surgical and oncological results [9].

The robotic platform combines the clinical advantages of a minimally invasive endoscopic approach with technical improvements such as full-HD three-dimensional with 10-time magnification of the surgical view, tremor elimination, motion scaling, precise articulated gesture, and comfort of the surgeon, which can enhance the safety and precision of the procedure. With the assistance of robotic system, identification and preservation of recurrent laryngeal nerves (RLNs) and parathyroid glands could be easier.

Three major remote access procedures have been described for thyroid surgery: transaxillary (TA), bilateral axillo-breast (BABA), and trans-oral (TO).

These different robotic accesses require long operative time and require a specific equipment, besides each procedure is related to different specific complications [10, 20].

For example, TA approach guarantees a clear and exposed surgical field with easier access to central lymph node dissection, but access to contralateral lobe is challenging and increases the risk of inadequate completeness in total thyroidectomy. A specific complication of this technique is the injury to the brachial plexus due to the hyperextension of the arm.

With the bilateral axillo-breast approach (BABA), it is possible to obtain a symmetrical view of both thyroid lobes and also a larger angle between the instruments

M. Piccoli (✉) · A. Francescato · B. Mullineris
Department of General, Emergency Surgery and New technologies, Baggiovara General Hospital, AOU Modena, Modena, Italy
e-mail: piccoli.micaela@aou.mo.it; francescato.alice@aou.mo.it; mullineris.barbara@aou.mo.it

S. Samreen et al. (eds.), *The SAGES Manual of Robotic Surgery*,
https://doi.org/10.1007/978-3-031-86927-3_30

to prevent robotic arms conflicts, thus facilitating the excision of large goiters and for total thyroidectomy, that though could require a further axillary incision for the extraction. Patients experienced transient sensory impairment due to postoperative adhesions.

Trans-oral (TO) approach could guarantee a real scarless approach with a completely invisible oral scar. With TO access, there is a good exposure of thyroid's lobes and central lymph node compartment, but flap elevation might be technically challenging. In TO access, it is also more difficult to control massive hemorrhage. Classic complications of this technique are mental nerve injury and postoperative infection due to oral environment.

Several different approaches to robotic thyroidectomy are described in literature; nevertheless, the ideal approach should be based on the patient and tumor characteristics and most importantly on the experience of the surgeon.

Our experience with robotic thyroidectomy started in 2010 tracing the experience of South Korean surgeons that firstly described the advantages of a gasless transaxillary access for the treatment of papillary thyroid cancer [8].

In this chapter, we describe our hybrid and swing technique for gasless unilateral transaxillary robotic thyroidectomy and parathyroidectomy with the use of the Da Vinci Xi System® (Intuitive Surgical, Inc., Sunnyvale), in combination with intraoperative nerve monitoring (IONM).

Indications and Contraindications

To date, robotic thyroidectomy isn't the gold standard technique; it is important to underline that robotic transaxillary thyroidectomy should be performed in high-volume centers with experience in both endocrine and robotic surgery [17].

Besides, according to international guidelines [5, 6, 11], robotic thyroidectomy and parathyroidectomy are reserved to highly selective nodules and patients.

Our indications for robotic remote access are benign nodules with a diameter inferior to 5 cm, little differentiated tumors and parathyroid adenomas superior to 3 cm.

Especially at the initial phase of learning curve, it is important to propose robotic transaxillary access to patients with benign nodule less than 4 cm and thin body habitus, without thyroiditis for the higher risk of hemorrhage.

Contraindications are large malignant nodules with enlarged lymph node involvement, large plunging goiters, patients with a pacemaker implant in the same side of the transaxillary unilateral access, and patients with history of neck surgery or radiotherapy. Relative contraindications are severe obesity, patients with thyroiditis and Graves' disease, or patients with previous surgery of the shoulder.

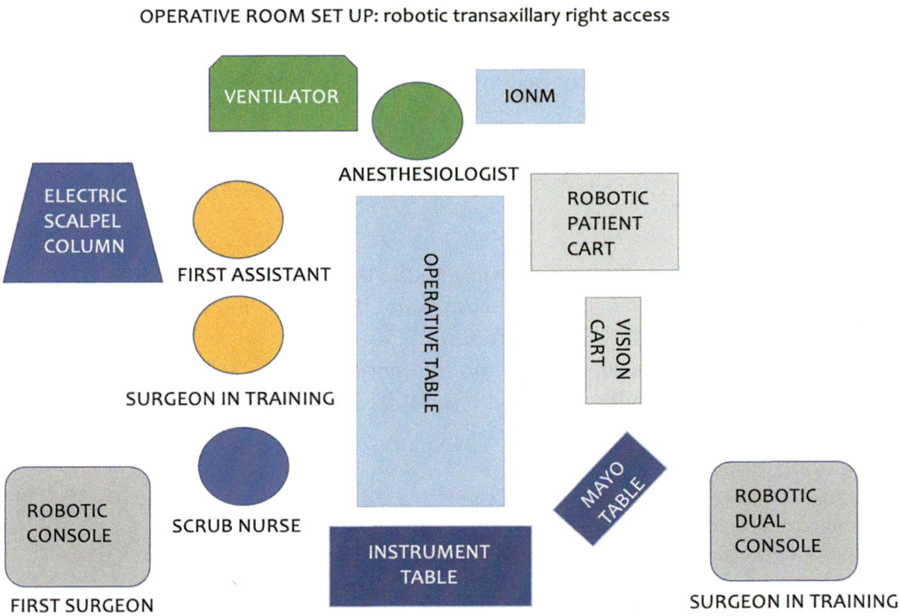

Fig. 30.1 Operative room setup for robotic transaxillary right access

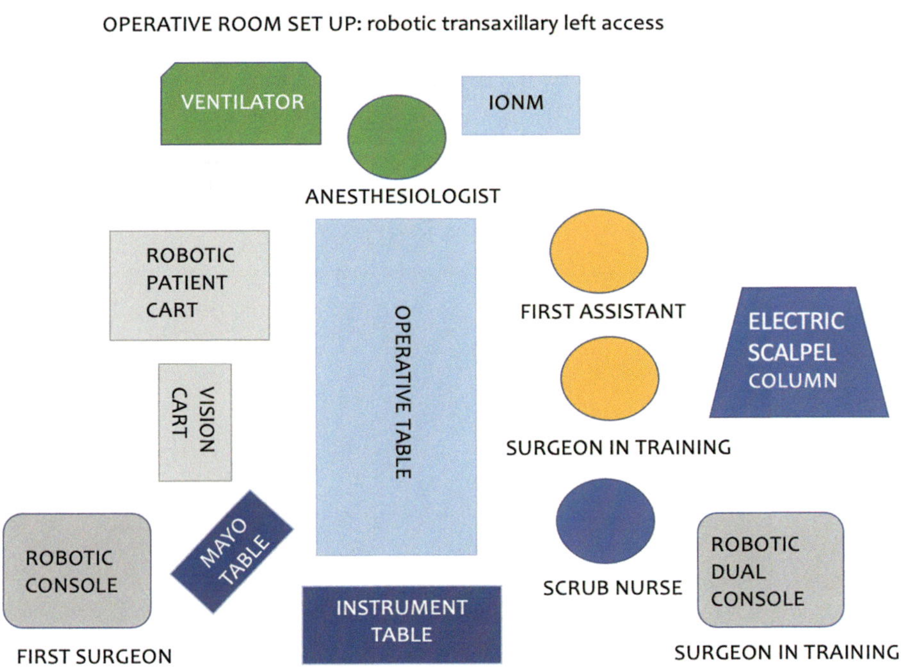

Fig. 30.2 Operative room setup for robotic transaxillary left access

Operative Room Setup

There is reported disposition of operative room setup for robotic transaxillary access for right and left access (Figs. 30.1 and 30.2).

Patient Position

Transaxillary access is chosen according to the target lesion or the lesion of largest dimension in case of total thyroidectomy for benign nodule, well-differentiated tumors, and target parathyroid adenomas.

Patient is placed in a supine position as reported in Fig. 30.3. To facilitate slight neck extension, a soft pillow under the shoulder is placed. The arm on the surgical

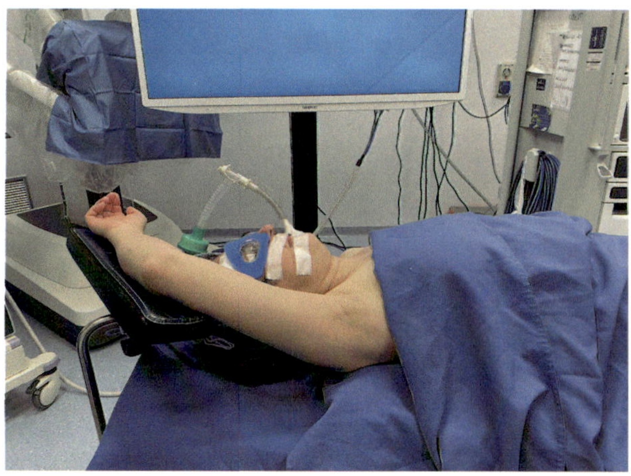

Fig. 30.3 Patient position for robotic transaxillary thyroidectomy right access

access side is raised upon the head with a 90° angle elbow abduction to minimize the distance between the axilla and the neck; arm position is checked while the patient is awake before undergoing general anesthesia to avoid wrong position, reducing the risk of consequent brachial plexus injury and postoperative shoulder discomfort. Another support is placed near the head to prevent any lateral movements during the procedures.

Surgical Procedure

The procedure is divided into three principal steps:

Step 1: Working space—A transaxillary subcutaneous tunnel is created with a laparoscopic view.
Step 2: Docking time—The robotic cart is positioned in the operative field and trocars are connected to the robotic arms.
Step 3: Console time—The planned operation is done by a surgeon sitting at the robotic console.

Step 1: Working Space

Following our experience of minimally invasive laparoscopic surgery, we have chosen the so-called "hybrid technique" for the tunnel's creation. The "hybrid technique" is a technique that uses the laparoscopic approach for the working space [1]

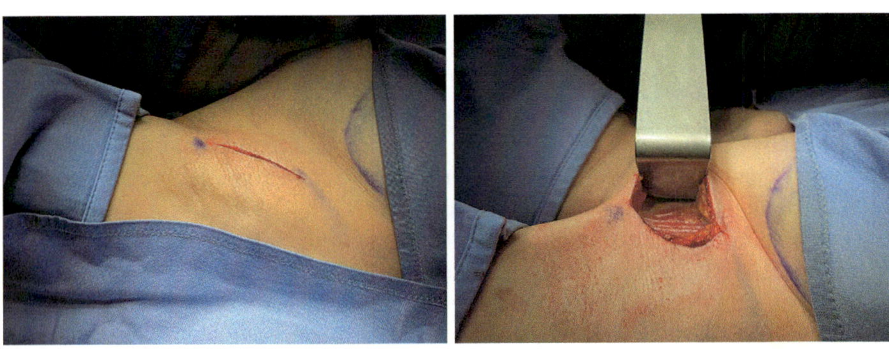

Fig. 30.4 Working space-incision and visualization of the MPM

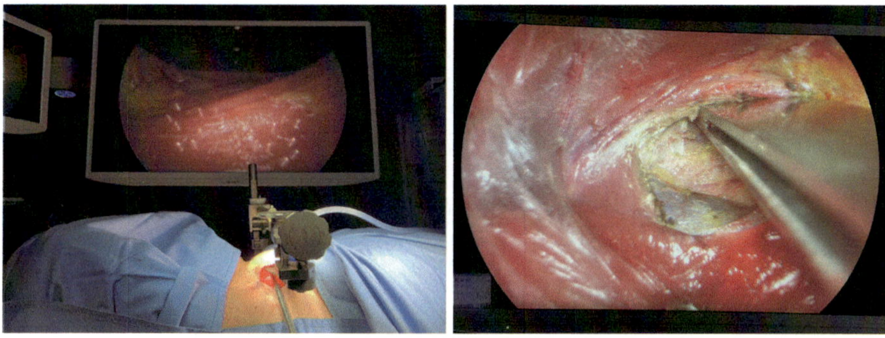

Fig. 30.5 Working space-SCM and up (Modena retractor) on the left; OHM and IGV on the right

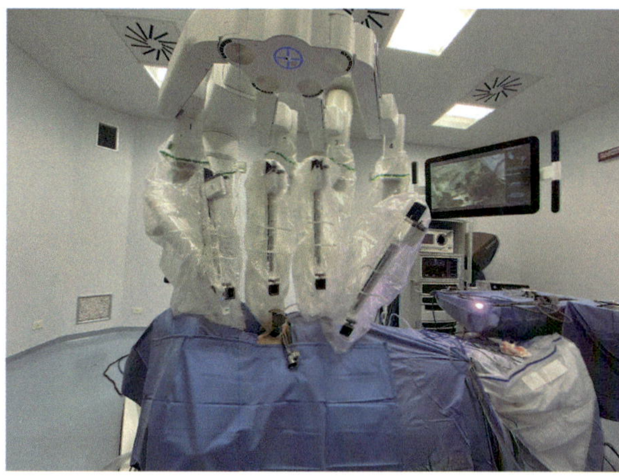

Fig. 30.6 Robot positioning and docking time in the right transaxillary access

and the robotic for the console time. With the laparoscopic approach, it is possible to minimize surgical trauma, making the surgical gesture more precise and also allowing all surgeons in the team to view the creation of the transaxillary tunnel and identify the anatomical landmarks, favoring the learning curve of these difficult step.

A 5 cm incision is performed in the axilla and a subplatysmal skin flap is created over the anterior surface of the major pectoralis muscle (MPM) till the anterior neck area (Fig. 30.4). Using laparoscopic hook and bipolar forceps, the sternocleidomastoideum muscle (SCM) is identified as the first landmark (Fig. 30.5), and then the sternal branch is lifted up with an external retractor, the so-called "Modena Retractor" (CEATEC® Medizintechnik) that is used from the beginning of flap dissection, to facilitate the suspension of skin flap and to reduce fogging. The superior anatomical landmark of the surgical field is represented by omohyoid muscle (OHM) (Fig. 30.5). The internal jugular vein (IGV) is dissected from the strap muscles. Finally, the Modena Retractor (CEATEC® Medizintechnik) is positioned beneath both the sternal branch of the SCM and the strap muscles and the thyroid is discovered. The contralateral strap muscles are identified and raised if a total thyroidectomy must be performed. During the flap creation, a conventional 30° laparoscopic high-definition camera and display system is used to magnify the image and make the surgical gesture more precise, reducing the risk of small hemorrhages.

Step 2: Robot Positioning and Docking Time

The Da Vinci Xi® robot is docked contralaterally to the axillary access (Fig. 30.6).

A four-arm procedure is illustrated [2]. It is possible to perform a three-arm procedure only if the learning curve is overcame (at least 20 robotic lobo-isthmusectomy have to be done), if the nodules diameter is less than 4 cm and if the target is a parathyroid gland.

Three robotic instruments are introduced into the axilla skin incision and one is inserted through an independent incision at the inferior part of the axilla incision.

If we consider the right approach as described in Fig. 30.6, port 1 is connected to Maryland forceps and port 2 holds the camera, port 3 a ProGrasp, and port 4 a Robotic Ultracision (Ethicon). During the console time, Maryland forceps, ProGrasp forceps, Robotic Ultracision, and 30° camera are all interchangeable (the swing technique).

Step 3: Console Time

The senior surgeon sits at the console and a junior surgeon sits at the operating table as assistant. All vessel dissections are performed using the Ultracision device. The middle thyroid vein is identified and dissected. The upper pole of the thyroid is drawn downward and medially using Maryland forceps or ProGrasp. The superior thyroid vessels are identified and divided close to the thyroid gland to avoid any injury of the external branch of the superior laryngeal nerve. The inferior thyroid

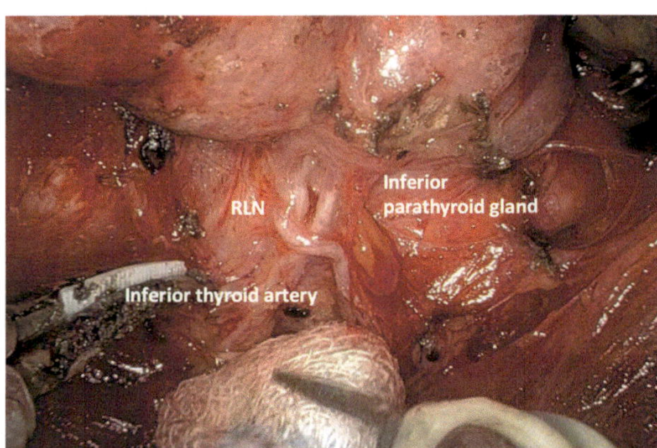

Fig. 30.7 Console time: correct identification of RLN, inferior thyroid artery, and parathyroid glands

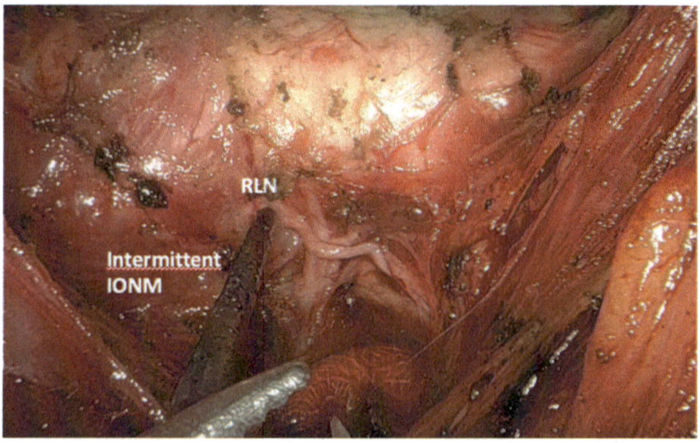

Fig. 30.8 Console time: correct identification of RLN and intermittent IONM

artery (ITA), the recurrent laryngeal nerve (RLN), and the parathyroid glands are identified (Fig. 30.7). The ITA is then divided close to the thyroid gland, and the whole cervical course of the RLN is traced and preserved. Correct identification and motility of the RLN is achieved with intermittent intraoperative nerve monitoring (IONM) (Fig. 30.8).

The thyroid lobe is dissected from the trachea and resected with the isthmus. The resected specimen is extracted through the axillary skin incision.

In case of total thyroidectomy, it will be performed using the same method with medial traction of the trachea and the thyroid. The identification of contralateral RLN is the challenging steps of this procedure because it is necessary to go beyond the trachea. The upper pole is the first step, with the dissection of the vessel direct to superior lobe with Ultracision device; afterwards, it is time to identify the RLN with the so-called "swing technique." During this procedure, a reusable handmade laparoscopic suction device is used to get a soft traction on the trachea in order to obtain a better vision of the RLN. With Da Vinci Xi® System that has 8 mm port, each instrument can be interchangeable, so the camera moves from arm 2 to arm 3 and to arm 4 to follow the correct path of the nerve and then can return to arm 2 at the end of the procedure. With this "swing technique," it is possible to dissect the inferior lobe following the whole cervical course of the RLN especially into the contralateral thyroid lodge. The dissection results are more precise and surgical completeness is achieved with direct and frontal vision of the trachea. The correct function of the contralateral RLN is checked with intermittent IONM. The contralateral thyroid lobe is then resected and extracted through the axillary skin incision.

In case of parathyroidectomy, the 30° camera is introduced in port 2. The thyroid gland is turned medially with a ProGrasp introduced in port 3. The middle thyroid vein is identified and dissected with Ultracision device in port 1. The parathyroid adenoma is then identified, dissected, and excised with the aid of Maryland forceps in port 4. The inferior thyroid artery (ITA) and the recurrent laryngeal nerve (RLN) are previously identified. The IONM is used.

After dissection steps, the venous bleeding is checked with the Valsalva maneuver. A closed suction drain is inserted through the separate incision under the axillary skin incision. The robotic arms are de-docked and the wound is cosmetically closed.

Discussion

During the last decade, there was an increasing incidence of thyroid carcinoma, and it represents the most common endocrine malignancy [16]. Different robotic remote access techniques for thyroidectomy have been described with the purpose to avoid a non-cosmetic anterior neck scar and also to overcome some limitations related to minimally invasive endoscopic procedure. In particular for robotic transaxillary gasless approach, several studies confirm feasibility and safety [17, 18], reporting a level 2a of evidence and a better cosmetic result when compared with open thyroidectomy [16].

Robotic transaxillary approach was widely used in East and Asian countries, and for long time, there has been a debate on its application in the Western population [3] because of difference in anthropometric characteristics, larger size of goiter, and also for elevated costs.

The operating time is undoubtedly increased if compared to the conventional technique, (working space and docking time). However, some authors have reported that the body mass index (BMI) does not influence the operating time; therefore, higher body mass index (overweight and obese patients) cannot be considered an exclusion criteria for the robotic transaxillary approach. Furthermore, overweight and obesity do not increase postoperative complication risk of flap hematoma, wound seroma, neck and chest paresthesia, and also shoulder discomfort, specific complications of transaxillary approach [7, 17, 18]. Operative time instead was found to be decreasing as the surgeon acquired experience [7].

Some controversies regarding surgical completeness and oncological safety have slowed the spread of the technique, but nowadays, several studies demonstrate comparable surgical completeness with open approach in malignant thyroid disease ([9, 12, 14, 16]).

Robotic transaxillary thyroidectomy allows compartment lymphectomy with good results in terms of lymph nodes sampling [9, 16]. In fact, our approach with Da Vinci Xi System, hybrid technique, and especially swing technique can enhance lymph nodes retrieval, RNL motility preservation, and parathyroids' functionality.

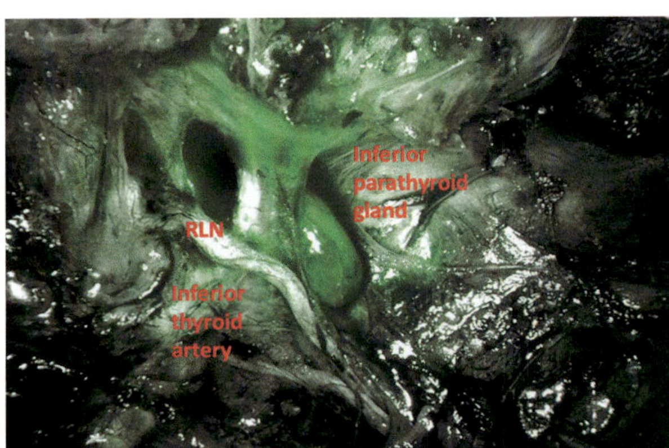

Fig. 30.9 Console time: intraoperative use of ICG for easier identification of parathyroid glands supply

Parathyroids identification is also facilitated with the application of intraoperative indocyanine green (ICG) [13]. Parathyroid surgery requires careful dissection to preserve blood supply to the gland and to reduce the risk of postoperative transient hypoparathyroidism. The intraoperative injection of ICG permits easier identification of vascular supply to the glands and also permits to test their perfusion after thyroid dissection (Fig. 30.9).

Recent systematic review also confirms safety and feasibility of robotic parathyroidectomy especially in patients diagnosed with primary hyperparathyroidism and preoperative localized parathyroid adenoma [15].

Regarding postoperative complications, several studies and meta-analysis confirm that remote access to thyroid glands is not inferior to cervical thyroidectomy with regard to length of hospital stay, transient RLN injury, permanent RLN injury, transient hypocalcemia, and permanent hypocalcemia [4, 19].

In conclusion, robotic transaxillary thyroidectomy and parathyroidectomy are safe and feasible in selected patients and nodules in high-volume center with experience in both robotic and endocrine surgery. The application of hybrid and swing technique, intraoperative nerve monitoring and ICG, could enhance the correct identification and preservation of RLNs and parathyroids.

References

1. Al Kadah B, Piccoli M, Mullineris B, et al. Modifications of transaxillary approach in endoscopic da Vinci-assisted thyroid and parathyroid gland surgery. J Robot Surg. 2015;9:37–44. https://doi.org/10.1007/s11701-014-0486-8.
2. Boggi U, Bianchi PP, Milone M, Troisi RI. Principi di tecnica in chirurgia robotica. Piccin; 2023.
3. Bonati E, Mullineris B, Del Rio P, et al. Mini-invasive video-assisted thyroidectomy vs robot-assisted transaxillary thryoidectomy: analysis and comparison of safety and outcomes. Updat Surg. 2024;76:573. https://doi.org/10.1007/s13304-023-01732-z.
4. De Vries LH, Aykan D, Lodewijk L, et al. Outcomes of minimally invasive thyroid surgery—a systematic review and meta-analysis. Front Endocrinol. 2021;12:719397. https://doi.org/10.3389/fendo.2021.719397.
5. Del Rio P, Polistena A, Chiofalo MG, et al. Management of surgical diseases of thyroid gland indications of the United Italian Society of Endocrine Surgery (SIUEC). Updat Surg. 2023;75:1393–417. https://doi.org/10.1007/s13304-023-01522-7.
6. Haugen BR, Alexander EK, Bible KC, et al. 2015 American Thyroid Association Management Guidelines for Adult Patients with Thyroid Nodules and Differentiated Thyroid Cancer: The American Thyroid Association Guidelines Task Force on Thyroid Nodules and Differentiated Thyroid Cancer. Thyroid. 2016;26:1–133. https://doi.org/10.1089/thy.2015.0020.
7. Kandil E, Akkera M, Shalaby H, et al. A single surgeon's 10-year experience in remote-access thyroid and parathyroid surgery. Am Surg. 2021;87:638–44. https://doi.org/10.1177/0003134820950300.
8. Kang S-W, Jeong JJ, Yun J-S, et al. Robot-assisted endoscopic surgery for thyroid cancer: experience with the first 100 patients. Surg Endosc. 2009;23:2399–406. https://doi.org/10.1007/s00464-009-0366-x.
9. Kang YJ, Stybayeva G, Hwang SH. Surgical completeness and safety of minimally invasive thyroidectomy in patients with thyroid cancer: a network meta-analysis. Surgery. 2023;173:1381. https://doi.org/10.1016/j.surg.2023.02.021.

10. Lee J, Kim S, Hoon; Hong, Hua. Comparison of various thyroidectomy approaches: a retrospective cross-sectional study. Surg Laparosc Endosc Percutan Tech. 2023;33(6):632–9. https://doi.org/10.1097/SLE.0000000000001243.
11. Marciniak C, Bihain F, Caiazzo R, Brunaud L. Robotic thyroidectomy. Recommendations of the AFCE (Association francophone de chirurgie endocrinienne) with the SFE (Société française d'endocrinologie) and the SFMN (Société française de médecine nucléaire). J Visc Surg. 2023;160:S127–9. https://doi.org/10.1016/j.jviscsurg.2023.04.006.
12. Matteucci V, Fregoli L, Papini P, et al. Comparison of surgical completeness in patients operated on conventional open total thyroidectomy (OT) or trans-axillary robot-assisted total thyroidectomy (RATT) by a single axillary approach. Updat Surg. 2023;75:1267. https://doi.org/10.1007/s13304-023-01510-x.
13. Pace-Asciak P, Russell J, Solorzano C, et al. The utility of parathyroid autofluorescence as an adjunct in thyroid and parathyroid surgery 2023. Head Neck. 2023;45:3157–67. https://doi.org/10.1002/hed.27538.
14. Papini P, De Palma A, Ginesini M, et al. Robot-assisted transaxillary surgery for thyroid cancer: Oncologic and surgical outcomes in long term follow-up. Robot Comput Surg. 2023:e2563. https://doi.org/10.1002/rcs.2563.
15. Paspala A, Spartalis E, Nastos C, et al. Robotic-assisted parathyroidectomy and short-term outcomes: a systematic review of the literature. J Robot Surg. 2020;14:821–7. https://doi.org/10.1007/s11701-020-01119-x.
16. Pavlidis ET, Psarras KK, Symeonidis NG, et al. Robot-assisted thyroidectomy versus open thyroidectomy in the treatment of well differentiated thyroid carcinoma. JSLS. 2021;25:e2021.00032. https://doi.org/10.4293/JSLS.2021.00032.
17. Piccoli M, Mullineris B, Gozzo D, et al. Evolution strategies in transaxillary robotic thyroidectomy: considerations on the First 449 cases performed. J Laparoendosc Adv Surg Tech. 2019;29:433–40. https://doi.org/10.1089/lap.2019.0021.
18. Piccoli M, Mullineris B, Santi D, Gozzo D. Advances in robotic transaxillary thyroidectomy in Europe. Curr Surg Rep. 2017;5:17. https://doi.org/10.1007/s40137-017-0180-7.
19. Xing Z, Qiu Y, Abuduwaili M, et al. Surgical outcomes of different approaches in robotic assisted thyroidectomy for thyroid cancer: a systematic review and Bayesian network meta-analysis. Int J Surg. 2021;89:105941. https://doi.org/10.1016/j.ijsu.2021.105941.
20. Yuan Y, Pan B, Tang E, et al. Surgical methods of total thyroidectomy for differentiated thyroid cancer: a systematic review and Bayesian network meta-analysis. Int J Surg. 2023;110:529. https://doi.org/10.1097/JS9.0000000000000819.

31 Robotic Pulmonary Lobectomy

Andrei I. Gritsiuta, Abbas E. Abbas, and Roman V. Petrov

Introduction to Robotic Lobectomy

Lung cancer remains the leading cause of cancer-related mortality in the United States, with over 56,000 lung cancer resection surgeries performed annually nationwide [47]. Following years of minimal progress, the combination of early detection and advancements in treatment over the past 10–15 years, along with better access to these treatments, has resulted in improved survival rates for lung cancer patients. However, despite these recent advances, the overall 5-year relative survival rate is still a concerning 23% [26]. In 2024, there are approximately 235,000 new cases of lung cancer expected, and the disease is projected to cause 125,000 deaths [54].

Anatomic lung resections remain the cornerstone of curative treatment for lung cancer, whether performed alone or as part of a multimodal approach. The first successful anatomic lung resection, a pneumonectomy for lung cancer, was performed by Evarts Graham in 1933, setting a precedent for the surgical approach [19]. The choice of anatomical unit to be resected—whether it be a segment, a lobe, or an entire lung—depends on multiple tumor and patient factors, including lesion location, size, histology, pulmonary function, comorbidities, and the performance status

A. I. Gritsiuta
Department of Surgery, University of Pittsburgh Medical Center, Pittsburgh, PA, USA
e-mail: gritsiutaai@upmc.edu

A. E. Abbas
Department of Thoracic Oncology, Warren Alpert School of Medicine at Brown University, Providence, RI, USA
e-mail: abbas_abbas@brown.edu

R. V. Petrov (✉)
Department of Cardiothoracic Surgery, John Sealy School of Medicine at University of Texas Medical Branch, Galveston, TX, USA
e-mail: rvpetrov@utmb.edu

S. Samreen et al. (eds.), *The SAGES Manual of Robotic Surgery*,
https://doi.org/10.1007/978-3-031-86927-3_31

of the individual. Safe surgical techniques require meticulous precision in dissecting hilar bronchovascular structures. Traditionally, this has been achieved through a thoracotomy, a large open incision, involving a division of extrathoracic muscles with rib spreading to allow adequate surgical exposure and effective bimanual dissection. However, this approach is associated with increased level of acute and chronic pain and impaired respiratory function, leading to increased rates of postoperative morbidity, especially pulmonary complications such as atelectasis and pneumonia. Therefore, thoracic surgeons have sought less invasive alternatives to traditional open procedures.

The first breakthrough in the field was the introduction of the video-assisted thoracoscopic surgery (VATS) technique in the 1990s [34]. VATS allows for lobectomies to be performed through small incisions using a video thoracoscope and modified instruments, significantly reducing patient morbidity and recovery time, compared to the traditional open thoracotomy. However, VATS lobectomy technique differs significantly from the thoracotomy approach. Due to ergonomic limitations and the transition of the viewing angle in VATS to a more anterior rather than superior position, all dissection of the hilum is performed in an anterior to posterior manner, leaving the division of the fissure for last. Posterior dissection, which is sometimes necessary, is particularly challenging with the VATS approach. Transition from an open technique to VATS requires significant changes in surgical strategies and a complete new set of skills. Surgeons face multiple challenges with the adoption of the new VATS technique, including impaired precision due to the distance and the use of, inflexible, "straight stick" instruments. The counterintuitive fulcrum motion of the instruments, fixated at the port site in the chest wall, and the antiparallel convergent optic position in the multiport approach further complicate the procedure. Even more challenges arise in the uniportal configuration, where the limited working area leads to space conflicts. These challenges extend the learning curve and impair adoption of the technique for lower-volume surgical centers. This has translated into relatively stagnant rates of VATS adoption for oncologic lung resections in thoracic surgery.

In contrast, robotic-assisted thoracic surgery (RATS) offers numerous advantages over traditional VATS approach, including three-dimensional (3D) binocular visualization, field magnification, scaled motion, tremor filtration, and wristed instruments with increased freedom of motion, thereby enhancing surgical field visualization, depth perception, and precise dissection. These advantages facilitate a smoother transition to minimally invasive robotic lung resections, allowing surgeons to more easily replicate traditional surgical techniques in the new environment. Unsurprisingly, robotic portal resection has been likened by some surgeons to a "virtual thoracotomy." This technique offers surgeons the visual illusion of viewing the lung through an open chest while allowing for natural bimanual wristed maneuvers to address the anatomy effectively [2]. Early clinical experiences reporting on safety and feasibility outcomes have generated significant interest in the robotic approach. Currently, the platform is widely accepted for providing all the benefits of a minimally invasive approach without the technical difficulties associated with VATS. However, it also raises questions regarding the learning curve, costs, and perioperative outcomes. Reports suggest that proficiency in robotic lobectomies can be achieved after 20 procedures, whereas VATS lobectomy proficiency ranges from 50 procedures for the multiportal approach to 140 for uniportal thoracic surgery [27]. As such, robotic technology may facilitate the expansion of minimally invasive lobectomies to surgeons who have not adopted traditional VATS techniques, making it more accessible to a broader cohort of surgeons and patients alike.

First robotic lobectomies were documented by Melfi et al., Morgan et al., and Ashton et al. as far back as 2002 and 2003, focusing initially on patients with early-stage lung cancer [3, 35, 36]. These pioneering procedures demonstrated the feasibility and potential benefits of robotic technology in thoracic surgery. Since then, robotic systems have significantly evolved. Early RATS closely mirrored the techniques used in VATS, with initial port placement strategies developed using nowadays obsolete da Vinci S/Si platforms. However, introduction of more versatile da Vinci Xi robot in 2016 further revolutionized port mapping strategy and the field of pulmonary lobectomy.

Despite growing popularity of robotic surgery among thoracic surgeons worldwide, ongoing debate regarding the optimal technique for lung resections remains unsettled. The four-arm, look-up-view method with low robotic ports placement in the seventh to ninth intercostal spaces provides a view of the intrathoracic cranial side from the caudal position and is currently the mainstream approach globally [43]. This method has evolved to incorporate adaptations such as utilizing fewer ports or skin incisions. Conversely, new approaches have emerged that align the patient's intrathoracic craniocaudal axis with the horizontal direction of the surgeon's console monitor. One notable innovation is the horizontal open thoracotomy view, or horizontal view approach [49]. These advancements reflect the continuous evolution and optimization of port placements in RATS, driven by technological progress and the refinement of surgical techniques.

Robotic technology evolution has also affected the stapling technology. A propensity score matching analysis of robotic lobectomies, identified in the Premier hospital database, compared perioperative outcomes, healthcare resource utilization, and costs between robotic and handheld staplers [63]. The analysis demonstrated that robotic staplers were associated with significantly lower risks of perioperative bleeding, conversion, possible air leaks, and overall complications without an increase in total costs of the procedure. Additionally, the robotic platform significantly facilitates teaching and training. A dual console enables two surgeons to operate together, allowing for seamless transfer of instrument control between an expert and a trainee as needed. Utilizing telestration, the faculty surgeon can guide the trainee through increasingly complex tasks while maintaining complete visual oversight and control of the procedure. Furthermore, surgical simulators have been developed to enhance trainees' proficiency with implementation of this advanced technology.

While robotic surgery provides numerous advantages, it also has certain limitations. The high initial capital costs represent a significant financial investment, rendering it inaccessible to many surgeons and patients in smaller communities, especially globally, in developing countries. A systematic review and meta-analysis indicated an increased cost of robotic lobectomies per patient: $16,645 compared to $13,310 for VATS [20]. This cost difference was largely attributed to the expense of robotic equipment, with no statistically significant differences in complication rates. Although some studies have demonstrated equivalence between RATS and VATS in terms of outcomes, most indicate that the overall direct cost of robotic lobectomy is higher by approximately $3000 to $5000 per procedure [42, 48, 55, 58]. When both direct and indirect costs are considered, the robotic procedure remains more expensive than VATS; however, both are less costly than an open thoracic procedure [37, 40]. Nonetheless, robotic surgery may become economically feasible and profitable in high-volume settings with distribution of the robotic capital costs. In an analysis of costs between RATS and VATS lobectomies across all hospitals, the robotic approach was found to be more expensive when hospital volume was not considered. This cost difference was primarily attributable to operating room and supply costs. However, for hospitals performing more than 25 annual lobectomies, there was no significant difference in total costs between these approaches [39]. A recent study indicated that positive net margins and profitability were achieved in robotic general thoracic surgical cases compared to other robotic surgery service lines and open thoracic procedures [1]. These financial benefits were largely due to managing variable costs associated with the length of stay. This finding was corroborated by another cost analysis comparing RATS and VATS [12]. In this analysis, total direct costs, including direct supply expenses, were not significantly different between two minimally invasive techniques ($6621 versus $6483; $P = 0.784$). On the other hand, median total operating costs and total unit support costs, both closely tied to length of stay, were lower in the RATS group. In a study involving 697 patients who underwent pulmonary lobectomy, an analysis utilizing propensity score adjustment by inverse probability of treatment weighting (IPTW), found that both RATS and VATS lobectomy demonstrated similar costs and enhanced clinical effectiveness compared to the open thoracotomy approach [24]. The IPTW-adjusted direct costs showed no significant differences between the groups (robotic $17,223 versus VATS $17,260 versus thoracotomy $18,075, $P = 0.48$). Furthermore, there were no significant differences in indirect costs or overall hospital charges among the three approaches. Conversely, robotic surgery for simple outpatient procedures may not be cost-effective at present [53]. Additionally, the setup time for robotic systems can be longer than other approaches. Surgeons also lose the palpable feedback during lung assessment, which is essential in lung resections, at least with previous generation robotic platforms. Moreover, the lack of haptic feedback means that surgeons do not receive tactile sensations that help them gauge tissue resistance and texture. However, the introduction of the new-generation surgical robot, Intuitive DV5, addresses some of these concerns. These considerations must be carefully evaluated when determining the most suitable surgical approach for each patient. Overall, the expected benefits of machine-surgeon interactions still need to be proven superior to challenges such as cost, operating room management complexity, and the difficulty of changing established surgical practices.

Current Evidence

Over the past two decades, numerous studies have supported the adoption of robotic lobectomy by demonstrating its safety, efficacy, and feasibility. Analysis of RATS and VATS outcomes has largely shown similar results. Both techniques are associated with overall improved surgical outcomes, particularly decreased blood loss, reduced postoperative pain, reduced chest tube durations and hospital stay, and overall fewer complications compared to an open lobectomy [7, 14, 23]. This was confirmed by analysis of the Premier hospital database, which evaluated 23,779 elective lobectomies from 2011 to 2015 [42]. The findings demonstrated a lower postoperative complication rate, shorter hospital stays, and decreased mortality in the RATS group. Additionally, patients in the robotic lobectomy group were more likely to be discharged home rather than to a transitional care facility. During this period, the authors noted an approximately threefold increase in the adoption of robotic techniques. When comparing RATS to VATS, the robotic group demonstrated a lower conversion rate to thoracotomy, a lower overall postoperative complication rate, and a shorter hospital stay. The postoperative mortality rates for RATS and VATS were similar, and there was no significant difference in iatrogenic injuries. Another study conducted on 33,095 cases of lobectomies and segmentectomies from 2008 to 2010 compared RATS with VATS [21]. The results indicated that RATS had lower mortality rates (0.2% versus 1.1%), shorter hospital stays (5.9 days versus 6.3 days), and fewer complications (43.8% versus 45.3%). However, these differences did not reach statistical significance, potentially due to the underpowered robotic group (only 430 patients in the RATS group versus 12,427 patients in the VATS group). Other studies demonstrated a higher number of lymph nodes harvested, improved postoperative and 30-day complication rates, and significantly lower incidence of conversion to an open surgery in the robotic group compared to VATS [29, 48]. Conversion rates from minimally invasive to open lobectomy were specifically examined using data from The Society of Thoracic Surgeons General Thoracic Surgery Database [52]. Analyzing 27,695 minimally invasive lobectomies, authors found that the conversion rate was higher in the VATS group (11%) compared to the RATS group (6%; $P < 0.001$). Anatomical challenges were identified as the primary reason for conversion in both the RATS and VATS groups, indicating that the robotic platform may offer enhanced ability of managing complex anatomical scenarios. However, it was noted that emergency conversions due to bleeding were significantly more frequent in the RATS group, often necessitating intraoperative blood transfusions. This finding suggests that surgeons might be more inclined to undertake complex cases with the robotic technology, potentially avoiding early conversion to thoracotomy. Despite these adverse outcomes, the data imply that surgeons may feel safer and more confident in pursuing a minimally invasive approach when utilizing the robotic platform.

Most studies, including systematic reviews and meta-analyses, suggest there is no difference in outcomes between the two techniques [13, 62]. A comprehensive meta-analysis of 145 studies encompassing 369,793 patients revealed no significant differences in terms of adverse events, the number of lymph nodes dissected, lymph node stations evaluated, or nodal upstaging between RATS and VATS [38]. However, when considering the cost of the procedure, RATS lobectomy proved to be more expensive. Another meta-analysis of 14 studies including a total of 7438 patients confirmed these results demonstrating comparable outcomes in terms of mortality rates, blood loss, operative time, ICU stay, chest tube duration, length of hospital stay, and complication profiles [30] although the study showed benefits of robotic lobectomy in terms of shorter duration of narcotic use and quicker time to return to regular activities. Similar findings were observed in a retrospective case-control analysis, which highlighted that patients in the RATS group required less narcotic analgesia and were able to resume normal activities sooner compared to those undergoing VATS [31].

In a comprehensive retrospective multicenter study examining Clavien-Dindo grade III or higher events in 1264 patients, an overall major complication rate of 4.3% was observed [5]. Pneumonia was the most common major complication, occurring in 1.2% of patients, followed by prolonged air leak, which occurred in 0.9% of patients. The overall mortality rate was 0.6%, with a 30-day mortality rate of 15% for those who developed major complications. Factors increasing the risk of major complications included male gender, lower FEV1 and DLCO, neoadjuvant therapy, and extended resections. Notably, the stage of the disease was not a significant risk factor for complications, although 74.1% of the patients were in clinical stage I. Naturally, the robotic approach has been shown to be beneficial for such a challenging surgical population as octogenarians, offering improved outcomes, including shorter hospital stays, fewer postoperative complications, and higher rates of discharge to home, compared to open thoracotomy according to a retrospective cohort study [50]. Cerfolio et al. highlighted the reliable performance of this platform in sublobar resections based on their initial experience with the first 100 planned robotic anatomic segmentectomies [6, 9, 10]. In this study, 79% of patients underwent curative lung cancer surgery using a fully robotic four-arm approach, achieving R0 resection with a median of 19 lymph nodes dissected. There were no conversions to open surgery, although 7% of the cases required an intraoperative conversion to lobectomy due to inadequate margins or difficulties with nodule localization.

As more surgeons receive training in robotic techniques and technology continues to advance, the rate of robotic lobectomies is expected to increase. This trend promises to offer patients a minimally invasive option that is likely to result in improved overall outcomes for surgical resections of lung cancer.

Surgical Technique

The authors previously described their preferred technique of the robotic lobectomy [46]. The procedure is performed using a completely portal-based, four-arm approach with a 10 mm Hg capnothorax. All ports are strategically placed in the eighth intercostal space along the midclavicular, anterior axillary, posterior axillary, and scapular lines, irrespective of the laterality or type of lobectomy being

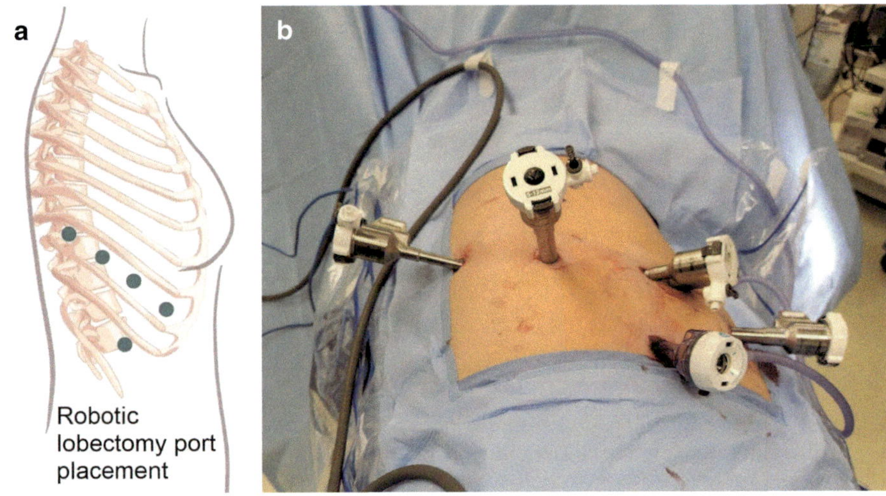

Fig. 31.1 Robotic port placement strategy. (**a**) Schematic depiction of the Xi robotic port placement for lobectomy. (**b**) Intraoperative image of the lobectomy ports

performed (Fig. 31.1a). Notably, a utility incision is not utilized in this technique (Fig. 31.1b). All assistance is provided through a 15 mm assistant port, advanced through a subcostal position in the projection of the tenth intercostal space. This port is utilized for specimen extraction (lymph nodes and pulmonary parenchyma at the end of the procedure), the delivery of various supplies and disposables (such as vessel loops and rolled gauze "cigars"), and clearing of the surgical field with a suction instrument. Authors avoid using assistant-controlled handheld staplers, exclusively relying on robotic technology controlled by the console surgeon. The benefits of the portal-based approach include the creation of a tension capnothorax, which results in an enlarged working space due to the contralateral shift of the mediastinum and downward displacement of the diaphragm with expansion of the intercostal spaces. In addition, this improves lung atelectasis and facilitates pneumodissection of the hilar planes, thereby enhancing the visualization and identification of anatomical structures.

For the standard pulmonary resection, we adopted a "minimalist" lean philosophy, popularized by R. Cerfolio [6, 9, 10]. We have eliminated the use of beanbags, axillary rolls, arm boards, epidurals, central lines, urinary catheters, and arterial lines (Fig. 31.2a). Following the induction of general anesthesia, lung isolation is achieved either with a bronchial blocker or a double-lumen tube (Fig. 31.3a, b). We have a strong preference for using a bronchial blocker for intraoperative lung isolation (Fig. 31.3b). The bronchial blocker's smaller profile allows for safer and easier airway dissection, facilitates pre- and post-procedure bronchoscopy by simply removing the blocker, and eliminates the need for potentially risky endotracheal tube exchanges when the patient requires prolonged intubation postoperatively [25]. We revert to using a double-lumen tube in cases of carinal resection, bilateral procedures, or instances of porcine bronchial anatomical variants during right-sided resections (Fig. 31.3a, c, and d). In the broader thoracic surgery community, there is

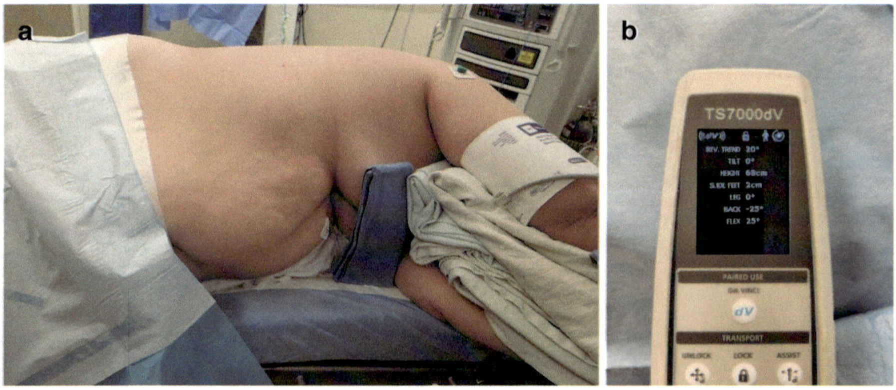

Fig. 31.2 Patient positioning. (**a**) Patient position on the OR table. Please note absence of bean-bag, axillary roll, and arm board. Gel rolls positioned along the chest and back, providing chest elevation and brachial plexus protection. Arms are secured on the blankets in swimmers' position (135° upward). (**b**) Bed control positions during robotic lung lobectomy

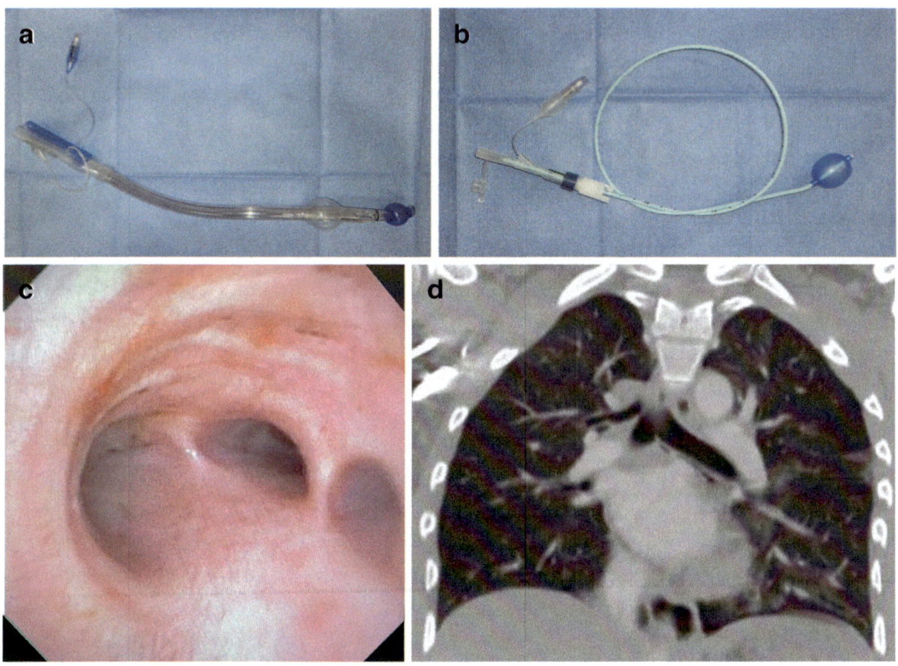

Fig. 31.3 Lung isolation strategy and limitation in anatomical variants. (**a**) Left-sided double-lumen endotracheal tube. (**b**) Fuji Uniblocker bronchial blocker device. (**c**) Porcine bronchus. Bronchoscopy view. Please note separate takeoff of the RUL bronchus from distal trachea, above RMSB. (**d**) CT image of the coronal reconstruction of the porcine bronchus anatomical variant

a reluctance toward the use of bronchial blockers due to perceived difficulties in their management. However, the use of the Fuji Uniblocker (Fuji Systems Corporation, Tokyo, Japan) mitigates the majority of these challenges due to the angled nature of its tip, which facilitates easier placement in the desired location compared to the more elaborate process required for Arndt blocker placement (Cook Medical, Bloomington, Indiana, USA). Additionally, the Rusch double EZ-blocker (Teleflex Medical, Morrisville, North Carolina, USA) further decreases the challenges associated with lung isolation, although the authors have limited experience with its use.

The patient is positioned on the contralateral side and secured on two medium gel rolls, which are placed along the chest and back (Fig. 31.2a). The bed is flexed at a point between the lower ribs and the iliac wing. The bed is then transitioned to a 20° reverse Trendelenburg position with a −25° back down position, resulting in approximately 155° flexion (Fig. 31.2b). The patient's arms are secured over folded blankets in a swimmer's position, angled at 135° toward the head. The patient is further secured with two straps of 3-inch tape applied directly to the skin without a towel, and a restraining belt is used for additional security. A lower body forced air warming blanket is also positioned to maintain the patient's body temperature (Fig. 31.2a).

Due to the rotational capability of the Xi and DV5 surgical platforms (Intuitive Surgical, Sunnyvale, California, USA), the patient cart can be positioned on either side of the patient. The authors prefer docking the robot from the back, as this facilitates better access for the bedside assistant to the chest. However, the robot's position remains unchanged regardless of the laterality of the procedure, as robot relocation significantly extends the turnover time between cases.

The first 8 mm camera port is placed at the anterior axillary line. To ensure safe initial air entry and avoid injury to the raised diaphragm due to lung isolation, a Kelly surgical clamp is inserted first. This is followed by the initiation of a 10 mm Hg capnothorax, resulting in visible downward displacement of the diaphragm. Subsequently, a 12 mm robotic port is inserted at the midclavicular and posterior axillary line locations. Finally, an 8 mm port is placed at the scapular line, along with the assistant port. Upon docking the robot, a 30° camera is placed in the anterior axillary port. Bipolar Maryland forceps are inserted into the midclavicular port, Fenestrated Bipolar Forceps into the posterior axillary line port, and a Tip-Up Fenestrated Grasper into the scapular port. These instruments are used for the hilar dissection. Robotic staplers are employed for all stapling applications, with the majority of the stapling performed through the midclavicular port. Occasionally, especially during right middle lobectomy procedures, the use of the stapler through the posterior axillary port can be advantageous. With the recent introduction of an 8 mm robotic stapler, 12 mm posterior axillary port may be replaced with a standard 8 mm port.

Once the initial inspection of the pleural cavity is performed and the decision to proceed with lobectomy is confirmed, the procedure begins with the inferior and posterior dissection of the hilum, regardless of the type of lobectomy. Bipolar energy is utilized for dissection and safe tissue division. Using the posterior arm as a static retractor, the lung is retracted cranially, and the inferior pulmonary ligament is divided up to the level of the inferior pulmonary vein (Fig. 31.4a). This maneuver

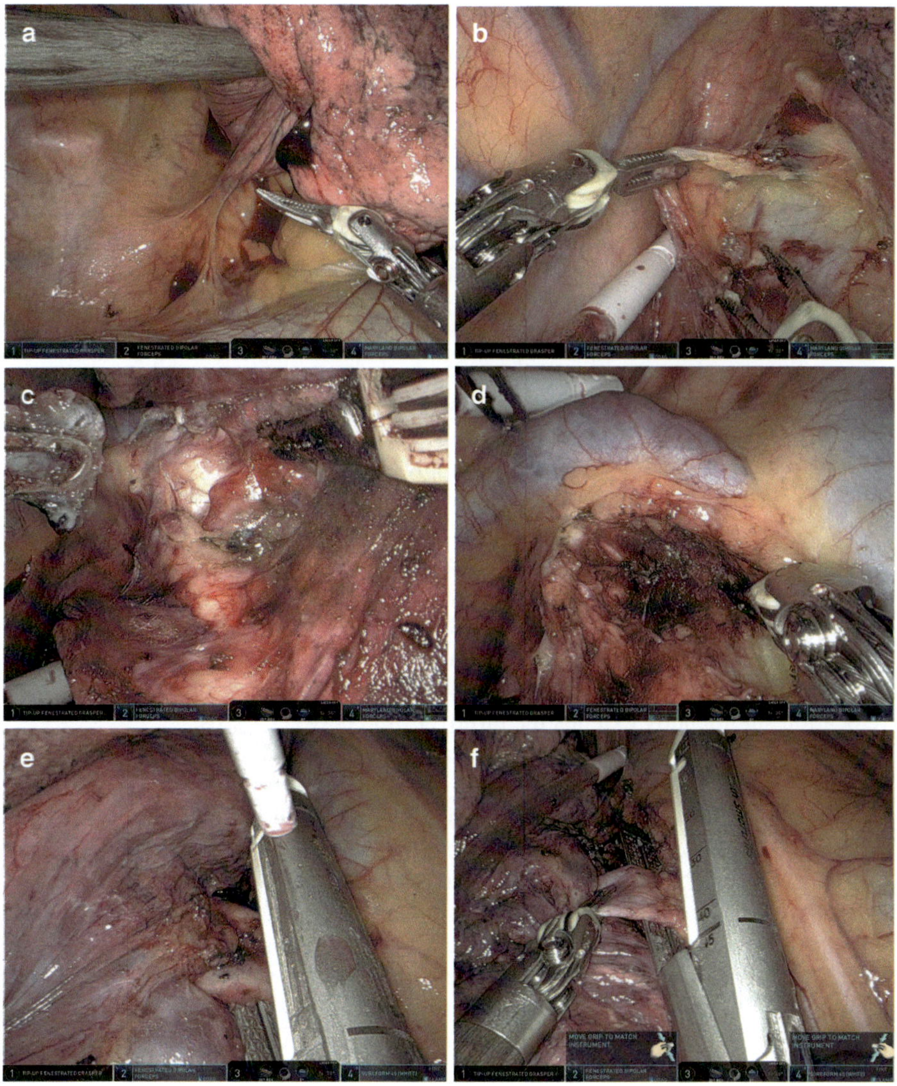

Fig. 31.4 Technical steps of the RUL. (**a**) Exposure and division of inferior pulmonary ligament. (**b**) Posterior hilar mobilization with dissection of the subcarinal LN. (**c**) Dissection of the bifurcation of the RUL and RBI with resection of the LN (Station 11R) and development of the plane between the bronchus and PA. (**d**) Superior hilar dissection with development of the plan between RUL bronchus and anterior apical trunk of the PA. (**e**) Dissection and division of the anterior apical trunk of the PA. (**f**) Division of the RUL tributary of the SPV. (**g**) Dissection and division of the posterior ascending branch of the PA after anterior apical trunk and SPV division. (**h**) Division of the RUL bronchus from the posterior approach. (**i**) Division of the parenchymal bridge of the minor and major fissures. (**j**) Placement of the specimen in Anchor tissue retrieval system. (**k**) Dissection of the paratracheal lymph node pocket (stations 2R, 4R, and 3). (**l**) Completion of the lobectomy with placement of the chest tube and visually confirmed lung reexpansion without torsion

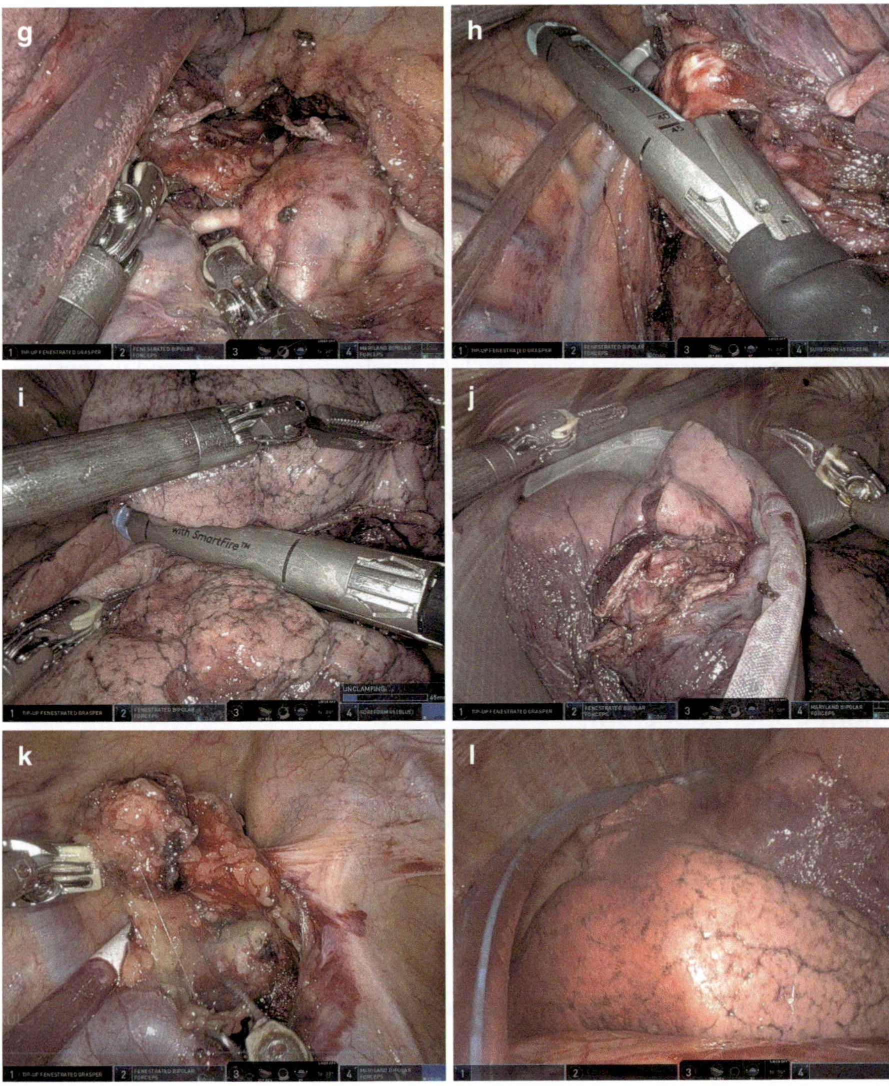

Fig. 31.4 (continued)

ensures exposure of the inferior pulmonary vein in cases of lower lobectomies and facilitates cranial displacement of the lung to accommodate the space after upper lobe resection. Subsequently, the lung is retracted anteriorly, and posterior hilum is mobilized. This dissection varies depending on the laterality of the procedure.

Techniques of Individual Lobectomies

Despite well-established surgical protocols outlining the sequential steps of various lobectomies, a certain degree of variability is acceptable in the conduct of each operation. Structures may be isolated and divided in an order that is most conducive to the patient's individual anatomy. Below, we present our preferred approach to these procedures, along with a description of the most common variants.

Right-Sided Resections

For the initial posterior dissection, the lung is retracted anteriorly, and the posterior hilum is mobilized (Fig. 31.4b). The subcarinal lymph node is exposed and dissected in its entirety, which may require mobilization of the esophagus from the overlying trachea and principal bronchi. The entire posterior airway is exposed, and the bifurcation of the right upper lobe bronchus and bronchus intermedius is dissected. A lymph node in this location is dissected and sent as station 11R, exposing the interlobar pulmonary artery and the takeoff of the posterior ascending branch (Fig. 31.4c). This dissection is carried all the way to the right tracheobronchial angle. Further dissection varies based on the specific lobectomy being performed.

Right Upper Lobectomy

- After the completion of the posterior hilar dissection, the lung is retracted inferiorly, and the superior hilar dissection is performed (Fig. 31.4d). The plane between the right upper lobe (RUL) bronchus and the anterior apical pulmonary trunk of the pulmonary artery (PA) is dissected.
- Next, the lung is reflected posteriorly to expose the anterior hilum. Anterior hilar dissection begins from the inferior pulmonary vein (IPV), exposing the superior pulmonary vein (SPV) and the bifurcation between the right upper and middle lobar veins. The RUL vein is dissected from the underlying interlobar pulmonary artery.
- The 10R lymph node, located in the space between the SPV, superior vena cava (SVC), and azygos vein, is removed.
- The anterior apical trunk is dissected circumferentially next. The previously developed plane between the PA and the RUL bronchus facilitates this dissection. The truncus branch of the PA is then divided with a vascular load stapler (Fig. 31.4e).
- Subsequently, the RUL pulmonary vein is divided with a vascular load stapler distal to the confluence with the right middle lobe (RML) vein (Fig. 31.4f).
- Division of the vein facilitates further posterior retraction of the RUL. This exposes the interlobar PA and the posterior ascending PA branch. This branch is circumferentially mobilized and divided with a vascular load stapler (Fig. 31.4g).

- Next, the RUL bronchus is approached from posterior. The lung is retracted anteriorly. The previous posterior dissection of the bifurcation between the RUL bronchus and RBI facilitates this step. Prior to the division of the bronchus, the absence of any catheters in the airway is confirmed through clear communication with the anesthesia team. Use of robotic staplers usually prevents firing in this situation by sensing excessive tissue thickness (Fig. 31.4h).
- After the division of the hilar structures, the RUL is retracted caudally, and the parenchymal bridge of the minor and major fissures is divided with serial firings of a blue stapler load starting anteriorly (Fig. 31.4i).
- The specimen is retrieved from the chest by placing it into a large Anchor Tissue Retrieval System (ConMed Corporation, Utica, New York, USA), delivered through the 15 mm assistant port. Some extension of the incision is usually required for specimen removal (Fig. 31.4j). After extraction, the assistant port is placed back, carefully avoiding subdiaphragmatic placement due to the rise of the diaphragm after the loss of the capnothorax, which is subsequently reinstated. The specimen is sent for frozen pathology for the inspection of resection margins.
- Attention is directed to the dissection of the paratracheal lymph nodes. The mediastinal pleura is incised vertically, posterior to the SVC, and horizontally, over the azygos vein, with meticulous care to preserve the integrity of the phrenic nerve. Maintaining the dissection plane along the vein wall, the dissection is extended to the tracheal wall, allowing for the complete resection of the tissue pocket containing lymph node stations 2R, 4R, and 3 (Fig. 31.4k).
- To prevent RML torsion following the division of the incomplete minor fissure, the tips of the right middle and lower lobes are approximated, and a small wedge resection is performed using a vascular stapler for pexy.
- Hemostasis is meticulously ensured. A single 24 French straight chest tube is placed through the anterior port, directed posteriorly toward the apex. The robot is then undocked, and the lung is observed to inflate under the Valsalva maneuver without evidence of torsion (Fig. 31.4l).
- *Most common variation of right upper lobectomy*:
  - The RUL vein can be divided prior to the anterior apical trunk of the PA to enhance arterial exposure. However, the authors prefer to divide the artery first to avoid parenchymal edema and difficulties during specimen extraction.
  - Due to the more distal takeoff of the posterior ascending branch, its dissection and division may necessitate the initial division of the RUL bronchus. In such cases, it is acceptable to divide the arterial branch together with the pulmonary parenchyma during fissure division.
  - The RUL bronchus can be approached anteriorly, though the authors prefer a posterior approach, as it better aligns the posterior membranous and cartilaginous portions of the airway wall.
  - Depending on the thickness of the parenchymal bridge, a white stapler load may be used for nearly complete fissures, while blue, green, and even black loads can be employed in cases of incomplete or absent fissures.

Right Lower Lobectomy

- After completing the posterior dissection, the lung is retracted posteriorly and superiorly. Anterior hilar dissection then begins at the IPV, exposing the SPV.
- The 10R lymph node station is dissected and removed.
- In the space between the superior and inferior pulmonary veins, dissection is initiated under the parenchymal bridge of the main fissure. Alternating between dissection and stapling, the division is carried posteriorly, eventually exposing the entire interlobar PA (Fig. 31.5a). In the gap between the superior segmental and posterior ascending arteries, the dissection enters the posterior plane of dissection between the RUL and right bronchus intermedius.
- Next, the lymph node over the PA, exposed during the previous step, is dissected and sent as a level 11R station specimen (Fig. 31.5b).
- The interlobar PA is circumferentially dissected and divided distal to the takeoff of the RML artery. Specific attention is paid to avoid narrowing or division of the RML PA branch (Fig. 31.5c).
- The IPV is divided flush with the pericardium to avoid a long stump, which could later serve as a nidus for clot formation (Fig. 31.5d).
- The right lower lobe (RLL) bronchus is isolated and divided with a green stapler load, taking care to avoid narrowing the RML bronchus takeoff (Fig. 31.5e). The specimen is extracted, and the completion steps are performed as described above.
- *Most common variation of the right lower lobectomy*:
  - If the RML vein is identified draining into the IPV during the anterior dissection, a more distal vein dissection is required for division above the RML vein confluence.
  - Depending on the anatomical relationship between the superior segmental and RML PA branches, the interlobar PA can be divided with a single stapler application or may necessitate separate division of the basilar trunk first, followed by the superior segmental branch.
  - Similarly, based on the relationship between the superior segmental and RML bronchi, the RLL bronchus can be divided with a single stapler application (green load). Alternatively, it may require separate division of the common basilar bronchus first (green load), followed by the superior segmental bronchus (blue load).

Right Middle Lobectomy

- Following the completion of the posterior dissection, the lung is retracted posteriorly and superiorly. The anterior hilar dissection begins at the IPV, exposing the SPV and the confluence of the right upper and middle lobar veins. The course of the RML vein is identified, as it can occasionally drain into the IPV.
- The 10R lymph node station, located in the space between the SPV, SVC, and azygos vein, is carefully removed.

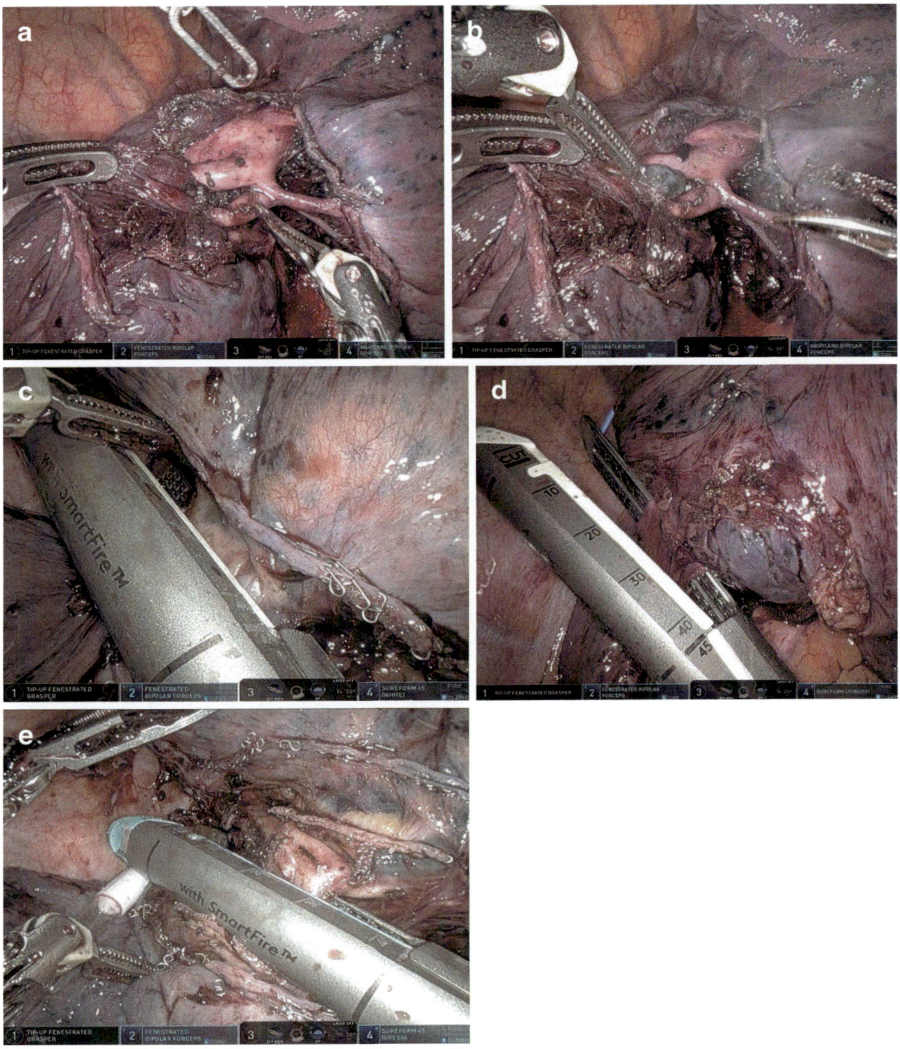

Fig. 31.5 Technical steps of the RLL. (**a**) Alternating dissection and division of the major fissure parenchymal bridge for exposure of the interlobar PA. (**b**) Dissection of the LN over the PA as station 11R. (**c**) Dissection and division of the interlobar PA below the takeoff of the RML branch. (**d**) Division of the inferior pulmonary vein. (**e**) Division of the right lower lobar bronchus

- Dissection between the superior and inferior pulmonary veins begins under the parenchymal bridge of the main fissure. Initially, the dissection is performed on top of the lymph node in this location. Once a tunnel is created, alternating dissection and serial firing of the vascular stapler are used to divide the parenchyma, completing the fissure. The division continues to the confluence of the minor and major fissures, or until the superior segmental and posterior ascending branches of the PA are exposed (Fig. 31.6a).

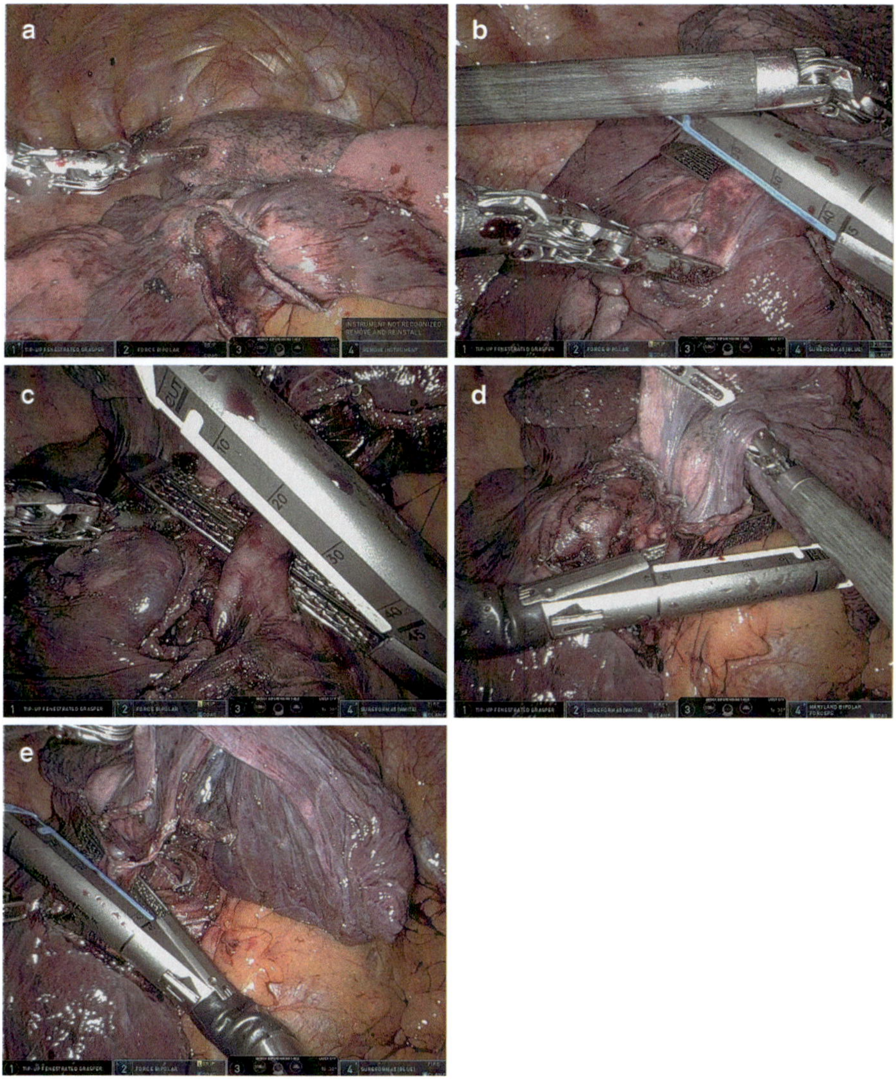

Fig. 31.6 Technical steps of the RML lobectomy. (**a**) Dissection and division of the parenchymal bridge of the major fissure until its fusion with the minor fissure. (**b**) Division of the minor fissure parenchyma until the previous plane of dissection. (**c**) Division of the RML PA. (**d**) Division of the RML tributary of the SPV. (**e**) Division of the RML bronchus at its takeoff from RBI. Please note use of blue load stapler

- Next, the lymph node over the PA, exposed during the previous step is dissected and sent as a level 11R station specimen.
- The SPV is then dissected from the underlying interlobar pulmonary artery, and the space between the RUL and RML venous tributaries is developed.

- Similarly, by maintaining the dissection plane over the PA, a tunnel is created under the minor fissure. Alternating dissection with serial firing of a vascular stapler load, the parenchyma is divided until it meets the major fissure, entering the previous plane of dissection, completing the minor fissure (Fig. 31.6b).
- These maneuvers lead to a wide exposure of the interlobar PA and the RML branch. The RML branch is circumferentially dissected and divided with a vascular stapler load (Fig. 31.6c). Utilizing the posterior axillary line for the stapler facilitates most of the steps in a middle lobectomy.
- Next, the RML vein is encircled and divided via the same port distal to the confluence with the RUL vein (Fig. 31.6d).
- The RML bronchus is then isolated, running underneath and around the interlobar PA. Careful dissection to its takeoff is required to avoid a long stump. The bronchus is divided with a blue stapler load. As a safety measure, the absence of a suction catheter in the airway prior to bronchus division has to be ensured (Fig. 31.6e).
- Once the specimen is resected, it is extracted from the chest as previously described. The paratracheal lymph node pocket is dissected, the chest tube is positioned, and the case is completed in the usual fashion.
- *Most common variation of the right middle lobectomy*:
  - The division of the minor fissure can be postponed until after the PA branches are divided. This approach may facilitate dissection from lateral to medial, potentially providing better exposure.
  - In cases where accessory RML PA branches are present, the division of the most anterior branch might be limited by the pulmonary parenchyma, necessitating the division of the minor fissure.
  - Prior to the division of the RML vein, its course needs to be verified, as it can occasionally drain into the inferior pulmonary vein.
  - The RML vein can be divided prior to the PA branches. This facilitates the dissection of the tunnel under the minor fissure. Due to the smaller size of the RML, concerns regarding edema and difficulties with extraction are less significant.

Left-Sided Resections

After takedown of the inferior pulmonary ligament (Fig. 31.7a), the lung is retracted anteriorly, and the posterior hilar dissection exposes the interlobar pulmonary artery. The dissection is then carried superiorly (Fig. 31.7b). The lymph nodes overlying the pulmonary artery in this location are sent as station 11 L. Deeper dissection under the interlobar artery leads to the subcarinal space, where, after dissecting the esophagus away, the subcarinal lymph node is dissected and sent as a specimen.

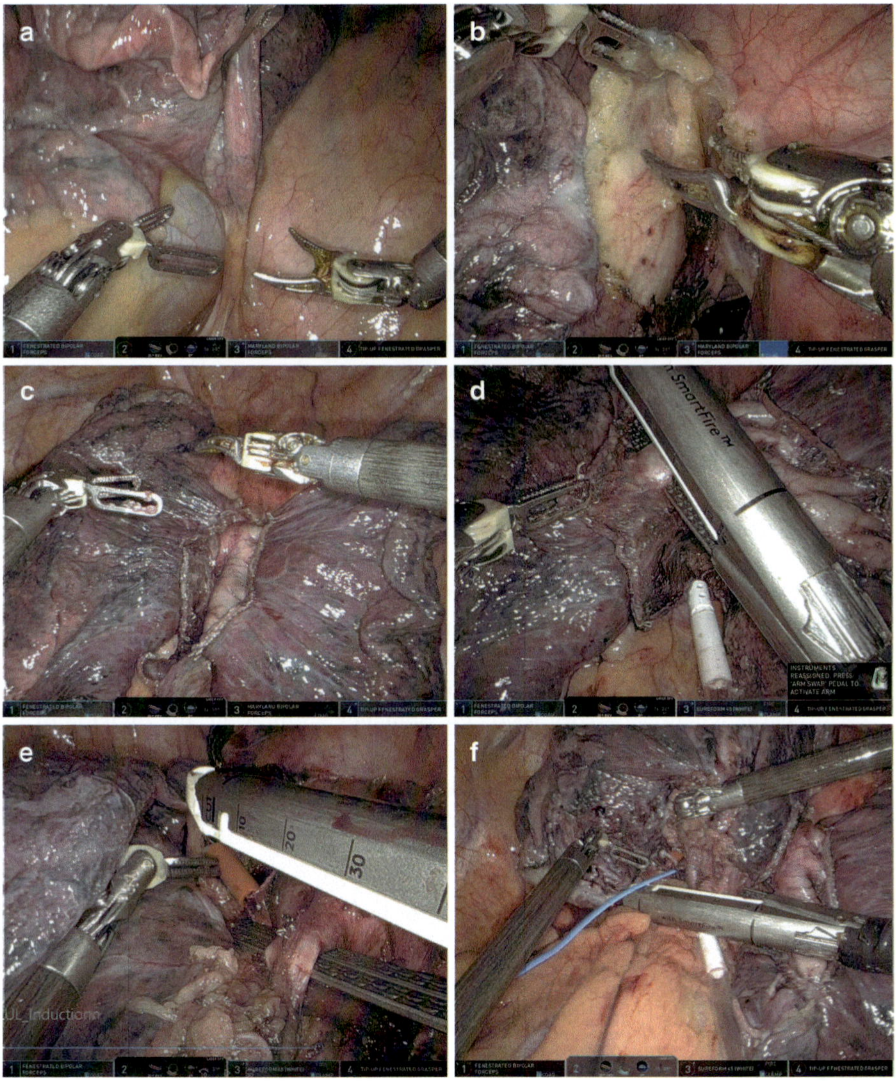

Fig. 31.7 Technical step of the LUL. (**a**) Exposure and division of the left inferior pulmonary ligament. (**b**) Posterior dissection of the left hilum with dissection of the interlobar PA and interlobar and subcarinal LNs. (**c**) Dissection and division of the fissural parenchyma for the exposure of the PA branches. (**d**) Dissection and division of the lingular branch of the PA. (**e**) Dissection and division of the anterior apical branch of the PA. Please note in the background prophylactic Rommel tourniquet in place in the neoadjuvant therapy case. (**f**) Division of the SPV. Rommel tourniquet and vessel loop are visible in the background. (**g**) Division of the LUL bronchus

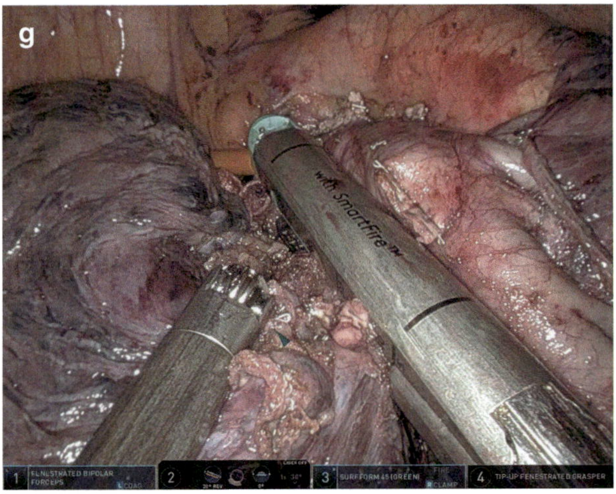

Fig. 31.7 (continued)

Left Upper Lobectomy

- After completion of the posterior dissection, the lung is retracted inferiorly, and the superior dissection is completed, exposing the branches of the PA to the left upper lobe (LUL).
- Next, the left lung is retracted posteriorly and superiorly, and the anterior hilar dissection starts from the IPV, exposing the SPV and joining with the superior dissection plane.
- In the space between the superior and inferior pulmonary veins, dissection is initiated under the parenchymal bridge of the fissure, staying on top of the lymph node in this area. Alternating dissection and division of the parenchyma with the stapler, the division of the parenchymal bridge of the fissure is carried posteriorly, eventually exposing the entire interlobar PA (Fig. 31.7c).
- The lymph node exposed during the previous step is dissected and removed as station 11 L.
- The branches of the PA to the LUL are circumferentially dissected and divided with a vascular stapler load, starting with the lingular branch (Fig. 31.7d), followed by the posterior apical branch, and subsequently the anterior apical branch (Fig. 31.7e). The posterior axillary line port is most useful for stapler placement during this step.
- Next, the SPV is circumferentially dissected and divided (Fig. 31.7f). Because the SPV can be fairly wide, consisting of lingular, intersegmental, and upper division branches, these may need to be dissected and transected separately.
- This maneuver leads to the exposure of the LUL bronchus. The bronchus should be encircled and divided with a green stapler load from the posterior axillary port for better apposition of the membranous and cartilaginous portions of the airway (Fig. 31.7g).

- The specimen is placed in a tissue retrieval system, extracted from the ches, and sent for frozen pathological assessment for margins. Enlarging of an assistant port site might be required.
- An assistant port is replaced for the maintanance of the capnothorax. Lymphadenectomy is completed by dissecting the aortopulmonary window and prevascular lymph nodes (stations 5 and 6). Dissection along the airway under the aortic arch can expose the left lower paratracheal lymph node (station 4 L) for resection.
- At the conclusion of the resection, the robot is undocked, and a 24 French chest tube is advanced to the apex posteriorly through an anterior port and secured to the skin. The lung is observed to inflate without torsion with the Valsalva maneuver.
- *Common variations of the left upper lobectomy*:
  - Dissection of the anterior apical branch from the back can be challenging if it is covered by the SPV, and initial division of the vein can be performed for better exposure.
  - After division of the SPV and the anterior apical branch of the PA, the LUL bronchus can be circumferentially dissected and divided from an anterior approach. This maneuver will expose the PA branches to the LUL and the parenchymal bridge of the fissure from the inside. The branches of the PA can be taken along with the parenchyma using this approach.

Left Lower Lobectomy

- After completion of the posterior dissection, the lung is retracted cranially and posteriorly and the parenchymal bridge of the fissure is divided as described previously.
- The lymph node, exposed during the previous step, is dissected and removed as station 11 L.
- The inferior lobar PA is circumferentially mobilized below the takeoff of the lingular branch and is divided from the anterior port with a vascular load stapler (Fig. 31.8a).
- After division of the artery, the lung is reflected cranially and posteriorly. The IPV is dissected and divided flush with the pericardium (Fig. 31.8b).
- The left lower lobe bronchus is isolated and divided from posterior axillary port with a green load stapler (Fig. 31.8c).
- *Common variations of the left lower lobectomy*:
  - In cases of a very distal takeoff of the last lingular branch, separate division of the basilar trunk of the left lower lobe PA and the superior segmental branch might be required.
  - In cases of early confluence of the pulmonary veins, clear identification of the IPV branch for division is necessary to avoid accidental pneumonectomy.

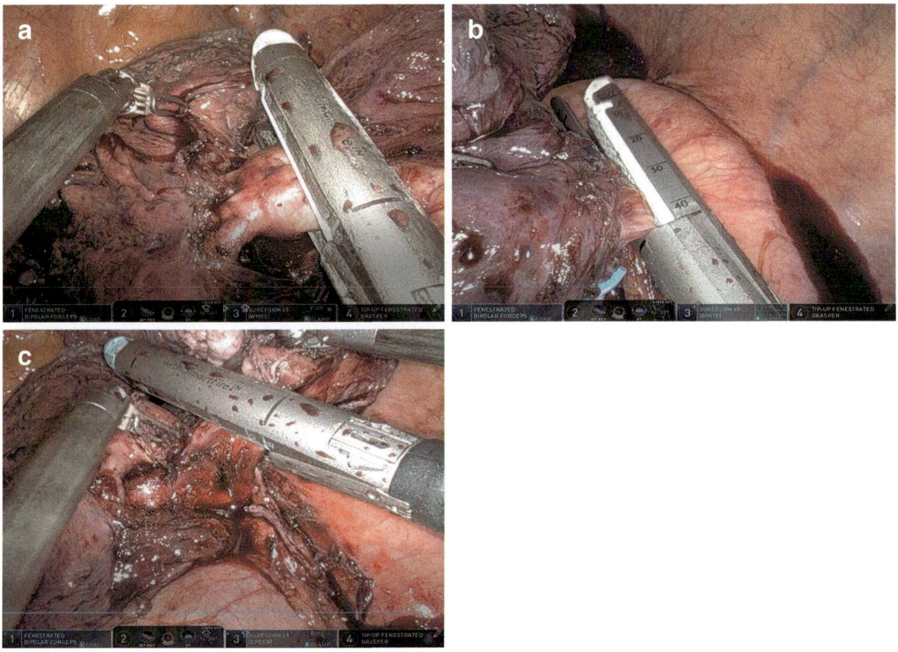

Fig. 31.8 Technical steps of the LLL. (**a**) After exposure of the PA in the fissure, interlobar PA is circumferentially dissected and divided below the takeoff of the most distal lingular branch. (**b**) Division of the IPV flush with the pericardium. (**c**) Division of the left lower bronchus

Tips and Tricks for Robotic Pulmonary Dissection

- *Lung Retraction*: To prevent parenchymal tears and prolonged air leak, a "passive" retraction should be used. This implies gentle pushing of lung parenchyma using a retractor, holding a gauze cigar instead of grasping and pulling on the pulmonary parenchyma directly.
- *Lymph Nodes Dissection*: Lymph nodes fill the spaces between tubular structures (vessels and bronchi). Initial dissection and removal of lymph nodes lead to identification of the anatomy, facilitating isolation and division of the hilar structures. Lymph nodes are fragile structures, and direct grasping can lead to their rupture and bleeding. To avoid this, retraction should be applied to the surrounding tissue, and the plane of dissection should be kept right on the hilar structures, gradually mobilizing and removing the nodes.
- *Vein Dissection and Division*: Veins are thin-walled and pliable structures and generally tolerate direct grasping well without excessive traction. They are divided using a vascular stapler load. Occasionally, mild bleeding can be observed from the staple line, which is usually controlled with gauze pressure for a few minutes.

- *Pulmonary Artery Dissection and Division*: Arteries are very fragile structures, and direct grasping, clamping, and retraction should be avoided at all costs. Instead, surrounding structures should be retracted and dissected away from the artery. While it may be tempting to avoid these critical structures during dissection, approaching them carefully but confidently, with the plane of dissection right on the arterial wall in the subadventitial plane, can lead to a more precise and quicker procedure.
- Using a curved tip stapler facilitates advancing the stapler and getting around the arteries for division. Forcing the stapler through can easily lead to injury and bleeding. If additional retraction is required for the passage of the stapler, a vessel loop placed around the vessel facilitates retraction and stapler advancement.
- In challenging dissections, such as in neoadjuvant cases, prophylactic placement of a Rommel tourniquet for quick bleeding control is advisable (Fig. 31.7e, f). These should be applied around the main pulmonary artery as it emerges from the mediastinum and both pulmonary veins. Alternatively, bulldog clamps can be applied. Tourniquets can be applied prophylactically and cinched in case of bleeding, whereas clamps are usually applied during temporary control of bleeding with pressure. Considering that the pulmonary artery is a low-pressure system, temporary control can almost always be obtained with pressure, applied with either a rolled gauze or lung tissue.
- Stapling of the pulmonary artery should be performed with full preparation for bleeding in case of stapler failure. The camera should be pulled away as far as possible to avoid loss of vision from blood jet. The free arm should either hold gauze or lung tissue for immediate tamponade of the bleeding vessel if that occurs. After completing the division, the stapler should be pulled back the way it was introduced rather than just lifted up to avoid avulsion of any tissue bands, which could lead to bleeding.
- *Dissection and Division of the Bronchi*: As with any tubular structure, the plane should be kept right on the bronchial wall. Notably, bronchi are often larger than they appear, and aggressive dissection can lead to perforation of the bronchial wall. In such cases, either the application of a suture for retraction of the tissue into the stapler or a complete division with subsequent suture closure can be a solution. For this purpose, we use a 6-inch 3–0 absorbable V-Loc 180 stitch (green color) (Medtronic, Minneapolis, MN, USA) with an absorption time of 180 days. During stapler firing, it is a good habit to confirm the absence of any foreign bodies (usually suction catheters) within the bronchus to avoid time-consuming and technically challenging repairs.
- *Division of the Pulmonary Parenchyma*: After the division of the hilar structures, the parenchymal bridge is divided along the anatomical fissures. Most of the time, the use of a white stapler load is sufficient for these purposes. However, for incomplete fissures, blue or even green loads might be required. In cases of completely absent fissures or segmentectomies, green or even black loads are usually used. Staple line reinforcement can sometimes be beneficial in patients with advanced emphysema and poor-quality parenchyma.

- *Dissection of the Fissure*: Authors avoid "fissure diving" for PA exposure and approach all dissection with extra fissural technique. Developing plane in the space between superior and inferior pulmonary vein leads the surgeon into the tunnel over the interlobar PA and under the parenchymal bridge of the major fissure. In a similar fashion, dissection in the space between the upper and middle lobar vein exposes the tunnel under the minor fissure.
- *Stapler Handling*: While many surgeons successfully utilize handheld staplers, this success is usually predicated on the availability of a consistent and experienced bedside assistant. The authors strongly prefer robotic staplers. In addition to providing full control of the device by the console surgeon, the tissue compression sensing SmartFire technology potentially can prevent some surgical mishaps, such as the division of the bronchus with a suction catheter in it.
- *Instrument Insertion and Removal*: During thoracic surgery, robotic instruments should initially be inserted under direct vision. Once safely positioned, instruments can be quickly and safely inserted or changed using the robot's memory feature, which automatically places new instruments 3 mm proximal to their last position. The new DV5 platform provides visual cues to aid in guided instrument exchange. Final removal of the robotic arms and undocking should be performed under direct vision to ensure good hemostasis upon relief of the capnothorax.
- *Specimen Drop Zone*: The safe "drop zone" for specimen transfer (mostly lymph nodes) should be established well away from the pulmonary artery to prevent injury during this process. Ideally, the same area should be used consistently to aid in developing muscle memory for the bedside assistant. The authors prefer to remove specimens in a cut glove finger to prevent rupture, loss, and potential contamination, particularly in cases of metastatic disease of the lymph nodes (Fig. 31.9).

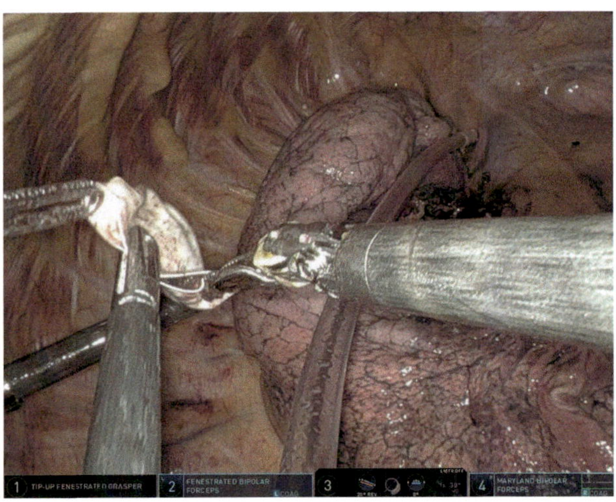

Fig. 31.9 Safe "drop zone" for specimen transfer for extraction away from hilar structures

- *Emergency Preparedness*: A rolled-up sponge should always be immediately accessible when working around vascular structures. In the event of an injury, the first step should be to tamponade the bleeding with the sponge or lung tissue. Minor injuries may respond to this packing alone with time, while preparations are made for an emergency thoracotomy. If previously placed, tourniquets may be cinched, or bulldog clamps applied. However, if bleeding is massive or continues, conversion will be necessary.
- *Protocol for Emergent Conversion*: Anatomical pulmonary resection is a high-risk procedure, with bleeding being the most dreadful complication. Regardless of a surgeon's level of skill, such complications will eventually occur with increasing number of cases. Gown and gloves for the surgeon, as well as a Finochietto retractor, should always be available on the table during any robotic anatomic lung resection. The authors' protocol for conversion is as follows:
- *Console Surgeon*:
  - Announces the massive bleeding scenario and the need for emergent conversion.
  - Clearly communicates to the bedside assistant which robotic arm is applying pressure on the bleeding vessel and should not be moved during robot undocking.
  - Requests an additional help from another faculty surgeon to the operating room immediately.
  - Emergently scrubs to transition to the bedside position and initiates emergent thoracotomy.
  - Once in the chest, the first move is to manually compress the main pulmonary artery upon its exit from the mediastinum.
  - If the patient remains stable, the application of a tourniquet or bulldog clamp can be undertaken.
  - After pulmonary artery control, subsequent control of veins is undertaken until bleeding subsides.
  - It is important to remember that due to bronchial artery circulation, there will always be low-intensity bleeding. This bleeding doesn't mean inadequate PA control and usually does not interfere with the repair, as the surgical field can be easily cleared with the suction.
  - In an unstable patient, after manual control of the main PA, packing of the chest with lap pads should be performed until anesthesia is able to catch up with volume and blood resuscitation.
- *Bedside Surgeon/First Assistant*:
  - Starts the immediate undocking process while maintaining visual control of the surgical field with the camera, transitioning into free handheld support.
  - Avoids manipulating the robotic arm exerting pressure and tamponade on the bleeding vessel.
  - If visualization is lost, immediately cleans the camera to reestablish visual control.
  - If control of the bleeding is lost, immediately undocks the robot and initiates emergent thoracotomy.

- *Surgical Technician*:
  - Requests another technician to scrub in for extra help.
  - Opens the thoracotomy tray in addition to the already available Finochietto retractor.
- *Circulating Nurse*:
  - Calls the charge nurse for help.
  - Requests additional faculty surgeons, circulators, surgical technicians, and anesthesia support.
  - Delivers blood to the anesthesia team.
  - Opens the thoracotomy tray.
  - Notifies the blood bank and requests 6 units of uncross matched blood.
  - Calls for a Massive Transfusion Protocol if requested by the faculty surgeon.
- *Anesthesia Team*:
  - Calls for a faculty physician to the room and requests additional help.
  - Starts blood transfusion.
  - Avoids lung inflation, which could lead to loss of exposure and access.
  - If lung inflation occurs, immediately disconnects the ventilator and starts bronchoscopy for repositioning of the double-lumen tube or bronchial blocker to reestablish the single-lung ventilation. Usually, the patient can tolerate several minutes of apnea while lung isolation is reestablished.
- It is essential to maintain proficiency in emergent conversion through regular team training and practice, including "dry runs" conducted before or after each case. Prior to each procedure, the steps of emergent conversion should be reviewed with the entire team. Implementing these protocols and strategies enhances the safety and efficiency of robotic thoracic surgery, ultimately ensuring better patient outcomes. As Benjamin Franklin wisely advised, "An ounce of prevention is worth a pound of cure."

Outcomes and Future Directions of Robotic Lobectomy

Despite the growing body of knowledge, there remains a paucity of long-term survival studies following robotic lobectomy. However, available data indicate that RATS provides oncologic outcomes that are comparable to, if not superior to, traditional methods, particularly for cancer-related procedures. A comprehensive retrospective analysis involving 6646 patients with clinical stages IA–IIIA was conducted across 21 centers in the United States, comparing long-term survival outcomes between open surgery and minimally invasive approaches [22]. Naturally, the study demonstrated advantages to minimally invasive techniques, with fewer in-hospital complications compared to open lobectomy. Postoperative length of stay in the robotic lobectomy group averaged 3 days, followed by the VATS group at 4 days and the open lobectomy group at 5 days. Conversion rates were notably lower in the robotic group (4%) compared to the VATS group (10%). Patients undergoing robotic lobectomy had the highest mean number of sampled N1 and N2 nodal stations (5.2 ± 1.5), compared to those undergoing VATS (4.5 ± 1.4) and open lobectomy

(4.6 ± 1.4), with the differences being statistically significant ($P < 0.0001$). The unadjusted 5-year overall survival rates were highest for open approach at 84%, followed by robotic at 81% and VATS at 74% ($P = 0.008$). These trends persisted after adjusting for inverse probability of treatment weighting. Multivariable Cox regression analyses indicated that robotic and open approaches provided statistically equivalent overall survival rates. However, VATS lobectomy was associated with a lower overall survival rate. The equivalent survival rates between RATS and thoracotomy for lung cancer have consistently been observed in most studies [24, 37, 57]. One notable study is a retrospective analysis of stage-specific survival involving 325 consecutive patients who underwent robotic lobectomy for non-small cell lung cancer across three centers (two in Italy and one in the United States) [44]. With a median follow-up of 27 months, the overall 5-year survival rate was 80%, broken down by stage as follows: 91% for stage IA, 88% for stage IB, and 49% for stage II. For patients with stage IIIA, the 3-year survival rate was 43%. These outcomes are at least comparable to those expected with VATS or thoracotomy. Another multicenter retrospective study reported outcomes following 1339 robotic lobectomies with promising oncologic results: The 5-year stage-specific survival rates were 83% for stage IA non-small cell lung cancer, 77% for stage IB, 68% for stage IIA, 70% for stage IIB, 62% for stage IIIA (with 73% of these patients having N2 disease), and 31% for stage IIIB excluding N3 disease [8]. The largest single-center case series with comparative data reported outcomes from 831 patients and demonstrated equivalent survival among all three surgical approaches without differences in morbidity, nodal upstaging, or mortality [37]. However, robotic lobectomy was associated with improved nodal harvest and decreased blood loss and length of stay.

Multiple retrospective database analyses have been conducted to compare the early outcomes of RATS lobectomy to those of VATS. One comprehensive retrospective study examined 774 patients with early-stage lung cancer, with 298 undergoing RATS versus 476 undergoing VATS [65]. After matching the groups using propensity scores, the analysis revealed no significant differences in operative time (RATS 147.91 minutes versus VATS 149.23 minutes; $P = 0.773$), blood loss (RATS 50 mL versus VATS 100 mL; $P = 0.177$), overall complications (RATS 17.9% versus VATS 14.8%; $P = 0.340$), and length of hospital stay (both RATS and VATS 4 days; $P = 0.417$) although RATS group had a significantly higher number of lymph node stations dissected compared to VATS group, which is essential for accurate pathological staging and adjuvant therapy. Additionally, a meta-analysis compared postoperative outcomes of anatomical resections performed by RATS and VATS, including a subgroup analysis for both lobectomy and sublobar resections [32]. In the lobectomy group, RATS approach was associated with lower conversion rate (OR = 0.50, 95% CI: 0.43–0.60, $P < 0.001$), greater number of harvested lymph nodes and dissected stations (WMD = 0.51, 95% CI: 0.15–0.86, $P = 0.005$), shorter postoperative chest tube duration (WMD = −0.61, 95% CI: 0.78–0.44, $P < 0.001$), lower overall complication rate (OR = 0.90, 95% CI: 0.83–0.99, $P = 0.020$), and reduced recurrence (OR = 0.51, 95% CI: 0.36–0.72, $P < 0.001$). However, these differences were not significant in the sublobar resection group. In another meta-analysis of 25 studies comparing the outcomes of RATS and VATS, a total of 50,404 patients were encompassed [60]. It was demonstrated that the RATS group had a significantly lower 30-day mortality rate (OR: 0.55; 95% CI: 0.38–0.81; $P = 0.002$) and longer disease-free survival (HR: 0.76; 95% CI: 0.59–0.97; $P = 0.03$), suggesting potential long-term survival benefits for the robotic approach compared to VATS. Nonetheless, the overall survival rates between the two techniques were similar (HR: 0.77; 95% CI: 0.57–1.05; $P = 0.10$). Similar findings were reported regarding long-term outcomes, indicating no significant difference in overall survival between the groups (95% CI: 0.90–1.02; $P = 0.22$) [64]. Conversely, slightly improved disease-free survival in the RATS group was observed (95% CI: 1.11–2.57; $P = 0.01$).

Lung resections after neoadjuvant therapy present additional challenges. The post-induction inflammatory state can create a risky surgical environment characterized by fibrosis and dense adhesions, significantly increasing the risk of major bleeding. Some studies comparing VATS with the open approach following induction therapy have found no significant differences in major outcomes such as survival and morbidity. However, a major concern is that the VATS group tended to have fewer lymph nodes dissected [15]. Cerfolio et al. investigated 223 patients with N2 disease who underwent RATS, with only 15.2% having received neoadjuvant therapy [6, 9, 10]. Among these patients, the complete resection rate was 98.1%, with no mortality reported. The major complication rate stood at 10.1%, comparable to that of patients without induction therapy. The conversion rate for resections after neoadjuvant treatment was 15%, primarily due to extensive mediastinal lymph node involvement. In a study conducted by Park et al., 428 patients with stages II–IIIA non-small cell lung cancer who underwent lobectomy after neoadjuvant therapy were reviewed [45]. Of these patients, 31 (7%) underwent minimally invasive surgery, with 17 (3%) utilizing the robotic approach. Although no direct comparison was made between VATS and RATS, there was no significant difference observed between the minimally invasive group and the open surgery group in terms of operative complications, extent of resection, and final pathological stage.

Neoadjuvant treatment combined with perioperative immunotherapy is increasingly gaining prominence in the field of thoracic oncology. A phase I trial examined the outcomes of 20 patients with stages I–IIIA lung cancer who received neoadjuvant nivolumab, and perioperative outcomes were analyzed [4]. Initially, a minimally invasive approach was attempted in 13 (65%) patients but was only successful in 46% of patients (3 VATS and 3 RATS). There was no perioperative mortality, and the morbidity rate was 50%, with atrial fibrillation being the most common complication. The primary reasons for conversion were hemorrhage, dense adhesions, and inflamed mediastinal and hilar nodal stations. A phase 2 study investigating neoadjuvant pembrolizumab in non-small cell lung cancer included 25 patients who underwent lung resections [56]. The majority (72%) had lobectomies. Of these patients, 92% initially underwent a minimally invasive approach, but 22% of these cases were converted to thoracotomy. An R0 resection was achieved in 88% of the patients. Another prospective randomized trial assessed perioperative outcomes of anatomic lung resections after neoadjuvant nivolumab (22 patients) or a combination of nivolumab and ipilimumab (17 patients) [51]. Lobectomy was performed in

89% of these cases, with 19% using the VATS approach and 8% using RATS. Conversion was necessary in 17% of the minimally invasive cases. All 37 patients achieved an R0 resection. Overall, the studies indicated that surgery following neoadjuvant immunotherapy, including minimally invasive approaches, is safe and effective, yielding perioperative outcomes similar to those achieved with chemotherapy or upfront resection. These reviews support increasing the adoption of the robotic approach for complex lung resections.

Robotic technology continues to evolve, bringing new and exciting advances to the field of thoracic surgery. The resulting rise in competition is expected to drive both the speed and variety of innovation while also reducing the costs of robotic technology. Uniportal robotic thoracic surgery represents a further advancement in minimally invasive surgical techniques, combining the benefits of robotic technology with the advantages of a single incision approach.

Yang et al. were the first to report a case of a right upper lobectomy performed using the uniportal RATS technique with a multiport platform [61]. In this procedure, a single 4.5 cm incision was created to accommodate three robotic arms and the assistant. They utilized 8 mm trocars for all robotic arms to fit within the limited incision space. However, this setup restricted the use of robotic staplers. Gonzalez-Rivas et al. have also reported on their uniportal RATS technique, utilizing robotic technology for more complex lung resections, including segmentectomies, pneumonectomies, and bronchoplasties [17]. Drawing from their extensive experience with uniportal VATS, the authors emphasized that a significant advantage of uniportal RATS is the ability to quickly convert to uniportal VATS or anterior thoracotomy in emergent situations. Authors of this chapter have performed limited number of uniportal RATS lobectomies. While technical challenges of the uniportal configuration are increased due to limited working space (Fig. 31.10a), patients had enjoyed fast recovery with decreased postoperative pain with relatively minor single incision (Fig. 31.10b).

The da Vinci Single-Port (SP) system after being trialed in thoracic surgery appears to be a practical tool for robotic lung resections and has recently received FDA clearance for thoracic surgery. This advancement holds promise for further enhancing the capabilities and flexibility of minimally invasive thoracic surgeries. The platform features a compact, circular design with instruments grouped together, which can be docked to a 2.5 cm trocar. The da Vinci SP system presents several potential benefits, such as alternative access points at the subxiphoid or subcostal locations. It also features double articulation of its instruments, with both wrist and elbow-like joints, which enhances the triangulation of instruments at the targeted anatomy. Additionally, the system offers an advanced perspective using an articulating 3D camera for a flexible view and includes a fourth arm that can be used for retraction [41]. Adapting this technology for use in the intercostal space posed several challenges. Initially, the SP system had several key differences from the multiport Xi system. It lacked a robotic stapler, requiring the bedside assistant to use a handheld stapler in conjunction with the SP system through a single access port. Additionally, the SP system was too large to be used through the intercostal space [33]. Wu et al. documented their preclinical experience using the da Vinci SP

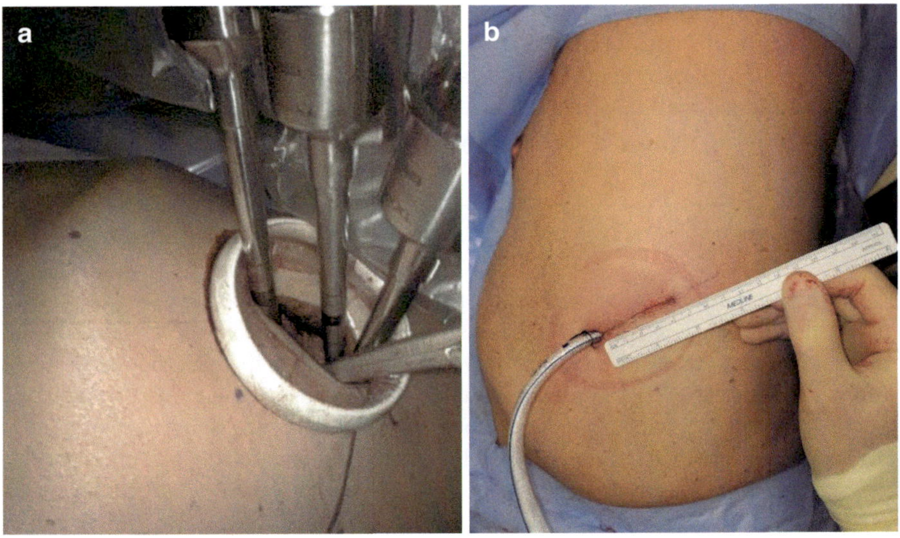

Fig. 31.10 Uniportal robotic lobectomy. (**a**) Position of the robotic ports in the 4 cm incision. (**b**) Postoperative view after the procedure

system for subcostal anatomic lung resections [59]. They highlighted the technology's ability to effectively dissect hilar structures and mediastinal lymph nodes. However, due to the absence of a robotic stapler, a handheld stapling instrument was necessary for transecting vital structures. In a different study, 25 patients with lung cancer underwent SP major subcostal pulmonary resections with no conversions to open thoracotomy, demonstrating its safety [28]. Another study involving 35 patients who underwent major anatomic lung resection using a single-port robotic system reported a conversion rate of 2.9% [11]. The median total operating time was 194 minutes (ranging from 63 to 405 minutes). The median number of harvested lymph nodes was 13 (ranging from 5 to 37), with a median of 6 nodal stations (ranging from 4 to 8). Median postoperative stay was 3 days with no in-hospital deaths.

With the advancement of SP robotic platforms, staplers can now be operated by the primary surgeon directly from the console. SP RATS provides the significant benefit of using robotic staplers through a single anterior incision, thereby avoiding the potential for rough maneuvers that can occur with VATS staplers in less experienced hands. This reduces the risk of vascular avulsion [18]. These technological improvements facilitate complex pulmonary resections, such as double-sleeve lobectomies following neoadjuvant immunotherapy, using a uniportal approach [16].

Another significant area of innovation in robotics is the development of virtual haptic feedback, which would allow surgeons to sense tissue characteristics, thereby enhancing their ability to localize lesions and perform delicate dissection. Additionally, a potentially revolutionary innovation is the ability to overlay reconstructed 3D imaging results (such as CT scans or MRIs) over the real-time intraoperative picture with AI enhancement. This capability would enable surgeons to more easily identify obscure anatomy, such as pulmonary vessels or difficult-to-locate nodules, thereby facilitating dissection. As technology continues to evolve, these techniques are likely to increase in adoption, further transforming the landscape of thoracic surgery and ultimately leading to better patient outcomes.

Conclusion

Currently, minimally invasive thoracic procedures include both VATS and robotic-assisted techniques. RATS lobectomy stands out as a state-of-the-art method that merges the advantages of minimally invasive surgery with the precision afforded by robotic technology. This approach enables further advancements in thoracic surgery, providing enhanced outcomes for patients undergoing lung resections. The decision between VATS and robotic techniques often depends on the surgeon's skill set and comfort level with each method. Current data indicate that the oncologic outcomes for both approaches are comparable. However, the superior 3D visualization and precise tissue handling provided by robotic surgery often make it the preferred choice. As technological advancements continue, RATS lobectomy is set to become an increasingly prevalent option in the surgical treatment of lung malignancies.

References

1. Abbas A, Bakhos C, Petrov R, Kaiser L. Financial impact of adapting robotics to a thoracic practice in an academic institution. J Thorac Dis. 2020;12:89–96. https://doi.org/10.21037/jtd.2019.12.140.
2. Abbas AE. Robotic portal lobectomy, surgery through a virtual thoracotomy. J Thorac Dis. 2017;9:2871–5. https://doi.org/10.21037/jtd.2017.08.84.
3. Ashton RC, Connery CP, Swistel DG, DeRose JJ. Robot-assisted lobectomy. J Thorac Cardiovasc Surg. 2003;126:292–3. https://doi.org/10.1016/s0022-5223(03)00201-0.
4. Bott MJ, Yang SC, Park BJ, et al. Initial results of pulmonary resection after neoadjuvant nivolumab in patients with resectable non-small cell lung cancer. J Thorac Cardiovasc Surg. 2019;158:269–76. https://doi.org/10.1016/j.jtcvs.2018.11.124.
5. Cao C, Louie BE, Melfi F, et al. Outcomes of major complications after robotic anatomic pulmonary resection. J Thorac Cardiovasc Surg. 2020;159:681–6. https://doi.org/10.1016/j.jtcvs.2019.08.057.
6. Cerfolio RJ, Bess KM, Wei B, Minnich DJ. Incidence, results, and our current intraoperative technique to control major vascular injuries during minimally invasive robotic thoracic surgery. Ann Thorac Surg. 2016;102:394–9. https://doi.org/10.1016/j.athoracsur.2016.02.004.
7. Cerfolio RJ, Bryant AS, Skylizard L, Minnich DJ. Initial consecutive experience of completely portal robotic pulmonary resection with 4 arms. J Thorac Cardiovasc Surg. 2011;142:740–6. https://doi.org/10.1016/j.jtcvs.2011.07.022.
8. Cerfolio RJ, Ghanim AF, Dylewski M, et al. The long-term survival of robotic lobectomy for non-small cell lung cancer: a multi-institutional study. J Thorac Cardiovasc Surg. 2018;155:778–86. https://doi.org/10.1016/j.jtcvs.2017.09.016.

9. Cerfolio RJ, Steenwyk BL, Watson C, et al. Decreasing the preincision time for pulmonary lobectomy: the process of lean and value stream mapping. Ann Thorac Surg. 2016;101:1110–5. https://doi.org/10.1016/j.athoracsur.2015.09.004.
10. Cerfolio RJ, Watson C, Minnich DJ, et al. One hundred planned robotic segmentectomies: early results, technical details, and preferred port placement. Ann Thorac Surg. 2016;101:1089–95.; Discussion 1095-6. https://doi.org/10.1016/j.athoracsur.2015.08.092.
11. Cheng C, Tagkalos E, Ng CB, et al. Subcostal uniportal robotic anatomic lung resection: A pilot trial. JTCVS Tech. 2024;25:160–9. https://doi.org/10.1016/j.xjtc.2024.01.024.
12. Coyan GN, Lu M, Ruppert KM, et al. Activity-based cost analysis of robotic anatomic lung resection during program implementation. Ann Thorac Surg. 2022;113:244–9. https://doi.org/10.1016/j.athoracsur.2021.01.053.
13. Emmert A, Straube C, Buentzel J, Roever C. Robotic versus thoracoscopic lung resection: a systematic review and meta-analysis. Medicine. 2017;96:e7633. https://doi.org/10.1097/MD.0000000000007633.
14. Falcoz P-E, Puyraveau M, Thomas P-A, et al. Video-assisted thoracoscopic surgery versus open lobectomy for primary non-small-cell lung cancer: a propensity-matched analysis of outcome from the European Society of Thoracic Surgeon database. Eur J Cardiothorac Surg. 2016;49:602–9. https://doi.org/10.1093/ejcts/ezv154.
15. Fang L, Wang L, Wang Y, et al. Video assisted thoracic surgery vs. thoracotomy for locally advanced lung squamous cell carcinoma after neoadjuvant chemotherapy. J Cardiothorac Surg. 2018;13:128. https://doi.org/10.1186/s13019-018-0813-7.
16. Fang Z, Li C, Bosinceanu ML, et al. Case report: Uniportal robot-assisted thoracoscopic double-sleeve lobectomy after neoadjuvant immunotherapy. Front Surg. 2024;11:1360125. https://doi.org/10.3389/fsurg.2024.1360125.
17. Gonzalez-Rivas D, Bosinceanu M, Motas N, Manolache V. Uniportal robotic-assisted thoracic surgery for lung resections. Eur J Cardiothorac Surg. 2022;62 https://doi.org/10.1093/ejcts/ezac410.
18. Gonzalez-Rivas D, Manolache V, Bosinceanu ML, et al. Uniportal pure robotic-assisted thoracic surgery-technical aspects, tips and tricks. Ann Transl Med. 2023;11:362. https://doi.org/10.21037/atm-22-1866.
19. Graham EA. The first total pneumonectomy. Tex Cancer Bull. 1949;2:2–4.
20. Keeney-Bonthrone TP, Frydrych LM, Karmakar M, et al. Robot-assisted vs. video-assisted thoracoscopic lobectomy: a systematic review of cost effectiveness. Video Assist Thorac Surg. 2020;5(4) https://doi.org/10.21037/vats.2019.12.07.
21. Kent M, Wang T, Whyte R, et al. Open, video-assisted thoracic surgery, and robotic lobectomy: review of a national database. Ann Thorac Surg. 2014;97:236–42; discussion 242–4. https://doi.org/10.1016/j.athoracsur.2013.07.117.
22. Kent MS, Hartwig MG, Vallières E, et al. Pulmonary Open, Robotic, and Thoracoscopic Lobectomy (PORTaL) study: survival analysis of 6646 cases. Ann Surg. 2023;277:1002–9. https://doi.org/10.1097/SLA.0000000000005820.
23. Kneuertz PJ, Abdel-Rasoul M, D'Souza DM, et al. Segmentectomy for clinical stage I non-small cell lung cancer: national benchmarks for nodal staging and outcomes by operative approach. Cancer. 2022;128:1483–92. https://doi.org/10.1002/cncr.34071.
24. Kneuertz PJ, Singer E, D'Souza DM, et al. Hospital cost and clinical effectiveness of robotic-assisted versus video-assisted thoracoscopic and open lobectomy: a propensity score-weighted comparison. J Thorac Cardiovasc Surg. 2019;157:2018–2026.e2. https://doi.org/10.1016/j.jtcvs.2018.12.101.
25. Kosarek L, Busch E, Abbas A, et al. Effective use of bronchial blockers in lung isolation surgery: an analysis of 130 cases. Ochsner J. 2013;13:389–93.
26. Kratzer TB, Bandi P, Freedman ND, et al. Lung cancer statistics, 2023. Cancer. 2024;130:1330–48. https://doi.org/10.1002/cncr.35128.
27. Lee EC, Lazzaro RS, Glassman LR, et al. Switching from thoracoscopic to robotic platform for lobectomy: report of learning curve and outcome. Innovations (Phila). 2020;15:235–42. https://doi.org/10.1177/1556984520911670.

28. Lee JH, Hong JI, Kim HK. Single-port robotic subcostal major pulmonary resection using the single-port robotic system. World J Surg. 2024;48:713–22. https://doi.org/10.1002/wjs.12051.
29. Li C, Hu Y, Huang J, et al. Comparison of robotic-assisted lobectomy with video-assisted thoracic surgery for stage IIB-IIIA non-small cell lung cancer. Transl Lung Cancer Res. 2019;8:820–8. https://doi.org/10.21037/tlcr.2019.10.15.
30. Liang H, Liang W, Zhao L, et al. Robotic versus video-assisted lobectomy/segmentectomy for lung cancer: a meta-analysis. Ann Surg. 2018;268:254–9. https://doi.org/10.1097/SLA.0000000000002346.
31. Louie BE, Farivar AS, Aye RW, Vallières E. Early experience with robotic lung resection results in similar operative outcomes and morbidity when compared with matched video-assisted thoracoscopic surgery cases. Ann Thorac Surg. 2012;93:1598–604; discussion 1604-5. https://doi.org/10.1016/j.athoracsur.2012.01.067.
32. Ma J, Li X, Zhao S, et al. Robot-assisted thoracic surgery versus video-assisted thoracic surgery for lung lobectomy or segmentectomy in patients with non-small cell lung cancer: a meta-analysis. BMC Cancer. 2021;21:498. https://doi.org/10.1186/s12885-021-08241-5.
33. Marshall MB, Wee JO. Robotic platform use in general thoracic surgery. JAMA Surg. 2019;154:1066–7. https://doi.org/10.1001/jamasurg.2019.3361.
34. McKenna RJ. Lobectomy by video-assisted thoracic surgery with mediastinal node sampling for lung cancer. J Thorac Cardiovasc Surg. 1994;107:879–81; discussion 881–2.
35. Melfi FMA, Menconi GF, Mariani AM, Angeletti CA. Early experience with robotic technology for thoracoscopic surgery. Eur J Cardiothorac Surg. 2002;21:864–8. https://doi.org/10.1016/s1010-7940(02)00102-1.
36. Morgan JA, Ginsburg ME, Sonett JR, et al. Advanced thoracoscopic procedures are facilitated by computer-aided robotic technology. Eur J Cardiothorac Surg. 2003;23:883–7; discussion 887. https://doi.org/10.1016/s1010-7940(03)00160-x.
37. Nelson DB, Mehran RJ, Mitchell KG, et al. Robotic-assisted lobectomy for non-small cell lung cancer: a comprehensive institutional experience. Ann Thorac Surg. 2019;108:370–6. https://doi.org/10.1016/j.athoracsur.2019.03.051.
38. Ng CSH, MacDonald JK, Gilbert S, et al. Optimal approach to lobectomy for non-small cell lung cancer: systemic review and meta-analysis. Innovations (Phila). 2019;14:90–116. https://doi.org/10.1177/1556984519837027.
39. Nguyen DM, Sarkaria IS, Song C, et al. Clinical and economic comparative effectiveness of robotic-assisted, video-assisted thoracoscopic, and open lobectomy. J Thorac Dis. 2020;12:296–306. https://doi.org/10.21037/jtd.2020.01.40.
40. Novellis P, Bottoni E, Voulaz E, et al. Robotic surgery, video-assisted thoracic surgery, and open surgery for early stage lung cancer: comparison of costs and outcomes at a single institute. J Thorac Dis. 2018;10:790–8. https://doi.org/10.21037/jtd.2018.01.123.
41. Oh DS. Innovations in robotic surgery and recent developments in the SP platform. Ann Cardiothorac Surg. 2023;12:126–7. https://doi.org/10.21037/acs-2022-urats-28.
42. Oh DS, Reddy RM, Gorrepati ML, et al. Robotic-assisted, video-assisted thoracoscopic and open lobectomy: propensity-matched analysis of recent premier data. Ann Thorac Surg. 2017;104:1733–40. https://doi.org/10.1016/j.athoracsur.2017.06.020.
43. Oh DS, Tisol WB, Cesnik L, et al. Port strategies for robot-assisted lobectomy by high-volume thoracic surgeons: a nationwide survey. Innovations (Phila). 2019;14:545–52. https://doi.org/10.1177/1556984519883643.
44. Park BJ, Melfi F, Mussi A, et al. Robotic lobectomy for non-small cell lung cancer (NSCLC): long-term oncologic results. J Thorac Cardiovasc Surg. 2012;143:383–9. https://doi.org/10.1016/j.jtcvs.2011.10.055.
45. Park BJ, Yang H-X, Woo KM, Sima CS. Minimally invasive (robotic assisted thoracic surgery and video-assisted thoracic surgery) lobectomy for the treatment of locally advanced non-small cell lung cancer. J Thorac Dis. 2016;8:S406–13. https://doi.org/10.21037/jtd.2016.04.56.
46. Petrov R, Bakhos C, Abbas A. Robotic portal lung resection. In: robotic surgery: clinical perceptions, approaches and challenges; 2019. pp. 3–15.
47. Potter AL, Puttaraju T, Sulit JC, et al. Assessing the number of annual lung cancer resections performed in the United States. Shanghai Chest. 2023;7:29. https://doi.org/10.21037/shc-22-7.

48. Reddy RM, Gorrepati ML, Oh DS, et al. Robotic-assisted versus thoracoscopic lobectomy outcomes from high-volume thoracic surgeons. Ann Thorac Surg. 2018;106:902–8. https://doi.org/10.1016/j.athoracsur.2018.03.048.
49. Sakakura N, Eguchi T. Port placement variations for robotic lung resection: focusing on their history, conventional look-up-view and horizontal open-thoracotomy-view techniques, and more. J Pers Med. 2023;13 https://doi.org/10.3390/jpm13020230.
50. Sarkaria IS, Gorrepati ML, Mehendale S, Oh DS. Lobectomy in octogenarians: real world outcomes for robotic-assisted, video-assisted thoracoscopic, and open approaches. J Thorac Dis. 2019;11:2420–30. https://doi.org/10.21037/jtd.2019.05.52.
51. Sepesi B, Zhou N, William WN, et al. Surgical outcomes after neoadjuvant nivolumab or nivolumab with ipilimumab in patients with non-small cell lung cancer. J Thorac Cardiovasc Surg. 2022;164:1327–37. https://doi.org/10.1016/j.jtcvs.2022.01.019.
52. Servais EL, Miller DL, Thibault D, et al. Conversion to thoracotomy during thoracoscopic vs robotic lobectomy: predictors and outcomes. Ann Thorac Surg. 2022;114:409–17. https://doi.org/10.1016/j.athoracsur.2021.10.067.
53. Shen J. Prof. Abbas E. Abbas: a robotic thoracic practice can provide both clinical and financial benefits for an academic institution. J Thorac Dis. 2017;9:E573–5. https://doi.org/10.21037/jtd.2017.04.72.
54. Siegel RL, Giaquinto AN, Jemal A. Cancer statistics, 2024. CA Cancer J Clin. 2024;74:12–49. https://doi.org/10.3322/caac.21820.
55. Subramanian MP, Liu J, Chapman WC, et al. Utilization trends, outcomes, and cost in minimally invasive lobectomy. Ann Thorac Surg. 2019;108:1648–55. https://doi.org/10.1016/j.athoracsur.2019.06.049.
56. Tong BC, Gu L, Wang X, et al. Perioperative outcomes of pulmonary resection after neoadjuvant pembrolizumab in patients with non-small cell lung cancer. J Thorac Cardiovasc Surg. 2022;163:427–36. https://doi.org/10.1016/j.jtcvs.2021.02.099.
57. Veluswamy RR, Whittaker Brown S-A, Mhango G, et al. Comparative effectiveness of robotic-assisted surgery for resectable lung cancer in older patients. Chest. 2020;157:1313–21. https://doi.org/10.1016/j.chest.2019.09.017.
58. Worrell SG, Dedhia P, Gilbert C, et al. The cost and quality of life outcomes in developing a robotic lobectomy program. J Robot Surg. 2019;13:239–43. https://doi.org/10.1007/s11701-018-0844-z.
59. Wu CF, Cheng C, Suen KH, et al. A preclinical feasibility study of single-port robotic subcostal anatomical lung resection and subxiphoid thymectomy using the da Vinci® SP system. Diagnostics (Basel). 2023;13 https://doi.org/10.3390/diagnostics13030460.
60. Wu H, Jin R, Yang S, et al. Long-term and short-term outcomes of robot- versus video-assisted anatomic lung resection in lung cancer: a systematic review and meta-analysis. Eur J Cardiothorac Surg. 2021;59:732–40. https://doi.org/10.1093/ejcts/ezaa426.
61. Yang Y, Song L, Huang J, et al. A uniportal right upper lobectomy by three-arm robotic-assisted thoracoscopic surgery using the da Vinci (Xi) Surgical System in the treatment of early-stage lung cancer. Transl Lung Cancer Res. 2021;10:1571–5. https://doi.org/10.21037/tlcr-21-207.
62. Ye X, Xie L, Chen G, et al. Robotic thoracic surgery versus video-assisted thoracic surgery for lung cancer: a meta-analysis. Interact Cardiovasc Thorac Surg. 2015;21:409–14. https://doi.org/10.1093/icvts/ivv155.
63. Zervos M, Song A, Li Y, et al. Clinical and economic outcomes of using robotic versus hand-held staplers during robotic lobectomy. Innovations (Phila). 2021;16:470–6. https://doi.org/10.1177/15569845211040814.
64. Zhang J, Feng Q, Huang Y, et al. Updated evaluation of robotic- and video-assisted thoracoscopic lobectomy or Segmentectomy for lung cancer: a systematic review and meta-analysis. Front Oncol. 2022;12:853530. https://doi.org/10.3389/fonc.2022.853530.
65. Zhang Y, Chen C, Hu J, et al. Early outcomes of robotic versus thoracoscopic segmentectomy for early-stage lung cancer: a multi-institutional propensity score-matched analysis. J Thorac Cardiovasc Surg. 2020;160:1363–72. https://doi.org/10.1016/j.jtcvs.2019.12.112.

32 Robotic-Assisted Cardiac Surgery

Amalia A. Jonsson and Michael E. Halkos

Introduction

Robotic technology has infiltrated into nearly every surgical domain over the past two decades, and cardiac surgery is no exception. This growth is driven by patient and referring cardiologist desire for less invasive options with safe and durable results. Despite the documented safety and efficacy of these techniques, adoption has been slow with less than 15% of robotic mitral valve repairs being performed robotically [1] and less than 1% of coronary bypass procedures being performed robotically [2]. This slow adoption is likely due to the high resource commitment required to start a robotics program and the steep learning curve for not only the surgeon but the entire team when learning these procedures.

Robotic-Assisted Coronary Artery Bypass

Minimally invasive coronary bypass has evolved significantly over the last decade. A wide variety of techniques from minimally invasive direct coronary artery bypass (MIDCAB) where the left internal mammary artery (LIMA) is harvested under direct vision to totally endoscopic robotic CABG (TECAB) where multivessel bypass is performed entirely endoscopically with the aid of the robot are currently performed. Robotic-assisted coronary bypass, our preferred minimally invasive technique, is an attractive option in the management of patients with isolated LAD disease or multivessel coronary disease providing the benefits of the left internal mammary artery (LIMA) to the left anterior descending (LAD) graft while avoiding

A. A. Jonsson (✉) · M. E. Halkos
Division of Cardiothoracic Surgery, Emory University School of Medicine, Atlanta, GA, USA
e-mail: Amalia.jonsson@emory.edu

S. Samreen et al. (eds.), *The SAGES Manual of Robotic Surgery*,
https://doi.org/10.1007/978-3-031-86927-3_32

the morbidity of a sternotomy. The procedure includes robotic LIMA harvest and a handsewn anastomosis performed through a small non-rib-spreading anterior mini-thoracotomy. For patients with multivessel coronary artery disease, this technique can be combined with percutaneous coronary intervention (PCI) to create a hybrid revascularization strategy.

Indications and Patient Selection

Robotic-assisted CABG can be used to treat patients with isolated LAD disease or can be applied to patients with multivessel coronary disease in conjunction with PCI in a hybrid revascularization (HCR) strategy. Absolute contraindications to this technique include prior cardiac surgery, severe lung disease which would preclude single lung ventilation, hemodynamic instability, or ongoing ischemia. Relative contraindications include truncal obesity and large ventricular size due to low ejection fraction. In terms of coronary anatomy, patients must have a segment of non-intramyocardial, noncalcified LAD. In the case of planned hybrid revascularization, non-LAD target vessels must have reasonable PCI options.

Operative Technique

Our technique requires that single lung ventilation be achieved using a double-lumen endotracheal tube or a bronchial blocker. A gel roll is placed underneath the left chest just inferior to the scapula so that the shoulder will gently fall away. Three 8 mm trocars are placed in the left chest, and CO^2 insufflation (8–12 mm Hg) is used. Instead of placing the camera port in a specific interspace, we always aim to put the camera port at the midpoint between the costal margin and the clavicle. Prior to placing the camera port, the chest is entered with a blunt instrument (Kelly clamp) so that there is minimal force needed to insert the camera port. This is almost always the fourth or fifth interspace and lies usually at or just posterior to the anterior axillary line. The superior port is placed two interspaces superior and slightly medial to the camera port and is placed after localizing with a spinal needle so the surgeon can appreciate the angle and location of entry. Placing this port too posteriorly will lead to conflict with the left shoulder. The inferior port is placed two or three interspaces below the camera port and should be slightly inferior to the apex of the heart. Similarly, a spinal needle can be used to identify the best location for port placement (Fig. 32.1). The da Vinci (Intuitive Surgical, Sunnyvale, California) robot is then used to harvest the LIMA in a semi-skeletonized fashion. We begin by removing the endothoracic fascia and transversus thoracic muscle to aid with exposure of the LIMA. The LIMA is harvested en bloc with the two mammary veins using the robotic clip applier to ligate large branches. A posterior pericardial window is made, and pericardial fat is removed from the anterior pericardium using electrocautery. Heparin is administered to achieve an ACT >300, and the LIMA is divided distally

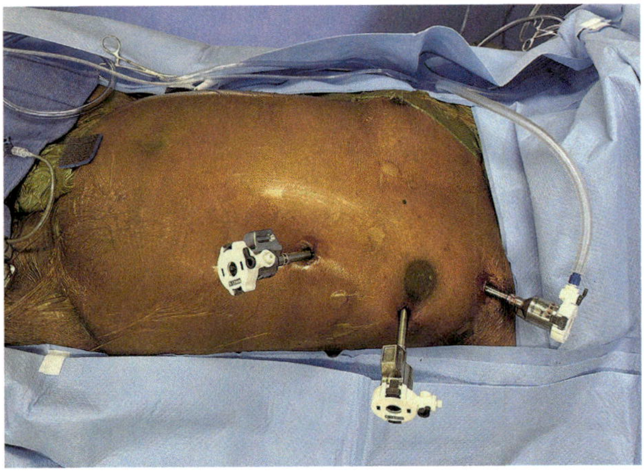

Fig. 32.1 Port placement for robotic-assisted CABG

between clips. The pericardium is opened longitudinally and the distal LAD target is identified. Care is taken to avoid injury to the phrenic nerve superiorly and inferiorly if the pericardiotomy is extended horizontally. The robot is then undocked and a 3–4 cm non-rib-spreading anterolateral thoracotomy is created after localizing the incision using a spinal needle and the endoscope. A spinal needle is inserted into either the fourth or fifth interspace and the carbon dioxide insufflation is disconnected to allow the heart to return to its normal position. With the endoscope, the surgeon is watching to see if the LAD at the planned site of anastomosis approaches the tip of the spinal needle. A soft tissue retractor (Edwards Lifesciences, Irvine, California) is used to provide gentle soft tissue retraction to expose the mid-distal third of the LAD. The Nuvo off-pump stabilizer (Medtronic Corp, Minneapolis, Minn) is inserted through the inferior robotic port site and used to stabilize the LAD at the planned site of the anastomosis (Fig. 32.2). The LIMA is retrieved from the chest and prepared in the usual fashion. A soft silastic vessel loop is placed around the LAD proximal to the planned site of the anastomosis and a period of test occlusion is performed for 3 min to ensure hemodynamic and electrical stability. After the LAD arteriotomy is completed, an appropriately sized intracoronary shunt is placed and a manual LIMA to LAD anastomosis is then performed off-pump using an 8-0 polypropylene suture. The shunt is removed prior to the final few sutures, and the vessel is tacked in place using a 6-0 polypropylene suture (Fig. 32.3). A 28 French Blake drain is left in the left pleural space via the inferior trocar site. The minithoracotomy incision is closed in multiple layers (Fig. 32.4).

Outcomes

This technique has yielded excellent results. In review of our first 1000 robotic-assisted CABG procedures, we demonstrated a 0.6% 30-day mortality and 0.5% stroke rate. Conversion to sternotomy was low (3.0%), as was repeat

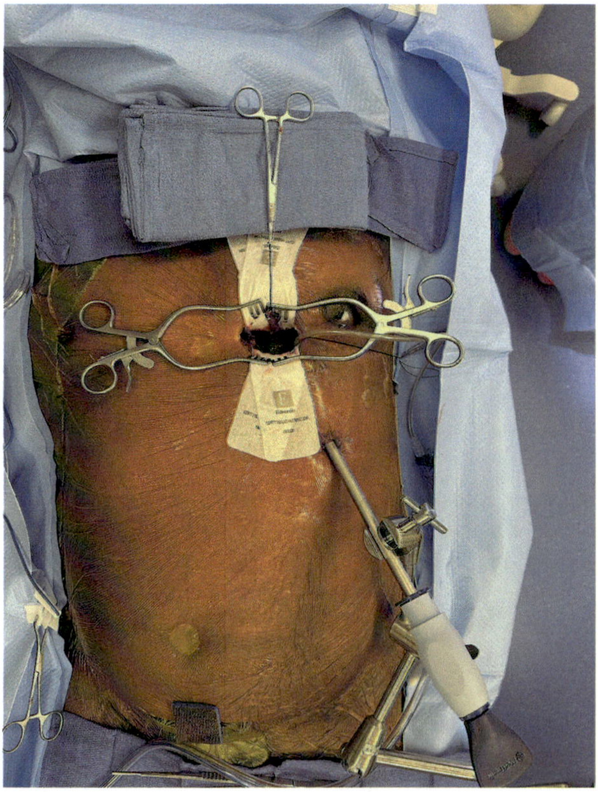

Fig. 32.2 Minithoracotomy and setup for anastomosis

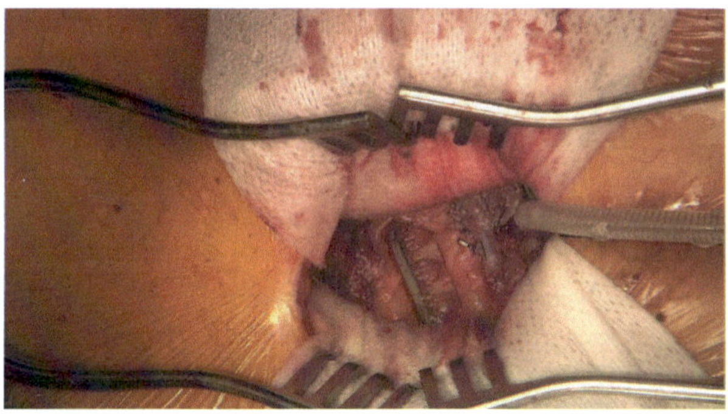

Fig. 32.3 Completed LIMA to LAD anastomosis

revascularization (1.0%), and left internal mammary to left anterior descending artery patency was high at 97% [3]. We recently developed a fast-track protocol where appropriate patients can bypass the ICU, cutting down on hospital length of stay as well as inpatient costs without affecting patient outcomes [4]. In addition to these positive clinical outcomes, patients also benefit from faster recovery and faster return to normal activities.

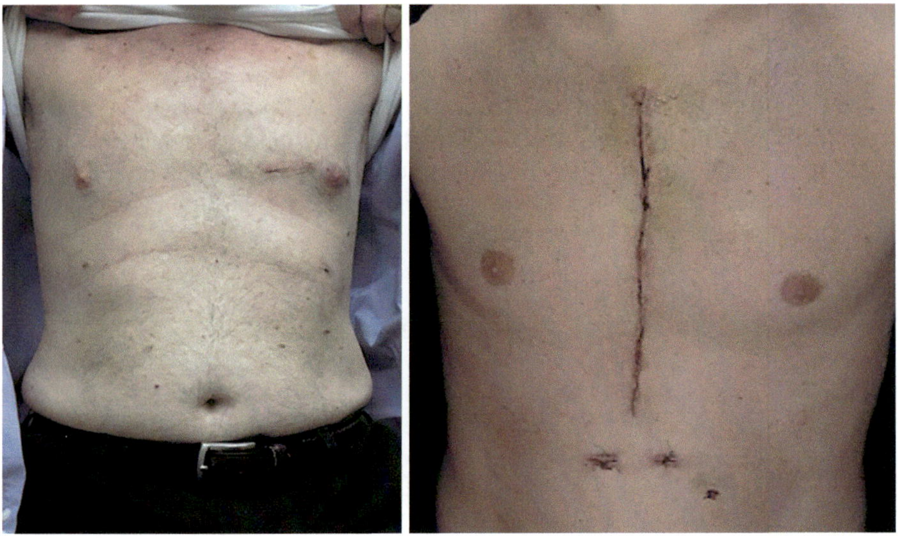

Fig. 32.4 Robotic-assisted CABG incisions (left) vs traditional sternotomy (right)

Robotic-Assisted TECAB

While robotic-assisted LIMA harvest is an excellent alternative to traditional CABG, some surgeons have transitioned to robot-assisted totally endoscopic coronary artery bypass (TECAB). The benefits of TECAB are even less tissue trauma because the need for a minithoracotomy is obviated, and the potential to perform multivessel bypass, including to the circumflex and right coronary territories. The first significant series, reported by Mohr and colleagues in 2001, described 27 patients who underwent LIMA harvest and endoscopic LIMA to LAD anastomosis using the da Vinci telemanipulation system [5]. In 2006, a multicenter FDA-sanctioned trial demonstrated the safety and efficacy of TECAB using the da Vinci system in 85 patients [6]. Since that time, select centers have begun to routinely perform multivessel TECAB with excellent results [7]. Unfortunately, the complexity of the operation and significant learning curve result in prolonged operative times and possibly increased complication rates early in a surgeon's experience [8, 9]. Despite overall good short-term results with TECAB, the aforementioned shortcomings have limited its widespread adoption.

Hybrid Coronary Revascularization (HCR)

With good outcomes for minimally invasive CABG surgery established, increasing demand for minimally invasive procedures, mediocre outcomes with saphenous vein grafts, and improved results with PCI using drug-eluting stent (DES), hybrid coronary revascularization (HCR) has garnered attention from surgeons, cardiologists, and patients. While many minimally invasive CABG techniques have been described, we feel that robotic-assisted CABG is ideally suited for this revascularization strategy in appropriate coronary anatomy. The robotic-assisted LIMA harvest is a relatively simple and short procedure and allows for versatility when combining with non-LAD PCI, which can be performed either before, after, or concomitantly with the surgical procedure. HCR has been repeatedly shown to be safe and effective [10–13] for many different patient populations. Although long-term outcomes with HCR are lacking, this strategy is quickly becoming an important option in the revascularization algorithm.

Robotic-Assisted Mitral Valve Surgery

Nonsternotomy approaches to the mitral valve range from a modestly sized right thoracotomy approach to total endoscopic techniques, some of which employ robotics. Our technique includes a double-lumen endotracheal tube and transesophageal echocardiography. The patient is positioned supine with a bump under the right side of the chest. Peripheral cannulation for cardiopulmonary bypass is utilized, most frequently femoral arterial and venous; however, axillary arterial cannulation can be used if there is a contraindication to femoral perfusion. The camera port is inserted in the fourth or fifth interspace and the endoscope is used to assess for any pleural adhesions. Three additional robotic 8 mm ports are placed in the right chest as well as a 3 cm service port through which the bedside assistant will work. Three angiocatheters are inserted as well which will be used for traction sutures (Figs. 32.5 and 32.6). Heparin is administered and the femoral vessels are cannulated using Seldinger technique and echo guidance. Typically, we place an additional cannula in the right internal jugular vein to achieve bicaval cannulation. The da Vinci Xi robot (Intuitive Surgical, Sunnyvale, CA) is then docked, and CO_2 insufflation is used for the entirety of the procedure. Cardiopulmonary bypass is initiated. The pericardium is opened using electrocautery and stay sutures are placed in the pericardium as well as in the diaphragm to aid with visualization. Aortic occlusion is

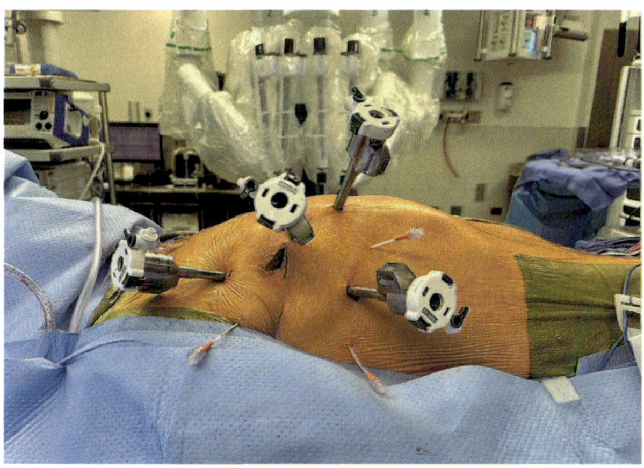

Fig. 32.5 Port placement for robotic mitral valve surgery

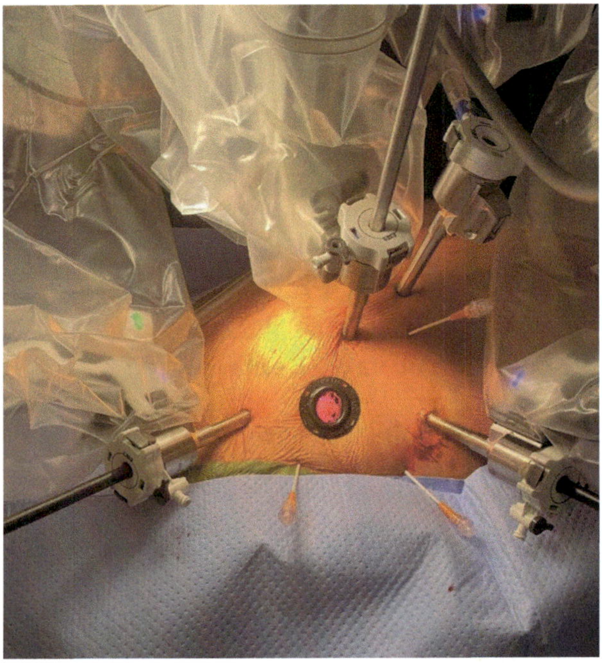

Fig. 32.6 Setup for robotic mitral valve surgery

achieved either with the endoaortic balloon (Edwards Lifesciences, Irvine, CA) or with a transthoracic clamp. Antegrade cardioplegia is delivered either via the endoaortic balloon's internal lumen or via an aortic tac inserted into the ascending aorta. Exposure of the mitral valve is achieved via left atriotomy using a robotic atrial retractor. Traditional mitral repair techniques including neocords, leaflet resection, plication, and annuloplasty are performed with the aid of the bedside assistant who uses long instruments introduced via the service port. When necessary, mitral replacement with either bioprosthetic or mechanical valves is performed. Concomitant procedures including atrial ablation, left atrial appendage closure, and tricuspid valvuloplasty are performed when indicated. This technique can also be used for resection of intracardiac tumors and ASD closures.

Patient Selection

There are very few absolute contraindications to robotic mitral valve surgery. As opposed to robotic coronary bypass in which a larger body habitus is a limitation, robotic mitral valve surgery is not contraindicated in these patients and exposure may even be easier than sternotomy and some right chest approaches for the morbidly obese patient. The only contraindications are dense right chest adhesions and vascular disease with no peripheral cannulation options. We have safely used this technique in patients who have had prior right chest cardiac surgery as well as prior cardiac surgery via sternotomy [14, 15].

Outcomes

Robotic intracardiac surgery can be performed with excellent safety and efficacy. Our technique has a less than 1% mortality and stroke rate, and at 6 years freedom from recurrent 2+ or greater MR was 85%, with only 3.9% of patients requiring reoperation for mitral repair failure [16]. Other experienced centers have published similar results [17, 18]. The safety of robotic mitral surgery is comparable to other approaches including thoracotomy and sternotomy and is associated with shorter length of stay and lower hospital readmissions [1].

Robotic Aortic Valve Replacement

One of the newest applications in robotic cardiac surgery is robotic aortic valve replacement. Although not yet widely performed, initial results from this technique are encouraging with less than 1% mortality and stroke rates [19]. Aortic valve replacement can be performed in conjunction with mitral valve procedures, ablations, and transaortic septal myectomy (Fig. 32.7).

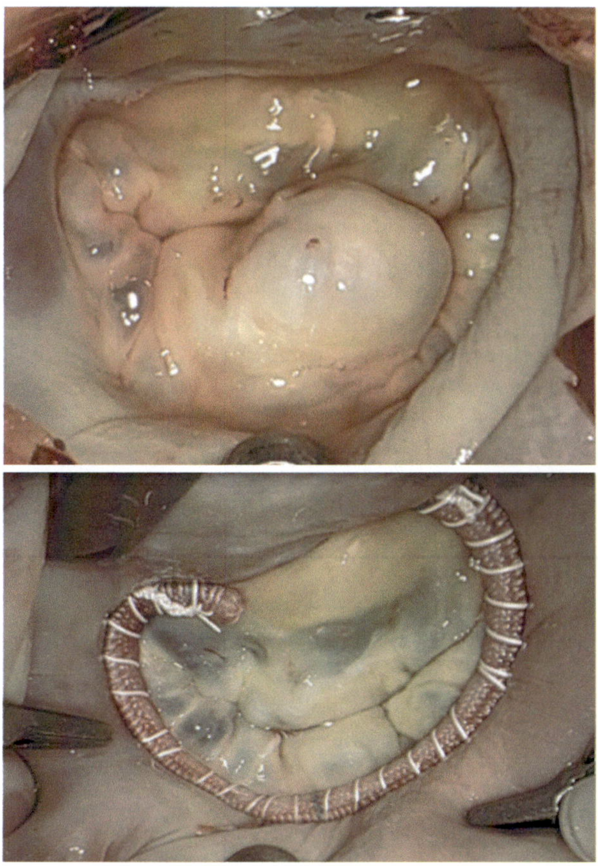

Fig. 32.7 Mitral valve before and after repair. This patient had posterior leaflet prolapse which was treated with neocords and annuloplasty

Conclusion

As demand grows for less invasive procedures, we must ensure that we can meet this demand without compromising short- or long-term patient outcomes. Robotic technology is a crucial tool for allowing surgeons to perform gold standard interventions through smaller incisions with minimal morbidity. Despite the slow early adoption in cardiac surgery, robotic cardiac surgical procedures are now routinely performed in many centers across North America and around the world.

References

1. Mori M, Parsons N, Krane M, Guy TS, Grossi EA, Dearani JA, Habib RH, Badhwar V, Geirsson A. Robotic mitral valve repair for degenerative mitral regurgitation. Ann Thorac Surg. 2024;117(1):96–104.
2. Whellan DJ, McCarey MM, Taylor BS, et al. Trends in robotic-assisted coronary artery bypass grafts: a study of the society of thoracic surgeons adult cardiac surgery database, 2006 to 2012. Ann Thorac Surg. 2016;102:140–6.
3. Jonsson A, Binongo J, Patel P, Wang Y, Garner V, Mitchell-Cooks D, Halkos ME. Mastering the learning curve for robotic-assisted coronary artery bypass surgery. Ann Thorac Surg. 2023;115(5):1118–25.
4. Edwards J, Binongo J, Mullin B, Wei J, Ghelani K, Kumarasamy M, Hanson P, Duggan M, Shoffstall J, Halkos M. Intensive care unit bypass for robotic-assisted single-vessel coronary artery bypass grafting. Ann Thorac Surg. 2023;115:511.
5. Mohr FW, Falk V, Diegeler A, Walther T, Gummert JF, Bucerius J, et al. Computer-enhanced "robotic" cardiac surgery: experience in 148 patients. J Thorac Cardiovasc Surg. 2001;121(5):842–53.
6. Argenziano M, Katz M, Bonatti J, Srivastava S, Murphy D, Poirier R, et al. Results of the prospective multicenter trial of robotically assisted totally endoscopic coronary artery bypass grafting. Ann Thorac Surg. 2006;81(5):1666–75.
7. Bonaros N, Schachner T, Lehr E, Kofler M, Wiedemann D, Hong P, et al. Five hundred cases of robotic totally endoscopic coronary artery bypass grafting: predictors of success and safety. Ann Thorac Surg. 2013;95(3):803–12.
8. Bonatti J, Schachner T, Bonaros N, Öhlinger A, Danzmayr M, Jonetzko P, et al. Technical challenges in totally endoscopic robotic coronary artery bypass grafting. J Thorac Cardiovasc Surg. 2006;131(1):146–53.
9. Bonaros N, Schachner T, Wiedemann D, Oehlinger A, Ruetzler E, Feuchtner G, et al. Quality of life improvement after robotically assisted coronary artery bypass grafting. Cardiology. 2009;114(1):59–66.
10. Harskamp RE, Williams JB, Halkos ME, Lopes RD, Tijssen JGP, Ferguson TB, et al. Meta-analysis of minimally invasive coronary artery bypass versus drug-eluting stents for isolated left anterior descending coronary artery disease. J Thorac Cardiovasc Surg. 2014;148(5):1837–42.
11. Kayatta MO, Halkos ME, Puskas JD. Hybrid coronary revascularization for the treatment of multivessel coronary artery disease. Ann Cardiothorac Surg. 2018;7(4):500–5.
12. Halkos ME, Vassiliades TA, Douglas JS, Morris DC, Rab ST, Liberman HA, et al. Hybrid coronary revascularization versus off-pump coronary artery bypass grafting for the treatment of multivessel coronary artery disease. Ann Thorac Surg. 2011;92(5):1695–701.
13. Gao C, Yang M, Wu Y, Wang G, Xiao C, Liu H, et al. Hybrid coronary revascularization by endoscopic robotic coronary artery bypass grafting on beating heart and stent placement. Ann Thorac Surg. 2009;87(3):737–41.
14. Murphy DA, Jonsson AA, Halkos ME. Endoscopic robotic mitral valve surgery in patients with previous sternotomy cardiac surgery. Innovations (Phila). 2022;17(4):297–303. 14

15. Murphy DA, Moss E, Miller J, Halkos ME. Repeat robotic endoscopic mitral valve operation: a safe and effective strategy. Ann Thorac Surg. 2018;105(6):1704–9.
16. Murphy DA, Moss E, Binongo J, Miller JS, Macheers SK, Sarin EL, Herzog AM, Thourani VH, Guyton RA, Halkos ME. The expanding role of endoscopic robotics in mitral valve surgery: 1,257 consecutive procedures. Ann Thorac Surg. 2015;100(5):1675–81.
17. Ramzy D, Trento A, Cheng W, De Robertis MA, Mirocha J, Ruzza A, Kass RM. Three hundred robotic-assisted mitral valve repairs: the Cedars-Sinai experience. J Thorac Cardiovasc Surg. 2014;147(1):228–35.
18. Mihaljevic T, Jarrett CM, Gillinov AM, Williams SJ, DeVilliers PA, Stewart WJ, Svensson LG, Sabik JF 3rd, Blackstone EH. Robotic repair of posterior mitral valve prolapse versus conventional approaches: potential realized. J Thorac Cardiovasc Surg. 2011;141(1):72–80. e1–4
19. Badhwar V, Pereda D, Khaliel FH, Poffo R, Darehzereshki A, Mehaffey JH, Yan TD, Melnitchouk S, Geirsson A, Arghami A, Navia JL, Raikar GV, Weber AC, Ramzy D, Černý Š, Vojáček J, Smith RL, Bonatti J, Thourani VH, Wei LM. Outcomes following initial multicenter experience with robotic aortic valve replacement: defining a path forward. J Thorac Cardiovasc Surg. 2024;S0022-5223(24):00078–3.

33 Mediastinal Procedures

Brittney Williams and Manu Sancheti

Introduction

Historically, resection of mediastinal pathology has required invasive surgical approaches via sternotomy, posterolateral thoracotomy, or anterolateral thoracotomy with or without transverse sternotomy (clamshell). Since the early 1990s, minimally invasive techniques have transformed mediastinal surgery, allowing for smaller incisions, shorter hospital stays, improved postoperative pain, and comparable oncologic outcomes when applicable [1, 2]. Video-assisted thoracoscopic surgery (VATS) has been utilized for various mediastinal pathologies including thymectomy for myasthenia gravis, thymoma and thymic carcinoma, germ cell tumors, neurogenic tumors, mediastinal cysts, lymphoma, and ectopic parathyroid and thyroid tissue [3].

Given the limited working space within the mediastinum and close proximity to great vessels, robotic-assisted thoracoscopic surgery has allowed for several advantages to navigation and dissection of the mediastinum. The benefits of robotics as compared to VATS include articulating instruments, three-dimensional visualization, scaling down of operative movements, and lack of tremor. Disadvantages include lack of tactile sensation, higher costs, initial learning curve, and lack of standardized approaches to robotic mediastinal procedures.

In this chapter, approaches to robotic mediastinal procedures are detailed, specifically categorized into three anatomical sections, the anterior, middle, and posterior mediastinum. The mediastinum is bounded laterally by the pleura, superiorly by the thoracic inlet, posteriorly by the thoracic spine, and inferiorly by the diaphragm. Within these boundaries, the mediastinum is further divided into anterior, middle, and posterior compartments. The anterior mediastinum is located between

B. Williams · M. Sancheti (✉)
Emory University School of Medicine, Atlanta, GA, USA
e-mail: manu.suraj.sancheti@emory.edu

S. Samreen et al. (eds.), *The SAGES Manual of Robotic Surgery*,
https://doi.org/10.1007/978-3-031-86927-3_33

the sternum and anterior border of the pericardium. The middle mediastinum lies between the anterior and posterior borders of the pericardium. The posterior mediastinum is the space between the posterior border of the pericardium and the anterior longitudinal ligament of the thoracic spine.

Preoperative Evaluation and Patient Selection

Preoperative evaluation for robotic mediastinal procedures is generally the same as open cases with several caveats. A thorough history and physical examination should be performed, particularly including history of prior chest surgeries that may indicate higher risk of conversion to an open procedure. Computed tomography (CT) with intravenous (IV) contrast is essential in evaluation of mediastinal lesions and their proximity to the great vessels and other important mediastinal structures as well as for planning port placement. Additional cross-sectional imaging can be useful in some circumstances, such as magnetic resonance imaging (MRI) in evaluating for local invasion and positron emission tomography (PET) for assessment of metastatic disease in malignant mediastinal pathologies. Histopathologic confirmation via percutaneous, transbronchial, or endoscopic biopsy can also be useful in cases where clinical, laboratory, or radiographic findings are inconclusive. Pulmonary function testing is recommended as poor pulmonary function may not allow for single-lung ventilation.

Patient selection plays a key role in successful completion of a robotic approach to mediastinal surgery as certain patient factors and past medical and surgery history can be prohibitive. In terms of patient factors, body habitus may preclude minimally invasive access to the anterior mediastinum. History of pleural space infections, malignancy, or prior instrumentation can result in chest wall adhesions that may require conversion to an open procedure. Inability to safely discern the appropriate anatomy for dissection is another common reason for conversion, which can be related to decreased working space from inability to tolerate carbon dioxide insufflation or single-lung ventilation. Other reasons for conversion to open include close proximity or involvement of vital mediastinal structures. The latter causes for conversion are largely avoided with appropriate preoperative workup.

General Port Placement and Robotic Positioning Considerations

Port placement and robotic positioning is a key aspect of successful mediastinal robotic operations. Positioning will vary depending on use of either the da Vinci Si or Xi surgical system (Intuitive Surgical, Sunnyvale, CA). In this chapter, the described approach will be based on use of the da Vinci Xi surgical system. In general, the camera port should be placed 10–20 cm away from the target anatomy.

Ports should be placed 6–10 cm apart (ideally 8 cm) to decrease conflict between the robotic arms. Preoperative imaging studies are key in determining appropriate port placement especially for masses in the middle mediastinum and posterior mediastinum where variability in tumor location is more common. Patient cart positioning will vary based on operating room layout.

Approach to Anterior Mediastinal Pathology

Anterior mediastinal pathologies for which robotic surgery has been utilized include thymus for myasthenia gravis, thymoma, lymphoma/lymph node excisional biopsy, germ cell tumors, and ectopic parathyroid and thyroid tissue. Specific preoperative consideration may be necessary for anterior mediastinal pathology. Myasthenia gravis patients have increased risks for general anesthesia requiring preoperative preparation with pyridostigmine, intravenous immune globulin (IVIG), or plasmapheresis. IVIG should be given 2 weeks prior to planned resection. Potential anesthetic-related issues include resistance to depolarizing paralytic agents, cholinergic crisis for neuromuscular blocking reversal agents, increased risks of aspiration, increased risks of respiratory failure, and continued requirements for intubation and ventilator use postoperatively. If the differential for the anterior mediastinal mass includes thymoma, screening for symptoms related to myasthenia gravis should be completed to direct further preoperative laboratory investigation to avoid potential anesthesia-related complications.

Indications for Robotic Anterior Mediastinal Mass Resection

Cross-sectional imaging, CT and/or MRI, is required to evaluate the association of an anterior mediastinal mass with its surrounding mediastinal structures to determine resectability of the lesion. In the case of a thymoma, complete resection is required for adequate treatment due to risk of recurrence. Therefore, Masaoka stage I tumors, enclosed within the thymic capsule, have been deemed acceptable for minimally invasive techniques [4]. Some data does suggest that minimally invasive resections of Masaoka stage I–III thymomas have equivalent rates of margin of positivity and similar 5-year survival, but longer-term follow-up is needed given the indolent nature of thymoma [5]. Robotic resections for anterior mediastinal germ cell tumors are indicated for mature teratomas and dermoid cysts. Seminomatous and non-seminomatous tumors are treated primarily with radiation and chemotherapy, respectively. If a mass persists after initial treatment, further medical treatment may be indicated or surgical resection if tumor markers AFP and beta-HCG are negative and remaining mass does not involve mediastinal structures. Excision of enlarged anterior mediastinal lymph nodes may also be appropriate for diagnosis of lymphoma or staging for other malignancies.

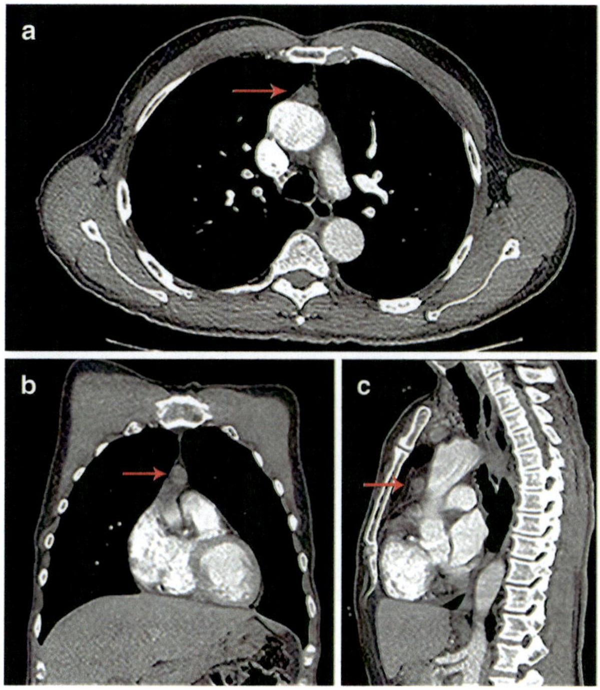

Fig. 33.1 Computed tomography scan for an anterior mediastinal mass. Red arrows point to the anterior mediastinal mass. (**a**) Axial, (**b**) coronal, (**c**) sagittal. Anterior mediastinal mass does not appear to involve surrounding mediastinal structures and appears to be encapsulated by thymus and surrounding thymic fat

Anterior Mediastinal Mass Example Case Scenario

A 67-year-old man undergoing workup for unintentional weight loss is found to have an incidental anterior mediastinal mass surrounded by thymus and thymic fat on CT (Fig. 33.1). He has no symptoms concerning for myasthenia gravis. Differential diagnosis included thymic hyperplasia, thymic carcinoma, thymoma, and lymphoma. The patient elected to undergo resection of the anterior mediastinal mass.

Surgical equipment used:

da Vinci Xi robotic system
da Vinci 0-degree camera
Long bipolar grasper
EndoWrist® Clip applier—small and large
EndoWrist® Cadiere forceps
Vessel sealer extend
8 mm instrument cannula × 3 (including one Optiview)
12 mm AirSeal trocar
5 mm Optiview trocar (optional)
5 mm 30-degree thoracoscope
Endo Catch bag
Kittner roll gauze sponges

Patient Positioning and Port Placement

Anterior mediastinal masses may be approached from either the right or the left side of the chest. In our example, a right-sided approach was used. A double-lumen endotracheal tube is inserted. The patient is placed in supine position with a jelly-roll, beanbag, or rolled sheet along the posterior midclavicular line to elevate the operative side. The arms are tucked with the arm on the operative side allowed to sit slightly below the OR table to allow more space for the robotic arms. The patient's entire chest is prepped and draped to allow access to the contralateral side if needed.

The right pleural space is accessed with an 8 mm Optiview trocar along the anterior axillary line at the midpoint of the sternum (typically the fifth intercostal space). The layers of the chest wall should be visualized during insertion to allow for safe entry into the pleural space (Fig. 33.2). After insufflation to 8 mmHg, two additional 8 mm ports are inserted under direct visualization along the anterior axillary line, port #1 in the third intercostal space and port #2 in the seventh intercostal space (Fig. 33.3). Port #1 can sometimes require bariatric length to clear the underlying arm. Finally, a 12 mm AirSeal is inserted in the midclavicular line as low as possible just above the diaphragm.

The robot is then driven into operative field from the contralateral side and perpendicular to the patient centered on the camera trocar. The ports are then secured into the robotic arms with the remote center of the three robotic ports just within the intercostal muscle of the chest wall. The 8 mm 0-degree da Vinci camera is passed into the center camera port. Under direct visualization, the Cadiere forceps are placed into the port #1 followed by the long bipolar grasper (or robotic vessel sealer) into port #2.

Anterior Mediastinal Mass Excision Operative Steps

The phrenic nerve is first identified along the pericardium, as this nerve must be preserved and defines the posterior border of the dissection. If unable to be visualized at any point in the operation, a 5 mm port can be placed on the contralateral side to allow the assistant to aid in visualization with a 30-degree thoracoscope. We use the long bipolar grasper to initiate the dissection of the mediastinal pleura just anterior to the phrenic nerve running along the superior vena cava (Fig. 33.4). The Kittner roll gauzes are inserted into the thoracic cavity through the access port to assist with absorbing minor bleeding and assist with retraction. The dissection of the mediastinal pleura is extended caudad to the inferior pole of the thymic tissue above the diaphragm denoting the right-sided inferior border of dissection. The mediastinal pleural incision is then extended cephalad to the innominate vein (Fig. 33.5). Care must be taken as the dissection nears the innominate vein, as clips may be necessary to divide vein branches to the thymus. Thymic tissue underneath the innominate is dissected free. The thymic tissues are dissected off the pericardium posteriorly to the mediastinal pleura on the left side which is incised at the same level as on the right side. The anterior dissection is started just medial to the

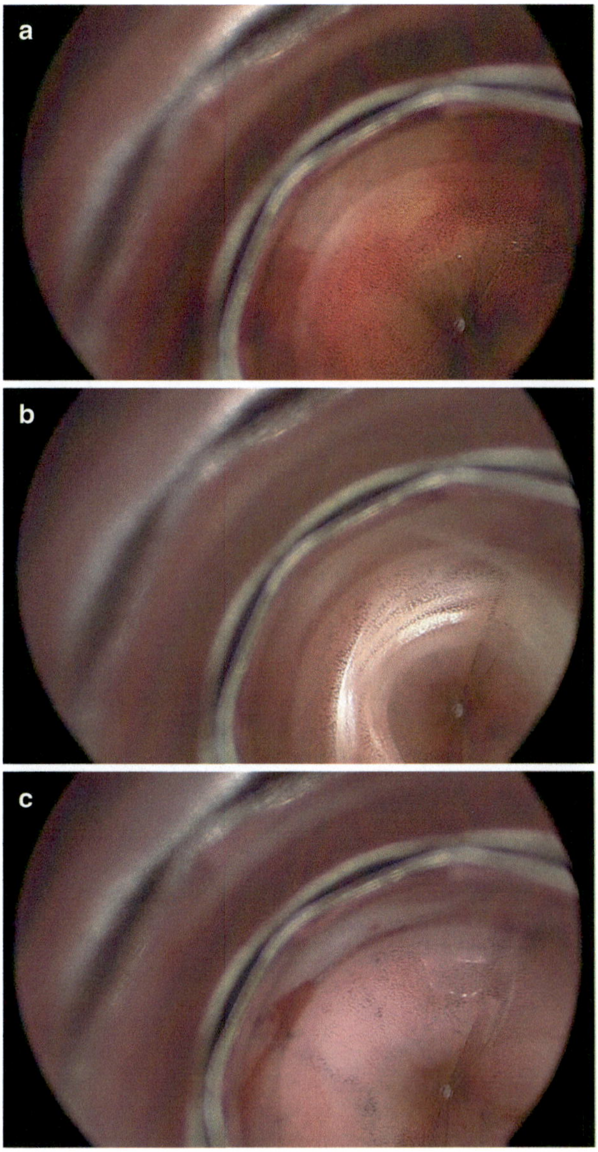

Fig. 33.2 Thoracic cavity entry using 5 mm Optiview trocar with 5 mm thoracoscope. (**a**) Subcutaneous fat layer, (**b**) muscle layer, (**c**) lung parenchyma visualized

internal mammary vessels (Fig. 33.6). Arterial branches may need to be clipped and divided supplying the thymus. The right-sided superior pole of the thymus is then dissected free using caudad and posterior traction (Fig. 33.7). A clip is usually necessary at the superior aspect of the pole to control bleeding. The dissection is then carried over to the left superior pole, which is similarly dissected away from the inferior neck (Fig. 33.8). The dissection is then carried over to the mediastinal pleura on the anterior aspect of the dissection along the sternum. The left pleural

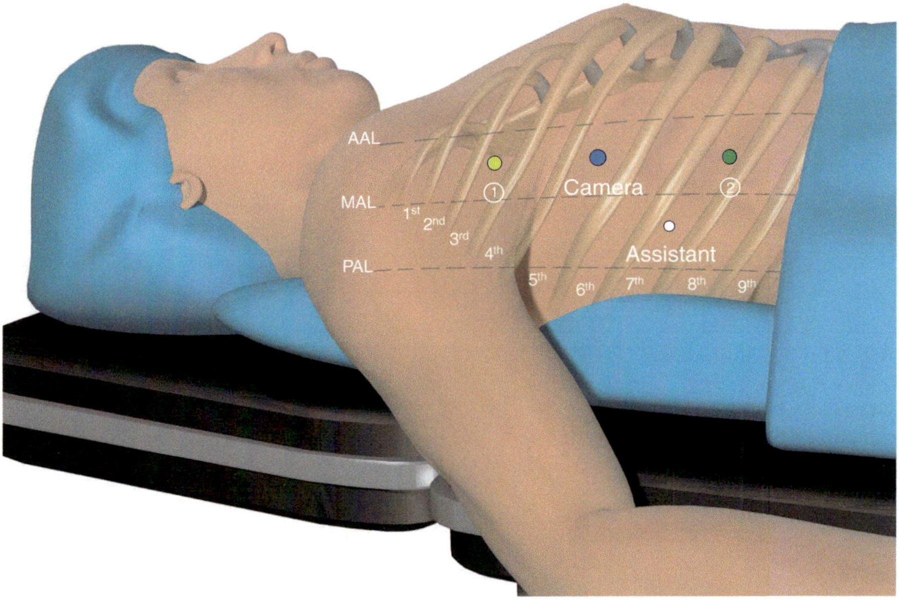

Fig. 33.3 Port placement for robotic anterior mediastinal mass resection. AAL (anterior axillary line), MAL (midaxillary line), PAL (posterior axillary line). Port sites are labeled blue for camera port, yellow for robotic port 1, green for robotic port 2

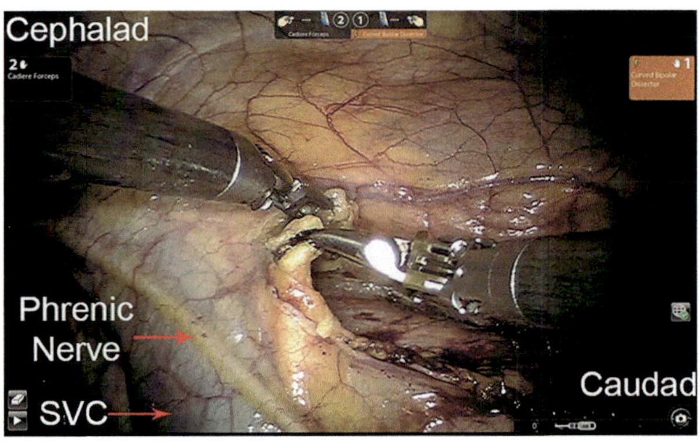

Fig. 33.4 Initial dissection plane for anterior mediastinal mass resection. The phrenic nerve and SVC (superior vena cava) are identified. The cephalad and caudad directions are denoted for orientation

space is entered anteriorly taking care not to injury the left internal mammary artery. The thymus is retracted over to the right side and the left lobe of the thymus is dissected free (Fig. 33.9). An Endo Catch bag is inserted through the 12 mm AirSeal port and the specimen is removed from the pleural cavity. The robotic instruments are then retracted and the robot disengaged from the ports. A 24 Fr chest tube is

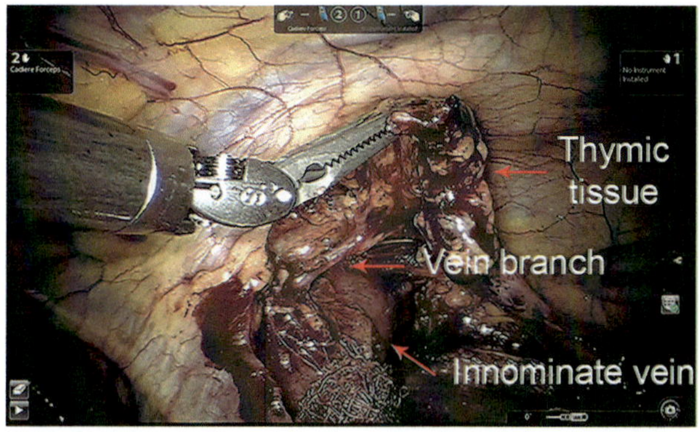

Fig. 33.5 Identification of the innominate vein. The innominate vein and vein branch draining the thymus is identified

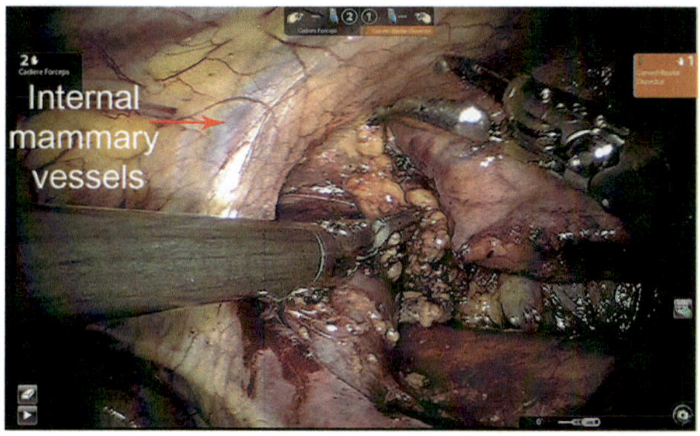

Fig. 33.6 Identification of the internal mammary vessels. Defines the superior and anterior dissection plane

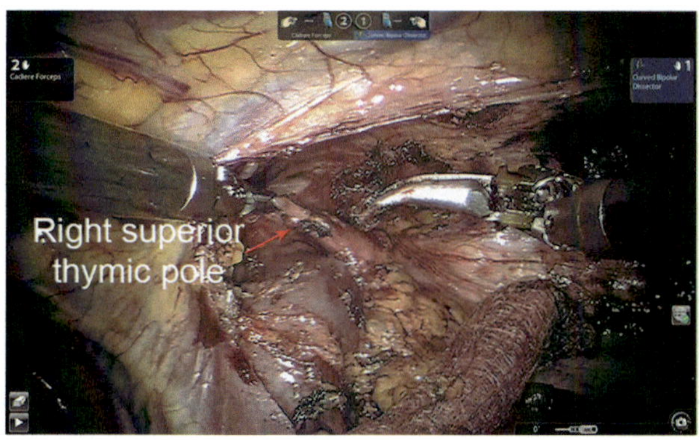

Fig. 33.7 Identification of the right superior thymic pole

inserted into the pleural cavity through the inferior incision. The right lung is then observed reinflating. The port sites are then closed with 3–0 Vicryl suture followed by 4–0 Monocryl subcuticular skin closure. The anterior mediastinal mass was found to be a thymoma, Masaoka stage I on pathology.

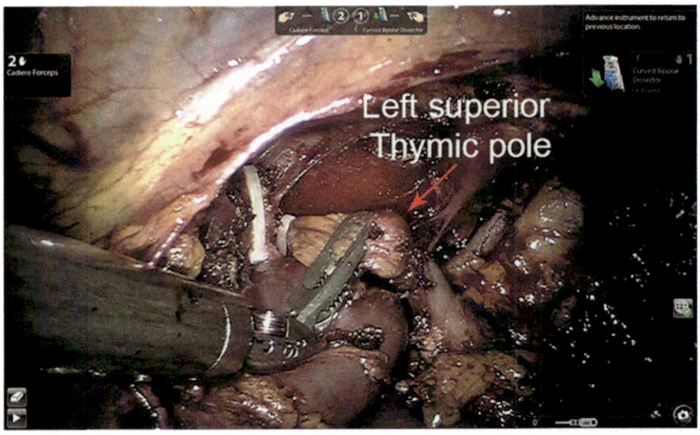

Fig. 33.8 Identification of the left superior thymic pole

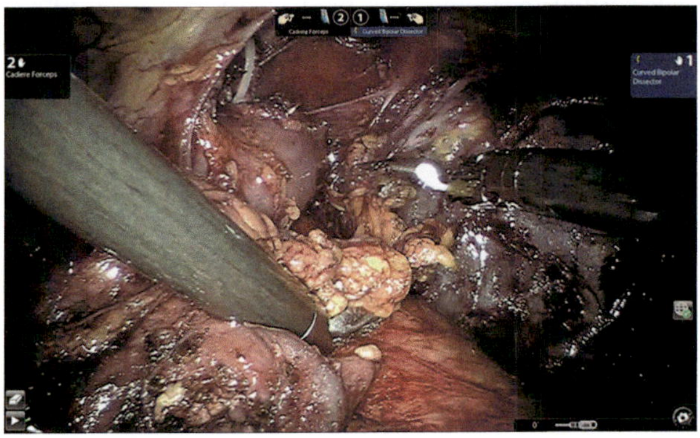

Fig. 33.9 Completion of the anterior mediastinal mass resection

Approach to Middle Mediastinal Pathology

Middle mediastinal masses include most commonly lymph nodes and congenital bronchogenic and pericardial cysts [6]. Lymph nodes in the middle mediastinum are addressed mainly via endobronchial ultrasound (EBUS), image-guided percutaneous biopsy, or less frequently mediastinoscopy. Lymph nodes not amenable to the aforementioned sampling approaches are often referred for robotic-assisted excisional biopsy. Bronchogenic cysts and pericardial cysts are rare congenital entities but have been addressed with robotic assistance in several case reports [7–9].

Indications for Resection

Bronchogenic cysts can be symptomatic due to extrinsic compression, infection, and rarely, transformation to malignant lesions [10]. Resection is indicated for lesions that are either symptomatic or asymptomatic but amenable to straightforward resection to avoid future complications. Surveillance of the lesion may be more appropriate for asymptomatic lesions in high-risk patients. Resection for diagnostic purposes is also indicated if the type of mediastinal cyst is in question. Pericardial cysts are benign lesions where resection is indicated for rare symptomatic lesions or for diagnostic purposes.

Middle Mediastinal Mass Example Case Scenario

The patient is a 66-year-old woman with history of mantle cell lymphoma who underwent computed tomography scan revealing an incidental middle mediastinal cyst in the aortopulmonary window that abutted the esophagus, trachea, pulmonary artery, and aorta (Fig. 33.10). Differential diagnosis included bronchogenic cyst, pericardial cyst, and less likely a foregut cyst. Observation versus resection was discussed with the patient, including discussion of risk of injury to the great vessels, trachea, esophagus, left vagus, and recurrent laryngeal nerve. The patient elected for resection due to her concerns with prior malignancy.

Surgical equipment used:

da Vinci robotic Xi system
da Vinci 30-degree camera
Long bipolar grasper

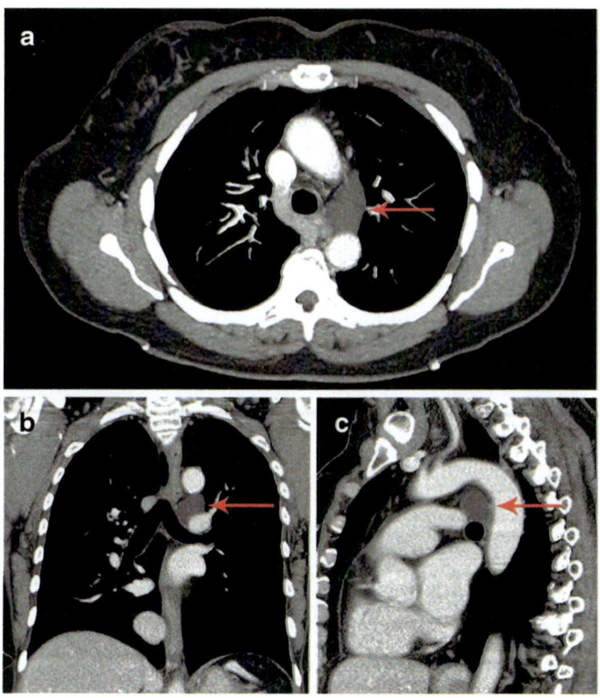

Fig. 33.10 Computed tomography scan for middle mediastinal cyst. Red arrow points to the cyst. The cyst abuts the aorta, pulmonary artery, esophagus, trachea, and left main stem bronchus. (**a**) Axial, (**b**) coronal, (**c**) sagittal

EndoWrist Cadiere forceps
Vessel sealer extend
8 mm instrument cannula × 3 (including one Optiview)
12 mm AirSeal trocar

Patient Positioning and Port Placement

For middle mediastinal masses, patient positioning will depend on the location of the tumor. In most cases, a right or left lateral decubitus position will be appropriate for resection. A right lateral decubitus position, left side up, on a reversed OR table was used for the example case due to the laterality of the lesion and to allow space for docking the robot.

The left pleural space is accessed with an 8 mm Optiview trocar in the eighth intercostal space along the posterior axillary line. The pleural cavity was then insufflated to 8 mmHg. Next under direct visualization, two additional ports were placed in the same intercostal space approximately 8 cm anterior (port #2) and posterior (port #1) to the camera port. Special care must be taken for posteriorly positioned ports to ensure the placement is anterior and lateral to the paraspinal muscles to avoid oozing. An assistant 12 mm AirSeal trocar was triangulated inferior to and between the camera and port #2. (Fig. 33.11).

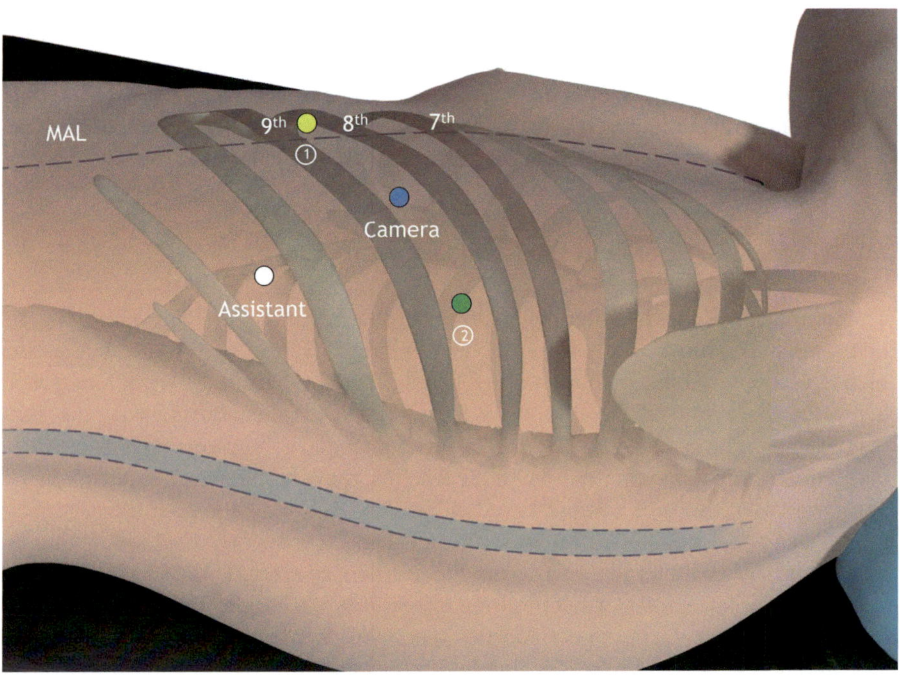

Fig. 33.11 Port placement for middle mediastinal cyst excision. Camera port is blue, robotic port 1 is yellow, robotic port 2 is green, and robotic port 3 is red. Assistant port is white

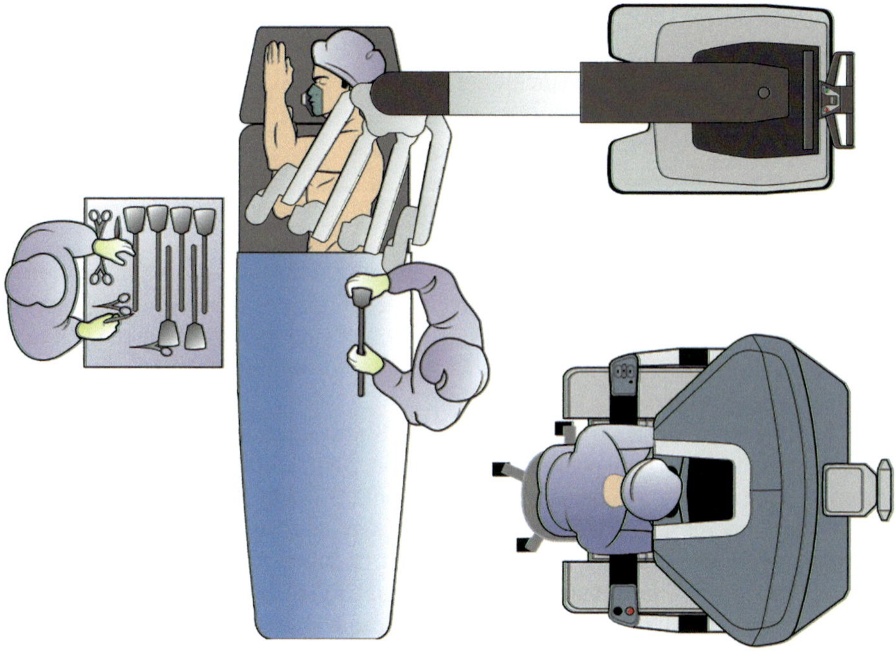

Fig. 33.12 Robot position in respect to the patient for middle mediastinal cyst resection

The robot is then driven into the operative field as depicted in Fig. 33.12. The ports are then secured into the robotic arms. The 8 mm 0-degree da Vinci camera is passed into the center camera port. The Cadiere forceps are placed in port #1 and the long bipolar grasper in port #2. The long bipolar grasper is chosen for dissection due to proximity of the left vagus nerve and recurrent laryngeal nerve.

Middle Mediastinal Cyst Excision Operative Steps

The lung is pushed away anteriorly using the robotic arm 3 with the Cadiere forceps instrument to expose the aortopulmonary window (Fig. 33.13). The mediastinal pleura was entered using robotic arms 1 and 2 centered around the camera port to begin the dissection of the cyst away from vital structures starting with the aorta (Fig. 33.14). The access port is used for suctioning and retraction assistance. As the dissection is carried medially toward the trachea, the left vagus and recurrent laryngeal nerve is visualized and preserved (Fig. 33.15). The cyst is then released from the trachea and esophagus. Blunt dissection is carried anteriorly while retracting the cyst anteriorly and laterally away from the pulmonary artery (Fig. 33.16). Once the cyst is fully released, a sterile cut glove finger was placed into the apex of the thoracic cavity via the access port and the specimen was then removed (Fig. 33.17). The middle mediastinal cyst was lined with mesothelial cells on pathology consistent with a pericardial cyst.

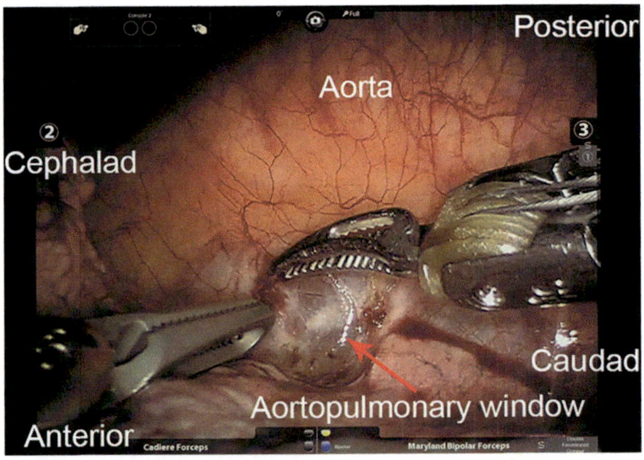

Fig. 33.13 Exposure of the aortopulmonary window. Red arrow points to the aortopulmonary window. Aorta is labeled. Cephalad, caudad, anterior, and posterior locations depicted for orientation

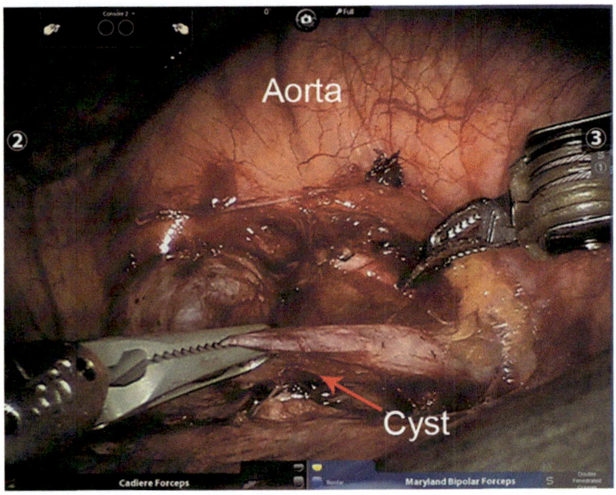

Fig. 33.14 Dissection of the middle mediastinal cyst away from the aorta. Aorta is labeled

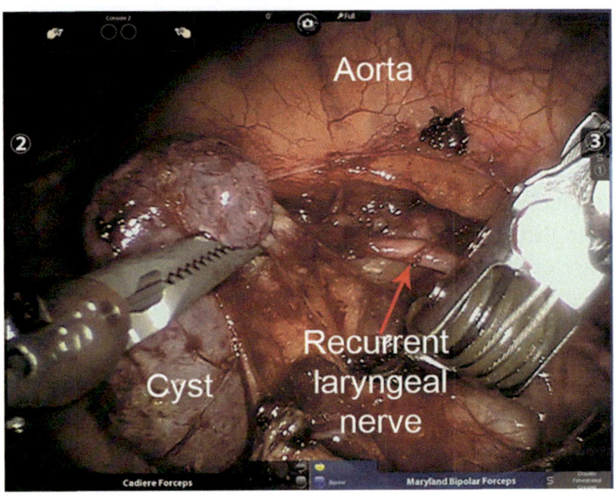

Fig. 33.15 Identification of the left recurrent laryngeal nerve for preservation. Red arrow points to the left recurrent laryngeal nerve. The aorta and middle mediastinal cysts are labeled

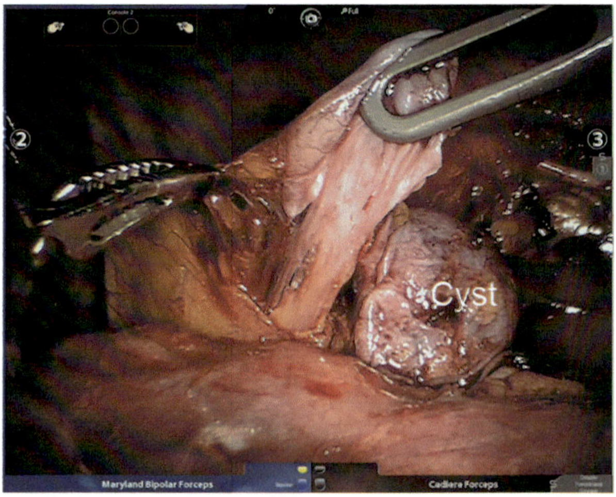

Fig. 33.16 Dissection of the cyst away from the pulmonary artery

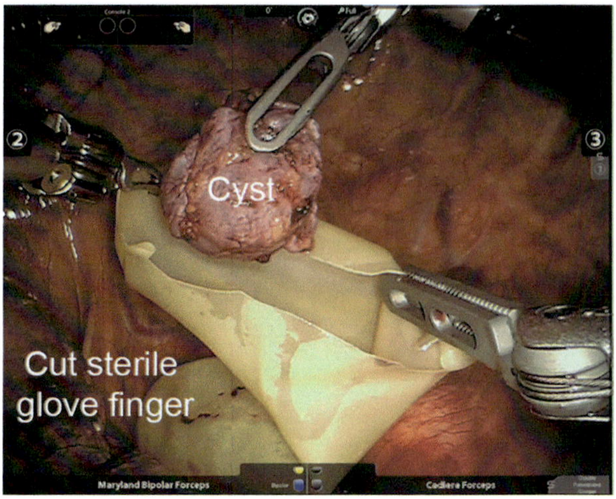

Fig. 33.17 Removal of the specimen using a cut sterile glove finger

Approach to Posterior Mediastinal Pathology

Posterior mediastinal pathologies for which robotic surgery has been utilized include neurofibroma, schwannoma, neuroganglioma, ganglioneuroblastoma, paraganglioma, and foregut duplication cysts. Mediastinal foregut duplications cysts are rare entities with case reports found in literature regarding the use of robotics in the pediatric population. Therefore, descriptions of such operations are outside the scope of this section. The most common adult posterior mediastinal masses are neurogenic in origin.

Indications for Robotic Posterior Mediastinal Mass Resection

Most adult neurogenic tumors are benign; however, resection is usually indicated in adults due to rare risk of malignancy [6]. There are preoperative considerations for posterior mediastinal solid tumors concerning for neurogenic origin. Patients with suspicious history of hypertension are evaluated for a functional paraganglioma with serum and urine catecholamine levels, as hypertensive crisis is a possible fatal intraoperative complication without the appropriate preoperative medical treatment [6]. Patients with neurogenic posterior mediastinal masses are screened for compressive spinal cord symptoms because such symptoms may indicate an intraspinal involvement of the tumor. Magnetic resonance imaging is the diagnostic study of choice in patients with neurogenic tumors, as this imaging modality is sensitive for identifying dumbbell or hourglass-shaped involvement of the intravertebral foramen [6]. If intraspinal involvement is detected, a combined robotic and posterior neurosurgical approach may be necessary for complete resection.

Posterior Mediastinal Mass Case Scenario

A 59-year-old man presents to the clinic with previously discovered posterior mediastinal mass that has grown in size on comparison computed tomography scan (Fig. 33.18).

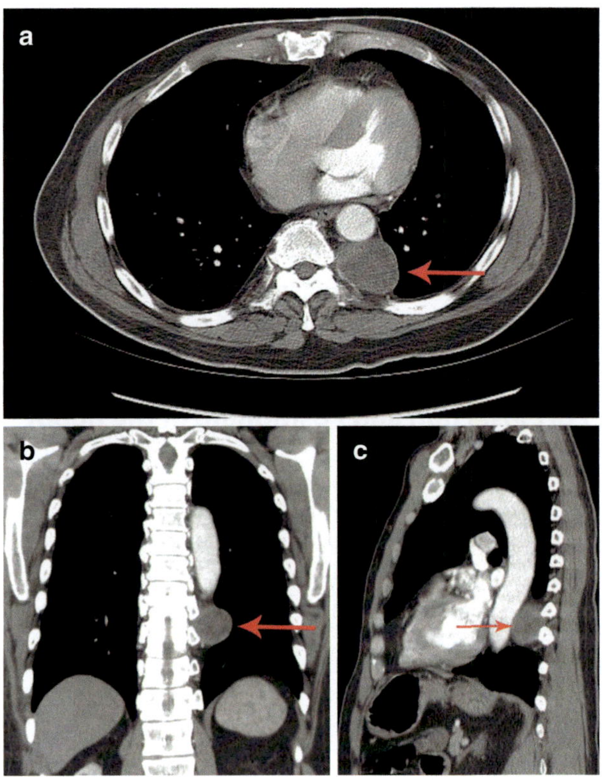

Fig. 33.18 Computed tomography scan of the posterior mediastinal mass. Red arrows point to the posterior mediastinal mass. The mass abuts the aorta. (**a**) Axial, (**b**) coronal, (**c**) sagittal

Past medical history was significant for previous lymphoma that had been in remission for over 5 years and well-controlled hypertension. The patient denied headaches, palpitations, or night sweats. He was referred for CT-guided biopsy of this mass with pathology consistent with schwannoma. Magnetic resonance imaging was obtained which did not identify involvement of the intravertebral foramen. After discussion about continued surveillance versus resection, the patient elected for surgical management.

Surgical equipment used:

da Vinci Xi robotic system
da Vinci 30-degree camera
EndoWrist® (Monopolar) permanent cautery spatula
Long bipolar grasper
Tip-Up fenestrated grasper
EndoWrist® Grasper—Cadiere forceps
EndoWrist® Clip applier—small and large
Kittner roll gauze sponges
8 mm trocars × 4
12 mm AirSeal
Endo Catch bag

Patient Positioning

Posterior mediastinal mass resections are approached from either right or left lateral decubitus position depending on the location of the mass. For the case example, the patient was placed in the right lateral decubitus position.

Port sites were determined by preoperative imaging studies (Fig. 33.18). In our example, a posterior mediastinal mass was found in the left pleural cavity at the level of the T9 vertebral body. The camera port was positioned along the posterior axillary line eighth intercostal space. Robotic port 1 was positioned anteriorly in the seventh intercostal space. Two additional ports were placed posterior to the camera, 7 cm apart, in the eighth intercostal space. The assistant port was marked for the tenth intercostal space triangulated between the camera and port 1 (Fig. 33.19).

Port Insertion and Positioning of the Robot

Entry into the thoracic cavity is accomplished using the Optiview technique as described in the anterior and middle mediastinal sections of this chapter. The pleural cavity is insufflated with carbon dioxide and assessed. The 8 mm reusable instrument cannulas were placed into the robotic port sites previously marked. The ports are then secured into the robotic arms. The 12 mm 30-degree da Vinci camera is

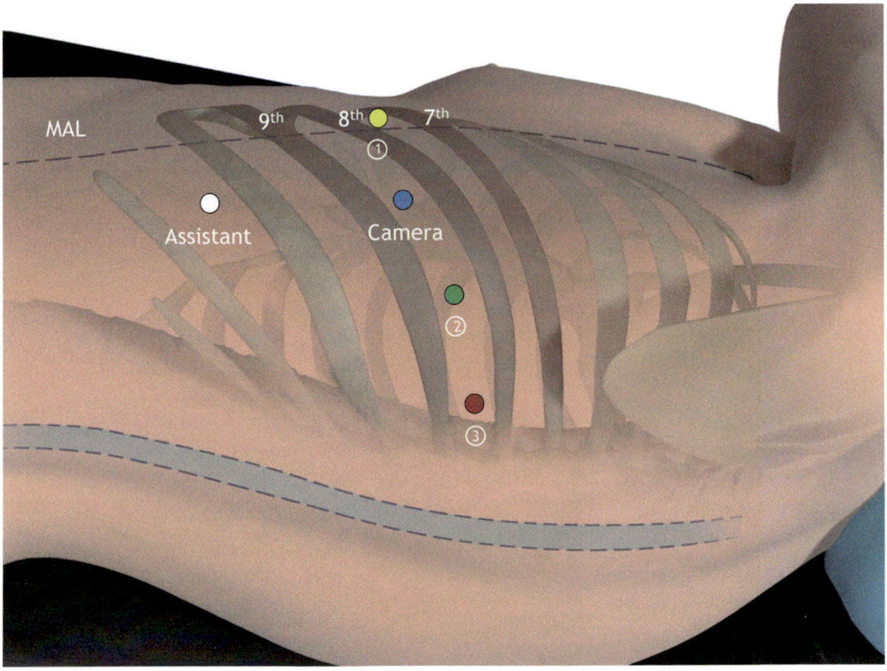

Fig. 33.19 Port placement for the posterior mediastinal mass resection. Camera port is blue. Robotic port 1 is yellow. Robotic port 2 is green. Assistant port is white

passed into the camera port. The monopolar cautery spatula was placed into the port site 2 followed by the Cadiere forceps into port site 1 and the Tip-Up fenestrated grasper in port site 3.

Posterior Mediastinal Mass Excision Operative Steps

The lung is retracted with the Tip-Up fenestrated grasper to expose the posterior mediastinal mass. Robotic arm 1 was used to retract the mass superiorly to initiate dissection of the mass along inferiorly using the monopolar cautery spatula (Fig. 33.20). Feeding vessels are identified during the dissection (Fig. 33.21). An intercostal artery branch was found feeding the tumor inferiorly requiring clips (Fig. 33.22). Long bipolar graspers were used once dissection became close to the vertebral foramina and decrease risk of nerve stimulation. The dissection is carried over medially with continued retraction using robotic arm 1 medially and anteriorly (Fig. 33.23). The anteromedial dissection is accomplished with retraction of the

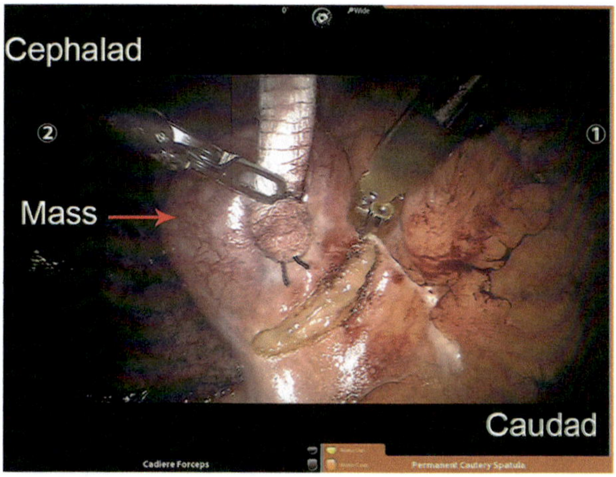

Fig. 33.20 Identification of intrathoracic mass and inferior dissection plane. Cephalad and caudad labeled for orientation

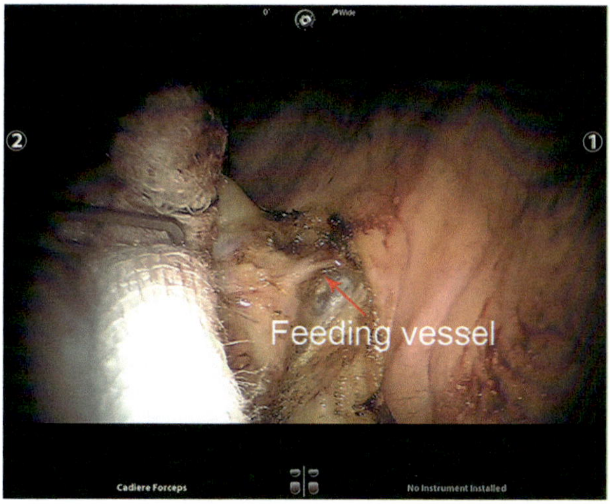

Fig. 33.21 Identification of a tumor-feeding blood vessel

aorta using robotic arm 1 and the assistant retracting the mass posteriorly (Fig. 33.24). A plane of dissection can be created easily along a rib when identified (Fig. 33.25). After the last tumor attachments are ligated in the superior and medial aspect of the dissection, the Endo Catch bag was placed into the assistant port with subsequent removal of the specimen after the trocar incision was enlarged (Fig. 33.26). Pathology revealed a schwannoma.

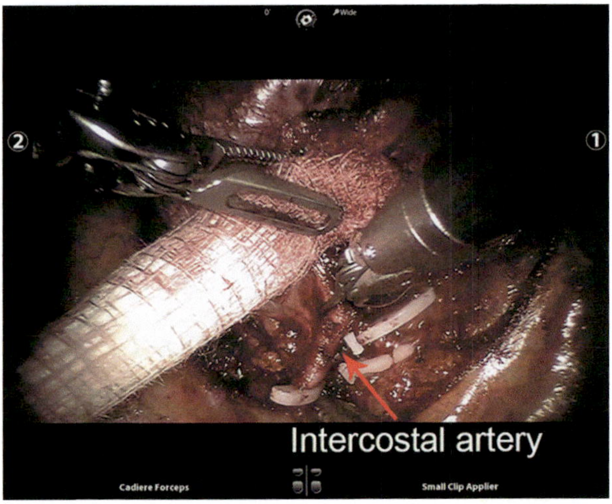

Fig. 33.22 Identification, dissection, and clipping of an intercostal artery feeding the tumor. Red arrow points to the intercostal artery off the aorta

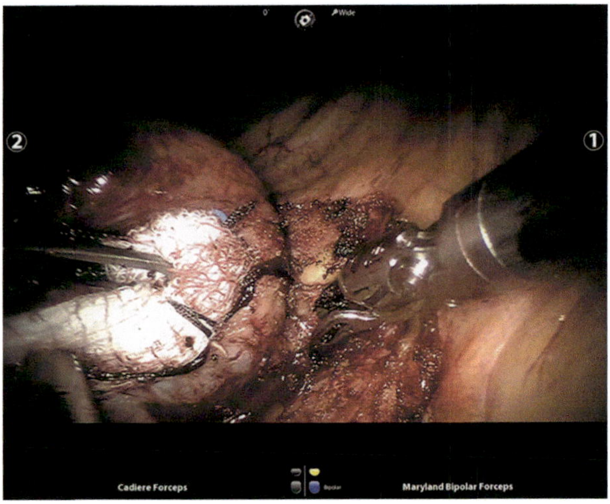

Fig. 33.23 Posterior and lateral dissection of the mass. The robotic arm retracts the mass anteriorly

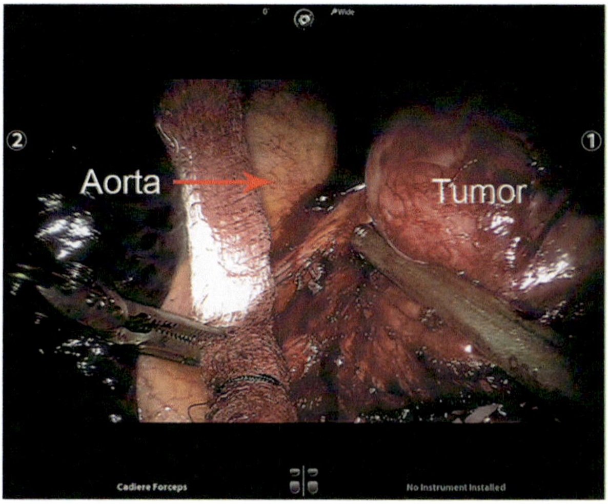

Fig. 33.24 Anterior and medial dissection of the mass. Aorta and mass are labeled. The robotic arm retracts the aorta anteriorly. The suction irrigator retracts the tumor posteriorly

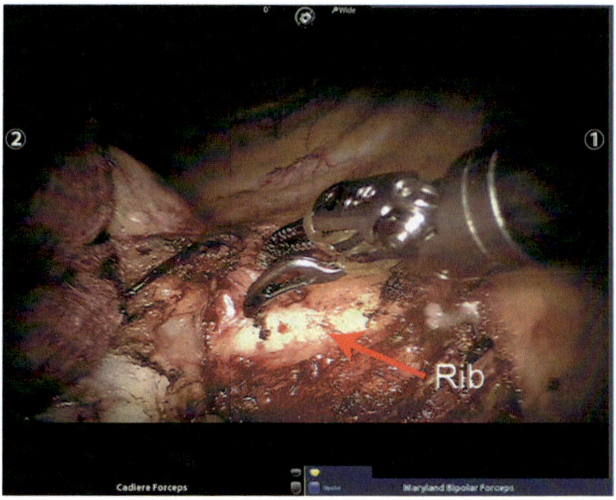

Fig. 33.25 Identification of a rib as a marker for the posterior dissection plane

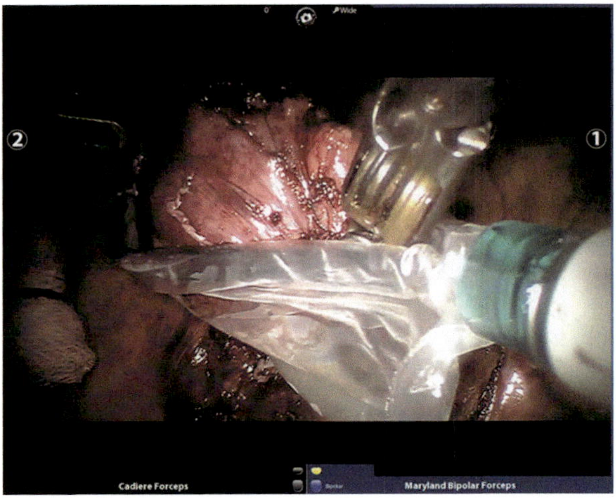

Fig. 33.26 Removal of the specimen using the Endo Catch bag through the access port

Summary

Robotic assistance is useful for navigating and dissecting the mediastinal space. In comparison to traditional open techniques, minimally invasive approaches have been shown to have superior short-term outcomes and comparable oncologic outcomes when applicable. Robotic-assisted mediastinal surgery has further enhanced existing VATS techniques given its three-dimensional visualization, improved dexterity with articulating EndoWrist technology, and elimination of tremor. Future advances such as haptic feedback would further increase the value of robotic assistance in delicate mediastinal operations. The most common indicated procedures were presented in detail for the anterior, middle, and posterior mediastinal lesions. The principles learned from these examples may be applied to a wide variety of mediastinal pathologies. Continued research on the efficacy of robotic-assisted mediastinal resections is needed as well as ongoing development of robotic surgical techniques and technology.

References

1. Manoly I, et al. Early and mid-term outcomes of trans-sternal and video-assisted thoracoscopic surgery for thymoma. Eur J Cardiothorac Surg. 2014;45(6):e187–93.
2. Straughan DM, Fontaine JP, Toloza EM. Robotic-assisted videothoracoscopic mediastinal surgery. Cancer Control. 2015;22(3):326–30.
3. Demmy TL, et al. Multicenter VATS experience with mediastinal tumors. Ann Thorac Surg. 1998;66(1):187–92.

4. Ye B, et al. Video-assisted thoracoscopic surgery versus robotic-assisted thoracoscopic surgery in the surgical treatment of Masaoka stage I thymoma. World J Surg Oncol. 2013;11:157.
5. Yang CJ, et al. A national analysis of open versus minimally invasive thymectomy for stage I to III thymoma. J Thorac Cardiovasc Surg. 2020;160(2):555–67.
6. Juanpere S, et al. A diagnostic approach to the mediastinal masses. Insights Imaging. 2013;4(1):29–52.
7. Asaf BB, Kumar A, Vijay CL. Robotic excision of paraesophageal bronchogenic cyst in a 9-year-old child. J Indian Assoc Pediatr Surg. 2015;20(4):191–3.
8. Toker A, et al. Resection of a bronchogenic cyst in the first decade of life with robotic surgery. Interact Cardiovasc Thorac Surg. 2014;19(2):321–3.
9. Bacchetta MD, et al. Resection of a symptomatic pericardial cyst using the computer-enhanced da Vinci Surgical System. Ann Thorac Surg. 2003;75(6):1953–5.
10. Ribet ME, Copin MC, Gosselin B. Bronchogenic cysts of the mediastinum. J Thorac Cardiovasc Surg. 1995;109(5):1003–10.

34 Liver Transplantation

Yee Lee Cheah, Gi Hong Choi, YoungRok Choi, and Kwang Woong Lee

Introduction

Living donor liver transplantation (LDLT) consists of two simultaneous operations where (1) a healthy living person donates a portion of their liver to a recipient on the liver transplantation waiting list and (2) the recipient has their diseased liver removed and the donated graft implanted. LDLT is possible due to the regenerative properties of the liver; in ideal situations, the remnant liver in the donor and the recipient may regrow to volumes close to 100% of original volume 1 year after surgery [1, 2].

The first successful living donor liver transplantation was performed in 1989, where the left lateral section of a mother was transplanted into her 18-month-old child with biliary atresia [3]. The selection of the lobe or section to be donated is the smallest portion of the liver that meets the requirement of the recipient (most

Supplementary Information The online version contains supplementary material available at https://doi.org/10.1007/978-3-031-86927-3_34.

Y. L. Cheah (✉)
JC Walter Jr Transplant Center, Sherrie and Alan Conover Center for Liver Disease and Transplantation, Houston Methodist Hospital, Houston, TX, USA

Department of Surgery, Houston Methodist Hospital, Houston, TX, USA
e-mail: ycheah@houstonmethodist.org

G. H. Choi
Division of Hepato-biliary and Pancreatic Surgery, Yonsei University College of Medicine, Seoul, South Korea

Y. Choi · K. W. Lee
Division of HBP Surgery, Department of Surgery, Seoul National University College of Medicine, Seoul, South Korea

S. Samreen et al. (eds.), *The SAGES Manual of Robotic Surgery*,
https://doi.org/10.1007/978-3-031-86927-3_34

common metric used is the graft to body weight ratio where the most conventional limit is ≥0.8) [4].

The majority of LDLT cases globally are performed in Asia, whereas only 658 out of 10,660 (6.2%) cases of liver transplantation in the United States were from living donor grafts in 2023 [5, 6]. Due to the technically complex nature of both the donor and recipient operations, these procedures are performed at highly specialized centers. Each potential living donor and recipient undergo an extensive evaluation process to determine suitability for LDLT.

In the United States, recipients who undergo living donor liver transplantation have improved survival rates at 1 year compared those who received grafts from brain-dead donors [7]. They also return to work earlier and have higher rates of returning to work for income. The availability of a living donor eliminates their need to wait for deterioration of their liver function to increase their chances of obtaining a deceased donor graft.

Robotic Donor Hepatectomy

The most common types of donor hepatectomy are right lobe, left lobe, and left lateral section resections. Most centers accept 30% as the minimum future liver remnant volume in the donor to allow for adequate regeneration. The differences between a donor hepatectomy and a hepatectomy for pathology are shown in Fig. 34.1.

Three-dimensional reconstruction of a potential donor's liver imaging is useful to detect (1) volumes of graft and remnant and (2) aberrant vascular anatomy, (3) gauge the length of hepatic artery and portal vein that will be available for recipient anastomosis and (4) the number of bile ducts that will need to be anastomosed, and

Resection for living donation vs resection for liver pathology

Living Donor Hepatectomy	Hepatectomy for pathology
• Resected lobe preserved for recipient implantation	• Resected lobe goes to pathology
• Adequate size for recipient GBWR ≥ 0.8	• Remnant size important
• Remnant has to be adequate for donor	• Option of Glissonian approach
• Dissection of HA, PV and HV branches to lobe	• Margins important in transection
• Accurate transection line reduces bleeding, aims for graft & remnant volumes as predicted	• Both inflow and outflow can be taken prior to transection
• Ideally NO inflow or outflow control during transection	• Segmental HVs ligated without issues
• Segmental HVs may need preservation and reconstruction	• No time or physical constraints to extraction of specimen
• Careful extraction of graft in a timely manner to reduce warm ischemic time	
• Preoperative workup more extensive	• Standard workup
• 3D liver anatomy reconstruction	
• Operating on a healthy person who wants to save recipient's life	• Patient needs resection for own cure and survival

Fig. 34.1 Differences between donor hepatectomy and hepatectomy for pathology

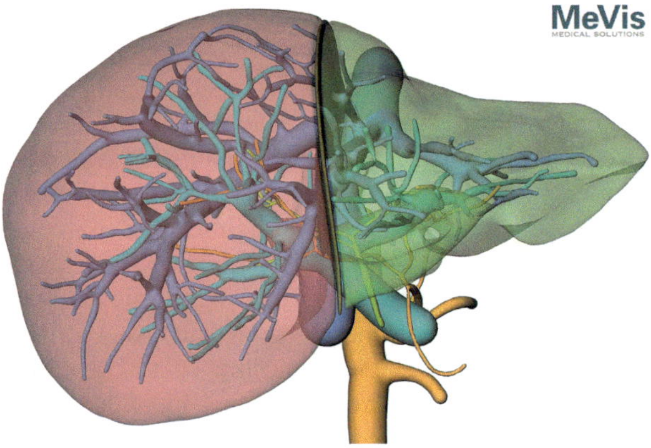

Fig. 34.2 Three-dimensional reconstruction of potential living donor liver with inflow and outflow vessels and proposed transection line. (Image courtesy of © 2024 MeVis Medical Solutions AG, Bremen, Germany)

(5) evaluate segmental hepatic venous drainage of the lobe to be donated (particularly important for right lobe grafts) to determine the need for reconstruction prior to implantation. Figure 34.2 demonstrates an example of a 3-D reconstruction of a donor liver created from a CT and MRI of the abdomen.

Donor safety is paramount in any LDLT, and informed consent is obtained prior to evaluation and surgery. Risks of a donor hepatectomy include but are not limited to bleeding, biliary complications, infectious complications, post-hepatectomy liver failure, and thromboembolic disease. Overall reported complication rates were 25–30% in right donor hepatectomy and 15–20% in left-sided grafts [8–10]. Mortality rates for LDLT in the United States has been quoted at up to 0.5% for right lobe donors and 0.1% for left-sided donors, though overall death rates appeared to have decreased in the last decade.

As living donors are healthy individuals willing to accept risks in order to save another's life, their well-being should be optimized. About 15% of donors reported donation-related issues including hernia (22%) and scar or adhesion problems (9%) and 22% could not perform physical activities as well as they did preoperatively, mainly due to limitations of abdominal wall strength. In a post-donation quality-of-life analysis, incisional discomfort was the most common symptom reported [11, 12]. This has spurred efforts by living donor teams to explore minimally invasive approaches to donor hepatectomy.

The first laparoscopic donor left lateral sectionectomy was reported in 2002 and the first laparoscopic right donor hepatectomy in 2013. The largest multicenter series from Korea reported a 10% overall and 4.9% serious complication rates. The emergence of the robotic approach in liver surgery prompted expansion of this modality in donor hepatectomy; the first robotic right donor hepatectomy was reported in 2012 (Chicago) [13], and first series in 2016 (Taiwan) [14]. Since then, larger series have been reported by a handful of highly specialized centers [15, 16]. Reported overall and serious complications rates have been better or comparable to open series.

Patient Selection

After completion of the standard evaluation process, determination of the suitability of the robotic approach is influenced by the experience of the surgical team and the anatomy of the graft. At the beginning of a center's experience with a robotic approach for donor hepatectomy, avoiding donors with previous upper abdominal laparotomy may be prudent. Straightforward graft anatomy should be selected (single hepatic artery and portal vein and few segmental veins requiring reconstruction) for right donor hepatectomy. Once the learning curve is achieved, these criteria may be relaxed. Liver anesthesia management should integrate enhanced recovery protocols in fluid management and low central venous pressure. Most living donors, who tend to be younger and healthy individuals, qualify for many aspects of an enhanced recovery protocol [17].

Patient Positioning and Port Placement

Positioning

Patients are placed in a split-leg position to enable the bedside surgeon to stand between the patient's legs (Fig. 34.3). One arm may be abducted to enable access by

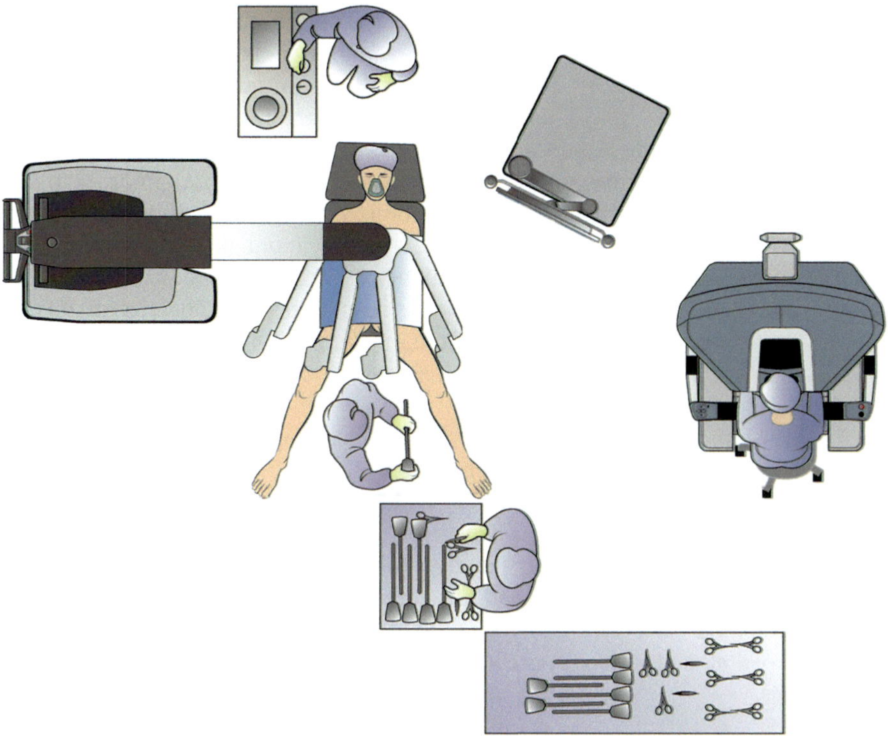

Fig. 34.3 Operating room setup for robotic donor hepatectomy

anesthesiologist to intra-arterial and intravenous cannulas during the operation. All pressure points are padded, and the patient is secured to the operating table at the hip and chest areas. Both legs are secured to the leg extensions and footrests are used to prevent slippage during positioning. Once all ports are placed, the patient is positioned at a 10-degree reverse Trendelenburg, and a slight right-side up rotation for donor right hepatectomy.

Port Placement

Recommended port placements for right versus left donor hepatectomy or left lateral donor sectionectomy are shown in Fig. 34.4a, b, respectively. The third arm is a right-handed instrument. Two laparoscopic assistant ports (12 mm and 5 mm) are inserted in the lower abdomen; their tracts are slanted toward the upper abdominal surgery. The grafts are retrieved from a Pfannenstiel incision. Pneumoperitoneum pressure is kept at or below 12 mm Hg.

Instruments

Basic Robotic Instruments for Dissection and Mobilization

1. Maryland bipolar (+ electrocautery)
2. Camera
3. Scissors (+ electrocautery)
4. Cadiere or ProGrasp forceps

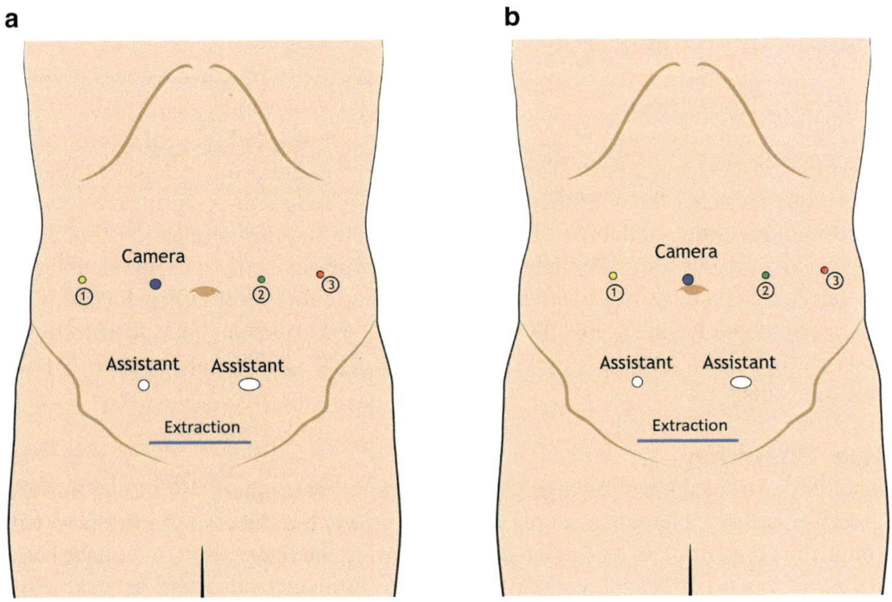

Fig. 34.4 (**a**) Port positions for right donor hepatectomy (**b**) Port positions for left or left lateral donor hepatectomy

Basic Robotic Instruments for Parenchymal Transection

1. Harmonic scalpel
2. Camera
3. Maryland bipolar (+ electrocautery)
4. Cadiere or ProGrasp forceps

Adjunct Robotic Instruments

1. Large needle driver or suture cut
2. Small, medium, and large clip appliers
3. Vessel sealer

Laparoscopic Instruments and Special Items

1. Laparoscopic suction irrigator
2. Laparoscopic grasper
3. Laparoscopic needle driver
4. Ultrasound with laparoscopic or drop-in probes
5. Bulldog clamps (e.g., Scanlan® Reliance Bulldog clamps, Scanlan International Inc., St. Paul, MN, USA)
6. Vessel loops
7. 4/0 and 5/0 polypropylene and 5/0 polydioxanone sutures
8. Surgicel™ Fibrillar™ (Ethicon, Raritan, NJ, USA)

A standardized stepwise technique is described below for right, left, and left lateral section donor hepatectomy.

Right Donor Hepatectomy

Falciform Dissection

The ligamentum teres and falciform ligamentum are divided up to the level of the hepatic vein-IVC confluence. The third arm is used to grasp the leaflets of the falciform ligament near the confluence and a gentle inferior and posterior retraction is used to expose the confluence. The peritoneal covering of the hepatic vein confluence is incised, exposing the three hepatic veins. The right coronary ligament lateral to the right hepatic vein is divided. The transection line follows the principal plane for a right donor hepatectomy; the superior end of the principal line is marked on the liver surface with electrocautery between the right (RHV) and middle (MHV) hepatic veins.

Hilar Dissection

The third arm cushioned by a gauze is used to retract segment 4B and gallbladder anterosuperiorly. The laparoscopic assistant retracts the duodenum inferiorly with blunt-tipped instrument or suction device exposing the liver hilum. A standard cholecystectomy is performed, with division of the cystic duct and artery between clips, and the gallbladder specimen is removed from the peritoneal cavity later. The clipped cystic duct stump is now ligated with 3/0 Vicryl/Silk tie or suture-ligated with 3/0 Vicryl/Silk sutures with tails left long. The tails are grasped by the third arm previously positioned at segment 4B, and using the forceps as a pulley, the cystic duct is retracted anteriorly and slightly to the patient's left, exposing the lateral and right posterior aspect of the common hepatic duct (CHD).

Dissection of Right Hepatic Artery

A standard right hepatic artery (RHA) usually courses posterior to the CHD and changes course toward the cephalad direction on the right side of the CHD. Lymphatic and nerve tissue covering the RHA are dissected free. As much of the length of the proximal RHA is separated from the posterior wall of CHD (taking care not to injure either the artery or the duct) to provide a good length for recipient anastomosis. If the RHA courses anterior to the duct, it will need to be dissected away from the anterior surface of the CHD (Fig. 34.5). The segment 4 hepatic artery may be encountered if it is a branch of the right hepatic artery; it is kept out of harm's way, and the future division point of the RHA will be distal to its' takeoff. Distally, the RHA is dissected away from the CHD and the distal right hepatic duct (which will be transected with the graft). Posteriorly, the RHA is freed from the portal vein. The RHA is then encircled with a vessel loop.

A replaced RHA from the superior mesenteric artery courses parallel to the lateral and posterior right wall of the common bile duct (CBD) and CHD. It is usually covered by the station 12b lymph node which may be excised to gain access to the RHA. The length of the replaced RHA is then dissected free from the bile ducts anteriorly and the portal vein posteriorly, and subsequently encircled (Fig. 34.6).

Dissection of the Right Portal Vein

The vessel loop of the RHA is grasped by the third arm and gentle retraction is used to expose the anterior surface of the portal vein and its bifurcation. The plane between the CHD and anterior surface of the portal vein (PV) is developed by

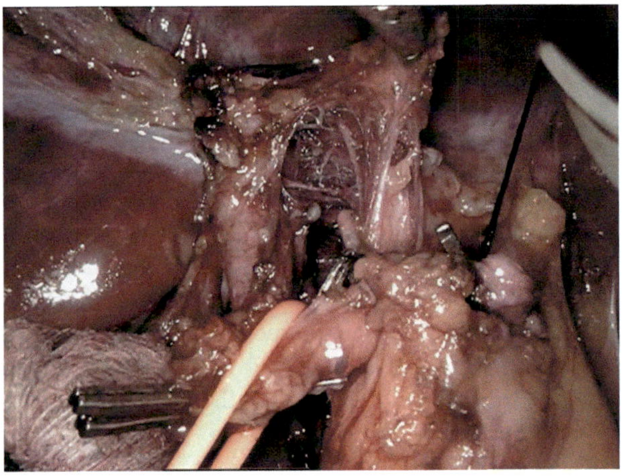

Fig. 34.5 Aberrant arterial anatomy with RHA (red vessel loop) coursing anterior to CHD

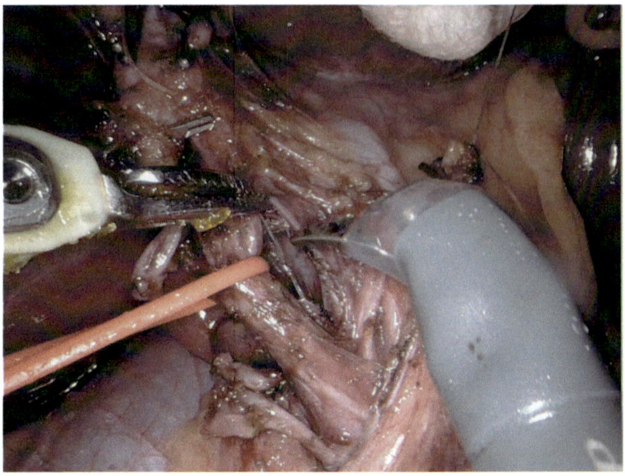

Fig. 34.6 Aberrant arterial anatomy with replaced RHA (red vessel loop) running along the posterior aspect of CBD

pushing the portal vein posteriorly off the attachments to the duct and RHA. Dissection proceeds cephalad until identification of the bifurcation is confirmed by visualization of the right, left, and main portal veins. The right portal vein (RPV) is then carefully teased off the hilar plate using the Maryland forceps and scissors.

Once the anterior and superior RPV is mobilized, the dissection of the posterior aspect of the RPV is performed. The peritoneal lining the posterior aspect of the RPV is divided and retracted posterior-inferiorly by the laparoscopic assistant. Caudate branches are visualized on the posterior RPV, and these are carefully encircled. The PV side of these branches are always ligated with a tie to avoid clips on the PV, which could hamper future clipping or stapling of the RPV, while the caudate side may be clipped prior to division.

Once all caudate branches are divided, the posterior RPV is then dissected off the hilar plate, moving cephalad until the dissection plane is met from the anterior side. Once this space is developed, the RPV is encircled with a vessel loop. A 5/0 Prolene stitch is placed superficially at the proximal RPV to mark the bifurcation (Fig. 34.7).

Mobilization of the Right Lobe

The third arm cushioned by a gauze is used to retract segments 5 and 6 superior-anteriorly, exposing the inferior layer of the right coronary and right triangular ligaments. These ligaments are divided and the bare area mobilized using the scissors or vessel sealer, taking care not to injure the diaphragm (Fig. 34.8). As more of the bare area is exposed, the third arm is moved sequentially superiorly and posteriorly to provide more retraction. The liver is mobilized off the right adrenal. We then turn our attention medially toward the retrohepatic inferior vena cava (IVC).

The peritoneal lining between the caudate and IVC is incised, and short caudate and hepatic veins draining directly to the IVC are serially divided between clips or vessel sealer. Dissection continues in a cephalad direction on the anterior surface of the retrohepatic IVC, mobilizing the liver from the IVC. Caudate process division from the right lobe at this point helps cephalad dissection of the IVC. Laterally, the

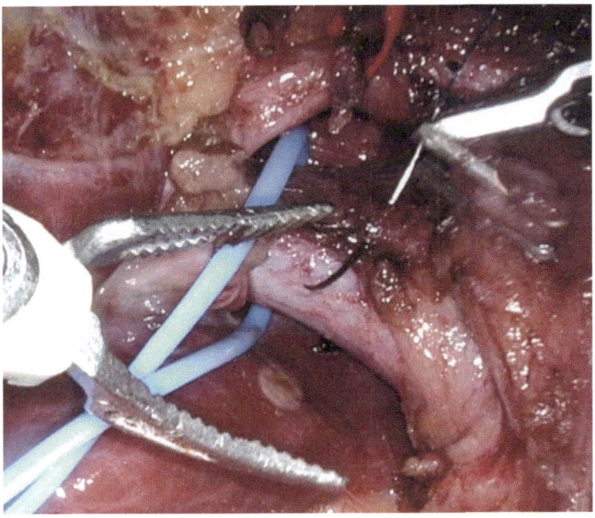

Fig. 34.7 Prolene suture placed superficially to mark PV bifurcation

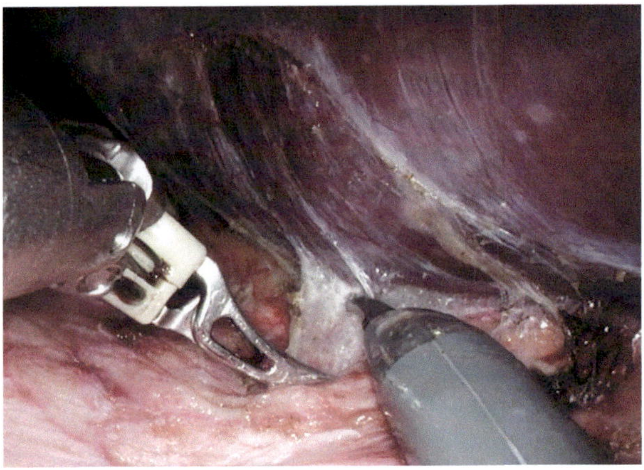

Fig. 34.8 Division of right triangular ligament and attachments to retroperitoneum

hepatocaval ligament is left intact as division of this ligament is easier after parenchymal transection. The liver is carefully mobilized from the IVC until the area near the right and middle hepatic veins is reached. This completes the right lobe mobilization, and the liver is returned to its anatomical position.

Demarcation

The third arm is used to retract segment 4B. The hilar plate is separated from the liver at the area of the bile duct bifurcation, and a small ball of Surgicel™ Fibrillar™ is inserted in this space to mark the hilar endpoint of the parenchymal transection. Bulldog clamps are placed on the RHA and RPV (Fig. 34.9). Indocyanine green dye (ICG) 2.5 mg is injected intravenously, and using the Firefly™ mode, demarcation of the perfused left lobe is augmented by fluorescence. The line of demarcation is

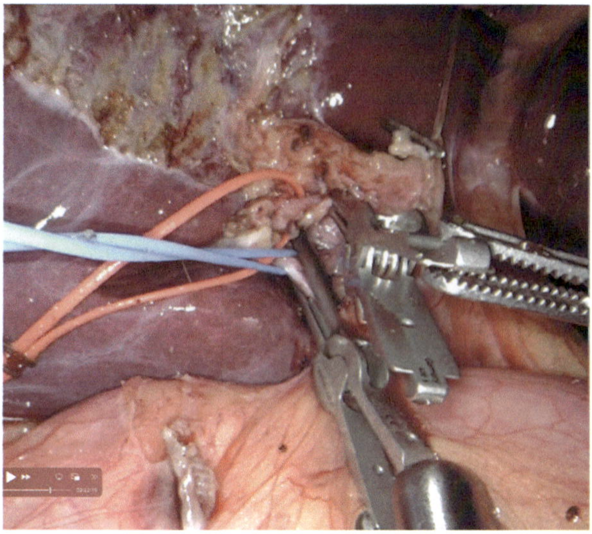

Fig. 34.9 Temporary clamping of RHA and RPV for demarcation

marked on the anterior and inferior liver surface using electrocautery. The clamps are removed. An ultrasound may be performed to mark the course of the MHV (which stays with the remnant) and segmental veins draining segments 5 and 8.

Parenchymal Transection

"Rubber Band" Retraction Technique

One rubber band is sutured to each side of the transection line at the tip of the liver. Each end of the rubber band is externalized on the respective sides of the upper abdomen and secured to the drapes. This technique takes advantage of the elasticity of the bands to provide contact retraction of the transection plane without having to use any of the robotic or laparoscopic arms or a liver retractor.

Parenchymal Transection

A Pringle maneuver is avoided unless necessary for hemostasis (details of a Pringle maneuver is described in Chap. 25). During the initial part of the parenchymal transection, the third arm cushioned by a gauze is used to gently lift the inferior surface of the liver off the hilum. Parenchymal transection is performed with harmonic scalpel and Maryland bipolar forceps. Small intervening vessels and oozing from the parenchyma are controlled with bipolar electrocautery. Larger vessels including segments 5 and 8 veins are divided between clips. If these veins are to be reconstructed in the recipient, an appropriate length of the vein stumps on the graft side will need to be preserved to enable anastomosis.

As more of the parenchyma is transected, the liver edges are continually retracted due to the elasticity of the rubber bands. These might need to be tightened as transection progress. Once most of the parenchyma has been transected, leaving about 2 cm of parenchyma anteriorly along the IVC, the right hepatic duct (RHD) is divided.

Division of Right Hepatic Duct

The parenchyma down to the level of the biliary bifurcation should be completely transected. An ICG cholangiogram is performed to visualize the biliary bifurcation using Firefly™. The location of RHD division is chosen based on the surgeon's interpretation of the cholangiogram. We usually aim to provide the recipient surgeon with as few ducts for anastomosis as possible while making sure not to impinge on the donor's biliary bifurcation.

There are two ways to transect the duct:

1. Clip-and-cut

   The Maryland forceps is used to encircle an umbilical tape around the entire hepatic duct with its surrounding hilar plate tissue. A large Hem-o-lock clip is then placed on the distal RHD ensuring that it does not encroach onto the bifurcation. The proximal RHD on the graft side is then sharply divided (Fig. 34.10). The stump of the distal RHD on the donor side is suture-ligated with a running 5/0 PDS.
2. Cut-and-clip/suture

   The posterior aspect of the RHD is examined to identify a crossing arterial branch, which, if seen, should be divided between clips. The RHD is then cut at the chosen point without cutting the hilar tissues This hilar plate tissue is divided between two small metal clips. The stump of the distal RHD is suture-ligated with a running 5/0 PDS.

The choice of the technique used is influenced by the length of the RHD and the thickness of the surrounding hilar tissue. The clip-and-cut option tends to take up an additional ~0.5–1 mm of RHD length, and it may be difficult to apply the Hem-o-lock clip on thick hilar tissues. The cut-and-clip/suture option may lead to fewer bile duct openings for recipient anastomosis.

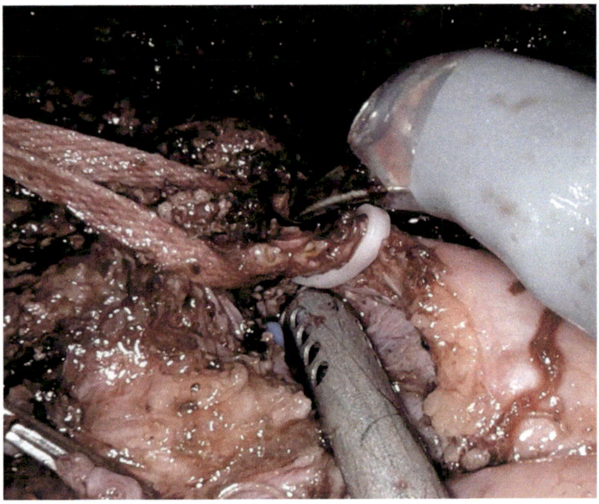

Fig. 34.10 Division of right hepatic duct using clip and cut technique

Completion of Parenchymal Transection

The remainder of the parenchyma is transected, from caudal to cephalad, with a vessel sealer while the assistant gently pushes the liver anteriorly off the IVC. The final piece of transection should be the parenchymal between the right and middle hepatic veins. Once completed, the right hepatic vein is encircled with an umbilical tape.

Cross-Clamp and Graft Extraction

The middle robotic arms are undocked. A Pfannenstiel incision is made. It is important not to injure the graft during extraction and to minimize the time between cross-clamp and flushing of the graft with preservation fluid on the backtable. There are two ways to extract the graft depending on the size of the graft and whether it fits in a laparoscopic retrieval bag:

1. Fits a laparoscopic retrieval bag
   The peritoneal lining at the Pfannenstiel is not opened at this point. The robot is redocked and the right lobe is partially placed into a laparoscopic retrieval bag that is inserted via the 12 mm assistant port. Cross-clamping is performed as described below and the graft is completely placed in the bag. The peritoneal lining is opened, the string of the bag is grasped, and the graft is extracted.
2. Does not fit a laparoscopic retrieval bag
   The peritoneal lining at the Pfannenstiel is opened and a Gelport (Applied Medical, Rancho Santa Margarita, CA, USA) is placed in the incision. The robot is redocked and a large retrieval bag is inserted via the Gelport and the graft partially placed in the bag. Cross-clamping is performed as described below and the graft is completely placed in the bag. The bag is grasped and extracted via the Gelport.

Cross-clamping commences when the RHA is doubly clipped and transected distal to the clips while preserving as much length as possible for recipient anastomosis. The RPV is transected with a stapler just distal to the stitch marking the bifurcation. The RHV and hepatocaval ligament are transected with separate firings of the stapler. The graft and gallbladder are then extracted as described above.

Closure

Hemostasis of the cut surface and hilum is performed. Bile leak is ruled out. The clips, staple, and suture lines are inspected. The left lobe is reattached to the falciform ligament to prevent torsion. A drain is placed in Morrison's pouch and externalized via one of the ports (Video 34.1).

Left Donor Hepatectomy

Falciform Dissection and Left Lobe Mobilization

Falciform dissection and exposure of the hepatic vein confluence is similar to the donor right hepatectomy. The superior end of the transection line is marked between the RHV and MHV (MHV is kept with the graft). The left triangular ligament is divided, and the left lateral segment is retracted toward the patient's right with the third arm exposing the gastrohepatic ligament.

If there is an accessory (10% of population) or replaced left hepatic artery (7.5%) arising from the left gastric artery (LGA), this vessel is carefully preserved. Oftentimes, this artery is dissected until its branch point from the left gastric artery. The LGA in this area is also dissected free of lymphatic tissues to enable procurement of a short segment of this artery during cross-clamp to form a branch patch for recipient anastomosis.

The Arantius ligament is located and divided at the superior pole of the caudate lobe, exposing the junction between the left hepatic vein and vena cava, which is marked by inserting a ball of Surgicel™ Fibrillar™. Dissection deeper into this area can be performed to encircle the middle and left hepatic veins but this step is not necessary. If the caudate lobe is to be procured as well, Spiegel's lobe is mobilized from the vena cava by incising the peritoneal attachments and dividing the short hepatic veins between clips or with a vessel sealer.

Hilar Dissection

The third arm is used to retract segment 4B to expose the hilum. A cholecystectomy is performed. The peritoneal covering over the left side of the hilum is opened.

Dissection of the Left Hepatic Artery

The left hepatic artery is dissected free from lymphatic and nerve tissue from the proper hepatic artery until the umbilical fissure. The station 12a lymph node may be excised to provide exposure. Medially, the artery is mobilized from the main and left portal vein and encircled with a vessel loop (Fig. 34.11). The location of the right hepatic artery is noted at all times and dissection close to this artery is avoided.

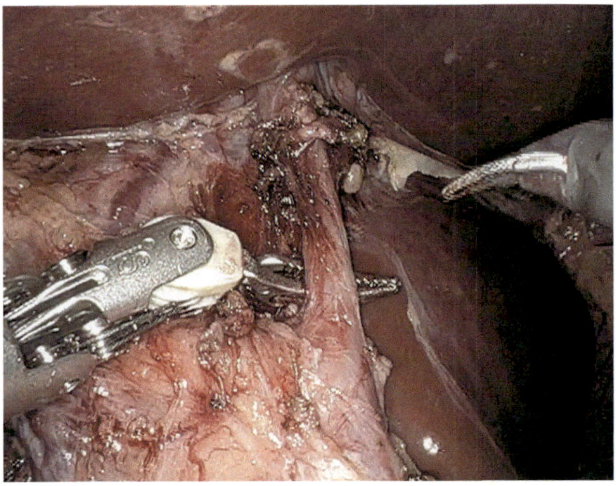

Fig. 34.11 Isolation of LHA

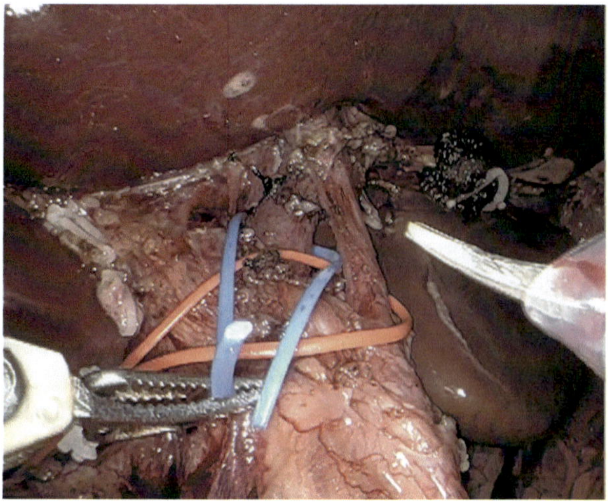

Fig. 34.12 LHA (red vessel loop) and LPV (blue vessel loop) encircled

Dissection of the Left Portal Vein

Gentle retraction on the vessel loop encircling the left hepatic artery toward the patient's left side will expose the left portal vein (LPV). The superior side of the LPV is mobilized from the left hepatic duct and hilar plate. Small branches to segment 4B in this area are divided between clips (the LPV side is ligated with ties to avoid clips obstructing future clipping or stapling of the LPV).

The artery is then retracted anteriorly exposing the posterior LPV. Several caudate LPV branches are usually seen near the umbilical fissure. If the caudate lobe is not to be procured with the graft, these caudate branches are dissected free and divided between clips (the LPV side is ligated with a tie). The LPV is then encircled with a vessel loop (Fig. 34.12). A 5/0 Prolene stitch is placed superficially at the proximal LPV to mark the bifurcation.

Demarcation

The hilar plate is separated from the liver at the area of the biliary bifurcation, and a small ball of Surgicel™ Fibrillar™ is inserted in this space to mark the hilar endpoint of the parenchymal transection. If preoperative imaging shows a hepatic duct branch to the right lobe coming off the left hepatic duct (LHD), the endpoint of the transection is shifted proximally on the left hepatic duct before the confluence of the right duct branch, and is usually divided just proximal to the umbilical fissure.

Bulldog clamps are placed on the LHA and LPV. Similar to the right donor hepatectomy, ICG 2.5 mg is injected intravenously, and using the Firefly™ mode, demarcation of the perfused right lobe is augmented by fluorescence. The line of demarcation is marked on the anterior and inferior liver surface using electrocautery. The clamps are removed. An ultrasound may be performed to mark the course of the MHV (which will be procured with the graft) and segmental veins draining segments 5 and 8 (Fig. 34.13).

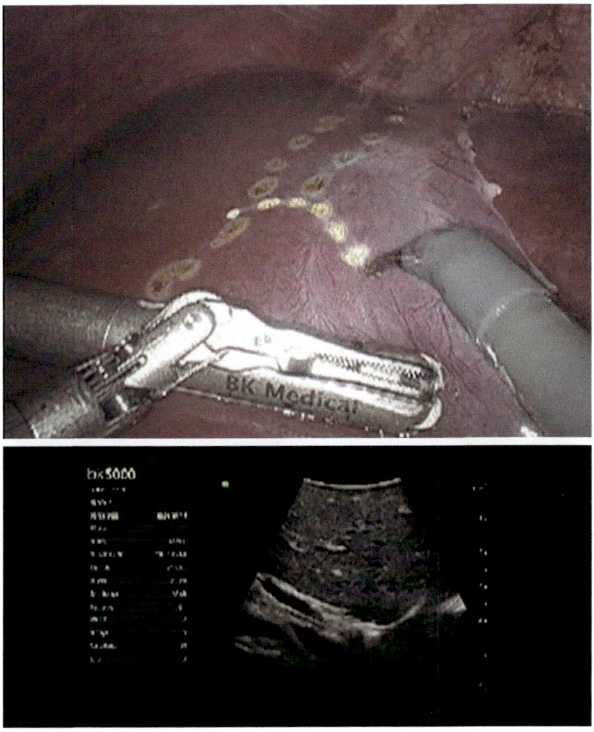

Fig. 34.13 Course of MHV, segment 4 and 5 hepatic venous branches marked on the surface using ultrasound guidance

Parenchymal Transection

"Rubber Band" Retraction Technique

The previously described rubber band retraction technique is used.

Parenchymal Transection

Parenchymal transection is performed as described above (Figs. 34.14 and 34.15). If the caudate is not to be procured, the sagittal parenchymal transection plane ends at the level of the caudate lobe and then curves along a horizontal plane dividing the left lobe from the caudate. If the caudate is to be procured, the caudate lobe is split, and the sagittal transection plane continues until the anterior IVC.

Division of the Left Hepatic Duct

Once all the parenchyma has been transected to the level of the biliary bifurcation, an ICG cholangiogram is performed. The biliary bifurcation is visualized, and the appropriate location chosen on the LHD for division (Fig. 34.16). The two techniques for bile duct division are described above.

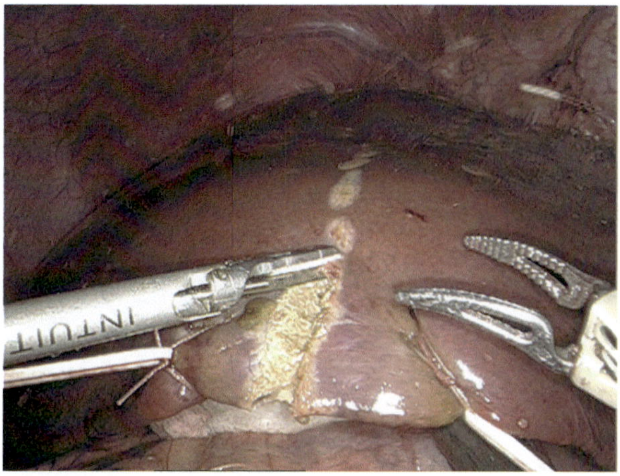

Fig. 34.14 Parenchymal transection using robotic energy devices

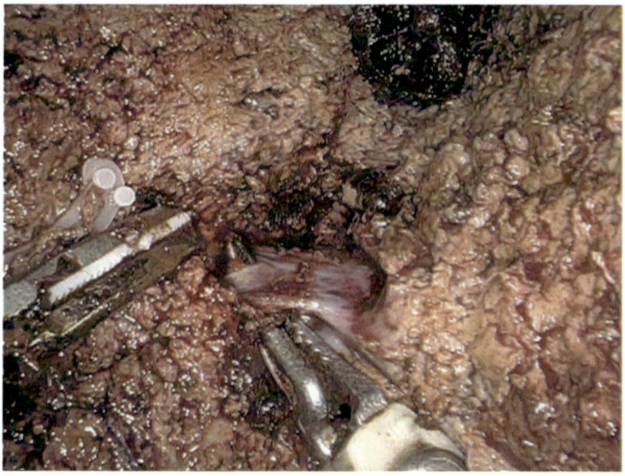

Fig. 34.15 Dissection of segment 5 hepatic vein branches

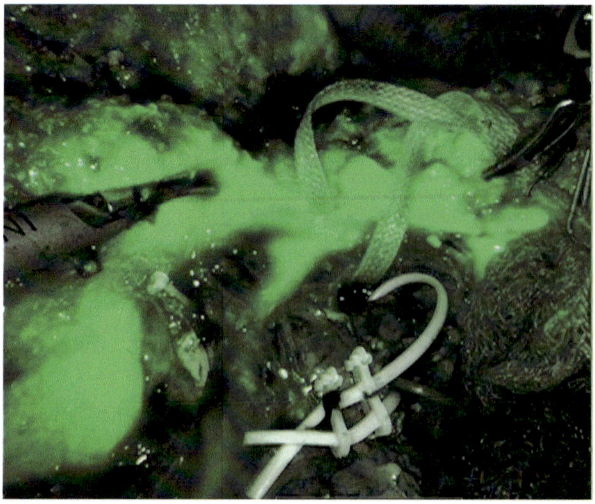

Fig. 34.16 ICG cholangiogram confirmation of biliary duct anatomy with umbilical tape around LHD

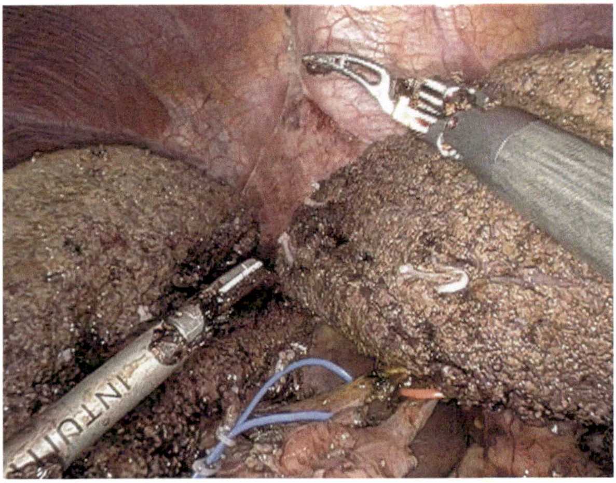

Fig. 34.17 Completion of parenchymal transection of left lobe graft (only attached to rest of liver by LHA, LPV, middle, and left hepatic veins)

Completion of Parenchymal Transection

Once the LHD is divided, the final portion of the parenchymal transection is performed. The transection proceeds cephalad until we encounter the area of the middle and left hepatic veins. This marks the end of the parenchymal transection for a left donor hepatectomy (Fig. 34.17). The middle and left hepatic veins are encircled with an umbilical tape if this was not previously done.

Cross-Clamp and Graft Extraction

The middle robotic arms are undocked. A Pfannenstiel incision is made. Left lobes should fit a laparoscopic retrieval bag, and this technique is described above.

The robot is redocked. Cross-clamping commences when the LHA is doubly clipped and transected distal to the clips while preserving as much length as possible for recipient anastomosis. The LPV is transected with a stapler or large clips just distal to the stitch marking the bifurcation. The middle and left hepatic veins are transected with a single firing of the stapler. The graft and gallbladder are then extracted as previously described.

Closure

Hemostasis of the cut surface and hilum is performed. Bile leak is ruled out. The clips, staple, and suture lines are inspected. A drain is placed at the cut surface and externalized via one of the ports.

Left Lateral Donor Sectionectomy

Falciform Dissection and Left Lateral Section Mobilization

This is similar to left donor hepatectomy except the superior end of the transection line is between the MHV and left hepatic vein (LHV). An accessory LHA from the LGA usually supplies segments 2 and 3 (this can be confirmed on preoperative imaging) and can be the sole arterial inflow to a left lateral section graft. The caudate lobe is not procured with a left lateral section graft.

Hilar Dissection

The third arm is used to retract segment 4B to expose the hilum. A cholecystectomy is performed. The peritoneal covering over the left side of the hilum is opened. Dissection of the left hepatic artery is similar to the left donor hepatectomy. The artery to segments 2 and 3 is usually a branch of the LHA and the length of the LHA is usually provided to the recipient for anastomosis. This is unnecessary if there is an accessory LHA from the LGA.

Demarcation

Demarcation of the left lateral section is usually not necessary as the transection line is guided by the falciform ligament (marked along the *right* side of the ligament and the umbilical fissure). Nevertheless, clamping of the inflow vessels and ICG injection as described above can be performed to ensure the right lobe is perfused and a cholangiogram is visible by the time of bile duct transection.

An ultrasound is performed to mark the course of the MHV (which will remain with the donor remnant) and the LHV (which is procured with the graft).

Parenchymal Transection

"Rubber band" Retraction Technique

The previously described rubber band retraction technique is used. One rubber band is sutured to each side of the transection line at the tip of the liver. Each end of the rubber band is externalized on the respective sides of the upper abdomen and secured to the drapes.

Parenchymal Transection

Parenchymal transection is performed as described above. Pedicles to segment 4 will be encountered during transection on the right side of the umbilical fissure. These are encircled and divided between clips. Transection is completed to the level of bile duct just to the right of the umbilical fissure.

Division of the Left Hepatic Duct

An ICG cholangiogram is performed. The biliary bifurcation and the left hepatic duct are visualized, and the appropriate location on the LHD just to the right side of the umbilical fissure is chosen for division. The two techniques for bile duct division are described above.

Completion of Parenchymal Transection

Once the duct is divided, parenchymal transection proceeds along the sagittal fissure (fissure for the ligamentum venosum) heading cephalad anteriorly along the previously marked line between the middle and left hepatic veins and posteriorly separating the caudate lobe from the left lobe. Transection is completed once the left hepatic vein is reached.

Cross-Clamp and Graft Extraction

This step of the procedure is similar to that described for a donor left hepatectomy, except for the outflow vessel; only the left hepatic vein is divided with a stapler and the middle hepatic vein is left with the remnant in the donor.

Robotic Recipient Transplantation

As accumulation of minimally invasive donor liver resection has mounted, minimally invasive recipient surgery (MIRS) has been attempted. However, in MIRS, there is a concern of massive bleeding due to coagulopathy, and the surgery is technically difficult [18–24]. MIRS can be classified into three different types: (1) small incisional open surgery, (2) laparoscopic or robotic mobilization followed by small incisional engraftment, and (3) totally laparoscopic, robotic, or laparoscopic and robotic hybrid engraftment. We aim to cover the indications and contraindications, preparation, requirements, operating room setup, port placement in hybrid and robotic recipient surgery, and surgical details for robotic LDLT.

Suitability Criteria for Robotic Recipient Surgery

Recipient Considerations

(i) *Cardiopulmonary stability*: The recipient must not have any cardiopulmonary dysfunction. This is crucial to withstand the reverse Trendelenburg position and the extended IVC clamping required during vascular anastomosis.

(ii) *Minimal inflammation and adhesions*: Candidates with a history of liver surgery, spontaneous bacterial peritonitis (SBP), or alcohol-associated cirrhosis often have unclear dissection planes or significant adhesions, making them less ideal for this procedure.

(iii) *Liver size*: Robotic surgery is not suitable for recipients with enlarged livers as seen in conditions like fulminant liver failure, primary biliary cirrhosis (PBC), or polycystic liver disease due to increased risk during surgery.

(iv) *Surgical complexity*: Ideal candidates should require minimal additional procedures such as thrombectomy of long segments, shunt ligation, or portal vein venoplasty.

(v) *Vascular stability*: Recipients with minor to moderate collateral circulation that can maintain stable vital signs during the anhepatic phase are preferable.

(vi) *ABO compatibility*: Recipients who are ABO incompatible are at a higher risk for diffuse intrahepatic biliary strictures (DIBS) due to longer warm ischemic times and are therefore not good candidates for robotic recipient surgery.

Graft (Donor) Considerations

(i) *Anatomical variations*: Donors with fewer anatomical variation are preferred to simplify the surgical procedure.

(ii) *Appropriate liver size matching*: The GRWR should be >0.8. More importantly, the size of the graft relative to the recipient's (right abdominal) cavity should facilitate ease of portal vein anastomosis.

(iii) *Liver quality and age*: The donor liver should be young and of high quality to endure the potentially longer warm ischemic times associated with robotic transplantation.

These criteria are essential to select the most suitable candidates for robotic liver transplantation, ensuring a higher success rate and minimizing complications. This approach leverages both recipient and donor characteristics to optimize the surgical outcomes.

Specific Preparation or Skill Requirements

Surgical Team

An experienced anesthesiologist skilled in laparoscopic operations and robotic liver resections is necessary, as changing positions during robotic procedures can be challenging and vital signs must be maintained consistently. A surgical team familiar with the robotic system and frequent arm changes should be involved. An expert surgeon should be present to assist, skillfully positioning and manipulating the liver graft for optimal access.

Equipment

Surgical equipment used in open procedures should be readily available in case of a necessary conversion to open surgery. A large Stansky or Chitwood DeBakey clamp (SCANLAN®) is required to securely clamp the inferior vena cava (IVC) during hepatic vein anastomosis, allowing for easy external control.

OR Setup

A patient is placed in a supine position with their legs apart, facilitating access for the surgery (Fig. 34.18). An assistant is positioned between the patient's legs, a common placement in robotic surgeries to aid with instrument handling and provide a better view of the surgical field. The operating table is set in a reverse Trendelenburg position at a 15-degree angle, elevating the patient's upper body. The scrub nurse stands on the right side of the patient, ready to assist by handling surgical instruments and maintaining sterility throughout the procedure.

Port Positioning

Laparoscopic and Robotic Hybrid LDLT

In hybrid laparoscopic and robotic LDLT, the laparoscopic ports are placed in typical positions used during a total hepatectomy (Fig. 34.19). An umbilical port is used for the laparoscopic camera, and four additional ports are used for the operator and assistant. During the engraftment phase, new robotic ports are configured. A 12 mm

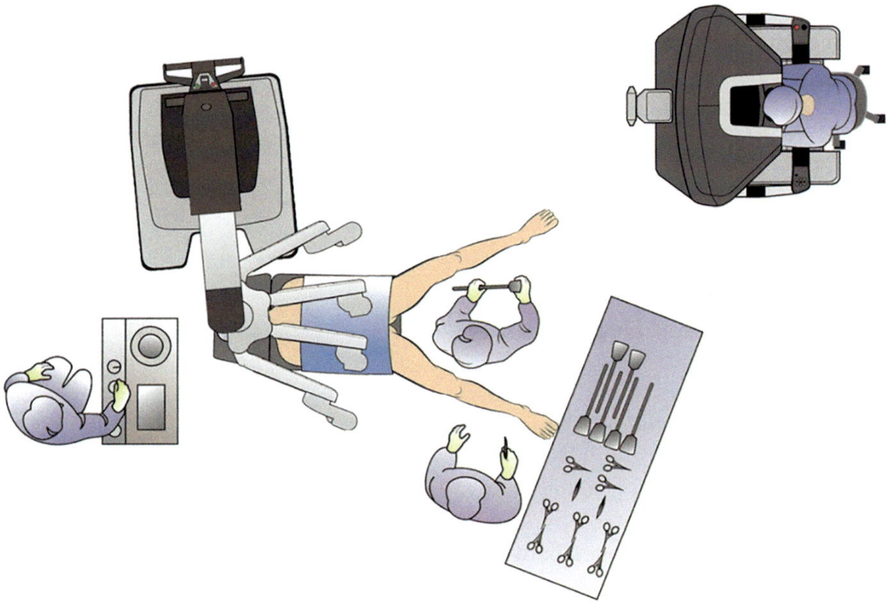

Fig. 34.18 Operating room setup for robotic recipient transplantation

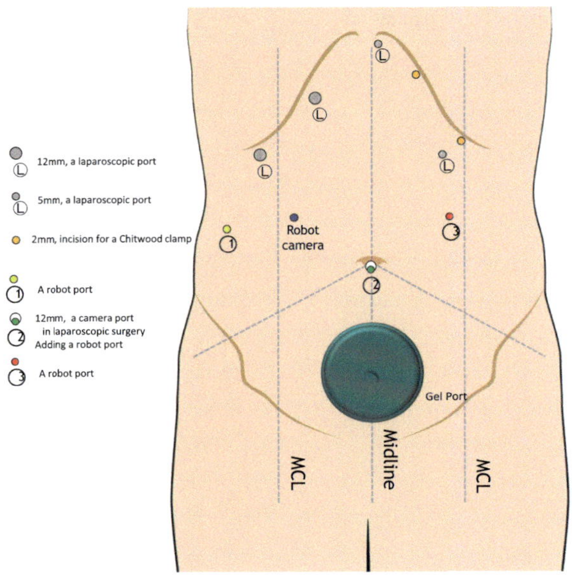

Fig. 34.19 Port placements for laparoscopic-robotic recipient transplantation

laparoscopic camera port is repurposed by inserting an 8 mm robotic port to connect the robotic arm. Three additional robotic ports are then added. Furthermore, two 2 mm incisions are made at the left subcostal margin to insert a Chitwood clamp for the total clamping of the IVC. A Gelport is also inserted through a low transverse incision to facilitate the removal of the diseased liver and the placement and adjustment of the liver graft.

Totally Robotic LDLT

For a completely robotic LDLT, the camera port is positioned about 15 cm below the midpoint between the hepatic vein and the portal vein (Fig. 34.20). The remaining ports are positioned approximately 8 cm from the camera port, along a line that is slightly tilted to the right.

Robotic Recipient Hepatectomy

Robot Arms Setup

Robot arm 1: Maryland bipolar forceps, fenestrated bipolar forceps
Robot arm 2: Camera
Robot arm 3: Hot shears, cautery hook, vessel sealer, HARMONIC ACE
Robot arm 4: ProGrasp forceps, suction/irrigator
Instruments are interchanged between arm 1 and arm 3 as needed.

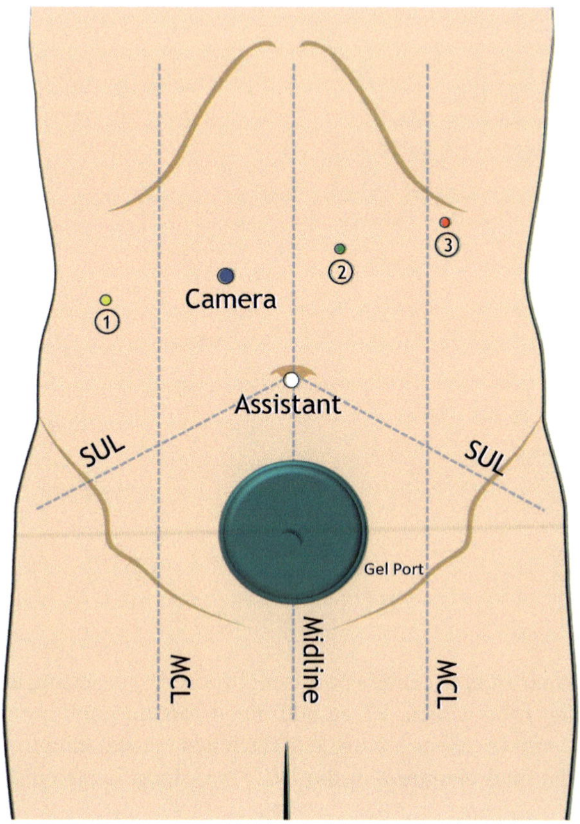

Fig. 34.20 Port placements for robotic recipient transplantation

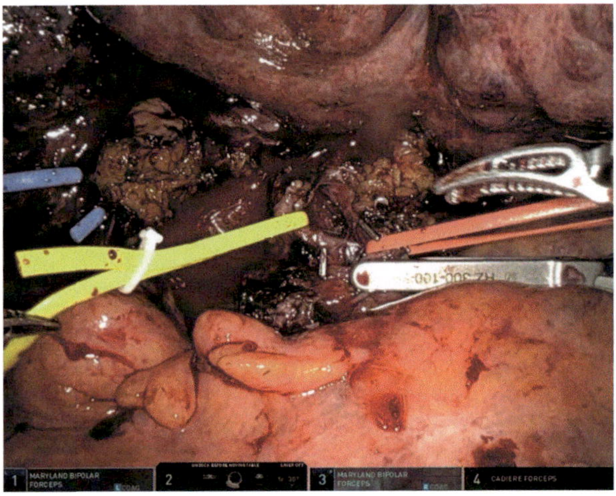

Fig. 34.21 Clamping of the proper hepatic artery for hilar dissection

Mobilization and Hilar Dissection

The surgery begins with port insertion followed by division of the falciform ligament. The right and left coronary ligaments are then dissected using scissors or a hook. The cystic duct and artery are resected, but the gallbladder remains attached for traction, aiding exposure of the hilar area. Complete cholecystectomy is performed after hilar dissection. The proper hepatic artery and main portal vein are clamped to minimize bleeding. The LHA, MHA, and RHA are carefully isolated and resected along with the extrahepatic bile duct resection at the hilum. Both RPV and LPV are clamped at the liver side and those are resected (Fig. 34.21).

Retrohepatic IVC Dissection

The lesser sac is opened, and the ductus venosus is ligated. The liver is mobilized from the right, detaching it from the adrenal gland. Dissection continues between the liver and the IVC, with short hepatic and right inferior hepatic veins being resected. The liver is lifted to separate it from the retrohepatic IVC (Fig. 34.22).

Hepatic Vein Division and Liver Removal

The common trunk of the LHV and MHVs is isolated and divided cranially using a stapler. The RHV is also stapled after dissection around the right IVC ligament. The diseased liver is then enclosed in a vinyl bag and removed through a Pfannenstiel incision, and a Gelport is applied (Fig. 34.23).

Backbench Graft Preparation

After the liver graft is flushed with organ preservation solution, typical backbench procedures are performed. The portal vein of the graft is elongated using the recipient's portal vein or a cadaveric iliac vein (Fig. 34.24). Additional sutures are placed for traction around the RHV, portal vein, and Glisson's capsule near the bile duct (Fig. 34.25). The hepatic artery is meticulously prepared, and the graft is wrapped in a vinyl bag with iced gauze. The graft is then inserted through the Pfannenstiel incision and positioned optimally for engraftment by an assistant surgeon.

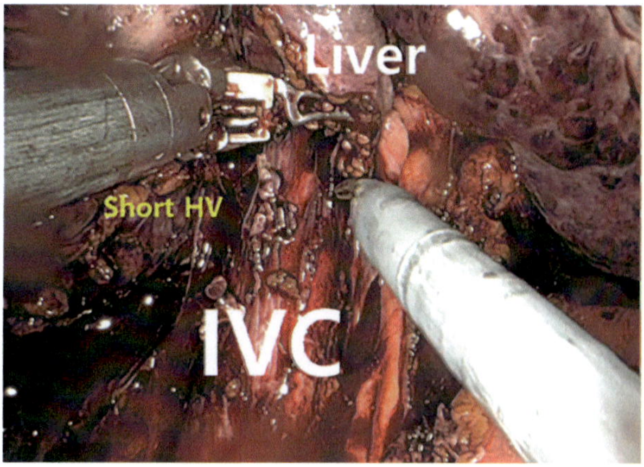

Fig. 34.22 Liver is lifted to separate it from the IVC

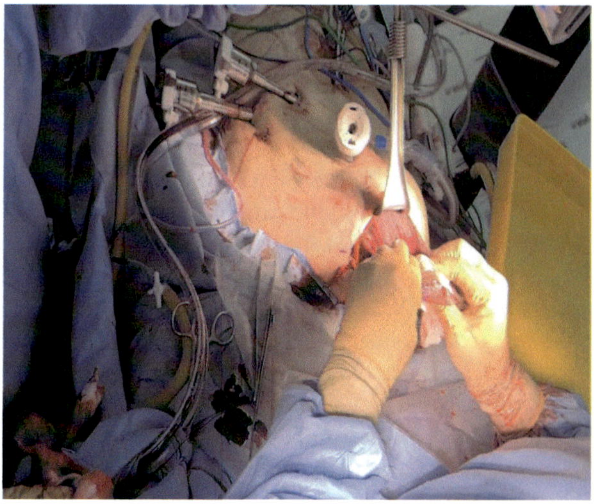

Fig. 34.23 Diseased liver removed via a Pfannenstiel incision

Graft Implantation

Robotic Arms Setup

- Robot arm 1: Maryland bipolar forceps or Cadiere forceps
  - Microsurgery: Black Diamond Micro forceps, DeBakey forceps, Maryland Bipolar forceps
- Robot arm 2: Camera
- Robot arm 3. Large SutureCut™ needle cut driver
  - Microsurgery: Black Diamond Micro forceps, Potts Scissors Large SutureCut™ needle cut driver, Hot Shears™
- Robot arm 4: ProGrasp forceps, suction/irrigator

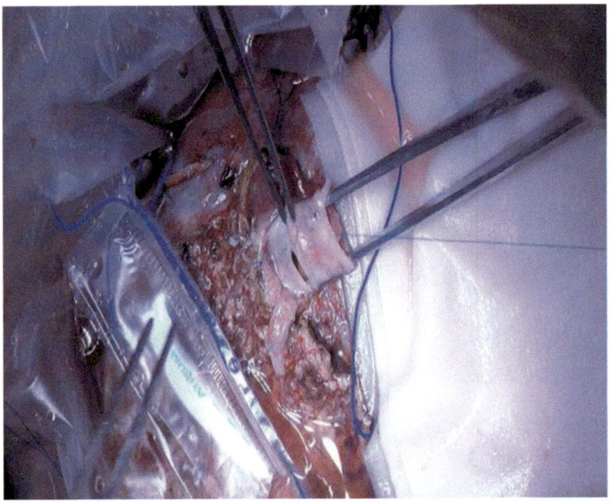

Fig. 34.24 The portal vein of the graft is elongated using the recipient's portal vein or a cadaveric iliac vein

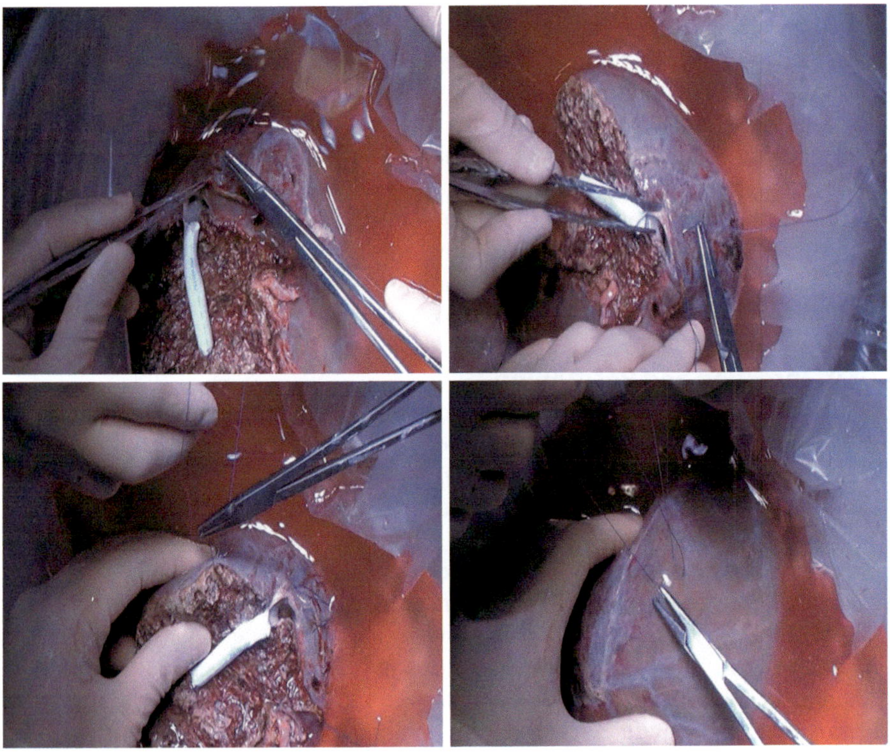

Fig. 34.25 Additional sutures are placed for traction around the RHV, portal vein, and Glisson's capsule near the bile duct

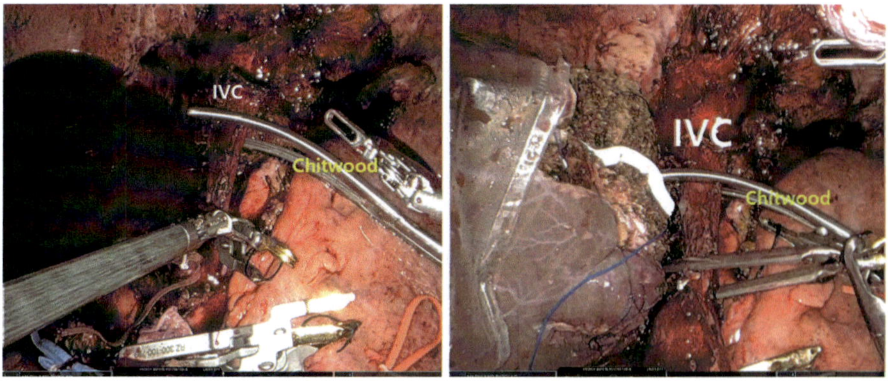

Fig. 34.26 A long segment of IVC must be isolated from surrounding tissues before applying a total clamp

Bleeding Control and Test Clamping of IVC

Given the challenges in controlling the graft's rotation and bleeding after implantation, meticulous bleeding management is imperative. Proper control of bleeding is particularly crucial around the right diaphragm, behind the right hepatic vein stump, adjacent to the adrenal gland, and in the retro-IVC region. For secure hepatic vein anastomosis, the long segment of IVC must be isolated from surrounding tissues before applying a total clamp. Similarly, even when using a partial clamp, separating the IVC ensures effective bleeding control and stabilizes the clamp during engraftment (Fig. 34.26). Subsequently, the effectiveness of the IVC clamp (Chitwood clamp for total clamping) is assessed by monitoring for any changes in vital signs before proceeding with the anastomosis.

Graft Insertion and Positioning

All robotic arms are removed to prevent damage to the graft. Ice-slushed gauzes are placed on the right diaphragm before the graft, encased in a vinyl bag, is inserted either through or without the Gelport. An assistant then helps to optimally position the graft for anastomosis (Fig. 34.27), after which the robotic system is reassembled.

Hepatic Vein and Portal Vein Anastomosis

The hepatic vein anastomosis is performed using Prolene 6-0 or Gore-Tex suture under IVC clamping, with Gore-Tex providing resistance against breakage by robotic instruments. Portal vein anastomosis is facilitated by vertically shifting the suture axis. If the axis is formed similarly to the white line in Fig. 34.28 when approximating the graft, it will put a lot of strain on the joints even if it is a robot system. Rotating the upper and lower tagging counterclockwise and moving the axis to the red line will allow for easier joint movement during anastomosis.

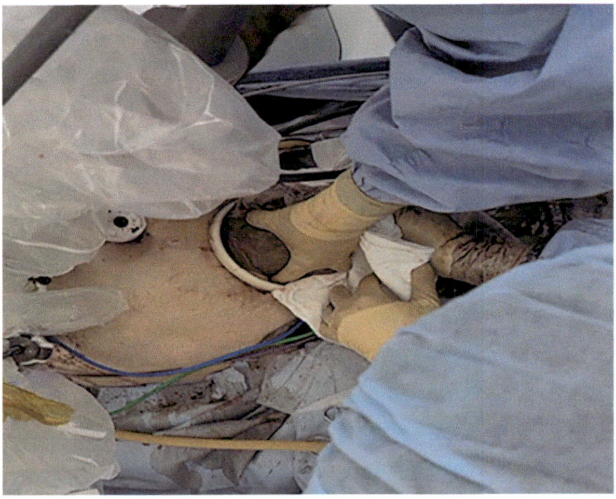

Fig. 34.27 An assistant inserts the graft via the Pfannenstiel and then helps to optimally position the graft for anastomosis

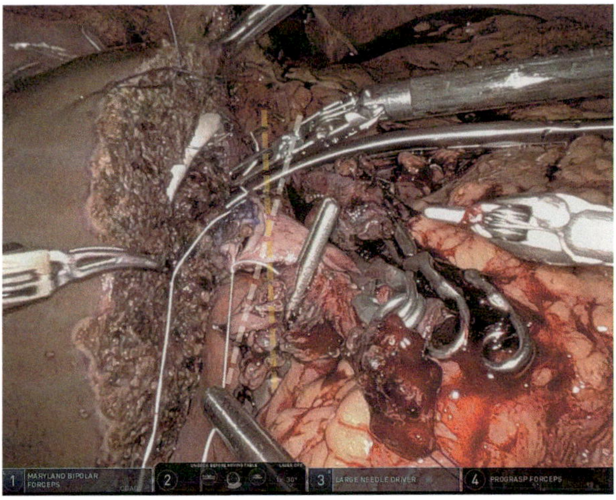

Fig. 34.28 If the PV anastomosis is performed parallel to the graft resection surface (the white line) using our proposed port placements, the operator's wrist might have to bend at an unexpected angle, making the anastomosis challenging. Conducting the anastomosis in the direction of the yellow line, while adjusting both ends of the portal veins with trimming and staying close to the IVC axis, will allow for a more comfortable wrist position

Hepatic Artery and Bile Duct Anastomosis

Microclamps are used on the hepatic artery, with interrupted or continuous sutures applied using Nylon 8-0 or 7-0 (Fig. 34.29a). Duct-to-duct anastomosis for bile duct reconstruction is achieved through posterior continuous and anterior interrupted sutures using Prolene 6-0 (Fig. 34.29b).

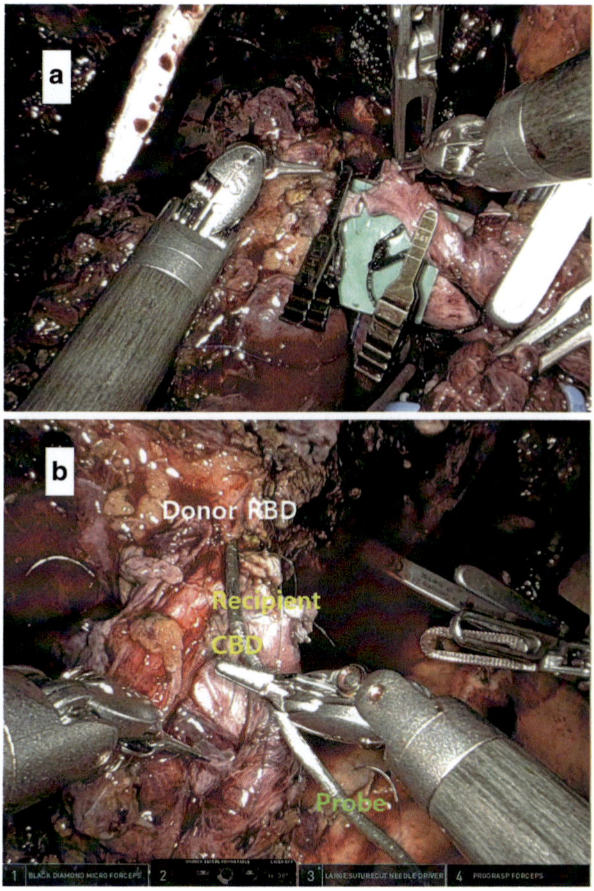

Fig. 34.29 (**a**) Hepatic artery anastomosis (**b**) Bile duct anastomosis

Pearls and Pitfalls

Robotic surgery offers ergonomic advantages, reducing surgeon fatigue and improving surgical precision through enhanced dexterity and tremor correction. Recipients benefit from minimally invasive techniques that result in smaller incisions, less pain, and potentially quicker recovery times. Despite its advantages, robotic surgery may result in slower surgical team response during emergencies compared to open or laparoscopic surgeries, potentially extending operation times and increasing the risk of graft injury. The limited number of specialized instruments and the absence of tactile feedback can complicate delicate tasks like vascular anastomosis, often leading to suture breakage.

Conclusion

Robotic donor hepatectomy offers a minimally invasive approach to this special group of patients who are undergoing major liver surgery for the benefit of another. Donor safety is paramount and centers planning to embark on a robotic donor hepatectomy program should have significant experience in both donor hepatectomy and robotic non-donor liver surgery. Robotic recipient surgery, particularly in the contexts of total hepatectomy and liver engraftment, represents a significant advancement in surgical technology, offering distinct benefits over traditional approaches. These ongoing advancements in robotic technology and technique refinement suggest that the future of robotic recipient surgery is promising. As surgeons gain proficiency and as the technology evolves to mitigate current limitations, robotic surgery is poised to enhance patient outcomes further and redefine standards in surgical care.

References

1. Olthoff KM, Emond JC, Shearon TH, Everson G, Baker TB, Fisher RA, Freise CE, Gillespie BW, Everhart JE. Liver regeneration after living donor transplantation: adult-to-adult living donor liver transplantation cohort study. Liver Transpl. 2015;21(1):79–88.
2. Haga J, Shimazu M, Wakabayashi G, Tanabe M, Kawachi S, Fuchimoto Y, Hoshino K, Morikawa Y, Kitajima M, Kitagawa Y. Liver regeneration in donors and adult recipients after living donor liver transplantation. Liver Transpl. 2008;14:1718–24.
3. Koido Y, Matsunami H, Lynch SV, Strong RW. Successful liver transplantation from a living donor to her son. N Engl J Med. 1990;322:1505–7.
4. Miller CM, Quintini C, Dhawan A, Durand F, Heimbach JK, Kim-Schluger HL, Kyrana E, Lee SG, Lerut J, Lo CM, Pomfret EA. The international liver transplantation society living donor liver transplant recipient guideline. Transplantation. 2017;101(5):938–44.
5. Hibi T, Wei Chieh AK, Chi-Yan Chan A, Bhangui P. Current status of liver transplantation in Asia. Int J Surg. 2020;82S:4–8.
6. Organ Procurement & Transplantation Network. March 25, 2024. National Data. https://optn.transplant.hrsa.gov/data/view-data-reports/national-data/
7. Black M, Gupta A, Asrani SK, Ma TW, Testa G, Wall A. Living donor liver transplantation versus donation after brain death and donation after circulatory death liver transplantation in the US. Proceedings (Bayl Univ Med Cent). 2022;35(3):273–7.
8. Acuna SA, Zhang W, Yoon PD, Ivanics T, Zhu MP, Claasen M, Zuckerman J, Anand G, Cattral MS, Sapisochin G. Right lobe versus left lobe living donor liver transplantation: a systematic review and meta-analysis of donor and recipient outcomes. Transplantation. 2022;106(12):2370–8.
9. Cheah YL, Simpson MA, Pomposelli JJ, Pomfret EA. Incidence of death and potentially life-threatening near-miss events in living donor hepatic lobectomy: a world-wide survey. Liver Transpl. 2013;19(5):499–506.
10. Cheah YL, Heimbach J, Kwon CHD, Pomposelli J, Rudow DL, Broering D, Spiro M, Raptis DA, Roberts JP, the ERAS4OLT.org Working Group. Influence of surgical technique in donor hepatectomy on immediate and short-term living donor outcomes – a systematic review of the literature, meta-analysis, and expert panel recommendations. Clin Transpl. 2022;36:e14703.
11. Dew MA, DiMartini A, Ladner DP, et al. Psychosocial outcomes 3 to 10 years after donation in the Adult to Adult Living Donor Liver Transplantation Cohort Study. Transplantation. 2016;100(6):1257–69.

12. Humphreville VR, Radosevich DM, Humar A, Payne WD, Kandaswamy R, Lake JR, Matas AJ, Pruett TL, Chinnakotla S. Long-term health-related quality of life after living liver donation. Liver Transpl. 2016;22(1):53–62.
13. Giulianotti PC, Tzvetanov I, Jeon H, Bianco F, Spaggiari M, Oberholzer J, Benedetti E. Robot-assisted right lobe donor hepatectomy. Transpl Int. 2012;25(1):e5–9.
14. Chen PD, Wu CY, Hu RH, Ho CM, Lee PH, Lai HS, Lin MT, Wu YM. Robotic liver donor right hepatectomy: A pure, minimally invasive approach. Liver Transpl. 2016;22(11):1509–18.
15. Rho SY, Lee JG, Joo DJ, et al. Outcomes of robotic living donor right hepatectomy from 52 consecutive cases: comparison with open and laparoscopy-assisted donor hepatectomy. Ann Surg. 2022;275(2):e433–42.
16. Broering DC, Elsheikh Y, Alnemary Y, et al. Robotic versus open right lobe donor hepatectomy for adult living donor liver transplantation: a propensity score-matched analysis. Liver Transpl. 2020;26(11):1455–64.
17. Joliat GR, Kobayashi K, Hasegawa K, Thomson JE, Padbury R, Scott M, Brustia R, Scatton O, Tran Cao HS, Vauthey JN, Dincler S, Clavien PA, Wigmore SJ, Demartines N, Melloul E. Guidelines for perioperative care for liver surgery: Enhanced Recovery After Surgery (ERAS) society recommendations 2022. World J Surg. 2023;47(1):11–34.
18. Dokmak S, Cauchy F, Sepulveda A, Choinier PM, Dondéro F, Aussilhou B, Hego C, Chopinet S, Infantes P, Weiss E, Francoz C, Sauvanet A, Paugam-Burtz C, Durand F, Soubrane O. Laparoscopic liver transplantation: dream or reality? The first step with laparoscopic explant hepatectomy. Ann Surg. 2020;272:889–93.
19. Suh KS, Hong SK, Hong K, Han ES, Hong SY, Suh S, Lee JM, Choi Y, Yi NJ, Lee KW. Minimally invasive living donor liver transplantation: pure laparoscopic explant hepatectomy and graft implantation using upper midline incision. Liver Transpl. 2021;27:1493–7.
20. Suh KS, Hong SK, Lee S, Hong SY, Suh S, Han ES, Yang SM, Choi Y, Yi NJ, Lee KW. Pure laparoscopic living donor liver transplantation: dreams come true. Am J Transplant. 2022;22:260–5.
21. Suh KS, Hong SK, Lee S, Hong SY, Suh S, Han ES, Yang SM, Choi Y, Yi NJ, Lee KW. Purely laparoscopic explant hepatectomy and hybrid laparoscopic/robotic graft implantation in living donor liver transplantation. Br J Surg. 2022;109:162–4.
22. Lee KW, Choi Y, Hong SK, Lee S, Hong SY, Suh S, Han ES, Yi NJ, Suh KS. Laparoscopic donor and recipient hepatectomy followed by robot-assisted liver graft implantation in living donor liver transplantation. Am J Transplant. 2022;22:1230–5.
23. Lee KW, Choi Y, Lee S, Hong SY, Suh S, Han ES, Hong SK, Yang SM, Yi NJ, Suh KS. Total robot-assisted recipient's surgery in living donor liver transplantation: first step towards the future. J Hepatobiliary Pancreat Sci. 2023;30:1198–200.
24. Broering DC, Raptis DA, Elsheikh Y. Pioneering fully robotic donor hepatectomy and robotic recipient liver graft implantation – a new horizon in liver transplantation. Int J Surg. 2024;110:1333–6.

Index

A
Abdominal wall reconstruction (AWR), 279
Achalasia
    botulinum toxin, 143
    calcium channel blockers and nitrates, 142
    clinical features, 140
    diagnosis, 141
    management, 139
    nitrates, 142
    pathophysiology, 140
    pharmacotherapies, 143
    pneumatic dilation, 143
    POEM, 144
    surgical management, 145
    surgical treatment, 144
Acute care surgery (ACS), 69
Adhesiolysis, 284
Adopting stage, 70–72
Adrenal tumor, 407, 412
Alarm icons, 49
American College of Surgeons (ACS), 114, 124
American College of Surgeons National Surgical Quality Improvement Program (ACS-NSQIP) database, 95
American Urological Association (AUA) Robotic Surgery Courses, 113
Anastomotic insufficiency, incidence, 160
Anchoring procedures for Robotic Surgery pathway, 124, 126
Annals of Surgery, 110
Annual SSF Robotics Course, 115
Anterior mediastinum, 471, 472
Antiplatelet therapy, 285
Antireflux surgery, 129, 228
Arm cart, 35
    design, 30
Arm clash, 54
Arm modes, 52
Articulating instruments, 23
Artificial intelligence (AI), 9, 17, 94
    automated surgery, 96
    patient care, 95, 96
    skills assessment system, 95
    surgical decision making, 94, 95
Artificial neural networks (ANNs), 94
Association of Program Directors for Colon and Rectal Surgeons Robotic Training Courses, 112
Atelectasis, 428
Augmented intelligence, 21, 28
Augmented reality/mediated reality (AR/MR) technology, 89
Automated endoscopic system for optimal positioning (AESOP), 6
Autonomous surgery, 17

B
Bariatric surgery, 185, 186
Barium esophagram, 141
Basic metabolic panel (BMP), 223
Bedside skills, 81, 82
Bedside units (BSUs), 56
Behind the Knife (BTK), 111
Bilateral axillo-breast approach (BABA) approach, 415
Bile duct injury, 322
Biliary disease, 300, 304
Biliary reconstruction, 321
Biliopancreatic diversion with duodenal switch (BPD-DS), 216
Billroth, 175
Bipolar Maryland Forceps, 435

S. Samreen et al. (eds.), *The SAGES Manual of Robotic Surgery*,
https://doi.org/10.1007/978-3-031-86927-3

BK5000 (R), 332
Botulinum toxin A (Botox®) injection, 264, 286
Bowel measurement, 219, 222
Bowel obstruction, 210
Braun enteroenterostomy, 182
Bronchi dissection, 448

C

Cadiere forceps, 259
Caresyntax, 93
Cholecystectomy, 299
  indications, 300
  patient positioning, 301
  robotic docking, 301, 302
  robotic equipment, 300
Choledochal cyst, 322
Common bile duct (CBD), 312
Complete mesocolic excision (CME), 351, 352
Complex abdominal wall, 280, 281
Complex incisional hernia, 281
Component separation techniques, 282
Conformité Européenne (CE), 39
Console screen, 46
Console training, 82
Continuing education, 114–115
  medical education opportunities, 114
  opportunities, 109
Coronary artery bypass surgery, 464, 467, 468
COVID-19 pandemic, 97
Credentialing, 84
Crowdsourced Assessment of Technical Skills (C-SATS), 111
Cumulative sum method (CUSUM), 162
Curriculum task force, 124

D

Da Vinci robotic platform, 109
Da Vinci SimNow, 112
Da Vinci Single-Port (SP) surgical system, 382, 454
Da Vinci Training Passport, 113
da Vinci Xi robot, 16, 429
Da Vinci XI Surgical System, 130, 232, 246, 330, 416
Deep vein thrombosis or pulmonary embolism, 211
Deep venous prophylaxis, 285
Defense Advanced Research Projects Agency (DARPA), 15
Delphi study, 281
Demarcation, 501
Digital surgery, 21, 101
  advanced visualization
    AR implementation, 90, 91
    AR/MR technology, 89, 90
    3-D visualization, 88
  connectivity, 96
  data analytics (*see also* Artificial intelligence (AI))
  data capture, 92
    from operative equipment, 93
    operating room and integrated operating room, 93, 94
    video data, 92
  elements of, 87
  enhanced instrumentation, 91
  growth of, 87
  robotic surgery platforms, 99
  telementoring, 97
    for clinical practice, 97, 98
    education, 97
  telesurgery, 98
Distal gastrectomy, 180, 181
Docking the arms, 37
Dor fundoplication, 152
Dor procedure, 151
Double tract reconstruction, 182
Drug-eluting stent (DES), 465
Dumping syndrome, 211
Duodenal dissection, 219
Duodenal switch (DS), 244
Duodenoileostomy, 220, 221
Dysphagia and definitive diagnosis, 139

E

Early recovery after anesthesia (ERAS), 348
Educational websites and platforms, 111
Endoscopic/endoluminal functional luminal imaging probe (EndoFLIP), 141, 142
Enhanced recovery pathways (ERPs) for perioperative care, 123
Enteroenterostomy, 222, 223
Ergonomics, 19
Esophageal myotomy, 149
Esophagectomy
  distant metastases, 159
  incidence rates, 159
  morbidity and mortality rates, 160
  reconstruction, 159
  types, 159

Established Program to Competitive Research (EPSCoR) program, 68
European Association for Endoscopic Surgery (EAES), 113
Eye tracking, 19, 25

F
Facebook groups, 113, 124–127
Falciform dissection, 310, 498
Fenestrated bipolar forceps, 435
First-time recurrent incisional hernia, 281
Fluorescence guided surgery (FGS), 88
Fundamentals of endoscopic surgery (FES), 123
Fundamentals of laparoscopic surgery (FLS), 80, 122
Fundamental use of surgical energy (FUSE), 122
Fundoplication, 135

G
Ganglioneuroblastoma, 484
Gastrectomy, 175, 177
Gastric bypass, 192
Gastric mucosal perforation, 153, 154
Gastric myotomy, 150, 151
Gastroduodenal artery (GDA), 180
Gastrointestinal stromal tumors (GIST), 176
Gastro-jejunal anastomosis, 200, 211
Gastrojejunostomy, 252
GelPort® Laparoscopic System, 64
Ghrelin, 193
Giant inguinoscrotal hernias, 264
GIBLIB, 112
Global evaluative assessment of robotic skills (GEARS), 82
Global robotic assisted surgery podcast (GRASP), 111
Graft implantation, 516–520
Graphics processing units (GPUs), 8

H
Hand-assisted laparoscopic surgery (HALS), 64
Hand controllers, 49
Hand detection, 48
Hand sewn anastomosis (HSA), 252
Haptic feedback, 19
Hasson technique, 131
Head Up Display (HUD), 47
Health and Medicine Division of the National Academies of Sciences, Engineering, and Medicine standards, 124
Heller myotomy, 145–150
Hepatobiliary surgery, 324
Hereditary non-polyposis colorectal cancer (HNPCC), 367
Hiatal dissection, 147–148
Hiatal hernias
  classification, 129, 130
  instruments, 132
  operating room setup, 131
  operative technique, 132–135
  pathophysiology, 129, 130
  port placement, 132
  post-operative care, 136
  surgical intervention, 130
High priority alarm icon, 49
Hilar dissection, 311, 318, 498
Hugo instruments, 36
The Hugo RAS™ system, 30, 31
Hybrid coronary revascularization (HCR), 462, 465, 466
Hybrid robotic TAR for lateral incisional hernia, 294
Hybrid robotic ventral hernia repair, 292
  extensive enterolysis and mesh removal, 292
Hybrid TAR for a complex incisional hernia, 293

I
Iatrogenic esophageal perforation, 153
Indocyanine green (ICG), 303
Indocyanine green (ICG) cholangiography, 88
Inferior mesenteric artery (IMA), 366, 394
Inferior thyroid artery (ITA), 422
Inferior vena cava (IVC), 335
ingle Anastomosis DuodenoIleal bypass with Sleeve gastrectomy (SADI-S)
  patient preparation, 217
Inguinal hernia repairs, 267
In Person Proctoring, 112
Institute for Research into Cancers of the Digestive System (irCAD), 112
Instrument adjust mode, 52
Instrument bedside units (IBSU), 45
Instrument change mode, 54
Instrument compatibility, 55
Intelligent surgical unit (ISU), 21, 25, 26
Internal herniation, 211

International Journal of Medical Robotics and computer assisted surgery, 110
Intra-abdominal access, 287
Intraoperative cholangiogram (IOC), 303
Intraoperative indocyanine green (ICG), 424
Intraoperative nerve monitoring (IONM), 416
Intrathoracic circular-stapled end-to-side esophagogastrostomy, 170
Intuitive Surgical Online Learning Platform (My Intuitive), 111
Intuitive telementoring, 112
Inverse probability of treatment weighting (IPTW), 430

J
Journal of Medical Insight (JOMI), 111
Journal of Robotic Surgery, 110

K
Key performance indices (KPIs), 73

L
Laparoendoscopic single-port surgery (LESS), 99
Laparoscopic adjustable gastric band (LAGB), 243, 250
Laparoscopic and robotic transabdominal approaches, 130
Laparoscopic cardiomyotomy, 145
Laparoscopic repairs, 130
Laparoscopic revisional procedures, 228
Laparoscopic sleeve gastrectomy (LSG), 244, 250
Laparoscopic ventral hernia repair (LVHR), 279
Learning management system (LMS), 127
Left hemicolectomy, 369, 371, 372, 374
  indications, 366, 367
  learning curve, 379, 380
  postoperative care, 379
  preoperative planning, 367, 368
  room setup, 368
Left hepatectomy, 317
Left internal mammary artery (LIMA), 461–463, 465
Left lateral sectionectomy, 320
Left renal vein, 336
Linea alba, 290
LinkedIn Groups, 113
Liver retraction, 147
Living donor liver transplantation (LDLT), 493
Lobe demarcation, 319
Locked mode, 52
Long bipolar grasper, 475
Loop of jejunum, 202
Low anterior resection, 388, 390, 393
Luna robotic surgical system, 28
Lung cancer
  anatomic lung resections, 427
  mortality, 427
  survival rates, 427
Lymphadenectomy, 176–178, 446
Lymph nodes dissection, 447

M
Major pectoralis muscle (MPM), 420
Manometry, 141
Master of Science in Robotic Surgery, 114
Masters Program, 122, 124
  clinical pathways, 120
  curriculum, 122, 127
  progression, 121
MASTERS Program logo, 120
Mayo Clinic Advanced Surgical Technologies and Robotics, 115
MBSAQIP Bariatric Surgical Risk/Benefit Calculator, 194
Mediastinal, 472, 473
Medical forward advanced surgical treatment (MEDFAST), 4
Metabolic and Bariatric Surgery (MBS), 215
Metric for Evaluating Task Execution in the Operating Room (METEOR), 93
Micronutrient deficiency, 211
Middle mediastinum, 472, 473, 479
Minimally invasive bariatric surgical procedures, laparoscopy, 192
Minimally invasive endoscopic approach, 415
Minimally invasive esophagectomy, 160, 161
Minimally invasive inguinal hernia repair (MI IHR), 257
  advantages, 258
  contraindication, 258
  post-operative complications of
    chronic pain, 265, 266
    mesh infection, 267
    recurrence rates, 266, 267
    seroma and hematoma formation, 265
    testicular ischemia, 267

preoperative evaluation, 257, 258
recurrence rate, 257
robotic TAPP
dissection, 259–262
instrumentation, 259
mesh fixation, 262, 263
patient positioning and preparation, 258, 259
peritoneal flap closure, 263
trocar placement and docking, 259
special cases
acute presentation, 264
inguinoscrotal hernias and loss of domain, 264
robotic-assisted radical prostatectomy, 265
TEP approaches, 258
Minimally invasive surgery (MIS), 69, 79
advantage of, 328
Minimally invasive techniques, 348
MIRA Surgical System, 64
advantage, 63
architecture of, 64
clinical data, 66, 67
indication, 64
on International Space Station, 68
mRASD arms
functions, 65
six degrees of freedom, 65
patient cart, 64, 65
six degrees of freedom, 66
surgeon console, 64, 65
surgical minibot and articulating camera, 64, 65
telesurgery, 67
workspace cross section, 65, 66
MIRO-trial, 161
Mobile army hospital (MASH), 4
Modena Retractor, 420
Modified Ventral Hernia Working Group (mVHWG), 281
Multivariable logistic regression, 186
Myotomy, 148, 149
with fundoplication, 145

N

Natural orifice transluminal endoscopic surgery (NOTES), 99
Networking, 113
Neurofibroma, 484
Neuroganglioma, 484
Nivolumab, 453
Non-adjustable gastric band (NAGB), 244, 250

O

Omohyoid muscle (OHM), 420
Open console, 29–31, 40
Open ventral hernia repair, 279
Operating room (OR), 72
Operationalizing stage, 73

P

Pancreatic cancer, robotic surgery, 328
Paraesophageal hernias, 129, 130
Paraganglioma, 484
Parathyroid adenomas, 416
Parathyroidectomy, 422, 424
international guidelines, 416
Parathyroid surgery, 424
identification using ICG, 423, 424
Parenchymal transection, 315, 502
Partial fundoplication, 150
Patient positioning, 475, 486
Percutaneous coronary intervention (PCI), 462
Per-oral endoscopic myotomy (POEM), 144
Pneumatic dilation, 143
Pneumonia, 428
Port insertion, 486
Port placement, 177
Port training mode, 52
Positioning, 176
Positron emission tomography (PET), 472
Posterior mediastinum, 471–473
Pringle maneuver, 320
Professional communities, 113–114
Professional networking, 109, 113–114
Professional organizations, 113
Proficiency Curriculum, 122
ProGrasp™ forceps, 259
Progressive pneumoperitoneum (PPP), 264
Proof-of-concept algorithms, 95
Proximal gastrectomy, 179
Pulmonary artery dissection, 448
Pulmonary lobectomy
da Vinci SP system, 454, 455
left lower lobectomy, 446, 447
left side resections, 443
left upper lobectomy, 444–446
long-term survival studies, 451
neoadjuvant therapy, 453
outcomes and future directions, 451–456
postoperative view after procedure, 454, 455
right lower lobectomy, 440, 441
right middle lobectomy, 440–443
right-sided resections, 436, 438
right upper lobectomy, 436, 438, 439
robotic port position, 454

Pulmonary lobectomy (*cont.*)
surgical technique, 435, 436
bed control positions, 434, 435
Fuji Uniblocker bronchial blocker device, 433, 434
lung isolation and limitation, 433, 434
patient placement and port placement strategy, 433
patient positioning, 434, 435
port placement, 433, 434
RUL steps, 435, 436
tips and tricks for, 447–451
uniportal robotic lobectomy, 454, 455
virtual haptic feedback, 455

R
RAMIE-trial, 161, 162
Reconstruction, 181
Rectus to defect ratio (RDR), 286
Recurrent incisional hernia after prior rectus abdominus flap, 292
Recurrent laryngeal nerves (RLNs), 415, 422
Reddit- r/Surgery, 114
Reflux disease, 194
Retromuscular dissection, 286, 290
Retromuscular repair, 291
Retromuscular ventral hernia repair, robotic technology, 294
Revisional bariatric surgery
adport placement, 246
classification, 242
complications after, 242
decisional flowchart based on index procedure, 243, 244
feasibility and safety, 243
Nathanson liver retractor, 246
outcomes, 254
patient selection for, 243, 244
port placement, 246
pre-operative assessment, 243
rate of, 242
risk of leak after, 249
setup, 244
success rate, 227
technical aspects of
adhesiolysis, 247, 248
anatomy take-down/reconstruction, 249, 250, 252
GI construction, 252, 253
hiatal hernia repair, 248
identification of surgical anatomy, 248
Revisional foregut surgery
access, 232
adhesiolysis, 233
advantages, 229
antireflux procedure
conversion to Roux-en-Y near esophago-jejunostomy, 240
redo fundoplication, 238, 240
wedge gastroplasty, 241
challenge, 228
circumferential dissection of esophagus, 234
crural dissection, 234
crural repair, 236
fundoplication take down, 235
indications for, 229
liver retraction, 232
mesh reinforcement, 237
operating room set-up, 231
options for, 229, 230
outcomes, 241, 242
patient positioning, 231, 232
for persistent or recurrent disease, 227
port placement, 232
postoperative complications, 228
pre-surgical care, 230
success rate, 227
Right hemicolectomy, 351, 356, 358–360
indications, 352
patient positioning, 353
preparation, 352, 353
recovery after surgery, 361
surgical technique, 355, 356, 360, 361
Right hepatic artery (RHA), 312, 499
Robot assisted approaches, 185
Robotic abdominal wall reconstruction technique, 280
Robotic adrenalectomy, 407, 410
docking, 409
left, 412
limitations, 413
patient positioning, 408
pertinent anatomy, 408
port placement, 411
postoperative care, 413
technique, 411, 412
Robotically assisted surgical (RAS) technology, 63
Robotic aortic valve replacement, 468
Robotic approach, 130
Robotic arms, 21
Robotic-assisted approaches, surgical community, 282

Robotic assisted colorectal training (RACT), 391
Robotic-assisted Ivor-Lewis esophagectomy, 162–166, 168, 169
 azygos arch, 166
 azygos vein, 166, 167
 creation of the gastric conduit, 164
 dissection of the thoracic duct, 168
 gastroesophageal junction, 163
 left gastric artery, 165
 mobilization of abdominal esophagus, 164
 parietal pleura, 167
 subcarinal lymph nodes, 169
 transverse colon and pancreas, 163
 trocar placement, 165
 trocar-placement for the abdominal phase, 163
 trocar-placement of the thoracic phase, 166
 wound protector, 169
Robotic assisted McKeown esophagectomy, 170–172
Robotic-assisted surgery (RAS), 98
Robotic-assisted thoracic surgery (RATS) lobectomy, 456
 advantages, 428
 anatomical resections, 452
 conversion rate, 431
 cost, 430
 outcomes, 431
 systematic reviews and meta-analysis, 432
 uniportal, 454
 vs. VATS, 452
Robotic-assisted transabdominal preperitoneal (r-TAPP), 271, 274, 275
Robotic curriculum, 121, 122
Robotic dissection, 302
Robotic donor hepatectomy, 494–496, 501, 507, 513, 519
 instruments, 497–498
 left donor hepatectomy, 505–507, 509
 left lateral donor sectionectomy, 509, 510
 parenchymal transection, 502–504, 510, 511
 patient selection, 496
 port placement, 497
 positioning, 497
 right donor hepatectomy, 498–504
Robotic enhanced view total extraperitoneal (eTEP) repairs, 286
Robotic gastric bypass, 192
Robotic intraperitoneal onlay mesh (r-IPOM), 271, 275, 276
Robotic liver resection, 307, 308
 patient selection, 308
 positioning, 308, 309
 right hepatectomy, 310, 311, 314–317
 standard robotic instruments, 310
Robotic lobectomy, 429
 analysis of, 429
 cost of, 430
Robotic mitral valve surgery, 467
Robotic recipient hepatectomy, 514–516
Robotic recipient transplantation, 511–513
Robotic retromuscular VHR with TAR, 290
Robotic Roux-en-Y gastric bypass
 absolute contraindications, 194
 anesthesia induction, 195
 behavioral modification, 194
 benefits and risks, 193
 DVT prophylaxis, 210
 gastro-jejunal anastomosis, 210
 indications, 193
 maximum medical optimization, 195
 monitoring parameters, 209
 operating room set-up and patient positioning, 195, 199–202, 204, 206, 209
 oral proton pump inhibitor, 210
 preoperative preparation, 194
 prophylactic Heparin, 210
 relative contraindications, 194
 restrictive and malabsorptive mechanism, 193
 T2D remission rates, 194
Robotics in bariatric surgery, contemporary role, 192
Robotic surgery (RS), 7–8, 69, 351, 395, 400
 adaption, 388, 389
 adoption of, 279
 commercialization, 6–8
 complexity and diversity, 109
 curriculum, 122, 123
 Da Vinci system, 83
 with educational programs and conferences, 113
 foundational knowledge through reviewing books, 109
 fundamentals, 82, 83
 genitourinary function, 392
 high-quality training resources, 109
 initial vision, 8
 journals and publications, 110
 network, 113
 operative procedure, 393
 origins, 3
 on patient outcomes, 282

Robotic surgery (RS) (*cont.*)
  perceived benefits, 282
  physical challenges, 192
  preoperative planning, 392
  surgeon ergonomics, 282
  technique, 394, 395, 399, 401
  three-dimensional optics, 282
  ventral hernia repair, rationality and adaptability, 281, 282
Robotic TAR
  absorbable, self-fixating sutures, 290
  application, 287
  bipolar grasper, 290
  blunt dissection, 290
  lateral decubitus position, 287
  optimal visualization, 289
  patient positioning strategies, 287
  port placement, 288
  preperitoneal mesh placement, 287
  substantial defects, 287
Robotic technology, 429
Robotic thyroidectomy
  development of, 416
  international guidelines, 416
Robotic total colectomy, 378, 381
Robotic training network (RTN), 83
Robotic transaxillary thyroidectomy
  contraindications, 416
  incidence, 423
  indications for, 416
  operative room set-up, right and left access, 417, 418
  patient position, 418, 419
  post-operative complications, 424
  safe and feasible, 424
  surgical procedure
    console time, 421
    Da Vinci Xi® robot positioning and docking time, 421
    hybrid technique for tunnel's creation, 419
    incision and visualization of MPM, 419, 420
    OHM and IGV, anatomical landmark of, 420
    SCM and Modena retractor, 420
    total thyroidectomy, 422
    working space, 419
Robotic ventral hernia repair (RVHR)
  advancing age and anticoagulant therapy, 285
  early postoperative pain and discomfort, 284
  economic impact, 283
  elevated costs, 283
  financial considerations, 283
  higher-grade complications and morbidity scores, 285
  increased operative time, 283
  increase in operative time, 283
  interdisciplinary protocols, 284
  intraperitoneal mesh, 284
  management, 284
  minimally invasive surgery, 283
  patient positioning, 288
  perioperative management, 284
  perioperative outcomes, 284
  port placement and docking, 289
  postoperative bleeding and thromboembolic events, 285
  postoperative hematomas, 285
  safety and feasibility, 284
  thromboembolic events and perioperative bleeding, 285
  utilization, 284
Robotic Whipple procedure, 327, 348
  "all in" approach, 330
  alternative to open surgery, 328
  complexity of, 330
  Da Vinci XI Surgical System, 330
  demanding anastomosis, 328, 329
  department and hospital administration, 330
  digital resources, 331
  evidence to support, 348
  high level proficiency, 330
  limitation, 328
  operating room setup and instrumentation, 332, 333
  patient selection, 331, 332
  postoperative care, 348
  predominant approach for, 330
  reconstruction phase, 343
    gastrojejunostomy, 344, 345
    hepaticojejunostomy, 344
    pancreaticojejunostomy, 343
  robotic hepatobiliary courses, 331
  surgeon working on, 329
  surgical steps
    basic plan, 335
    by console surgeon, 335
    creating tunnel for pancreatic transection, 340
    diagnostic laparoscopy, 334
    docking of, 335
    entering lesser sac and colon mobilization, 335
    falciform flap, 345
    falciform ligament suturing to abdominal wall, 338

gallbladder suturing to abdominal wall, 338
hepatic artery lymph nodes removal, 339
hilar dissection, 338, 339
infra-pancreatic neck dissection, 337
ligament of Treitz dissection, 336
pancreatic neck division with scissors, 340
patient position, 334
Pfannenstiel incision closure, 345
port placement, 334, 335
SMA exposing IVC and LRV, 335, 336
SMV exposed under pancreatic neck, 337
supra-pancreatic/Hilary dissection, 338
uncinate dissection, 337, 341, 343
vascular resections, 345–347
Roux-en-Y gastric bypass (RYGB), 182, 216, 244, 251

S

SAGES Robotics Resident & Fellows Courses, 112
SAGES Surgical Multimodal Accelerated Recovery Trajectory (SMART) Initiative, 123
Schwannoma, 484
Senhance connect, 27
Senhance surgical system, 19, 21, 24
surgeon console, 21, 22
Side docking technique, 131
Simulation training, 112
Simultaneous localization and mapping (SLAM) technique, 90
Single anastomosis duodenoileal bypass, 216
Single anastomosis duodenoileal bypass with Sleeve gastrectomy (SADI-S)
bowel measurement, 219
duodenal dissection, 219
duodenoileostomy, 220
surgical technique, 217, 218
Single-port robotic cholecystectomy (SPRC), 305
Single-site robotic surgery, 381, 382
Sleep mode, 52
Sleeve gastrectomy, 219
Bougie or Visigi positioning, 188
vs. conventional laparoscopy, 185
diluted methylene blue or Indocyanine Green, 189
gastrocolic ligament, 188
gastrosplenic ligament, 187
vs. laparoscopic sleeve gastrectomy, 186
metabolic procedure, 185
operative technique, 186
perceived safety profile, 185
Xi platform, 186
port position, 187
reverse Trendelenburg position, 187
stapling the stomach, 189
Sliding hiatal hernia, 129
Smart tissue anastomosis robot (STAR), 96
Social media and networking, 113, 114
Society of American Gastrointestinal and Endoscopic Surgeons (SAGES), 80, 111, 113
educational content, 123
evidence-based recommendations for surgeons, 124
Guidelines Committee, 124
MASTERS program, 127
Society of Laparoscopic and Robotic Surgeons (SLS), 114
Society of Robotic Surgery (SRS), 113
Sovato App, 68
Standardization, 73–75
Standardizing stage, 74
Sternocleidomastoideum muscle (SCM), 420
Superior vena cava, 475, 477
SureForm60™, 249
The surgeon console, 31–33
Surgeons console design, 29, 30
Surgical coaching skills, 127
Surgical Council on Resident Education (SCORE), 111
Surgical Endoscopy, 110
Surgical Innovation (SRI), 110
System connections, 58
System design, 44
System tower, 34, 35

T

Telementoring, 97, 112
for clinical practice, 97, 98
education, 97
Telepresence surgery system, 3, 15, 17
Telesurgery, 9, 67, 98
Thoracotomy, 428
3D high-definition vision (3DHD), 55
Thymoma, 473, 478
Thyroid carcinoma, incidence of, 423
Thyroid surgery
bilateral axillo-breast approach, 415
transaxillary approach, 415
trans-oral (TO) approach, 416

TIGER-protocol, 161
TilePro™, 249, 253
Tip-Up Fenestrated Grasper, 435
Total colectomy, 366, 375
Total gastrectomy, 181
Totally endoscopic coronary artery bypass (TECAB), 465
Totally endoscopic robotic CABG (TECAB), 461
Totally extraperitoneal (TEP) approaches, 258
Total mesorectal excision (TME), 389, 390
Transabdominal preperitoneal (TAPP), 258
Transaxillary (TA) approach, 415
TransEnterix, 43
Trans-oral (TO) approach, 416
Trans-thoracic approaches, 130
Transthoracic esophageal resection, 160
Transthoracic esophagectomy
  with abdominal and thoracic lymph node dissection, 160
  with gastric pull-up reconstruction, 160
Traumapod, 5, 8
TrueWrist instruments, 28

U
Uniportal robotic thoracic surgery, 454
Unlocked mode, 52
Upper endoscopy, 141
  with retroflexion, 152
Upper gastrointestinal endoscopy, 243
Upper-GI Robotic Association (UGIRA) Congress, 161

V
Vagal nerve injury, 153–155
Ventral hernia repair techniques
  AWR procedures, 279
  clinical and economic outcomes, 282
  clinical benefits, 280
  ergonomic challenges, 280
  evolution of, 279
  incidence, 271
  IPOM, 275, 276
  minimally invasive approach, 280
  operating room set up, 274
  outcomes, 276
  patient positioning, 272
  patient preparation, 272
  port placement, 273, 274
  pre-operative heparin, 286
  preoperative considerations, 271, 272
  preoperative preparation, 285
  robot docking, 273
  R-TAPP, 274, 275
  surgical environment and patient safety, 285
  urinary drainage, 286
Versius arm, 50
Versius surgical robot, 44–46
Vertical banded gastroplasty (VBG), 244, 251
Video-assisted thoracoscopic surgery (VATS) lobectomy, 428, 471
  anatomical resections, 452
  challenges, 428
  conversion rate, 431
  cost effective, 430
  function, 428
  vs. open approach, 453
  outcomes, 431
  proficiency ranges, 429
  vs. RATS, 452
  uniportal, 454
  vs. thoracotomy approach, 428
Virtual haptic feedback, 455
Virtual Incision, 63
Virtual simulation, 81
Virtual Surgical Assist, 98
Virtual thoracotomy, 428

W
Web-based training, 81
WebSurg, 111
Wedge gastroplasty, 241
Weight loss, 216
Wind up icon, 48

9783031869266